Handbook of Experimental Pharmacology

Continuation of Handbuch der experimentellen Pharmakologie

Vol. 80

Cadmium

Contributors

A. Bernard · A. C. Chang · M. M. El-Amamy · M. D. Enger
J. H. Exon · E. C. Foulkes · K. Fuwa · C. E. Hildebrand
I. S. Jamall · L. D. Koller · S. J. Kopp · R. Lauwerys
K. Matsumoto · K. Nomiyama · A. L. Page · M. Piscator
JC. Seagrave · J. C. Smith · R. A. Tobey · M. Webb

Editor

E. C. Foulkes

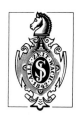

Springer-Verlag Berlin Heidelberg New York Tokyo

Professor ERNEST C. FOULKES, Ph.D.
University of Cincinnati, College of Medicine
Department of Environmental Health (56)
3223 Eden Avenue
Cincinnati, OH 45267, USA

With 59 Figures

ISBN 3-540-16025-6 Springer-Verlag Berlin Heidelberg New York Tokyo
ISBN 0-387-16025-6 Springer-Verlag New York Heidelberg Berlin Tokyo

Library of Congress Cataloging-in-Publication Data. Main entry under title: Cadmium. (Handbook of experimental pharmacology; vol. 80) Includes bibliographies and index. 1. Cadmium–Toxicology. 2. Cadmium–Physiological effect. 3. Cadmium–Environmental aspects. 4. Cadmium–Analysis. 5. Metallothionein. I. Bernard, A. II. Foulkes, Ernest C., 1924– . III. Series: Handbook of experimental pharmacology; v. 80. [DNLM: 1. Cadmium–adverse effects. W1 HA51L v. 80/QV 290 C1239] QP905.H3 vol. 80 615'.1 s [615.9'25662] 85-27658 [RA1231.C3] ISBN 0-387-16025-6 (U.S.).

Typesetting, printing and bookbinding: Brühlsche Universitätsdruckerei, Giessen
2122/3130-543210

List of Contributors

A. BERNARD, Université Catholique de Louvain, Faculté de Médecine,
   Unité de Toxicologie Industrielle et Medicale du Travail, 30.54 Clos
   Chapelle-aux-Champs, Boite Postale 3054, B-1200 Bruxelles, Belgium

A. C. CHANG, University of California, Department of Soil and Environmental
   Sciences, Riverside, CA 92521, USA

M. M. EL-AMAMY, University of California, Department of Soil and
   Environmental Sciences, Riverside, CA 92521, USA

M. D. ENGER, Department of Zoology, Iowa State University of Sciences
   and Technology, Science Bldg. 11, Ames, IA 50011, USA

J. H. EXON, School of Veterinary Medicine, University of Idaho, Moscow,
   ID 83843, USA

E. C. FOULKES, University of Cincinnati College of Medicine, Department of
   Environmental Health (56), 3223 Eden Avenue, Cincinnati, OH 45267, USA

K. FUWA, Department of Chemistry, Faculty of Science, The University
   of Tokyo, Bunkyo-Ku, Tokyo, 113, Japan

C. E. HILDEBRAND, Genetics Group, Life Sciences Division, University of
   California, Los Alamos Scientific Laboratory, P.O. Box 1663, Los Alamos,
   NM 87545, USA

I. S. JAMALL, Toxicology Program, College of Pharmacy and Allied Health
   Professions, St. John's University, Grand Central and Utopia Parkways,
   Jamaica, NY 11439, USA

L. D. KOLLER, University of Idaho, Idaho Faculty, WOI, Regional Program,
   Veterinary Medicine, Moscow, ID 83843, USA

S. J. KOPP, Department of Physiology and Nuclear Magnetic Resonance
   Laboratory, Chicago College of Osteopathic Medicine, 1122 East 53rd Street,
   Chicago, IL 60615, USA

R. LAUWERYS, Université Catholique de Louvain, Faculté de Médecine, Unité de Toxicologie Industrielle et Medicale du Travail, 30.54 Clos Chapelle-aux-Champs, Boite Postale 3054, B-1200 Bruxelles, Belgium

K. MATSUMOTO, Department of Chemistry, School of Science and Engineering Waseda University, Okubo, Shinjuku-ku, Tokyo, 160, Japan

K. NOMIYAMA, Department of Environmental Health, Jichi Medical School, Minamikawachi-Machi, Kawachi-Gun, Tochigi-Ken 329-04, Japan

A. L. PAGE, University of California, Department of Soil and Environmental Sciences, Riverside, CA 92521, USA

M. PISCATOR, Department of Environmental Hygiene, Karolinska Institute, P.O. Box 60400, S-10401 Stockholm, Sweden

JC. SEAGRAVE, Genetics Group, Life Sciences Division, University of California, Los Alamos Scientific Laboratory, P.O. Box 1663, Los Alamos, NM 87545, USA

J. C. SMITH, Agricultural Research Services, United States Department of Agriculture, Western Regional Research Center, 800 Buchanan Street, Berkeley, CA 94710, USA

R. A. TOBEY, Genetics Group, Life Sciences Division, University of California, Los Alamos Scientific Laboratory, P.O. Box 1663, Los Alamos, NM 87545, USA

M. WEBB, Toxicology Unit, Medical Research Council Laboratories, Woodmansterne Road, Carshalton, Surrey SM5 4EF, Great Britain

Preface

The toxic properties of cadmium compounds have been well recognized in many species. There is little evidence to suggest a physiologic role for the metal. Rather, because of its long biologic half-life, cadmium acts as a cumulative poison, and even at quite low ambient concentrations, it can accumulate in mammals to values not insignificant in terms of critical toxic levels.

The problem of cadmium toxicity has become especially important, as cadmium concentrations in the environment have begun to rise owing to a variety of human activities such as mining, the metallurgical industry, coal combustion, and the use of cadmium-containing fertilizers. It seemed appropriate, therefore, to assemble in one volume an up-to-date analysis of the mechanism of action of cadmium on biologic systems. Aspects of this field have repeatedly been reviewed in the past, and particular reference must be made to the volumes prepared by FRIBERG and collaborators from Sweden. Much outstanding work on cadmium has also been reported from Japan, and I am happy that investigators from both countries were able to contribute to the present volume.

Obviously, this volume does not report a consensus by its contributors. The purpose of the work was to permit leading investigators in the field to present a critical review with sufficient documentation to support their interpretations and conclusions. A certain amount of overlap and disagreement between chapters was therefore unavoidable. The result, I hope, will be a useful state-of-the-art discussion.

My thanks go to the collaborators, to the publishers, whose continuous help was essential, and to Mrs. Annette Townsley here in Cincinnati who put it all together.

Cincinnati   E. C. FOULKES

Contents

CHAPTER 1

The Estimation of Cadmium in Biological Samples
K. MATSUMOTO and K. FUWA. With 19 Figures 1

A. Brief Survey of Cadmium Chemistry 1
B. Analytic Methods for Cadmium 3
    I. Atomic Absorption and Emission Spectrometry 4
    II. Polarography 16
    III. X-Ray Fluorescence Analysis 23
    IV. Neutron Activation Analysis 26
    V. Isotope Dilution Method 28
References 31

CHAPTER 2

**Cadmium in the Environment and its Entry into Terrestrial
Food Chain Crops.** A. L. PAGE, M. M. EL-AMAMY, and A. C. CHANG . . . 33

A. Introduction 33
B. Natural Occurence 34
C. World Production 35
D. Consumption 36
    I. Electroplating 38
    II. Pigments and Chemicals 38
    III. Alloys 38
    IV. Other Uses 38
E. Cadmium in Noncontaminated and Contaminated Soils 39
    I. Natural Levels in Soils 39
    II. Sources and Extent of Cadmium Contamination of Soils 41
    III. Soil Factors Influencing the Accumulation of Cadmium
        by Food Chain Crops 47
F. Phytotoxic Effects of Cadmium 53
G. Concentrations of Cadmium in Food Chain Crops 54
H. Human Intake of Cadmium 60
J. Methods to Control the Entry of Cadmium into Food Chain Crops . 62
K. Summary 64
References 65

CHAPTER 3

Absorption of Cadmium. E. C. FOULKES. With 6 Figures 75

A. Introduction 75
B. Routes of Exposure 75
    I. Lungs 75
    II. Skin 76
    III. Intestine 76
C. Mechanism of Intestinal Cd Absorption 77
    I. General 77
    II. Methods of Study 79
    III. Kinetics 82
    IV. Role of the Brush Border 83
    V. Interaction Between Cd and Other Metals 84
    VI. Conclusions 90
D. Control of Cd Absorption 91
    I. Introduction 91
    II. Endogenous Factors 91
    III. Influence of Diet 94
E. Summary 95
References 97

CHAPTER 4

**The Chronic Toxicity of Cadmium: Influence of Environmental
and Other Variables.** K. NOMIYAMA. With 16 Figures 101

A. Introduction 101
B. Environmental Pollution with Cadmium and Health Effects 101
    I. Itai-Itai Disease 101
    II. An Episode in Annaka District, Japan 102
    III. Other Episodes in Japan 104
    IV. Episodes in Europe 105
C. Renal Effects 106
    I. Renal Effects Among Residents in Cadmium-Polluted Areas
      in Japan 106
    II. Mortality Study on Residents in Cadmium-Polluted Areas . . . 108
D. Skeletal Effects of Cadmium 109
    I. Itai-Itai Disease 109
    II. Epidemiologic Studies on Residents in Cadmium-Polluted Areas . 109
    III. Animal Experiments 110
    IV. Discussion at the International Conference on Cadmium-
      Induced Osteopathy 110
E. Blood Pressure, Cerebrovascular Disease, and Heart Disease 111
    I. Depressed Blood Pressure 111
    II. Epidemiologic Studies on Mortality from Cerebrovascular Disease
      and Heart Disease 112
F. Recovery from Cadmium-Induced Health Effects 112

G. Chemical Forms of Cadmium in Food and Health Effects 114
H. Elevated Sensitivity to Cadmium 114
    I. Aging 114
    II. Protein-Calorie Malnutrition 116
    III. Environmental Temperature 116
    IV. Combination of Hot Environment and Protein-Calorie
        Malnutrition 116
J. Metal Shift in Cadmium Intoxication 117
K. Biologic Monitoring of Cadmium Exposure. 120
    I. Urinary Cadmium. 120
    II. In Vivo Determination of Organ Cadmium 122
L. Estimation of Allowable Intake of Cadmium 122
    I. Biologic Half-Life of Cadmium in the Renal Cortex 123
    II. Critical Concentration of Cadmium in the Renal Cortex 123
References. 128

CHAPTER 5

Effects of Cadmium Exposure in Humans. A. Bernard and R. Lauwerys . 135

A. Introduction 135
B. Human Exposure to Cadmium 135
    I. Environmental Exposure 135
    II. Industrial Exposure 137
    III. Tobacco Smoke 140
C. Metabolism 140
    I. Absorption 140
    II. Distribution 141
    III. Excretion 143
    IV. Evaluation of Cadmium Exposure 143
D. Acute Toxicity 144
    I. Acute Toxicity by Inhalation 144
    II. Acute Toxicity by Ingestion 145
E. Chronic Toxicity 145
    I. Effects on the Bones 146
    II. Effects on the Lung. 147
    III. Effects on the Kidney 150
    IV. Effects on the Cardiovascular System: Hypertension 159
    V. Carcinogenicity 161
    VI. Other Effects 163
    VII. Dose-Effect and Dose-Response Relationships 164
References. 168

CHAPTER 6

The Nephropathy of Chronic Cadmium Poisoning. M. Piscator 179

A. Introduction 179
B. Uptake, Storage, and Turnover of Cadmium in the Kidneys 180

C. Effects on Tubular Function 182
  I. Proteinuria 182
  II. Glucosuria and Aminoaciduria 184
  III. Disturbances in Mineral Metabolism 185
D. Effects on Glomerular Function 187
E. Diagnosis 188
F. Prognosis 189
G. Prevention 190
References 190

CHAPTER 7

Cadmium and the Cardiovascular System. S. J. KOPP. With 7 Figures . . . 195

A. Preface 195
  I. Regulatory Aspects of Cardiovascular Function:
     Intrinsic Considerations 195
  II. Extrinsic Considerations 198
B. Historical Overview 200
C. Actions of Cadmium on the Myocardium 203
  I. Actions of Cadmium Affecting Myocardial Inotropism 204
  II. Actions of Cadmium Affecting Cardiac Excitability 225
D. Vascular Actions of Cadmium 233
  I. Introduction 233
  II. Vascular Responses to Cadmium 234
  III. Reactivity of Vascular Tissue Following Chronic
       or Acute Cadmium-Treatment 241
E. The Cadmium Hypertension Controversy 243
  I. Experimental Animal Studies 244
Appendix A 251
Appendix B 259
References 270

CHAPTER 8

Role of Metallothionein in Cadmium Metabolism. M. WEBB

With 4 Figures 281

A. Introduction 281
B. Historical Background and Chemistry of the Metallothioneins 282
C. Determination of Metallothionein Concentrations in Mammalian
   Tissues 285
D. Metallothionein and the Metabolism of Cadmium 287
E. Metallothionein Synthesis in Relation to the Chronic Toxicity
   of Cadmium 298
F. Metallothionein Synthesis in Relation to the Acute Toxicity
   of Cadmium 304
  I. Normal Animals 304
  II. Cd-Pretreated Animals 306

G. Kidney Uptake, Metabolism and Toxicity of Exogenous
   Metallothionein 310
H. Function of Metallothionein in the Transport of Cd from the Liver
   to the Kidney 313
 J. Normal Functions of Metallothionein and the Interactions of Cd
   with these Functions 315
K. Function of Metallothionein in the Reproductive Toxicology of Cd:
   Role in Perinatal Development 318
L. Metallothionein: A Limiting Factor in the Chelation Therapy of Cd
   Intoxication 323
References 325

CHAPTER 9

Immunotoxicity of Cadmium. J. H. Exon and L. D. Koller 339

A. The Immune System 339
B. Immunoassays 340
C. Effects of Cadmium on Immune Responses 341
     I. Host Resistance 341
    II. Antibody Synthesis and B-Cells 342
   III. Cell-Mediated Immunity and T-Cells 344
    IV. Macrophage Function 346
     V. Other Immunologically Related Effects 347
D. Summary 348
References 348

CHAPTER 10

The Effect of Dietary Selenium on Cadmium Cardiotoxicity
I. S. Jamall and J. C. Smith 351

A. Introduction 351
B. Cadmium and the Heart 351
C. Selenium Deficiency and Cardiomyopathy 352
D. Cadmium-Selenium Interactions 352
E. Cadmium-Copper Interactions 353
F. Cadmium-Metallothionein Studies 354
G. Investigations into the Mechanism of Cadmium Cardiotoxicity . . . 354
     I. The Idea 354
    II. The Experiment 354
H. Physiologic Studies 357
 J. Conclusions 358
References 359

CHAPTER 11

Cellular Resistance to Cadmium. M. D. Enger, C. E. Hildebrand,
JC. Seagrave, and R. A. Tobey. With 7 Figures 363

A. Introduction 363
B. Cultured Cell Systems for Studying Cd Metabolism 363
   I. Use of Cultured Cell Systems to Study the Roles of Metallothionein
      in the Cellular Response to Cd 364
  II. Cd Uptake 370
 III. Use of Cultured Cell Systems to Study Cd Responses Other than
      Uptake or Cytotoxicity 371
  IV. Use of Freshly Cultured Blood Cells to Study Variation
      in Human Response to Cd 372
C. Role of Metallothionein in Cellular Cd Resistance 373
   I. Metallothionein Production is Regulated at Several Levels . . . 375
  II. Role of Metallothionein in Cellular Cd Resistance in Cultured
      Human Blood Cells 380
D. Non-Metallothionein Mechanisms of Cellular Cd Resistance 380
E. Models Describing Cd Metabolism and the Role of Metallothionein
   and Other Factors in Resistance and Sensitivity 383
F. Future Directions 383
   I. Models 383
  II. Cd Toxicity Targets 384
 III. Gene Expression Domains 384
  IV. Non-Metallothionein Protective Mechanisms 385
   V. Role of Cd in Altered Gene Expression: Possible Involvement
      in Carcinogenesis 386
  VI. Extracellular Factors and Cd Responses 387
 VII. Role for Genetic Polymorphisms in Altered Cellular Responses
      to Cd 387
VIII. Tissue-Specific Regulation of Expression of Metallothioneins
      and Other Factors 388
  IX. Strategies for Derivation of New Cell Systems to
      Define Mechanisms of Cellular Cd Resistance 388
   X. Variation in Human Response 390
G. Summary 390
References 390

Subject Index 397

CHAPTER 1

The Estimation of Cadmium in Biological Samples

K. Matsumoto and K. Fuwa

A. Brief Survey of Cadmium Chemistry

Cadmium has a relatively low abundance in nature (the Clarke number is 5×10^{-5}), but it has long been known because it is easily extracted from its ores. Although cadmium minerals are scarcely found in nature, it occurs widely by isomorphous replacement of zinc in sphalerite (Zn, Fe)S, which usually coexists with galena PbS. This substitution is due to the similar chemical properties of Zn and Cd, both in group IIb. Zinc and lead are commonly recovered simultaneously by a blast furnace method. Cadmium is invariably a by-product and is usually separated from zinc by distillation or by precipitation from sulfate solutions by inc dust. The reaction corresponds to the following equation

$$Zn + Cd^{2+} = Zn^{2+} + Cd \qquad E = +0.36 \text{ V.}$$

Cadmium is a white lustrous metal. The structure of cadmium metal deviates from perfect hexagonal close packing by elongation along the sixfold axis. The metal is remarkably volatile for a heavy metal. It reacts readily with nonoxidizing acids to produce hydrogen and the divalent ion, but does not dissolve in alkali solution. Cadmium reacts readily when heated with oxygen to give the oxides. It also reacts directly with halogens, S, Se, P, etc.

With regard to complex formation, cadmium is classified as an intermediate metal according to the so-called soft–hard classification. Complex anions with halides are formed by both cadmium and zinc, but the formation constants for the former are usually 3–7 orders of magnitude larger than those for the latter and both are many orders of magnitude smaller than those of mercury (Table 1). Zn^{2+} tends to form stronger bonds to F and O, whereas Cd^{2+} is more strongly bound to Cl, S, and P ligands.

The cadmium complex with dithiocarbamate is an important species, extracted from an aqueous into an organic layer; it is widely employed in analytic chemistry for concentrating cadmium. The compound $[Cd(S_2CNEt_2)_2]$ is a dimer, as shown in Fig. 1, and each cadmium is pentacoordinated by sulfur atoms.

The complexes formed by cadmium with sulfur-containing amino acids have been compared in detail with those of zinc and mercury. This is due partly to the important biologic role of zinc(II) and partly to the very toxic nature of cadmium(II) and mercury(II). Interest in the differences in their chemical properties have been further enhanced by the recognition that D-penicillamine (Fig. 2) is very effectively employed for the treatment of mercury poisoning, whereas it proves

Table 1. Equilibrium constants for halides of Zn, Cd, and Hg[a]

X	K		
	Zn^{2+}	Cd^{2+}	Hg^{2+}
Cl^-	1	10^3	10^{16}
Br^-	10^{-1}	10^4	10^{22}
I^-	10^{-2}	10^6	10^{30}
NH_3	10^9	10^7	10^{19}
CN^-	10^{21}	10^{19}	10^{41}

[a] The equilibrium constant is defined as $K = [MX_4]^{2-}/[M^{2+}][X^-]^4$ for a reaction $M^{2+} + 4X^- = [MX_4]^{2-}$

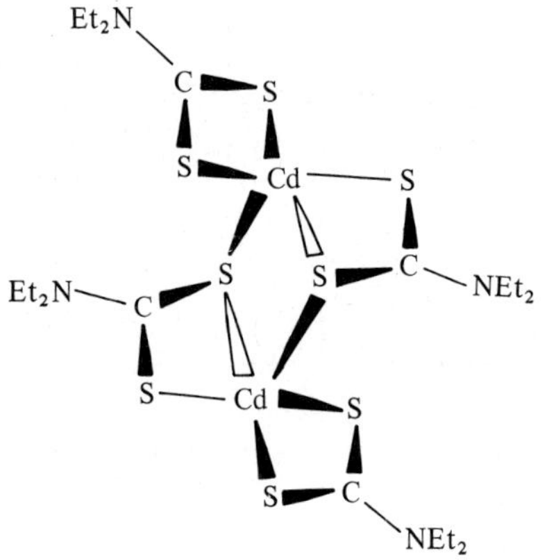

Fig. 1. Structure of cadmium dithiocarbamate, $[Cd(S_2CNEt_2)_2]_2$

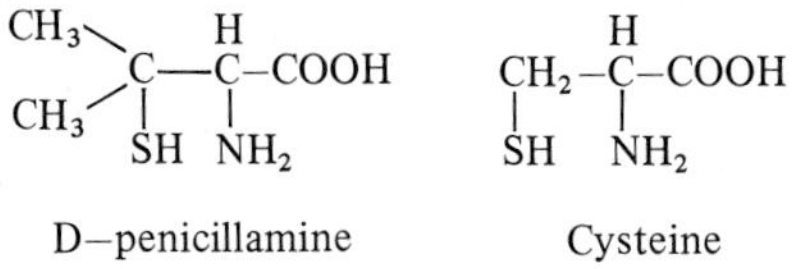

Fig. 2 a, b. Structures of **a** D-penicillamine and **b** cysteine

ineffective in the case of cadmium. The details of this study are outlined in the recent review edited by Sigel (1979) a summary of which is given here.

Most of the publications dealing with zinc(II) complexes of cysteine and penicillamine come to the general conclusion that zinc forms only the complexes ZnA and ZnA_2, where the ligands coordinate to the metal through S and N. The formation of protonated and polynuclear complexes is assumed in these systems.

Concerning the cadmium(II)–L-cysteine and cadmium(II)–D-penicillamine systems, several workers came to the conclusion that complexes of the type MA are formed, where cysteine and penicillamine act as tridentate ligands using S, N, and O. In an X-ray study of the 1:1 Cd(II)–D-penicillamine complex, the cadmium ion is hexacoordinated, being surrounded by two sulfur atoms, three oxygen atoms, and one nitrogen atom. In glutathione complexes of Zn and Cd, stronger coordination of sulfur is indicated for Cd than for Zn by NMR studies.

Zinc plays an important role in living matter as an active site in metalloenzymes, such as carbonic anhydrases, carboxypeptidases, dehydrogenases, and alkaline phosphatases. In contrast, cadmium is usually toxic to humans, probably partially owing to cadmium substitution of zinc in those enzymes.

B. Analytic Methods for Cadmium

There are several methods for cadmium determination as shown in Table 2. Each method has its advantages and disadvantages compared with other methods. For instance, X-ray fluorescence analysis, neutron activation analysis, and isotope dilution analysis can be applied to either solid or liquid samples, whereas atomic absorption spectrometry and polarography are limited to liquid samples. From the comparison of detection limits, atomic absorption spectrometry, neutron activation analysis, and isotope dilution methods seem advantageous over other methods.

In terms of accuracy, the isotope dilution method is extremely reliable, since it is an absolute method, using no standard samples for calibration. Turning to

Table 2. Detection limits and dynamic ranges of various analytic methods for cadmium

	Method	Detection limit	Dynamic range
Atomic absorption spectrometry	Flame	1 ppb	0.01 –0.5 ppm
	Graphite furnace	0.008 ppb	0.008–0.2 ppb
Polarography	Direct current	0.6 ppm	0.6 –10^3 ppm
	Alternating current	1 ppm	1 –10^3 ppm
	Square wave	0.01 ppm	0.01 –10^3 ppm
X-ray fluorescence analysis	Wavelength dispersive	5 ppm	5 –10^4 ppm
	Energy dispersive	50 ppm	50 –10^4 ppm
Neutron activation analysis		1 ppb	1 –10^5 ppb
Isotope dilution method		10 ppb	10 –10^5 ppb
Inductively coupled plasma emission spectrometry		1 ppb	1 –10^6 ppb

the more practical points of the analytic methods, for instance ease of operation and cost of the instrument, atomic absorption spectrometry and polarography are advantageous. Although each method has its own advantages, atomic absorption spectrometry is the most widely used technique for cadmium determination and therefore the method will be described in more detail than other methods in the following section. As a nondestructive in vivo analytic method, mobile prompt gamma in vivo activation analysis has recently been developed. The details will be given in Sect. B.IV.3 of this chapter.

I. Atomic Absorption and Emission Spectrometry

Atomic absorption spectrometry is probably the most widely applied method for cadmium determination, owing to its high sensitivity and the metal's relatively high volatility (the detection limits are 1 ppb for flame atomic absorption spectrometry and 0.008 ppb for graphite furnace atomic absorption spectrometry), as well as the relative ease of operation of the method. The instrumental details and the practical procedures in sample preparation and measurement are described in the rest of this section.

1. Principles of Atomic Absorption Spectrometry

Atomic absorption spectrometry utilizes absorption intensities for determining analyte concentrations and therefore the instrument has many similarities to that of colorimetry. Although both methods are based on the measurement of how much the light from a source is decreased by passing through the analyte, the basic difference is that whereas, in colorimetry, absorption by molecules in solution is measured, in atomic absorption spectrometry, absorption by atoms produced at high temperature is the object to be measured. Therefore, the molecules dissolved in a sample solution must be converted to atoms by some means. The usual methods for this conversion is heat decomposition by use of chemical flames or an electrically heated carbon furnace cuvette. The other difference is that as a general feature of atomic absorption, spectral bandwidth is very narrow,

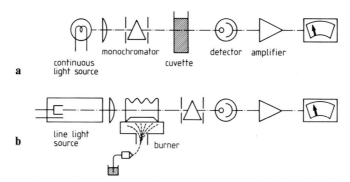

Fig. 3 a, b. Comparative illustration of **a** a colorimetric spectrophotometer and **b** an atomic absorption spectrophotometer

less than 0.1 Å. Therefore, a light source emitting a line spectrum is necessary. Summing up all these similarities and differences, an atomic absorption spectrophotometer can be considered basically as a colorimetric spectrophotometer whose cuvette is replaced by a flame burner or a carbon furnace and the continuous light source (usually a tungsten or a D_2 lamp), by a line source. Schematic diagrams of a colorimetric spectrophotometer and an atomic absorption spectrophotometer are shown in Fig. 3. In Fig. 3, the arrangement of sample cuvette and monochromator is reversed in an atomic absorption spectrophotometer, because, in colorimetry, monochromatic light irradiates the sample solution so as not to decompose the sample by direct irradiation of strong polychromatic light. In atomic absorption, the monochromator is placed after the flame, since detection of flame emission must be avoided. A comprehensive description of the method including both theoretical and instrumental details is given in the textbooks by WELZ (1976), L'VOV (1970), and SLAVIN (1976); therefore, only the minimum basic principles and practical sample treatment procedures are described in this section.

2. Instrument

a) Light Source and Background Correction

Although the absorption spectral width of atoms in a high temperature medium differs from element to element, it is less than 0.1 Å for all elements. Therefore, a monochromatic light source with less than 0.1 Å spectral width, either from a continuous light source monochromated by a monochromator with long focal length, or from a monochromatic light source, is necessary. The former method requires a light source with high intensity, since the light intensity is greatly reduced by the monochromator and, therefore, is not suitable for practical use. For the latter purpose, a hollow cathode lamp or an electrodeless discharge lamp is used. Although an electrodeless discharge lamp is more luminous than a hollow cathode lamp, its use is limited to volatile elements and the sensitivity is sometimes lower than that of the latter; it is not as widely used as the hollow cathode lamp.

Light intensity is a function of discharge current and increases linearly with current over 2–3 orders of magnitude. However, with the increase of the current, sputtered atoms are increased, which results in the increase of nonexcited nonemitting atoms in the front region of the cathode. These nonexcited atoms absorb Cd atomic emission light and reduce the light intensity (self-absorption). In this current region, the light intensity does not increase significantly with increasing current. Moreover, as a result of the self-absorption, the line profile is varied; this is disadvantageous for analytic work, and the sensitivity decreases as shown in Fig. 4. As a general rule, analytic sensitivity is higher as the current is decreased; however, at very low currents, stability of the light intensity decreases and the relative noise is increased. Moreover, continuous operation of a hollow cathode lamp at high currents greatly reduces the life span of a lamp. Therefore, optimum current occurs in the intermediate current region.

A D_2 lamp is a continuous light source which is used for correction of the background absorption due to coexisting molecules in the matrix of the solution;

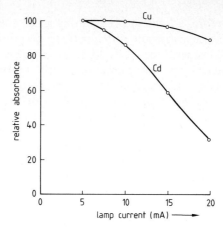

Fig. 4. Relationship between the analytic sensitivity and the lamp current of a hollow cathode lamp

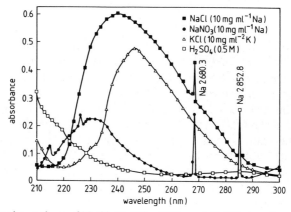

Fig. 5. Molecular absorptions of NaCl, NaNO₃, KCl, and H₂SO₄ in a flame

these are not completely atomized even at high temperatures in the flame or a carbon furnace. In sample analyses, absorption is often observed even when no analyte element exists in the sample solution. This is due to molecular absorption of the matrix molecules or molecules formed from them in the flame. As an example of these molecular absorptions, spectra of NaCl, NaNO₃, KCl, and H₂SO₄ in a flame are shown in Fig. 5. An apparent background absorption is sometimes also observed, which is due to light scattering by the particles. Whatever the real cause of the background absorption may be, accurate estimation of the background absorption is necessary to obtain the correct atomic absorption intensity. Background absorption due to molecular absorption is an especially serious problem, since NaCl absorption overlaps the Cd 228.8 nm line. In order to estimate the molecular absorption, the following method is employed. The spectral bandwidth of molecular absorption is usually large (more than 10 Å), compared with that of atomic absorption (less than 0.1 Å). Therefore, the molecular absorption can be

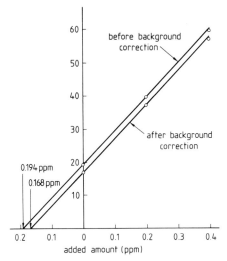

Fig. 6. Calibration curves before and after background correction

estimated by the absorption measurement using a D_2 lamp with a wide slit (usually a spectral bandwidth of 20–30 Å). In this case, the contribution of the atomic absorption to the observed total absorption is negligibly small because of the small atomic spectral width (less than 0.1 Å). Therefore, accurate atomic absorption can be estimated by subtracting the molecular absorption obtained by a D_2 lamp from the total absorption, which is measured with a hollow cathode lamp. This operation is called background correction and several measurement systems for both light intensities exist in commercially available instruments. Mechanical chopper systems are available, permitting alternate measurement of both light intensities. Figure 6 shows how a calibration curve of Cd is corrected by background correction.

b) Atomization

The emission spectrum from the atoms produced in the light source is passed through an absorption cell in which a portion of the incident light is absorbed by analyte atoms produced by thermal dissociation of the molecules in the sample solution. Accordingly, the most important function of the absorption cell is efficiently to produce metal atoms in the ground state from the ions or molecules present in the sample solution. For this purpose, chemical flames in a burner or electrical heating in a carbon furnace is adopted in commercial atomic absorption spectrophotometers.

α) Chemical Flames and Nebulizers. To atomize a sample in a flame, the sample solution is usually sprayed into the flame by means of a pneumatic nebulizer. Methods have also been described in the literature in which solid samples are introduced directly or as suspensions into the flame. However, these methods are designed for special purposes and require further detailed study. By using a nebulizer to spray the sample into the flame, a steady, time-independent signal is ob-

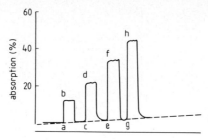

Fig. 7. Chart profiles of standard solutions in flame atomic absorption spectrometry

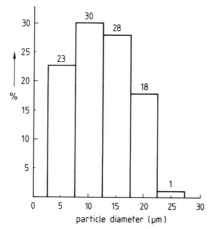

Fig. 8. Particle size distribution of the mist produced by a venturi nebulizer

tained, as shown in Fig. 7, whose height is proportional to the concentration of the element analyzed; the signal continues as long as the sample solution is aspirated and sprayed.

Atomization by means of a chemical flame includes the process of spraying of the sample solution, desolvation of the sample mist, and production of solid sample particles, which at last are atomized by thermal dissociation. These processes must be carried out in a very short period (of the order of 0.002 s). To spray the solution, a venturi tube is widely used. The particle size distribution in the mist from the spray is widely spread as shown in Fig. 8. Those particles with relatively large diameter are difficult to atomize in flames and cause light scattering. In a "premixed" or "laminar" burner, these large particles are removed before entering the flame. On the other hand, in a "total consumption" burner, all the particles enter the flame. In the latter case, the large undecomposed particles cause relatively large light scattering, which causes apparent absorption of the incident light. Therefore, careful attention should be paid to the correction for light scattering. Since the use of a total consumption burner is limited to special cases, the following description is focused on a premixed burner. A typical structure of a premixed burner is depicted in Fig. 9. The disperser is a glass sphere of 7 mm diameter. When large particles collide on the disperser, they are dispersed into a

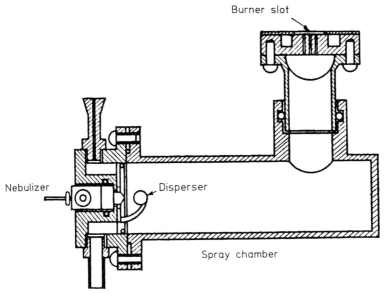

Fig. 9. Structure of a premixed burner for flame atomic absorption spectrometry

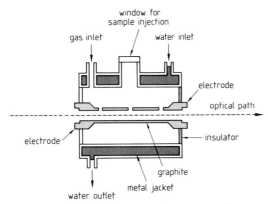

Fig. 10. Structure of an electrically heated carbon furnace atomizer

mist of smaller diameter particles and, accordingly, the nebulization efficiency is increased.

It is expected that the analytic sensitivity increases with increase of the amount of mist introduced into the flame. However, a flame has its own heat capacity and introduction of too much mist decreases the temperature of the flame; this decreases the atomization efficiency in the flame and also increases the interference of the coexisting salts. The nebulizer gas is usually also used as an oxidant of the flame and, therefore, two independently controlled oxidant gas flows are provided in the usual commercial atomic absorption spectrophotometers and the amount of mist and flame oxidant gas can be adjusted independently.

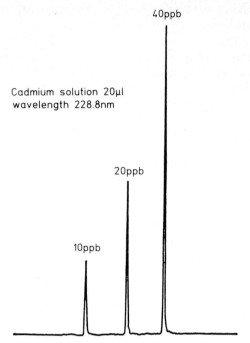

Fig. 11. Chart profiles of signals obtained with an electrically heated carbon furnace atomizer

The fuel gas, oxidant gas, and sample mist are mixed homogeneously before they reach the burner head. The conventional fuel gases are acetylene, hydrogen, or propane; oxidant gases are air or N_2O_5. Cadmium is a relatively easily atomizable element and an air–acetylene flame is employed.

β) Electrically Heated Furnace. An electrically heated furnace for atomization was first developed by L'vov and Massman (see L'vov 1970). It is made of carbon or heat-resistant metal, and the atomization of the sample is carried out by electrical heating of the furnace. The maximum temperature obtained with these furnaces is 2,800 °C, which, although slightly lower than that of a N_2O_5–acetylene flame, can atomize most metals with the aid of the reducing power of carbon. A schematic diagram of a typical carbon furnace is shown in Fig. 10. The carbon tube is shielded by Ar flow in order to prevent air oxidation of the tube. The tube is usually cooled with water and 10–100 μl sample solution is injected into the furnace from an entrance port located in the center of the tube.

The furnace temperature is dependent on the voltage applied to the furnace. The temperature is first gradually elevated to around 100 °C, while the solution is dried. After drying is completed, the furnace is continuously and gradually heated to higher temperatures. At these temperatures all the organic materials are removed by ashing. Finally, the temperature is suddenly elevated to 2,000 °– 2,800 °C; this atomizes the sample and, at the same time, the absorption peak is observed. Since the atomic atmosphere produced in the furnace is blown off by

Ar gas soon after the atomization occurs, the absorption profile is a transient signal and a sharp absorption peak is observed as in Fig. 11. The peak height is usually used for calibration.

Carbon is most frequently used as a furnace material, but sometimes a heat-resistant metal filament, such as tungsten or tantalum may be employed. Commercially available furnace atomic absorption spectrophotometers are provided with an operating unit which controls the increase of temperature as a function of time and enables automatic repetitive analyses of many samples.

In electrically heated furnace atomic absorption spectrometry, the atomic atmosphere of the sample is confined in a relatively small cavity of the furnace and a high atomic density is obtained. Accordingly, detection limits are improved 10–100 times compared with those of flame atomic absorption spectrometry.

3. Selection of Optimum Conditions

For cadmium determination, an acetylene–air flame is usually employed. The optimum gas flow rates are determined as follows. Nebulizing a cadmium solution of suitable concentration into a flame, the flow rates of both fuel and oxidant gases are varied to the optimum point. The optimum flow rates are usually 2–6 l/min for acetylene and 8–15 l/min for air. When an organic solvent is introduced, baseline fluctuation is usually larger than that of an aqueous solution. In that case, the fuel gas flow rate must be decreased to obtain the highest sensitivity. After optimum flow rates are determined, burner position is varied vertically and horizontally to find the flame position where the absorbance is maximum and, therefore, the highest sensitivity is obtained.

The cadmium line with the highest sensitivity is 228.8 nm. However, when the cadmium concentration is high and the absorbance is outside the dynamic range, the less sensitive cadmium line at 326.1 nm is used. Since the line width of a hollow cathode lamp increases with the lamp current, which in turn decreases the sensitivity and also decreases the lamp life span, it is desirable to operate the lamp at the lowest possible current provided the current noise causes no trouble. The lamp current optimum for cadmium determination is 4–10 mA.

Since a hollow cathode lamp emits ionic lines of the analyte element and atomic and ionic lines of the sheath gas (Ar or Ne), besides an analytic line, a monochromator is used to exclude these undesired lines. The slit width is usually selected as large as possible without detecting the neighboring undesired lines, so that background correction can be done simultaneously, measuring the absorption with a hollow cathode lamp and a D_2 lamp.

A carbon furnace is more difficult to operate in optimum conditions than a flame. The reason is the fact that commercial carbon furnaces differ in size, shape, and the gas flow route. Moreover, the furnace temperature-controlling system is different from instrument to instrument. In some instruments, the temperature is regulated only by the current, in which case the temperature may gradually vary with time according to the change of the electrical resistance of the furnace owing to gradual deterioration over repetitive measurements. On the other hand, other instruments are provided with a temperature detector, which regulates the current and therefore the temperature. Owing to this diversity of commercial instruments, and also the fact that the sensitivity critically depends on how the sample is dried, ashed, and atomized, the conditions are drastically different, depending on the instrument and also on how much matrix the sample contains.

The widely accepted, general procedure for determining optimum conditions is as follows. First, ashing temperature is varied by 100 °C from 400° to 1,300 °C, while sensitivity is compared, the drying and atomizing temperature being kept constant. Using the optimum ashing temperature thus obtained, drying temperature is next varied from 90° to 120 °C with both ashing and atomizing temperatures kept constant. In the final stage, the atomizing temperature is optimized with the other two temperatures kept constant. The atomizing temperature is usually varied from 1,900° to 2,700 °C.

A commercial carbon furnace atomizer is provided with a temperature controller and the temperature increase can be programed for repetitive measurements. Usually, the temperature can be raised in two modes: one is the "step mode", in which the temperature is jumped discontinuously to a preset value; and the other mode is the "ramp mode". In the ramp mode, the temperature is linearly increased with time and the temperature gradient can be varied by a temperature controller.

In an analysis of a simple solution, the optimum rate of temperature increase can be easily determined with the procedure described. However, in analyses of complex samples, the optimum temperature increase is often substantially different from that for a simple solution. This is due to the fact that, in the ashing stage, most of the coexisting molecules must be removed so that no serious interference occurs in the atomizing stage. Since the coexisting matrix substances differ from sample to sample, the optimum ashing temperature and ashing period must be determined according to how much organic and inorganic matrix substances the sample solution contains or how easily they are ashed and removed in the ashing stage.

4. Experimental Procedure

With the optimum conditions determined according to the procedure described in the previous section, the dynamic range in flame atomic absorption spectrometry is 0.01–0.5 ppm for an organic solution and 0.03–1.0 ppm for an aqueous solution. In electrically heated carbon furnace atomic absorption spectrometry, the dynamic range is 0.008–0.2 ppb. The precision of repetitive measurement is usually 2%–10%.

Although the method is highly sensitive, cadmium concentrations in biologic samples are usually low (for instance, the concentration is about 5 ppb in whole blood), and therefore concentration procedures are necessary. The most commonly used procedure is solvent extraction. This procedure is advantageous in that it eliminates interfering elements in the sample solution, besides concentrating the analyte element. Several common extraction procedures are described.

a) Dithizone Extraction

About 1 g sample is decomposed in a 100-ml beaker or a Kjeldahl flask by adding 6–8 ml HNO_3 and 3–4 ml H_2SO_4 and gently heating. After the sample is completely decomposed and a clear solution is obtained, it is made up to 100 ml and a portion of the solution (containing 1–12 µg cadmium) is placed in a separating funnel. NaOH solution (10 w/v%) is added to neutralize the solution, using bromothymol blue as an indicator, 1 ml hydroxylamine hydrochloric acid solution (20 w/v%), 5 ml ammonium citrate solution (10 w/v%),

Table 3. Typical measurement conditions for flame atomic absorption spectrometry[a] of Cd

		Aqueous solution	Organic solution
Wavelength (nm)		228.8	228.8
Lamp current (mA)		6	6
Acetylene gas	Pressure (kg/cm^2)	0.5	0.5
	Flow rate (l/min)	2.5	2.0
Air	Pressure (kg/cm^2)	1.8	1.9
	Flow rate (l/min)	14	13.5

[a] The instrument is a Hitachi 518 atomic absorption spectrophotometer

10 ml NaOH solution (10 w/v%), and 1 ml KCN solution (1 w/v%) are added and the solution is shaken vigorously. Then 10 ml dithizone–chloroform solution (0.005 w/v%) is added and the solution is shaken vigorously for 1 min. After separation, the chloroform layer is transferred to another 100-ml separating funnel. The extraction is repeated once with 10 ml and once with 5 ml chloroform. The combined chloroform layer is next processed for backtitration into acidic aqueous solution. The procedure is as follows.

First, 10 ml HCl solution (1 : 50 dilution of concentrated HCl) is added to the chloroform layer, which is shaken for 2 min and the aqueous layer is separated. This backextraction is repeated twice more with 10 and 5 ml HCl solution and the aqueous layers are combined and made up to 25 ml. This aqueous solution is subjected to the measurement. For calibration, standard solutions are prepared by dissolving Cd metal in HNO$_3$. The calibration line is prepared within the range 0.03–0.5 ppm. Table 3 summarizes the conditions when using the Hitachi 518 flame atomic absorption spectrometer, as a typical example of an aqueous solution analysis.

b) Sodium Diethyldithiocarbamate (DDTC) Extraction

The sample is decomposed with HNO$_3$ and H$_2$SO$_4$ as described in the previous section. An aliquot of the solution (containing 0.3–8 µg Cd) is placed in a separating funnel and 10 ml ammonium citrate solution (10 w/v%) and a few drops of *m*-cresol purple solution (0.1 w/v%) are added. Aqueous ammonia (1 part concentrated NH$_4$OH + 1 part H$_2$O) is gradually added until the solution changes to light purple, and the solution is made up to a constant volume; 5 ml DDTC–butyl acetate solution (1 w/v%) is added and the solution is shaken. After 20 ml butyl acetate is added, the solution is vigorously shaken for 1 min and the butyl acetate layer is separated. The extraction is repeated by adding 5 ml butyl acetate and all the butyl acetate is collected and made up to 25 ml, which is used for measurement. An example of the optimum conditions of measurement for an organic solution is shown in Table 3.

c) Calibration Methods

Standard solutions with known concentrations are most frequently used for obtaining a calibration curve. However, such standard solutions differ in the matrix constitution from that of the sample solution, which sometimes results in a difference in the slope of the calibration curves. The interference of the matrix elements can be removed by extraction with organic solvents. However, in electrically heated carbon furnace atomic absorption spectrometry, the sensitivity is so high that the sample can sometimes be analyzed without such preconcentration procedure. The acid-decomposed solution is used directly for measurements. In such cases, the interference from the matrix elements must be eliminated by some means. Even though the method is provided with a background correction function using a D_2 lamp, this is not sufficient to remove all the effects due to coexisting materials. In order to remove these undesired matrix effects, the standard solutions are usually prepared by adding major elements and acids that constitute the sample solution besides the analyte element. The slope of the calibration curve obtained with such standard solutions is much closer to that of the sample solution than a simple standard solution containing only the analyte element. The other calibration method is the conventional standard addition procedure.

5. Plasma Emission Spectrometry

In the last 10 years, plasma emission spectrometry has been rapidly developed and it has replaced atomic absorption spectrometry in certain areas of spectrochemical analysis of trace metals. It uses the high temperature plasma of rare gases such as argon or helium and provides a simultaneous multielement analysis. Cadmium can be analyzed at the level of ppb, which is about equal to atomic absorption.

Table 4 gives the types of plasma which have been investigated in this field. Among various types of plasma listed, those most commonly used, namely the radiofrequency inductively coupled argon plasma (ICP) and DC plasma jet, are selected and described briefly.

a) Inductively Coupled Plasma Emission Spectrometry

A schematic diagram of ICP produced at the tip of a quartz torch is shown in Fig. 12. The torch consists of three coaxial quartz tubes, which are from the inside: (a) for Ar gas carrying the sample aerosol (1–2 l/min); (b) for Ar plasma gas (1 l/min); and (c) for coolant Ar gas (15–20 l/min). At the top of the torch, 2–4 turns of the induction coil are set, through which radio frequency of 27.12 MHz and 0.5–2.5 kW is supplied.

When the high frequency current is coupled with the argon gas, an alternating magnetic field is produced, around which the eddy current accelerates the electrons; these, in turn, excite argon atoms, which induces the high temperature ($\sim 6,000$ K) plasma state. The temperature is highest at 2–3 mm from the center, producing a so-called doughnut-shape structure.

The sample aerosol carried through the inner tube goes into the lower temperature center of the doughnut, which effectively spreads into the higher temperature excitation zone, without losing the unused part of the sample. The electron

Table 4. Rare gas plasma for emission spectrometry

1. DC plasma
   a) DC plasma jet
   b) Stabilized arc
2. Induction plasma
   a) Radiofrequency inductively coupled plasma
   b) Capacitively coupled microwave plasma
   c) Microwave induced plasma

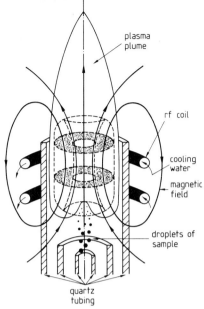

Fig. 12. Schematic illustration of ICP and its excitation mechanism

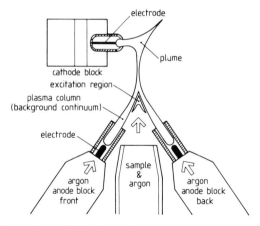

Fig. 13. Schematic illustration of DC plasma jet

density of the plasma is as high as 10^{15}–10^{16} cm^{-3}, and the metastable argon atoms, Ar^{m} 11.71 eV, are also available for the excitation of the sample atoms.

The production of the sample aerosol resembles that in atomic absorption spectrometry, namely, the compressed argon carrier gas atomizes the aqueous sample solution through the atomizer inside the atomizer chamber. The sensitivity for cadmium is approximately 1 ppb, which is similar to that of flame atomic absorption.

b) Direct Current Plasma Emission Spectrometry

The DC arc, the original type of emission spectroscopy, has been modified and a DC plasma jct such as shown in Fig. 13 is now available as a direct reading argon plasma emission source. The main feature is that both DC electrodes are placed at an angle of approximately 60°, argon gas (~ 10 ml/min) is injected through the holes of both electrodes, through which DC current is supplied. The highest temperature at the mixing point of both gas flows is approximately 6,000 K with the highest excitation. A separate argon gas flow carries the sample aerosol from the lower part of the arc and injects it into the high temperature region. Excitation of sample atoms takes place after the decomposition of compounds. The sensitivity for cadmium is approximately 1 ppb. Systems for simultaneous analysis of 30–60 elements have been built using these plasma emission sources, but single element systems are also available.

II. Polarography

Cadmium exhibits a typical reversible polarographic wave, and it is one of the elements that can be determined relatively easily by polarography. The analytic dynamic ranges are from 10^{-2} to approximately 5×10^{-6} M for direct current polarography, to approximately 10^{-5} M for alternating current polarography, and to about 10^{-7} M for square wave polarography. The accuracy of repetitive measurement is usually 2%–10%. Besides these high sensitivities, polarography possesses the great advantage that several elements can be determined with one measurement.

1. Principles of Direct Current Polarography

Figure 14 is a schematic illustration of a basic circuit for direct current polarography. It consists of a potentiometer drum, a direct current power supply, an ammeter, and a recorder for measuring the electrolytic current. The anode is a large

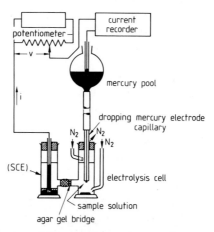

Fig. 14. Schematic illustration of direct current polarography

saturated calomel electrode or a large mercury pool electrode and the cathode is dropping mercury, whose surface area is neglibibly small compared with that of the anode and the surface is always kept clean by the continuous dropping of the mercury. This dropping mercury is the main feature of the method, which makes the method applicable to trace element analysis.

The potentiometer drum is first adjusted to set the voltage to a suitable value (usually 2.0 V). As the electrolysis is initiated and the contact point is gradually and linearly shifted, the voltage applied between the electrodes increases and the potential of the dropping mercury cathode decreases to negative values. In the course of this potential scan, the current is recorded. The diagram showing the relation between the electrolysis current and the voltage is called a polarogram. As a typical example, the polarogram for a 0.1 M KCl solution is shown in Fig. 15. The potential is scanned from zero to negative values. The electrolysis current is negligible (curve A) when the applied voltage is higher than -1.8 V. However, when the voltage reaches -1.8 V, an abrupt increase of the current is observed. This current increase is due to the reduction of potassium cation. The polarogram for a solution containing 10^{-3} M Cd in addition to 0.1 M KCl is shown in Fig. 15 (curve B). The current is also negligible down to -0.5 V. However, when the potential reaches -0.5 V, reduction of cadmium begins and the current suddenly increases with decreasing voltage. After the steep increase of the electrolysis current, it reaches a plateau and no more increase is observed. When the potential sweep is further continued and reaches -1.8 V, the reduction of potassium cation begins and the current again increases rapidly. In Fig. 15, a small residual amount of current (ir) is observed, even when neither Cd nor K is being reduced. The current id, which is due to cadmium reduction, is called the limiting current. The potential where the current is half the limiting current is called the halfwave potential. Since the polarographic wave in Fig. 15 is based on cadmium reduction, it is called the reductive wave. When the reaction at the dropping mercury electrode is oxidation, the current is in the opposite direction and the wave is called the oxidative wave. Electrolyte material like KCl in Fig. 15, which does not participate in the redox reaction of the analyte element at the electrode, but is added to the solution at relatively high concentration to maintain the conductivity of the solution, is called the supporting electrolyte.

As mentioned earlier, the fact that the working electrode is dropping mercury whose surface area is very small compared with that of the mercury pool counterelectrode is an indespensable factor for the control of the electrode potentials and also for maintaining a clean electrode surface, thus providing stability for analytic work. The voltage between the two electrodes E is expressed as Eq. (1)

$$E = E_a - E_c + iR,\qquad(1)$$

where E_c is the potential of the cathode (dropping mercury), E_a is the potential of the anode (mercury pool), and R is the total resistance of the circuit, including that of the electrolyte solution. Since the electrolytic current is usually less than 10 μA and R is around 100 Ω, the voltage drop iR is ~ 1 mV and is negligible compared with E_a and E_c. Since the surface area of the mercury pool electrode is very large compared with that of a dropping mercury electrode and an equivalent amount of redox reactions take place at both electrodes, the concentration

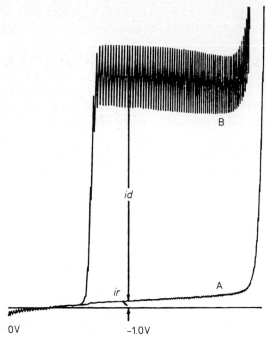

Fig. 15. Polarograms of 0.1 M KCl solution (curve A) and of Cd^{2+} in 0.1 M KCl solution (curve B)

change of the solution owing to the electrolyte reaction at the electrode surface is negligible at the mercury pool electrode. This means that the potential of the mercury pool anode is considered constant during the potential scan and the applied voltage is rewritten as Eq. (2)

$$E = -E_c + \text{const}. \tag{2}$$

Equation (2) means that the cathode potential varies linearly and negatively with the applied voltage and the voltage – current diagram shown in Fig. 15 is therefore equivalent to the cathode potential – current diagram.

Besides the fact that the surface is kept clean and therefore no hysteresis is observed, the dropping mercury electrode is advantageous in that the overvoltage of mercury for hydrogen evolution is large and therefore it can be used in the negative potential region, even in acidic solutions. Moreover, the amount of the electrolyzed substance is negligibly small and the concentration of the solution is unchanged even after the measurement. Therefore, the solution may be repeatedly used for measurements.

2. Limiting Current

The electrode reaction at the cathode is expressed as Eq. (3)

$$Ox + ne \rightarrow Red, \tag{3}$$

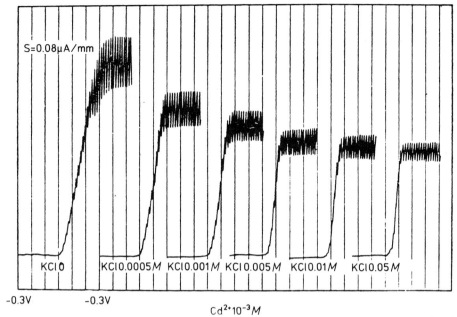

S=0.08μA/mm

KCl 0   KCl 0.0005M KCl 0.001M KCl 0.005M KCl 0.01M KCl 0.05M

-0.3V   -0.3V

Cd²⁺10⁻³M

Fig. 16. The effect of the supporting electrolyte concentration on the limiting current of cadmium

where Ox is the oxidant, Red is the reductant, and n electrons are transferred. As the electrolysis proceeds, Ox is consumed at the electrode surface and its concentration is decreased. In contrast, the concentration of Red is increased. Therefore the concentrations of Ox and Red at the electrode surface are different from those in the solution itself. The situation is called concentration polarization, where the concentration of Ox at the electrode is slightly lower than that of the solution and the concentration of Red is slightly higher than that of the solution. As a result, Ox migrates from the solution to the dropping electrode surface, and Red moves from the electrode surface to the solution. When metal ion is reduced at the electrode surface, as is the case in most polarography, the resulting metal migrates into the dropping mercury, forming amalgam. In order to maintain continuous electrolysis, Ox must be supplied from the solution to the electrode surface. The electrolytic current is determined either by the rate of the Ox supply to the electrode surface or the reduction rate of Eq. (3). For those potential regions where the limiting current is observed, Ox reaching the electrode is immediately reduced, and therefore Ox concentration at the electrode is zero. In this case, the current is determined only by the Ox supply rate. Although the reaction rate of Eq. (3) is increased with increased negativity of the potential, the electrolytic current does not increase since the current is determined only by Ox supply rate; this is the reason for the occurrence of the limiting current.

Generally, the Ox supply to the electrode surface is provided either by diffusion down the concentration gradient between the solution itself and the electrode surface, by electrophoresis due to the potential difference, or by solution convection. In polarography, where the solution is not stirred, solution convection is negligible. Neither is electrophoresis a main factor for supplying Ox, since the solution is provided with excess of supporting electrolyte; this greatly reduces the solution resistance, and the potential gradient in the solution is very small. Therefore, Ox supply to the electrode surface is mostly achieved by diffusion and the limiting current in such a case is called the diffusion current. Figure 16 shows the effect of the supporting electrolyte concentration on the limiting current of cadmium. The limiting current is large when the electrolyte concentration is small, owing to the contribution of electrophoresis. This additional current is called migration current. Supporting electrolyte is usually added in 50–100 times the concentration of the analyte.

3. Diffusion Current and Ilkovic Equation

The limiting current in polarography oscillates around the average value labelled i_d in Fig. 15. The periodic current change is due to the growth of the mercury drop, and the diffusion current $(i_d)_t$ at time t is expressed as Eq. (4)

$$(i_d)_t = 708 \, nm^{2/3} t^{1/6} D^{1/2} {}^*C. \tag{4}$$

In Eq. (4), n is the number of electrons participating in the electrode reaction, m is the rate of flow of mercury (mg/s), t is the time after the initiation of the mercury drop formation (s), D is the diffusion coefficient (cm^2/s), and $^*C$ is the analyte concentration of the bulk solution. The growth and dropping rate of the mercury electrode is constant and the diffusion layer around the dropping mercury electrode is destroyed on every drop. Therefore, the current change with growth of the mercury drop is exactly repeated on every drop and the average current i_d is unchanged for a substantial period; this is a great advantage over the usual solid electrodes. The average current i_d is calculated as Eq. (5),

$$i_d = \frac{1}{\tau} \int_0^\tau (i_d)_t dt = \frac{6}{7} i_{max}, \tag{5}$$

where τ is the lifespan of a mercury drop. Combining Eqs. (4) and (5) gives Eq. (6).

$$i_d = 607 \, nm^{2/3} \tau^{1/6} D^{1/2} {}^*C. \tag{6}$$

Equation (6) is called the Ilkovic equation and provides a basis for quantitative analysis. The polarogram is expressed by Eq. (7)

$$E = E_{1/2} + \frac{RT}{nF} \ln \frac{i_d - i}{i}, \tag{7}$$

where $E_{1/2}$ is the halfwave potential, E is the potential, i is the current, and n is the number of electrons involved in the redox reaction. $E_{1/2}$ is expressed as Eq. (8) and is a specific value for the analyte in a given supporting electrolyte solution

$$E_{1/2} = E^0 + \frac{RT}{nF} \ln \frac{D_R^{1/2}}{D_0^{1/2}} \sim E^0, \tag{8}$$

E^0 is the standard potential, D_0 and D_R are the diffusion coefficients of the depolarizer (analyte) and the reduction product, respectively. $E_{1/2}$ is slightly dependent on the electrolyte composition, but is independent of the concentration of the analyte, which provides the basis for qualitative analysis by polarography.

4. Limitations of Direct Current Polarography

Although direct current polarography provides rapid analysis for trace metals, it has several limitations, e.g., trace analytes in large amounts of matrix substance which is electrolyzed before the analyte can be determined, since the analyte trace current overlaps the large limiting current of the matrix substance. The maximum permissible excess of matrix in such a case would be 50 times the amount of analyte. Since mercury is used for the working electrode, those positive potential regions where mercury is oxidized can not be used for measurement. Although mercury is advantageous in that its overpotential for hydrogen is large and therefore it can be used as a working electrode down to -1.0 V (saturated calomel electrode), even in acidic solution, it can be used in the positive direction only to 0.4 V owing to mercury oxidation.

In order to circumvent these disadvantages, several modifications of the method have been developed. These include differential polarography, alternating current polarography, square wave polarography, high frequency polarography, pulse polarography, and oscillographic polarography. The development of these methods has been based on the progress of electronic technology. Most of these methods can effectively eliminate the undesired residual current and the effect of the predischarging substance, so that sensitivity is expanded down to 10^{-7} or 10^{-8} M. Moreover, recent development of solid electrodes enables the measurement in potential regions more positive than 0.4 V. However, the details of these methods are not described here.

5. Qualitative Analysis

As mentioned previously, the halfwave potential $E_{1/2}$ is specific for the depolarizer, that is, the analyte, at a given supporting electrolyte concentration and pH of the solution. This provides the basis for qualitative analysis. The halfwave potential is obtained graphically as shown in Fig. 17. The potential obtained in this

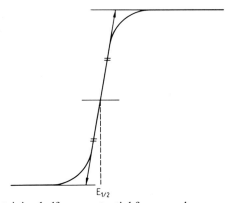

Fig. 17. Method of obtaining halfwave potential from a polarogram

way is the value compared with the counterelectrode and therefore the potential of the counterelectrode must be measured against a suitable reference electrode, such as the saturated calomel electrode (SCE). In another procedure, a suitable reference ion with known halfwave potential is added to the sample solution and the potential of the analyte is measured against that known potential. Tl^+ is used for this purpose, since the halfwave potential is substantially constant (-0.46 V vs SCE) in various supporting electrolyte solutions.

6. Quantitative Analysis

The quantitative basis of the method is that the limiting current is proportional to the concentration of the depolarizer (analyte) as shown in Eq. (6). A calibration line is obtained by measurement of several standard Cd solutions whose matrix component is matched with the sample solutions. The calibration method can be used even when the calibration line does not cross the origin or the line is slightly curved.

For sample solutions with complex matrix composition, for which standard solutions with the same matrix component are diffucult to prepare, the standard addition method is often employed. This method is based on the assumption that the calibration line is strictly linear and crosses the origin. After measurement of the sample solution, a known amount of the analyte is added and the measurement repeated. The analyte concentration C_1 is calculated by Eq. (9)

$$C_1 = \frac{i_1 C_2 v}{i_2(V+v) - i_1 V} \tag{9}$$

where V is the volume of the sample, i_1 and i_2 are the limiting currents before and after the addition, v is the addition volume of the standard solution, and C_2 is the concentration of the standard solution. It is desirable that the standard solution be as concentrated as possible so that the matrix composition is not changed by the addition procedure.

7. Experimental Procedure

A dropping mercury electrode consists of a glass capillary which is connected to a mercury pool. The capillary is about 15 cm long and is either of uniform inner diameter (0.03–0.05 mm) or with gradually reduced diameter toward the exit (0.01 mm). With either capillary, the cutoff plane must be perpendicular to the capillary axis. The optimum configuration is such that, when the mercury pool is at a height of about 70 cm, the dropping period is 4–7 s. The requirements for cell design are: the mercury counterelectrode is placed at the bottom of the cell and is connected to the outer electrical circuit; the cell is usually provided with a tube for degassing in order to remove dissolved oxygen.

In order to obtain a good polarogram, a 50- to 100-fold excess of supporting electrolyte must be added to the solution. Typical and most frequently used supporting electrolytes and the halfwave potentials of cadmium in them are summarized in Table 5.

Table 5. Effect of the supporting electrolyte composition on cadmium halfwave potential compared with standard calomel electrode at 25 °C

Supporting electrolyte	Halfware potential (V)
0.1 M HCl	−0.599
0.1 M KCl	−0.599
1 M HCl	−0.642
1 M KCl	−0.642
1 M HNO$_3$	−0.586
1 M KNO$_3$	−0.586
0.5 M H$_2$SO$_4$	−0.586
1 M H$_3$PO$_4$	−0.59
1 M KI	−0.74
1 M KCN	−1.18
1 M NH$_4$OH + 1 M NH$_4$Cl	−0.81
0.5 M sodium tartrate (pH 4–8)	−0.64

Samples for analysis are prepared as follows: 1 g sample is accurately weighed, placed in a platinum dish or a Teflon beaker, and 10 ml HNO_3 and 3–5 ml $HClO_4$ are added and the sample is completely decomposed by gently heating. If the decomposition is incomplete, additional HNO_3 and H_2SO_4 is added (2–3 ml) and the heating is continued. After complete decomposition, 8 ml 6 M HCl and about 20 ml H_2O are added, followed by 5 ml hydroxylamine hydrochloride (10 w/v%) with heating in order to reduce Fe^{3+} to Fe^{2+}. After cooling, 2.5 ml gelatin or Triton X-100 solution (0.2 w/v%) is added and the solution is adjusted to 50 ml. The addition is made only for direct current polarography, not for alternating current polarography or square wave polarography. A portion of the solution is transferred to an electrolysis cell and the dissolved oxygen is removed by passing N_2 gas. The potential is scanned from −0.4 to 0.8 V against SCE to obtain the polarogram.

When the sample solution contains substantial amounts of organic materials, extraction with DDTC or dithizone and backextraction with dilute HCl as described in Sect. B.I.4 are employed in the sample preparation. After gelatin or carboxymethylcellulose (CMC) solution is added, the solution is subjected to measurement.

III. X-Ray Fluorescence Analysis

1. Principles

When a sample is irradiated with X-rays, the atoms in the sample emit characteristic X-rays, whose wavelength is specific for each element and is related to the atomic number by Moseley's law, and whose intensity is proportional to the concentration of each element. These are the bases for qualitative and quantitative analysis with X-ray fluorescence spectrometry. The instruments are basically divided into two systems: wavelength dispersive and energy dispersive systems. In the former system, the X-rays are monochromated by a crystal and measured by

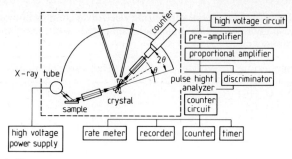

Fig. 18. Schematic illustration of a wavelength dispersive X-ray fluorescence spectrometer

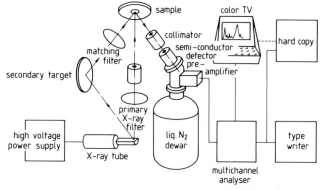

Fig. 19. Schematic illustration of an energy dispersive X-ray fluorescence spectrometer

moving a proportional counter or a scintillation counter to the angle where the Bragg equation is satisfied by the analyte wavelength; a schematic drawing of the system is given in Fig. 18. In the latter system, X-rays are detected nondispersively by a semiconductor detector, that is, there is no crystal for monochromation. Instead, the detector fulfills the functions of both energy discrimination and intensity measurement; a schematic diagram is shown in Fig. 19. Although the energy dispersive system provides simultaneous multielement analysis, the detection limits are usually higher by a factor of 10–100 than those of wavelength dispersive systems. Therefore, in this section, application of the latter system to cadmium analysis will be described. Details of each component in both systems are described in the textbook by BERTIN (1975) and will not be discussed here any further.

Although X-ray fluorescence analysis can be applied to either solid, powder, or liquid samples and, what is more advantageous, solid samples can be analyzed nondestructively, the sensitivities are usually poorer compared with those of other techniques of atomic spectrometry, such as atomic emission or absorption spectrometry. The detection limit for cadmium is 10 ppm at best. Therefore, some preconcentration treatment must be employed. Biologic samples are usually decomposed and cadmium is concentrated either on chelating resin or homogeneously precipitated on a film. Some typical procedures are described in the next section.

Table 6. Typical experimental conditions for cadmium in wavelength dispersive X-ray fluorescence analysis

	Cd K_a	Cd L_a
Tube target	Tungsten	Chrome
Tube voltage (kV)	50	50
Tube current (mA)	40	40
Crystal	LiF	Graphite
Detector	Scintillation counter	Scintillation counter
X-ray pass	Air	Vacuum
2θ	15.30°	72.38°
Background 2θ	15.00°–15.80°	71.50°–73.26°
PHA condition	Integral	Differential
PHA gain ($\Omega/100\,pF$)	60	30–60
Measurement time (s)	40	40

PHA = pulse-height analyzer

In X-ray fluorescence analysis, selection of the X-ray tube anode, excitation voltage, monochromating crystal, and detector all critically affect the sensitivity. Some typical selections for wavelength dispersive systems are listed in Table 6.

2. Experimental Procedure

Several preconcentration methods for cadmium and their detection limits and precisions are tabulated in Table 7. As one of the typical and most sensitive preconcentration methods, preconcentration by DDTC precipitation is described below.

About 2 g sample is accurately weighed and is decomposed by adding about 13 ml acid mixture ($HClO_4$ 1.5 : H_2SO_4 1.5 : HNO_3 10) in a 250-ml Erlenmeyer flask. The flask is immersed in boiling water until the sample is completely decomposed to give a clear solution. If necessary, some additional HNO_3 is added to the sample. After decomposition, the sample solution is made up to 100 ml. The solution is transferred to a beaker and the pH is adjusted to about 8 with NH_4OH. At this stage, 1 ml 100 ppm Cu solution is added to the sample solution, which greatly increases the cadmium precipitation by DDTC below cadmium concentrations of 1 ppm. The DDTC solution (2 w/w%) is prepared by dissolving 2.6 g sodium diethyldithiocarbamate in 100 ml H_2O; 5 ml DDTC solution is added to the sample solution and the resulting precipitate is filtered by a membrane filter. For X-ray fluorescence analysis, the filter must be thin to reduce X-ray background and be as free from impurities as possible; the surface must be flat. The membrane filter HAWP 04700 (pore size 0.45 μm, thickness 0.1 mm, diameter 47 mm, Millipore Company), satisfies these requirements and is used for filtration of the precipitate. After filtration, the filter is air dried and is subjected to X-ray measurement.

Table 7. Detection limits and precision of several preconcentration methods in X-ray fluorescence analysis

Method	Detection limit (μg)	Precision (%)
Ion exchange film	0.3	6
Ion exchange paper	0.77	10
DDTC precipitate	0.081	3.6

IV. Neutron Activation Analysis

1. Principles

Neutron activation analysis is based on measurement of γ-rays produced as a result of a nuclear reaction. A sample is irradiated with thermal neutrons in a nuclear reactor and the γ-rays emitted by the radioactive isotope produced in the reactor are measured, usually with a γ-ray pulse-height analyzer or a Ge(Li) semiconductor detector. The detection limit is ~ 1 ppb.

The intensity of the γ-rays at time t is expressed as Eq. (10).

$$A_t = N_A f \sigma_{act} (1 - e^{-\lambda t}) e^{-\lambda t}. \tag{10}$$

In Eq. (10) A_t is the intensity of the γ-ray (dis/s), N_A is the number of analyte atoms, σ_{act} is the activation cross section (cm), λ is the decay constant of the radioactive isotope, and f is the flux of the thermal neutrons. Although absolute analysis by calculating the analyte amount from Eq. (10) is possible, it is not usually used, since it is difficult to obtain accurate values of f and also to maintain f constant. Therefore, in real analysis, calibration with standard samples is employed.

Cadmium ($Z=48$) has stable isotopes: ^{106}Cd (isotope ratio 1.22%), ^{108}Cd (0.87%), ^{110}Cd (12.39%), ^{111}Cd (12.75%), ^{112}Cd (24.07%), ^{113}Cd (12.26%), ^{114}Cd (28.86%), and ^{116}Cd (7.58%). The isotopes utilized for neutron activation analysis and the corresponding radioactive isotopes and half-lives are shown in Table 8. The most frequently used nuclear reaction is

$$^{115}\text{Cd (54 h)} \xrightarrow[(n,\gamma)]{} {}^{115\,m}\text{In (45 h)}$$

and the γ-ray intensity at 523 KeV is measured.

The advantage of the method over other analytic methods is that interfering elements are completely different from those of other methods, since the interference elements, depends on their energies and half-lives. No chemical reactions are involved in the interference. Another advantage is that in some cases the sample can be analyzed without decomposition. This is especially useful for biologic samples and for clinical applications, since it enables in vivo determination of cadmium and not only reduces the analysis time, but also provides much informa-

Table 8. Isotopes of cadmium utilized in neutron activation analysis

Nuclear reaction	Produced Isotope	Half-life	Saturated radioactivity (dis min^{-1} µg^{-1})	Relative radioactivity after 1 h irradiation (dis min^{-1} µg^{-1})
^{114}Cd (n,γ)	^{115m}Cd	43 days	2.4×10^3	$<1 \times 10$
	^{115}Cd	54 h	1.3×10^3	1.2×10
^{116}Cd (n,γ)	^{117m}Cd	2.9 h	1.0×10^5	1.3×10^3
	^{117}Cd	50 min	3.8×10^4	8.4×10^3

tion about the clinical status of the sample. In this regard, the recently developed mobile prompt gamma in vivo neutron activation analysis system greatly facilitates the application of neutron activation analysis in the medical field. The details of the instrument and its application will be described in Sect. B.IV.3.

2. Experimental Procedure

a) Pretreatment

An accurately weighed sample (2–15 mg) is sealed in a quartz ampule, which is then placed in an aluminum capsule for irradiation. A typical size of the quartz ampule is 1.0 cm inner diameter, 1.3 cm outer diameter, and 20 cm length. The aluminum capsule covering the quartz tube would be 1.5 cm in diameter and 125 cm long. As a standard for calibration, 5–10 μg cadmium is dropped onto a filter paper ($\sim$ 1 cm^2) as cadmium sulfate solution (5–10 μl) with a pipet. This paper is sealed in a quartz ampule, as is the sample. Both the sample and the standard are irradiated with thermal neutrons under identical conditions and the resulting γ-ray intensities are measured and compared.

b) Irradiation

Both the sample and the standard are irradiated for 3–5 days with a thermal neutron flux of about 5×100^{11} n cm^{-1}s^{-1}. After irradiation, the sample is left standing for several hours so that short half-life isotopes can decay. The sample is then processed after the following chemical treatment.

c) Preparation of the Sample for Measurement

A 10-ml sample of 1 mg/ml Cd solution (2.282 g CdSO$_4 \cdot 8/3$ H$_2$O dissolved in 1 l H$_2$O) is placed in a 300-ml beaker and evaporated to dryness; 5 ml fuming nitric acid is added to the beaker and the sample in a quartz ampule is placed in the beaker. The ampule is crushed with a glass rod and the contents are heated gently until the sample is decomposed and the solution becomes clear. The solution is transferred to a 150-ml Erlenmeyer flask, and the total volume is adjusted to about 120 ml. The solution is further treated according to the following purification procedure.

The pH of the solution is adjusted to 1–2 by adding 3 M HCl, through which H$_2$S is bubbled and cadmium is precipitated as CdS. The solution and the precipitate is then centrifuged (3,000 rpm) for 10 min. The supernatant solution is discarded. The residual precipitate is dissolved by adding 3 M HCl in the centrifuge tube, which is heated in a water bath to drive off all H$_2$S.

An anion exchange column is prepared by pouring 10 g Dowex IX-8 anion resin (200–400 mesh) in 3 M HCl into a column with approximate diameter 1.5 cm. The centrifuged solution free of H$_2$S is poured onto the column at approximately 1 ml/min. Cadmium is trapped in the resin as CdCl$_3$ anion in 3 M HCl. Other metal elements which do not form chloroanions in 3 M HCl are removed by this procedure. After the sample solution is poured through the column, 150 ml 3 M HCl is again poured into the column and all the eluate is discarded. In order to remove those metals which are adsorbed on the resin and whose stability constants for chlorocomplexes are relatively small, 150 ml 0.1 M HCl is poured onto the column and the eluate is also discarded. After these procedures, cadmium is eluted with 100 ml water. The eluate is collected in a 300-ml beaker. The eluate is adjusted to pH 1 $\sim$ 2 by adding a few drops of 1 M HCl and H$_2$S gas is passed through to precipitate CdS. Again the precipitate and the solution is centrifuged for 10 min at 3,000 rpm and the supernatant is discarded. The precipitate is completely dissolved with 3 M HCl and 5 mg Cu^{2+} (1 ml of a solution prepared by dissolving 2 g CuSO$_4 \cdot 5$ H$_2$O in 100 ml H$_2$O) and 5 mg Sb^{3+} (1 ml of a solution prepared by dissolving 1 g SbCl$_3$ in 100 ml 3 M HCl) is added, which is precipitated as sulfide by the H$_2$S remaining in the solution. Additional H$_2$S is further passed and the precipitation is completed. The precipitate is centrifuged and the supernatant solution is transferred to a 300-ml beaker. The solution is boiled to remove all the H_2S and, after cooling, 10 mg Fe^{3+} (1 ml of a solution prepared by dissolving 2.5 g $FeCl_3 \cdot 6H_2O$ in 100 ml H_2O) is added, which is precipitated as $Fe(OH)_3$ by adding 1 M ammonia. The precipitate is removed by centrifugation at 3,000 rpm, and the supernatant is transferred to another centrifuge tube. A few drops of 1 M HCl are added to acidify the solution to pH 1–2, and CdS is precipitated with H_2S. After centrifugation, the supernatant is discarded and the precipitate is dissolved with 3 M HCl. The solution is evaporated to dryness, and the residue dissolved with 3 ml 3 M HCl for γ-ray measurement.

d) Measurement and Concentration Calculation

The solution prepared as described in the previous section is transferred to a polyethylene tube with a diameter of 1 cm and the 523 KeV γ-rays from ^{115}Cd (half-life 54 h) are measured with a γ-ray pulse-height analyzer or a Ge(Li) semiconductor detector. After γ-ray measurement, the cadmium recovery with regard to the previously described chemical treatment is determined by chelatometric titration. The procedure is as follows.

The solution in a polyethylene test tube is transferred to a 300-ml beaker, and 10 ml NH_4Cl–NH_3 buffer solution (prepared by dissolving 67.5 g NH_4Cl and 570 ml aqueous ammonia of specific gravity 0.9 in 1 l water), 2 ml 10% KCN solution, 5 ml formaldehyde (1:9), and 0.1 ml Eriochrome Black T indicator solution (0.5 g reagent and 4.5 g hydroxylamine hydrochloride dissolved in 100 ml methanol) are added. The solution is titrated with 0.01 M EDTA. The end point is the color change from red to blue; 1 ml 0.01 M EDTA solution corresponds to 1.124 mg cadmium.

The recovery of the added 10 mg cadmium is calculated from the titration. The true count for ^{115}Cd in the sample is calculated by dividing the experimental γ-ray count by this recovery value. The concentration of cadmium is obtained by calibration against a standard sample, which is prepared as described previously and chemically treated in the same way as for the sample.

3. Mobile Prompt Gamma In Vivo Activation Analysis

Although neutron activation analysis has a capability of nondestructive analysis which facilitates in vivo analysis, the necessity of a nuclear reactor as an activation source has so far limited its wide application in the medical field. As a compact mobile apparatus which overcomes this disadvantage, an instrument for mobile prompt gamma in vivo activation analysis has recently been developed and the in vivo determination of liver and kidney cadmium has been actually carried out for some patients in European countries and the United States. A neutron beam emitted from ^{238}Pu induces the nuclear reaction, converting ^{113}Cd to ^{114}Cd and the γ-rays at 559 KeV are measured with a Ge(Li) semiconductor detector. The use of the radioisotope as a neutron source reduces the instrument size and makes it mobile. The ^{238}Pu neutron source is placed in a tungsten container covered with epoxy resin and is installed under a bed. The epoxy cover is removed before the neutron beam is used. Since the amount of radiation is only 0.6 rem, and the induced activity decays rapidly, the method is not at all hazardous. However, laws concerning the treatment of radioactive materials still limit the transport of the instrument and the method has so far been used to a very limited extent. Further details of the method and its medical applications are described in the references by Harvey et al. (1975) and Vartsky et al. (1977).

V. Isotope Dilution Method

1. Principles

The isotope dilution method is based on the measurements of isotope ratios before and after a sample is spiked with the element to be analyzed; the added element possesses a different isotope composition from that of the sample. The isotope ratio measurement is carried out either by a mass spectrometer when a stable isotope is added or by radioactivity measurement when a radioactive isotope is used as a spike.

When a sample having x atoms of the element to be analyzed, whose isotope ratios are $a_1, a_2 \ldots.. a_n \left(\sum_{i=1}^{n} a_i = 1 \right)$, is spiked with y atoms of the element, whose isotope ratios are $b_1, b_2, \ldots.. b_n \left(\sum_{i=1}^{n} b_i = 1 \right)$, and is well mixed, the ratio, C_i/C_k, for any two isotopes (i and k) is given by Eq. (11)

$$C_i/C_k = (xa_i + yb_i)/(xa_k + yb_k) .\qquad (11)$$

Therefore, the number of atoms, x originally present in the sample, is given by Eq. (12)

$$X = y \frac{B_{ik} - C_{ik}}{C_{ik} - A_{ik}} \frac{b_k}{a_k} ,\qquad (12)$$

where A_{ik}, B_{ik}, and C_{ik} are the relative isotope ratios of i and k for the sample, the spike, and the mixture, respectively, and are expressed as $A_{ik} = a_i/a_k$, $B_{ik} = b_i/b_k$, and $C_{ik} = c_i/c_k$. For usual analytic purpose, it is more convenient to express the amount of the element in grams, X and Y for the sample and the spike, respectively. These are calculated by Eq. (13) using the atomic weights, $M_x = \sum_{i=1}^{n} a_i M_i$ and $M_y \sum_{i=1}^{n} b_i M_i$, for the sample and the spike, respectively

$$X = Y \cdot \frac{B_{ik} - C_{ik}}{C_{ik} - A_{ik}} \cdot \frac{b_k}{a_k} \cdot \frac{M_x}{M_y} .\qquad (13)$$

In order to obtain satisfactory analytic results, it is necessary that the spike be completely equilibrated with the sample. Also it is desirable that the chemical forms of the element are the same both for the sample and the spike, and, in order to achieve this chemical similarity, chemical treatment including chemical separation is carried out before measurement. When the measurement is achieved by mass spectrometry, the separation need not always be quantitative, since only the relative isotope ratios are used for calculation, and even the chemical separation is not necessary if no interference occurs.

In the case of the use of a radioactive isotope and γ-ray measurement, the amount W_x of the element originally present in the sample is given by Eq. (14)

$$W_x = \left(\frac{S_1}{S_2} - 1 \right) W_1 ,\qquad (14)$$

where S_1 and S_2 are specific radioactivities of the spike and the mixture, repectively and W_1 is the added amount of the spike. When $W_1 \ll W_x$, Eq. (14) can be rewritten as Eq. (15)

$$W_x = \frac{S_1}{S_2} W_1 = \frac{A_1}{A_2} W_2 ,\qquad (15)$$

where $A_1 (= S_1 W_1)$ and $A_2 (= S_2 W_2)$ are the radioactivities of the spike and the mixture $(W_2 \text{ g})$, respectively.

2. Spike

The isotope composition of the spike should be as different as possible from natural abundance. These concentrated isotopes are manufactured by Oak Ridge National Laboratory (United States), UKAEA Harwell (England), or the Weizmann Institute (Israel), and are available for most elements.

The concentrated isotopes are used in trace amounts, and are sometimes contaminated with impurities, which leads to analytic errors. Therefore, the accurate isotope concentrations must be determined before using them in spikes. The experimental procedure for determining their isotope concentrations are as follows. A solution with appropriate concentration of the isotope is spiked with a standard solution of natural isotope abundance and the accurate concentration is determined by the isotope dilution method.

Although for cadmium analysis either stable or radioactive isotope is used as a spike, the use of radioactive isotope and γ-ray measurement provides more rapid and convenient analysis than the combination of stable isotope and mass spectrometry. Therefore, in this section, cadmium determination with ^{109}Cd as a spike is described. ^{109}Cd decays by electron capture with a half-life of 470 days, emitting γ-rays of 0.0880 MeV.

3. Experimental Procedure

About 2 g sample is accurately weighed and placed in a 250-ml Erlenmeyer flask, to which 13 ml acid mixture ($HClO_4$ 1.5 : H_2SO_4 1.5 : HNO_3 10) is added. The sample is completely decomposed by immersing the flask in boiling water and, if necessary, adding additional HNO_3. The clear solution is cooled to room temperature and neutralized with 6 M ammonia. The neutral point is confirmed with bromthymol blue test paper A 5×10^{-6} M $CdCl_2$ solution of ^{109}Cd is prepared as follows. A commercial concentrated ^{109}CdCl$_2$ solution (containing $CdCl_2$ 4 mg/ml) is added dropwise to a 5×10^{-6} M $CdCl_2$ solution to a radioactivity of about 10,000 cpm/ml. Then, 3 ml of the ^{109}CdCl$_2$ solution thus prepared is added to the sample solution and 3 M HCl is added to pH 1–2. The solution is transferred to a 100-ml separating funnel and 5 ml 10^{-4} M dithizone–chloroform solution is added. After vigorous shaking, the organic layer is discarded; 2 ml 20 w/v% sodium tartrate solution, 2 ml 20 w/v% urea solution, and 3 ml dimethylglyoxime–NaOH solution (1 g dimethylglyoxime dissolved in 100 ml 0.1 M NaOH) are added to the aqueous layer, which is then adjusted to 1 M NaOH by adding an equal volume of 2 M NaOH. Then. 5 ml 10^{-4} M dithizone–chloroform solution is added and the solution is vigorously shaken for 5 min. By this procedure, Cd is extracted to an organic layer, which is then transferred to another separating funnel. After 10 ml 2.5 M NaOH is added to the organic layer and the solution is shaken, the organic layer is further transferred to another separating funnel and is washed with 10 ml H_2O. The organic layer is again transferred to a 100-ml separating funnel and is shaken after addition of 5 ml 0.01 M HCl. Cadmium is backextracted into the aqueous layer by this procedure. The aqueous layer in the separating funnel is completely transferred to a 100-ml beaker by washing with a small amount of water and is neutralized with 0.01 M ammonia. The solution is then made up to 20 ml with a 0.2 M CH_3COONH_4–NaOH buffer solution of pH 10.7. The solution is transferred to a 100-ml separating funnel and is vigorously shaken after addition of 2 ml 5×100^{-6} M dithizone–chloroform. After the organic layer is evaporated to dryness on an aluminum dish with a diameter of 2 cm, the radioactivity is measured with a Geiger–Müller counter. The net count is obtained by subtracting the background count, which is obtained by processing $CdCl_2$ solution in exactly the same way as described, except that no $^{109}CdCl_2$ is added.

The standard sample for calibration is prepared by dropping 0.3 ml 5×10^{-6} M $CdCl_2$ solution onto 1 cm^2 filter paper, which is then processed according to the same procedure as for the sample. Alternately, the standard addition method is used and a known amount of $CdCl_2$ is added to the sample solution, and processed and measured as usual. The detection limit for cadmium by this method is 0.15 µg and the precision is ± 0.01 µg.

References

Bertin EP (1975) Principles and practice of X-ray spectrometric analysis. Plenum, New York

Harvey TC, McLellan JS, Thomas BJ, Fremlin JH (1975) Measurement of liver-cadmium concentrations in patients and industrial workers by neutron-activation analysis. Lancet II:1269–1272

L'vov BV (1970) Atomic absorption spectrochemical analysis. Hilger, London

Sigel H (1979) Metal ions in biological systems, vol 9. Dekker, New York

Slavin W (1976) Atomic absorption spectroscopy. Wiley, New York

Vartsky D, Ellis KJ, Chen NS, Cohn SH (1977) A facility for in vivo measurement of kidney and liver cadmium by neutron capture prompt gamma ray analysis. Phys Med Biol 22:1085–1096

Welz B (1976) Atomic absorption spectroscopy. Verlag Chemie, Weinheim

CHAPTER 2

Cadmium in the Environment and its Entry into Terrestrial Food Chain Crops

A. L. PAGE, M. M. EL-AMAMY, and A. C. CHANG

A. Introduction

Cadmium (Cd) is regarded by many as one of the most toxic trace elements in the environment. The increased emissions from production, use, and waste disposal combined with long-term persistence in the environment, and its relatively rapid uptake and accumulation by food chain crops contribute to its potentially hazardous nature. Cadmium originating from different sources may find its way to parts of the human population through food and beverages, drinking water, air, and cigarette smoking. Although acute Cd toxicity caused by food consumption is rare, chronic exposure to high Cd levels in food could significantly increase the accumulation of Cd in certain body organs. When the concentration in the human body reaches levels considered to be harmful (>200 µg per gram wet weight in the renal cortex; KJELLSTROM and NORDBERG 1978), cadmium-induced kidney damage, skeletal disorders, as well as other diseases may result.

The most highly publicized episode of Cd poisoning of humans was first reported in Japan in the mid-1950s (TSUCHIYA 1978). In this case, the source of excessive Cd in the affected individuals was rice grown on paddies which had been irrigated with water contaminated by nearby Zn mining operations. The Cd concentrations of the rice, sediments from the river, and the soil in which the high-Cd rice was grown were considerably greater than that found in uncontaminated regions.

Even for populations not subjected to a Cd-contaminated environment, the main source of the human body burden of Cd is also food. Drinking water and ambient air usually contribute considerably less to the daily intake. Concentrations of Cd in domestic water supplies rarely exceed a few micrograms per liter, and at a water consumption of 1–2 l/day the daily intake would not exceed a few micrograms (FRIBERG et al. 1974; TSUCHIYA 1978; PAHREN et al. 1979). Cadmium concentrations of ambient air rarely exceed 0.01 µg/m^3, and at an intake of 20 m^3 air per day, the daily Cd intake would not exceed 0.2 µg. Cigarette smoking, however, adds considerably to Cd input via inhalation. FRIBERG et al. (1974) estimate a daily intake of 2–4 µg Cd from smoking one package of cigarettes per day. They estimate that the daily ingestion of Cd for most of the world's population ranges from 25 to 75 µg/day. On the basis of market basket surveys over a 7-year period, the US Food and Drug Administration (MAHAFFEY et al. 1975) showed an average intake of 39 µg/day Cd for 15- to 20-year-old males. If the figure is adjusted by the recommended daily caloric intake for various age groups, the average intake from birth to age 50 years would be 33 µg/day for men and 26 µg/day for women (PAHREN et al. 1979). These values, however, were based upon minimum quantitative levels of 20 μg/kg for the market basket food items analyzed. More recent data based upon fecal excretion give figures of 18–21 μg/day for teenage males (RYAN et al. 1982; KOWAL 1984).

This information illustrates the significance of Cd in the food chain to the accumulation of Cd in the human body. The concentration of Cd in foods is in turn controlled by its concentration in the plant-growing substrate and by the physical and chemical nature of the substrate. In the following sections, natural and anthropogenic sources of Cd, concentration of Cd in foods produced from natural and Cd-contaminated soils, as well as the soil and plant factors influencing the Cd accumulation are reviewed.

B. Natural Occurrence

Cadmium is a relatively rare metal not found in the pure state in nature. It was discovered in 1817 as a constituent of smithsonite ($ZnCO_3$) obtained from a zinc ore by a German chemist, F. Stromeyer. The new metal was named cadmium (from *Kadmia,* the ancient Greek name for calamine or zinc carbonate) (NRIAGU 1980). Cadmium is a soft, ductile, silver-white metal with a specific gravity of

Table 1. Abundance of cadmium in common rocks[a]

Rock type	Cadmium content (μg/g)	
	Mean	Range
Igneous		
Granite	0.09	0.001– 0.60
Basalt	0.13	0.006– 0.60
Ultramafic	0.026	0.001– 0.03
Metamorphic		
Gneisses	0.04	0.007– 0.26
Schists	0.02	0.005– 0.87
Eclogite	0.11	0.04 – 0.26
Sedimentary		
Limestone	0.065	0.001– 0.50
Sandstone	0.02	0.01 – 0.41
Shale, clay	0.03	0.02 – 11.0
Red clay	0.56	
Organic mud	0.39	
Deep ocean sediments	0.5	0.05 – 17
Oceanic manganese oxides	8.0	< 3.0 – 21
Phosphorites	25	<10 –500
Recent sediments		
Lake sediments	0.91	0.02 – 6.2
Stream sediments	0.16	0.03 – 0.40

[a] Based on compilations by FLEISCHER et al. (1974), GONG et al. (1977), WAKETA and SCHMITT (1970), HORN and ADAMS (1966), and MAROWSKY and WEDEPOHL (1971)

8.642, and melting point of 320.9 °C. The atomic weight of 112.40 is derived from a mixture of eight stable isotopes with mass numbers 106, 108, 110–114, and 116. Cadmium is concentrated in sulfide minerals and found mainly in zinc, lead–zinc, and lead–copper–zinc ores. It is recovered as a by-product from the smelting and refining of zinc concentrates at a rate of 0.02%–1.4% with a median recovery of 0.3% (FLEISCHER et al. 1974).

The average concentration of cadmium in the lithosphere is 0.098 µg/g (HEIN-RICHS et al. 1980). It is rarer than mercury and about 1/700 as abundant as zinc (whose crustal abundance averages 70 µg/g). The ranges and mean concentra-tions of cadmium for some common igneous, sedimentary, and metamorphic rocks are presented in Table 1. There are very small differences in the overall abundance of cadmium in mafic and granitic rocks. It tends to accumulate in sed-imentary environments, as indicated by the high concentrations (0.001–11.0 µg/g) in sedimentary rocks. Certain shales are unusually high in Cd (WEDEPOHL 1968). Along the Pacific Coast in the United States, the Monterey shale formation in some locations contained as much as 90 µg Cd per gram (LUND et al. 1981). Amounts of cadmium in marine sediments in the Atlantic and Pacific Oceans range from 0.1 to 1.0 µg/g (MULLIN and RILEY 1956). Marine manganese nodules (5.1–8.4 µg/g) and marine zinc-bearing phosphorite (60–340 µg/g) are unusually high in cadmium (MULLIN and RILEY 1956; GOLDSCHMIDT 1958; AUER 1977).

C. World Production

The first reported production of metallic cadmium on an industrial scale was in 1829 in Upper Silesia (CHIZHIKOV 1966). The annual production of cadmium never exceeded 100 kg until 1871 because no commercial uses of the metal were known. After 1871, production of the metal expanded rapidly, owing to its use in paint pigments. By the turn of the century, approximately 20 tonnes were pro-duced annually with about 90% of the supply coming from sources in Ger-many.

Production in the United States commenced in 1906, and by 1919 the United States became the principal producer of cadmium. During the 1940s, the United States produced approximately 70% of the total world supply (Table 2). During the 1960s, marked increases in cadmium production occurred in Japan and the Soviet Union. In 1969, the United States produced approximately 34% of the world's supply, while Japan and the Soviet Union produced 16% and 14%, re-spectively. Since 1975, the Soviet Union has been the world's leading producer.

Between 1940 and 1944, worldwide cadmium production increased by 22% in response to the greater demand for the metal for military purposes (NRIAGU 1980). Cadmium production during the 1910s and 1920s increased at an annual rate of 44.4% and 43.2%, respectively. The average annual increase was 7.3%, 5.3%, 6.6%, and 3.1% for the 1930s, 1940s, 1950s, 1960s, and 1970s, respectively (Table 2). Since 1970, the concern regarding the health effects of cadmium re-sulted in a downward trend of cadmium production and consumption. Approx-imately 65% of the cumulative world production has occurred within the last 20 years.

Table 2. Trends in the world smelter production of cadmium by decade[a]

Country	Cadmium production (tonnes)								
	Total for 10-year periods							Total	
	1910s	1920s	1930s	1940s	1950s	1960s	1970s	Country	Continent
North America									248,763
Canada		574	2,316	3,792	7,217	9,995	12,272	36,166	
Mexico			5,268	8,334	8,047	7,358	17,525	46,532	
United States	456	3,204	15,241	34,962	42,940	47,380	21,882	166,065	
South America									6,758
Peru				22	387	1,593	4,756	6,758	
Europe									114,919
Austria					44	199	294	537	
Belgium		10	2,270	1,108	5,623	7,839	11,971	28,821	
Finland							3,569	3,569	
France		191	1,216	350	1,401	3,933	6,352	1,344	
Germany	521	86	1,860	1,407	2,149	3,896	11,725	21,644	
Italy			418	853	1,844	2,636	4,463	10,214	
Netherlands					131	697	2,609	3,427	
Norway			1,204	313	1,014	967	1,046	4,544	
Poland			1,132	1,803	2,340	4,034	5,918	15,227	
Spain				10	72	556	2,065	2,703	
United Kingdom		29	415	1,460	1,377	1,676	2,946	7,903	
Yugoslavia					84	718	2,075	2,877	
USSR			115	223	2,290	17,668	26,550	46,846	46,846
Asia									47,756
Japan			206	620	2,921	14,478	27,243	45,463	
North Korea						313	1,300	1,613	
South Korea							675	675	
Africa									21,284
Congo/Zaire				178	1,979	3,638	2,450	8,245	
South-West Africa			764	1,537	7,969	1,500	1,072	12,842	
Zambia						129	68	197	
Oecania									20,015
Australia		1,220	1,895	2,171	3,094	4,529	7,106	20,015	
Totals	977	5,314	34,320	59,143	92,923	135,732	177,932		506,341
Estimated total world production	977	5,314	28,288	49,094	74,999	124,207	163,300		446,179

[a] Derived from US Bureau of Mines (1965–1980)

D. Consumption

Six countries, France, Germany, Belgium, Japan, the United Kingdom, and the United States, accounted for over 70% of the cadmium consumed during the last decade (Table 3). The various uses of cadmium in these countries are given in Table 4. Approximately 90% of all the cadmium went into electroplating (29%), stabilizers (25%), pigments (23%), and batteries (13%). During the 1960s and

Table 3. Cadmium consumption (tonnes) in western countries and Japan[a]

Year	United States	Federal Republic of Germany	France	Bel- gium	United King- dom	Japan	Total Con- sumption	% of Total world pro- duction
1965	4,679	1,419	806	1,008	1,270	787	9,969	83.8
1970	4,107	1,800	1,028	1,758	1,313	1,485	11,491	69.1
1973	6,267	2,225	1,087	1,793	1,519	1,651	14,542	84.7
1974	6,050	2,195	1,431	2,008	1,148	1,480	14,312	82.8
1975	3,055	1,241	923	1,033	1,023	1,186	8,461	55.5
1976	5,381	1,938	738	1,741	1,394	1,059	12,251	72.1
1977	3,818	2,050	1,283	1,641	1,484	2,060	12,336	67.6
1978	4,510	1,863	1,084	1,461	1,310	2,420	12,648	73.0
1979	4,928	1,898	946	1,797	1,525	2,446	13,540	73.2

[a] Derived from US Bureau of Mines (1965–1980)

Table 4. End uses of cadmium in some of the industrial countries[a]

Country	Year	Percentage of total use					Total use by Country (tonnes)
		Electro- plating	Pigment	Stabili- zers	Bat- teries	Others[b]	
United States	1965	52.3	24.8	8.2	6.0	8.7	4,679
	1970	45.0	14.3	26.3	3.3	6.1	4,107
	1974	48.5	17.8	16.2	9.7	7.8	5,605
	1980	33.3	10.0	17.2[c]	20.0	20.0	3,532
Federal Republic of Germany	1965	14.8	19.7	8.5	7.2	49.8	1,419
	1970	15.0	24.4	10.6	12.2	37.8	1,800
	1974	14.9	32.7	14.4	15.0	23.0	2,016
France	1965	42.9	29.7	8.4	27.8	4.8	806
	1970	29.2	34.0	5.8	24.3	6.6	1,028
	1974	24.1	44.7	6.9	20.6	3.7	1,454
United Kingdom	1965	38.8	21.4	10.7	9.2	19.9	1,270
	1970	37.3	25.5	12.8	8.4	16.0	1,313
	1974	31.7	28.9	14.4	12.5	12.5	1,441
Japan	1965	21.3	23.5	20.5	6.5	28.2	787
	1970	9.1	29.9	23.0	11.9	26.1	1,485
	1974	0.5	27.2	18.7	34.5	19.1	927

[a] Based on data published by STUBBS (1978) and US Bureau of Mines (1965–1980)
[b] Includes alloys, solders, and other uses (the 1980 figure was reported for trans- portation)
[c] Estimated

1970s, amounts of cadmium used in alloys and solders showed a declining trend, while uses for pigments and chemicals showed an increasing trend. The trend in pigments and chemicals is attributed to increased uses in the plastics industry. Since 1955, the amounts of cadmium used in electroplating reveal no consistent trend, but the percentage of the total consumption appears to be declining.

I. Electroplating

Cadmium is coated over iron, steel, copper alloys, and aluminum alloys by electrodeposition, dipping, or hot spraying. Products coated with cadmium are many and varied (PAGE and BINGHAM 1973). These include nuts, bolts, screws, rivets, nails, washers, fasteners, automotive and aircraft parts, household appliances, tools, industrial machinery, and many others. For most uses, coatings only 7.6 μm thick are satisfactory (LANSCHE 1958).

II. Pigments and Chemicals

Compounds of cadmium are used extensively for imparting high quality red, maroon, yellow, and orange colors to such materials as paints, enamels, rubber, glass, ceramic glazes, textiles, artist's colors, leather, printing ink, and plastics. Pigments of cadmium are unaffected by heat, light, and moisture, and resist weathering by both acids and bases. Cadmium sulfide is one of the best known and widely used compounds in pigments. Depending upon its method of preparation, its colors range from yellow ($CdS–BaSO_4$) to orange ($CdS–BaSO_4–ZnS$) to dark red ($CdS–BaSO_4–CdSe$). These are referred to as cadmium lithopones and contain 15%–27% cadmium (GABBY 1950). Inorganic and organic cadmium compounds are currently widely used as coloring agents and stabilizers in plastic materials.

III. Alloys

Cadmium-containing alloys are used in the production of bearings for aircraft and other internal combustion engines, for solders, and low melting and brazing alloys. Low melting temperature alloys of cadmium are used for fire prevention sprinkler systems, fire detection apparatus, and safety plugs for tanks and cylinders containing compressed gases. Certain alloys of cadmium with tin, bismuth, lead, and indium have melting points below the boiling point of water. These alloys can be used to solder tin, lead, iron, zinc, and brass in hot water. Silver solders containing cadmium in amounts ranging between 15% and 23% are used to join both ferrous and nonferrous metals.

IV. Other Uses

Cadmium usage in batteries constitutes the largest single use outside the areas of electroplating, pigments, chemicals, and alloys. Growth in the production of products which utilize cadmium batteries has increased substantially during the last two decades. Cordless household items such as brushes, electric shavers, flashlights, and communication equipment utilize sealed nickel–cadmium batteries. Vented batteries on the other hand, are used in aircraft, buses, and diesel locomotives. Other cadmium uses include fungicides, phosphorescent dials, compounds in photography, lithography, process engraving, curing rubber, and miscellaneous uses.

E. Cadmium in Noncontaminated and Contaminated Soils

I. Natural Levels in Soils

The concentrations of Cd in cultivated and noncultivated soils not subjected to contamination are governed by the quantities of Cd found in the parent materials, plus amounts added through atmospheric deposition, fertilizers, pesticides, and irrigation water, minus amounts removed by leaching, erosion, and in harvested crops. Based upon Cd concentrations reported for common rocks, one would expect that, on the average, soils of similar age derived from igneous rocks would be lowest in total Cd, soils derived from metamorphic rocks would be intermediate, and soils derived from sedimentary rocks would contain the largest quantities of Cd.

The most extensive survey of natural levels of Cd in soils from the continental United States is that recently completed by the US Department of Agriculture–Soil Conservation Service. The survey involved the collection of 3,305 soil samples from major crop-producing areas in 36 states. Great care was taken to insure that the sites sampled were free from any known sources of contamination and to insure the utmost analytic accuracy. Concentrations of Cd in surface soils ranged from 0.005 to 2.4 mg/kg with the mean and median concentrations of 0.27 and 0.24 mg/kg, respectively (HOLMGREN et al. 1985). A summary of the results by geographic region is presented in Table 5. On average, Cd concentrations in soils from the western and north central states are greater than those from the northeastern and southern states. Lower concentrations in soils from the south and northeast United States may be due to higher rainfall and greater leaching in these regions.

Results from a national survey in Japan showed mean Cd concentrations for nonpolluted rice paddies (2,746 samples), farmland (722 samples), and orchard soils (268 samples) of 0.4, 0.3, and 0.3 µg/g, respectively (YAMAGATA 1978). Maximum concentrations of Cd for the nonpolluted rice paddies, farmland, and orchard soils were, respectively, 7.1, 1.0, and 1.2 µg/g.

Reports of less extensive studies than those of YAMAGATA (1978) and HOLMGREN et al. (1985), from Sweden (ANDERSSON 1977), Norway (ALLEN and STEINNES 1979), United States (PIERCE et al. 1982; KLEIN 1972; LOGAN and MILLER 1983), Denmark (TJELL and HOVMAND 1978), USSR (ORESHKIN et al. 1979), England (MOORCROFT et al. 1982), and Canada (DUDAS and PAWLUK 1977) also show soil Cd concentrations within the range mentioned. Thus, it appears that typical soils contain 0.05–1.0 µg/g with a median concentration of a few tenths of a microgram Cd per gram. However, as much as 30 µg/g have been observed in

Table 5. Concentrations of cadmium in noncontamined soils

Country	Sample description	No. of samples	Cd (µg/g) Range or maximum	Mean	References
Japan	Rice paddy	2,746	7.1	0.4	YAMAGATA (1978)
	Farmland	722	1.0	0.3	
	Orchard	268	1.2	0.3	
Sweden	Cultivated	186	0.03– 2.3	0.22	ANDERSSON (1977)
	Noncultivated	175		0.22	
Norway	Noncultivated humus layer	500	0.27– 1.07[a]	0.42[b]	ALLEN and STEINNES (1979)
United States					
California	Agricultural	177	0.05–10.1[c]	1.24[c]	BURAU et al. (1973)
Minnesota	Agricultural	16 soil series	0.06– 0.74	0.17	PIERCE et al. (1982)
Michigan	Residential	70		0.41	KLEIN (1972)
	Agricultural	91		0.57	
Western	Agricultural	742		0.33	HOLMGREN et al. (1985)
North Central	Agricultural	937		0.37	
Northeast	Agricultural	293		0.17	
Southern	Agricultural	1,230		0.15	
Ohio	Agricultural	235	<0.1 – 2.9	0.2	LOGAN and MILLER (1983)
Denmark	From 25 locations	51	0.05– 0.55	0.26	TJELL and HOVMAND (1978)
USSR	Virgin and cultivated Gray Forest Chernozem Podzolic soils	44	0.015–0.8	0.24	ORESHKIN et al. (1979)
England	Garden soils	235	0.1 – 6.8	0.8	MOORCROFT et al. (1982)
Canada	Chernozems	12		0.23	DUDAS and PAWLUK (1977)
	Luvisols	6		0.09	
	Humic gleysols	18		0.34	
	Solonetz	18		0.15	

[a] Range of the means from twelve districts throughout Norway
[b] Mean of means from twelve districts throughout Norway
[c] A number of soils from this region are developed from parent material unusually high in Cd

nonpolluted soils derived from Monterey shale in the coastal ranges in southern California (LUND et al. 1981). A survey of soils from the Salinas Valley in California, where outcrops of Monterey shale are common, showed a range of 0.05–10.1 µg/g (BURAU et al. 1973). A summary of Cd concentrations in the surface of nonpolluted cultivated and noncultivated soils is presented in Table 5.

Although there are considerable data in the literature on concentrations of Cd in uncontaminated soils, there is only very limited information to relate Cd concentrations in soils to their morphological properties. PIERCE et al. (1982) present data for the metal concentrations of soils developed on seven parent materials in Minnesota. The Cd concentrations of all soils were relatively low and ranged from 0.06 to 0.74 µg/g (Table 5). The highest total concentrations occurred in calcareous soils developed in lacustrine sediments and generally in soils with free carbonates. ORESHKIN et al. (1979) also reported higher concentrations of Cd in soils with free carbonates (chernozems). The content of Cd in the eluvial horizons of Chernozem soils averaged 0.4 µg/g while that of Gray Forest soils average 0.27–0.30 µg/g. The upper horizons of the Chernozem and Gray Forest soils were about 3–6 times richer in Cd than the lower horizons. PIERCE et al. (1982) also present data which show levels of Cd in surface horizons substantially greater than that found in subsurface horizons. Mean Cd concentrations for surface soils were 0.39 µg/g, compared with a mean of 0.23 µg/g for subsurface samples. Higher concentrations in surface soils are probably the result of atmospheric deposition and the cycling of Cd from lower horizons to upper horizons by vegetation. SPOSITO and PAGE (1985) show that particulates in air from remote, rural, and metropolitan regions are all enriched in Cd relative to typical soils.

II. Sources and Extent of Cadmium Contamination of Soils

Soils may be contaminated with cadmium by fallout from aerial sources, by application of water, fertilizers, or pesticides which contain cadmium, or by the discharge of liquid or solid cadmium-containing waste materials from industrial, metallurgical, or urban activities.

1. Levels Near Mining and Smelting Operations

Processing of industrial metals is an important source of emission of trace metals, including Cd, into the atmosphere. Smelting and sintering of nonferrous metals result in Cd contamination of the nearby environment. The major sources of emission are the ore-smelting furnaces in which metals enter the flue-gas stream as fine particulate or volatile material, are discharged from the stack, and eventually are deposited onto soils and vegetation. Airborne dusts and fumes from charging furnaces, transporting metal ores, and from sintering and metal-reducing furnaces are also sources of metals found in and near the operations.

Soils contaminated by smelting operations show high Cd concentrations in the upper horizons. However, the concentrations at a depth of about 30–40 cm are close to background levels. Elevated cadmium concentrations (> 50 mg/kg) in the surface soils near cadmium-emitting industries have been reported (FULKERSON and GOELLER 1973; BUCHAUER 1973; CARTWRIGHT et al. 1976; NWANKO and ELINDER 1979; MUNSHOWER 1977; RAGAINI et al. 1977; MERRY and TILLER 1978; MARPLES and THORNTON 1980). Cadmium contamination of soils from these sources is usually greatest near the point of discharge and in the direction of the prevailing winds. Following the prevailing wind direction, contamination of soil may extend to distances as great as 20–30 km. Data derived from the U.S. ENVIRONMENTAL PROTECTION AGENCY (1972) are representative of the extent of airborne contamination which may occur (Table 6). The data, obtained adjacent to a lead smelter which began operations in 1888, show high levels of contamina-

Table 6. Cadmium concentrations in surface and subsurface soils adjacent to an industrial smelting complex[a]

Depth of sample	Direction from source	Distance from source (km)			
		1	2	4	8
(cm)		Cd (µg/g)			
0 – 2.5[b]	Northeast	158	44	11	2.7
2.5–10[c]	East-Northeast	51	20	7.7	3.0
	North-Northeast	45	17	6.0	2.2
	Northwest	23	11	5.1	2.4
10 –26	East-Northeast	8.3	4.7	2.6	1.5
	North-Northeast	1.9	1.4	1.1	
	Northwest	2.3	1.7	1.3	

[a] Derived from the US Environmental Protection Agency (1972)
[b] From cultivated field
[c] From uncultivated field

tion near the plant site. The extent of contamination is greatest in the surface soil and occurs at distances of at least 8 km from the source. BUCHAUER (1973) has made similar observations adjacent to a zinc smelter in Pennsylvania. Within 1 km of the smelter in the direction of the prevailing wind, concentrations of Cd in the surface organic horizon as great as 750 mg per kilogram soil were reported. The Cd accumulated in soils decreased logarithmically with distance, and levels exceeding the background were observed up to 21 km from the source. Near presently operating or abandoned mining operations, the contamination may also be caused by tailings blown onto soils or from mine water leaching through soils (DAVIS and associates 1970; LAGERWERFF and BROWER 1975; THORNTON 1983). JOHNSON et al. (1975) reported concentrations which ranged between 2.5 and 61 mg/kg in the upper horizon of soils in the Coeur d'Alene mining district in Idaho. The surface soils in a village (Shipham, Somerset, United Kingdom) built on slag heaps from old abandoned zinc mines, which were worked in the eighteenth and nineteenth centuries, have cadmium concentrations up to 800 mg/kg with a median concentration of about 80 mg/kg (THORNTON et al. 1981).

2. Disposal or Recycling of Municipal Sewage Sludges

Sewage sludges from municipalities are frequently applied to soils in disposal operations, as soil conditioners, or as a source of plant nutrients. The concentrations of Cd in sewage sludge always exceed those normally found in soils. Municipal sewage sludge contains approximately 2–3,500 µg Cd per gram sludge, with median values of the order of 5–20 µg/g (PAGE 1974; SOMMERS 1977; LOGAN and CHANEY 1984). Application of sludge as a nitrogen fertilizer can elevate the cadmium level in surface soils. A 5 tonnes/ha application of sludge with a Cd content of 10–15 mg/kg may result in an increase of cadmium concentration by as much as 10%–15% in the surface soil (background level 0.22 mg/kg). The applied cadmium may remain available to plants for an extended period of time; however, the annual loading appears to be of greater importance than the cumulative amount added (PAGE et al. 1981).

Cadmium added to soils, regardless of the chemical form at the time of application, tends to remain at or near the depth of incorporation. ANDERSSON and NILSSON (1972) reported data which PAGE (1974) used to show that, following application of the equivalent of 0.7 kg Cd per hectare in the form of sewage sludge over a 12-year period, all of the cadmium remained in the surface 20 cm. Similar observations following six annual additions of as much as 9 kg Cd per hectare per year in the form of sewage sludge were made by CHANG et al. (1984). Likewise, WILLIAMS et al. (1980) observed essentially no movement of Cd beyond the depth of incorporation following massive annual applications (up to 225 tonnes/ha) of sewage sludge over a period of 3 years. Because of the possible entry of the land-disposed Cd into the human food chain via crops grown on contaminated soils, considerable research has been focused on studying soils which have received waste in either recycling or disposal operations. A number of monographs and review articles summarizing the impact of trace elements, including Cd, in waste applied to land have been published (LOEHR 1977; ELLIOTT and STEVENSON 1977; MCKIM 1978; LEEPER 1978; PAGE 1974, 1981; COUNCIL FOR AGRICULTURAL SCIENCE AND TECHNOLOGY 1976, 1980; CEP CONSULTANTS LTD 1979, 1981, 1983; BITTON et al. 1980; D'ITRI et al. 1981; SOPPER et al. 1982; LEPP 1981; PAGE et al. 1984).

3. Phosphorus Fertilizers

Phosphorus fertilizers frequently contain greater concentrations of Cd than are typically found in soils. Depending on the source, commercial fertilizers produced in the United States contain from a few to 200 mg Cd per kilogram fertilizer, with median values from 2 to 20 mg/kg (U.S. ENVIRONMENTAL PROTECTION AGENCY 1978). In Sweden, levels of cadmium in triple superphosphate (TSP) fertilizer cited by ANDERSSON and HAHLIN (1981) ranged from 20 to 24 mg Cd per kilogram TSP (98–118 mg Cd per kilogram phosphorus in TSP). Over the period 1971–1978, the fertilizer industry in Sweden has reduced the average content of Cd in phosphate fertilizers from about 160 to 60 mg Cd per kilogram phosphorus in the fertilizer material (GUNNARSSON 1980). The amount of cadmium is usually related to the amount of phosphate (HUTTON 1982). Although the amounts of Cd added through normal phosphorus fertilization practices are small, their long-term use can cause accumulations of Cd in surface soils. For example, the application of 50 kg P per hectare from rock phosphate $[Ca_{10}F_2(PO_4)_6]$ which contained 20 mg Cd per kilogram introduce 5.4 g Cd to the soil. Results presented in the literature demonstrate that the long-term continuous use of phosphorus fertilizers does, in fact, cause increased concentrations of Cd in surface soil (WILLIAMS and DAVID 1973, 1976; MULLA et al. 1980; ANDERSSON and HAHLIN 1981). Data presented by WILLIAMS and DAVID (1973, 1976) show that applications of Australian super-phosphate containing concentrations of Cd less than 50 mg/kg resulted in 0.212 mg Cd per kilogram topsoil versus 0.046 mg Cd per kilogram topsoil in similar soils which received no phosphorus fertilizer. Likewise, MULLA et al.

(1980) reported a tenfold increase in the Cd concentration of surface soil as a result of 36 years of phosphorus fertilization.

4. Atmospheric Deposition

The estimated total annual emission of cadmium to the atmosphere is approximately 8,000 metric tonnes. Only 10% of the total is derived from natural sources, whereas the remaining 90% is derived from anthropogenic sources (NRIAGU 1980). Volcanic activities account for 62% of natural emissions. Other natural sources include decaying vegetation (25%), airborne soil particles (12%), and forest fires (2%) (NRIAGU 1980).

Nonferrous metal production contributes approximately 73% of the total anthropogenic cadmium. This includes zinc operations (40%), copper smelting (20%), lead and cadmium smelting (5%), and secondary nonferrous metals (8%). Waste incineration generates 20% of the anthropogenic cadmium. The remaining 7% is contributed by iron and steel production, industrial applications (electroplating, pigments, alloys, and batteries), coal, oil, and wood combustion, phosphate fertilizers, and rubber tire wear (Table 7).

Air in urban and industrial areas on the average contains greater concentrations of Cd than air in rural areas. The Cd in air originates from salvage and industrial activities, combustion of fuels, urban trash incineration, and wear of products containing Cd. Based upon an extensive review of data pertaining to

Table 7. Worldwide anthropogenic emissions of cadmium 1975–1976[a]

Source	Cadmium emitted (tonnes/year)
Zinc mining operations	2.8
Primary nonferrous metal production	
Zinc operations	2,800
Copper smelting	1,580
Lead smelting	230
Cadmium extractions	111
Secondary nonferrous metals	595
Iron and steel production	72
Industrial applications	
Electroplating	8.5
Pigments, plastics, etc.	38
Alloys and batteries	6.4
Inadvertent sources	
Coal combustion	62
Oil combustion	2.8
Wood combustion	200
Waste incineration	1,350
Rubber tire wear	10
Phosphate fertilizers	118
Total	7,186

[a] Adapted from NRIAGU (1980)

measurements of atmospheric concentrations of Cd in various regions, NRIAGU (1980) has estimated that air in remote and rural areas generally contains Cd at levels less than 1.0 ng/m^3 and that in urban areas Cd concentrations in air commonly range from 1 to 50 ng/m^3. Levels of Cd in air presented by NRIAGU (1980) are in general agreement with measurements published more recently. ALKEZWEENY et al. (1982), for example, reported concentrations of Cd in air from remote regions of northern Michigan, ranging from less than 0.1 to 4.3 ng/m^3 with an average of 2.2 ng/m^3. Likewise, HARRISON and WILLIAMS (1982) reported Cd concentrations in two rural sites in northwest England which range from 0.1 to 8.2 and 0.2 to 6.8 ng/m^3. Mean cadmium concentrations at the two sites were 2.13 and 1.55 ng/m^3.

Near point emission sources such as Pb–Zn–Cu smelting operations, the concentrations of Cd in air may be considerably greater. In a city in Belgium where the major metal industries are concentrated, Cd concentrations in air between 1972 and 1975 ranged from 5 to 715 ng/m^3 with a mean of 35 ng/m^3. Adjacent to a smelter in Montana, during the fall of 1969 the average 24-h concentrations of cadmium in air were between 60 and 290 ng/m^3 (U.S. ENVIRONMENTAL PROTECTION AGENCY 1972; RUPP et al. 1978). LAGERWERFF and BROWER (1975) presented data which show Cd concentrations in aerosols in the vicinity of a zinc smelter (now abandoned) in Kansas, from 20 to 140 ng/m^3.

The extent of contamination of soil arising from deposition from air in rural and urban regions, except near point emission sources, amounts to a few grams per hectare per year. For example, data derived from HUNT et al. (1971) for 77 cities in the midwestern United States show annual Cd deposition of 1.2, 1.9, and 2.2 g/ha in residential, commercial, and industrial areas, respectively (PAGE and CHANG 1979). Utilizing data in BOWEN (1979) and a deposition velocity of 0.5 mm/s obtained from LANNEFORS and HANSSAN (1983), SPOSITO and PAGE (1985) computed that, on the average, amounts of Cd deposited onto soil in rural regions of Europe and North America are 0.8 and less than 0.2 g Cd per hectare per year. In a rural region of Tennessee, LINDBERG et al. (1981) reported a deposition of 0.9 g Cd per hectare per year. Data derived from HARLER and BARBER (1979) show a deposition of 2.6 g Cd per hectare per year for rural regions of England and 13 g Cd per hectare per year for the city of London. For ten stations within the Federal Republic of Germany, data derived from ROHBOCK et al. (1981) show amounts of Cd deposited onto soil which range from 3.65 to 13.5 g Cd per hectare per year. Based upon the data available, it appears that annual deposition of Cd onto soils in rural regions is of the order of a few grams per hectare per year, and approximately equal to the amounts which would be added to soil through the annual application of phosphorus fertilizers. In metropolitan regions that are distant from any point emission sources, amounts of Cd deposited onto land from air are of the order of 2–20 times greater than those deposited onto land in rural regions.

Adjacent to point emission sources, concentrations of Cd in air are considerably greater. Consequently, amounts deposited onto land surfaces are also greater. Data derived from RUPP et al. (1978), for example, show annual deposition of Cd of 170, 89, 46, and 23 g/ha at distances of 1.6, 3.2, 6.4, and 12.8 km downwind from a smelter.

Although information on amounts of Cd deposited onto land is informative, it does not show the extent to which the Cd concentration of soil may be increased as a result of atmospheric deposition. Increases of Cd concentrations in soil resulting from atmospheric deposition can be estimated from the amount deposited, the depth of soil to which the deposited Cd is mixed, and the bulk density of the soil. Assuming a soil bulk density of 1.33×10^3 kg/m^3 (typical for a silt loam soil), a deposition of 2 g Cd per hectare per year (representative of a rural region), and depth of mixing of 15 cm (representative of a tilled agricultural soil), the increase in the concentration of Cd in soil would amount to 1 µg per kilogram per year. The typical natural level of Cd in soil, according to BOWEN (1979), is approximately 350 µg/kg. Therefore, if all of the Cd deposited onto a rural agricultural soil from the atmosphere were to remain in the surface 15 cm of soil, it would increase the Cd concentration of the layer by 0.3% per year. This deduction points out that the extent of soil contamination in rural regions arising from atmospheric deposition on an annual basis is rather small.

In metropolitan regions and in regions close to point emission sources, particularly under conditions where the Cd deposited from the atmosphere remains in the surface few centimeters, the percentage increase in soil Cd would be substantially greater. Utilizing data presented by RUPP et al. (1978), an annual Cd deposition of 170 g/ha would increase the concentration of Cd in the surface 15 cm of soil by 85 µg/ha, or a 23.6% annual increase in soil concentration.

5. Water

Until recently, reliable data on the distribution of cadmium in natural waters have been scarce. Oceanic surface waters contain 0.004–0.02 µg/l, whereas concentrations at mid-depth range between 0.02 and 0.7 µg/l (MARTIN et al. 1976; BOYLE et al. 1976; BRULAND et al. 1978; NRIAGU 1980). A typical concentration in ocean water at the surface is 0.01 µg/l, while the concentration at mid-depth is approximately 0.07 µg/l (FORSTNER 1980; NRIAGU 1980). It is believed that cadmium is depleted from the surface water as a result of its uptake by marine organisms, and enriched in the deep waters owing to the sinking of debris.

The amounts of cadmium in fresh waters range from 0.01 to 0.1 µg/l (NRIAGU 1980). KENNEDY and SEBETICH (1976) reported concentrations of 0.01–0.03 µg/l for remote California streams. The Mississippi contained 0.1 µg/l (TREFRY and PRESLEY 1976) and the Amazon contained 0.07 µg/l (BOYLE et al. 1976). Lake waters contain amounts of cadmium similar to those found in rivers. Based on data from several studies, concentrations in lake waters are typically 0.02 µg/l (BEAMISH 1976; SCHELL and NEVISSI 1977; NRIAGU 1980). The average cadmium concentration in groundwater is 0.1 µg/l (NRIAGU 1980).

Ground and surface waters of regions where cadmium ores are processed or cadmium-containing products are manufactured have been observed to contain high concentrations of cadmium. In Japan, drainage from a mined area contained 5–61 µg/l; on one occasion water (pH 2.8) containing 4,130 µg/l has been reported (YAMAGATA and SHIGEMATSU 1970). Upstream from the mine, the Zinzu river contained < 1 µg/l cadmium, whereas mine drainage elevated the content of the downstream water to 1–9 µg/l (YAMAGATA and SHIGEMATSU 1970). High concentrations of cadmium were also reported in some Missouri river drainage waters (McKee and Wolf 1971). Lieber and Welsh (1954) reported cadmium contamination of groundwater to the extent of 3,200 µg/l in Long Island, New York as a result of wastes from electroplating industries.

III. Soil Factors Influencing the Accumulation of Cadmium by Food Chain Crops

The two most important factors governing the accumulation of Cd by crops are the soil pH, and the concentration of Cd in the soil. Factors of less importance include the time following Cd addition to the soil, soil temperature, content of hydrous oxides of iron and manganese in soils, redox potential in soil, and interactions with other metals. In the remainder of the chapter, a wide variety of crops will be referred to by their common names. To avoid unnecessary duplication, the scientific names of these crops are summarized in Table 8.

1. Soil pH Effects

If other soil conditions remain unchanged, the Cd concentration of plant tissue decreases as the pH of the soil increases. Bingham et al. (1980) show a progressive decrease of Cd in rice grain as the pH of the soil on which the plants were grown

Table 8. Common and scientific names of listed crops

Common name	Scientific name
Barley	*Hordeum vulgare*
Bean	*Phaseolus vulgaris*, c.v. *Sankt Andreas*
Snap bean	*Phaseolus* spp.
Broccoli	*Brassica oleracea botrytis*
Cabbage	*Brassica oleracea captitata*
Cantaloupe	*Cucumis melo*
Carrot	*Daucus carota sativa*
Corn	*Zea mays*
Eggplant	*Solanum melongena*
Lettuce	*Lactuca sativa*
Oat	*Avena sativa*
Pea	*Pisum sativum*
Pepper	*Capsicum* spp.
Potato	*Solanum tuberosum*
Radish	*Raphanus sativus*
Rape	*Brassica napus*
Rice	*Oryza sativa*
Ryegrass	*Lolium* spp.
Sorghum	*Sorghum vulgare*
Soybean	*Glycine soja*
Squash	*Cucurbita* spp.
Swiss chard	*Beta vulgaris* var. *cicla*
Tomato	*Lycopersicon esculentum*
Wheat	*Triticum* spp.

Table 9. Influence of soil pH and cadmium concentration on the cadmium concentration of Swiss chard and oat grain[a]

Treatment	Soil Cd (mg/kg)	Soil pH	Cd (mg/kg)[b] Swiss chard	Oat grain
Control				
Farm 1	0.18	4.9	3.34	0.104
Farm 2	0.10	5.3	2.65	0.076
Farm 3	0.22	5.4	1.48	0.034
Farm 4	0.07	5.9	0.44	0.051
Mean			1.98	0.066
Control + lime				
Farm 1	0.15	6.4	0.94	0.052
Farm 2	0.10	6.1	0.37	0.064
Farm 3	0.16	6.4	0.63	0.025
Farm 4	0.07	6.3	0.33	0.044
Mean			0.57	0.046
Sludge-treated				
Farm 1	1.66	4.9	94.8	1.96
Farm 2	9.10	5.5	54.3	2.24
Farm 3	0.98	4.9	3.24	0.209
Farm 4	3.26	5.5	9.51	0.299
Mean			40.5	1.18
Sludge-treated + lime				
Farm 1	2.10	6.3	2.20	0.259
Farm 2	7.02	6.2	5.34	0.277
Farm 3	0.94	6.0	0.82	0.065
Farm 4	4.50	6.2	3.68	0.193
Mean			3.01	0.198

[a] Data from paired plots on sludge utilization farms in four northeastern United States cities; derived from data presented by Council for Agricultural Science and Technology (1980)
[b] Dry weight basis

was increased stepwise from pH 5.5 to 7.5. CHANEY et al. (1975) also report decreasing Cd concentrations in soybean leaves as the pH of the soil substrate is increased from 5.3 to 7.0. Similar observations have been extended to rape fodder (ANDERSSON and NILSSON 1974), wheat (LINNMAN et al. 1973; HYDE et al. 1979), corn (HYDE et al. 1979; COUNCIL FOR AGRICULTURAL SCIENCE AND TECHNOLOGY 1976), lettuce (MAHLER et al. 1978; GIORDANO et al. 1979; JOHN et al. 1972), Swiss chard (MAHLER et al. 1978; SIKORA et al. 1980), oats (SIKORA et al. 1980), barley (CHANG et al. 1982a, 1983; SINGH and STEINNES 1976), and sorghum (CHANG et al. 1979). Data selected from results published in a report by the COUNCIL FOR AGRICULTURAL SCIENCE AND TECHNOLOGY (1980), illustrate Cd accumulation by Swiss chard and oat grain in relation to soil pH (Table 9). The mean concentration of Cd in Swiss chard grown at control plots of four farms with soil pH values ranging from 4.9 to 5.4 was 1.98 mg/kg while that of the paired control plots whose soil pH had been raised to values between 6.1 to 6.4 by liming was 0.57 mg/kg. Liming the same soils, which are contaminated with Cd from land application of municipal sewage sludge, reduced the mean Cd concentration of the Swiss chard from 40.5 to 3.01 mg/kg. Similar results reported by CHANEY et al. (1975) showed a reduction in the Cd concentration of soybean leaves from 33 to 5 mg/kg when the pH of the soil on which the plants were grown was increased by liming from 5.3 to 7.0. These data and others demonstrate that one of the most effective means of minimizing the absorption of Cd by plants grown on acid soils is to raise soil pH by liming.

2. Effect of Substrate Cadmium Concentration

Under similar chemical, physical, biologic, and mineralogic conditions in the soil, amounts of Cd absorbed by plants tend to increase as the concentration of Cd in the soil increases (VALADARES et al. 1983; CHANG et al. 1983). However, the increased Cd concentration in plants may or may not be proportional to the increased concentration in the soil. Also, repeated annual applications of fertilizers or soil conditioners which contain Cd (e.g., municipal sewage sludges), even though they increase the concentration of Cd in the soil each year, may or may not increase the content of Cd in the crop from year to year. Repeated applications alter the soil conditions and subsequently the availability of Cd to plants. Perhaps the factors which control the availability of Cd to the crop are not necessarily the same each year. Additional information on the availability of Cd to crops following repeated applications of Cd to soil can be obtained from CHANG et al. (1982c) and the COUNCIL FOR AGRICULTURAL SCIENCE AND TECHNOLOGY (1980). These reports demonstrate that the magnitude of increased concentrations of Cd in plants is not always consistent with cumulative amounts applied to soil, and depends upon a wide variety of environmental factors.

Both field and greenhouse experiments have been conducted to evaluate the effect of Cd level in soil on its concentration in plants. Plants grown on Cd-enriched soils in containers in the greenhouse tend to absorb more Cd than the same plants grown on the same soil supplemented with identical amounts of Cd in the field (PAGE and CHANG 1978; DE VRIES and TILLER 1978). The extension of the field plant roots beyond the contaminated layer results in less Cd absorption and accumulation in the plant tissues (PAGE et al. 1981).

The data presented in Table 10 illustrate the relationship between the increased Cd added to soils during one cropping season and the corresponding Cd concentration in a variety of vegetables (PAGE et al. 1981). Progressive increases in concentration of Cd in foliage and the edible part of carrot, radish, and lettuce were observed as the amounts of Cd added to the soil in the form of municipal sewage sludge was increased from 0.8 to 6.4 kg/ha. Results derived from field experiments conducted by GIORDANO et al. (1979) also show increased Cd concentrations in a wide variety of vegetable crops, except for potato, upon addition of Cd to soil at a rate equivalent to 11.2 kg/ha (Table 11). Additional data on the accumulation of Cd in crops in relation to amounts applied in the form of sewage sludge are presented in a review by SOMMERS (1982).

Table 10. Concentration of cadmium in various vegetables in relation to cadmium added to soil[a]

Crop	Tissue	Cd application rate (kg/ha)				
		0	0.8	1.6	3.2	6.4
		Cd content (µg/g)[b]				
Carrot	Foliage	0.5	1.64	2.52	3.89	3.91
	Edible part	0.44	0.91	1.64	2.44	2.61
Radish	Foliage	0.48	0.70	1.86	2.81	5.01
	Edible part	0.19	0.36	0.63	0.88	1.88
Swiss chard	Foliage	0.2	0.5	0.7	2.1	2.6
Lettuce	Foliage	0.5	2.2	3.1	4.4	

[a] Cadmium added in the form of municipal sewage sludge; crops grown under field conditions in a calcareous soil
[b] Dry weight basis

Table 11. Influence of cadmium applications to soils on the cadmium concentrations of various vegetable crops[a]

Crop	Tissue	Cd application rate (kg/ha)[b]	
		0	11.2
		Cd content (µg/g)[c]	
Lettuce	Edible part	0.83	4.44
Broccoli	Edible part	0.27	0.89
Eggplant	Foliage part	0.81	2.02
	Edible part	0.54	1.64
Tomato	Foliage part	1.11	3.61
	Edible part	0.52	1.04
Potato	Foliage part	0.80	0.69
	Edible part	0.11	0.10
Corn	Foliage part	0.29	16.3
	Edible part	0.10	1.83
Squash	Foliage part	0.15	1.40
	Edible part	0.15	0.27
Pepper	Foliage part	0.90	7.51
	Edible part	0.24	1.08
Bean	Foliage part	0.16	0.72
	Edible part	0.07	0.21
Cabbage	Edible part	0.18	0.27
Carrot	Edible part	0.84	1.77
Cantaloupe	Edible part	0.21	0.63

[a] Derived from data published by GIORDANO et al. (1979)
[b] Cadmium applied in the form of municipal sludge
[c] Dry weight basis

Numerous studies indicate that the chemical form of Cd will also influence the amount absorbed by plants (KORCAK and FANNING 1978; LOGAN and CHANEY 1984). MAHLER et al. (1978) added $CdSO_4$-spiked sludges to soil to produce concentrations of Cd in soil equal to 10 and 20 kg/ha. They reported concentrations of Cd in Swiss chard plants of 15 and 26 µg/g whereas PAGE and CHANG (1978) reported, respectively, 4.8 and 6.6 µg Cd per gram plant tissue when plants were grown under similar conditions, but with Cd added to the soil entirely in the form of composted sewage sludge. Similarly, KORCAK and FANNING (1978) reported that the Cd accumulation by corn foliage, from a soil supplemented with $CdSO_4$, is 5–18 times greater than Cd accumulation by foliage from a soil treated with sewage sludge to contain the same amount of Cd.

In soil solution, cadmium may form relatively strong complexes with chloride and sulfate ions. Different chemical species of cadmium in solution may be different in their availability to plants. Using Swiss chard as the indicator plant, BINGHAM et al. (1983, 1984) tested the availability of cadmium under the influence of various chloride concentrations in a series of greenhouse pot experiments. They found that total concentration of cadmium in soil solution increased with chloride concentration in soil and it was present principally as Cd^{2+} and $CdCl^+$. Leaf cadmium content of Swiss chard was, however, primarily a function of Cd^{2+} concentration. These data point out that an assessment of availability of cadmium should be made on the basis of the various chemical species of cadmium present, rather than on the total concentration of soluble cadmium.

3. Influence of Time Following the Application of Cadmium to Soil

A number of studies suggest that the length of time during which soils treated with Cd are incubated affects the availability of Cd to crops. BATES et al. (1975) followed the Cd concentrations from successive planting of crops grown on soils which were treated with the same amount of Cd prior to each planting. They reported that the concentrations of Cd in the first crop of ryegrass were essentially the same as their concentrations in the following three crops, suggesting that residual Cd from previous applications is no longer available to plants. HINESLY et al. (1978), DOWDY et al. (1978), and COKER et al. (1982) reported similar observations with corn, snap beans, and herbage (mixture of oats and ryegrass), respectively. HINESLY et al. (1979 a) also studied the availability of Cd to corn plants for a 5-year period after the last application of Cd (in the form of sewage sludge). They reported a gradual decline in the Cd concentration in leaves and grain with time following cessation of Cd inputs. In the fifth year, the concentration of Cd in corn grain decreased to background levels. Although the Cd concentration of the corn foliage also decreased progressively, it did not approach the background level at the end of the 5-year period. Results presented by VIITASALO (1973) for oats and barley are similar to those of HINESLY et al. (1979 a) in that concentrations of cadmium in the crops diminished with time over a 30-month period following sludge application. Observations made by STREET et al. (1978), CHANEY et al. (1977), CHANG et al. (1982 b, 1983) are somewhat contrary to those of HINESLY et al. (1978, 1979 b), BATES et al. (1975), and DOWDY et al. (1978). After a 16-week incubation period, STREET et al. (1978) observed that the availability

of Cd to corn seedlings decreased when Cd was added to soils in the form of inorganic salts ($CdSO_4$), but the uptake increased when it was added through
sludge applications. They suggested that increased availability of Cd to plants
grown in soils treated with sewage sludge as incubation time increased was due
to the release of organically absorbed Cd through microbial decomposition of organic matter. CHANEY et al. (1977) and CHANEY and HORNICK (1978) reported elevated concentrations of Cd in plants grown on soils long after the soil was
treated with sludge. Likewise, CHANG et al. (1982b, c, 1983) observed essentially
no change in the availability of Cd to barley, radish, tomato, and Swiss chard each
year for a period of 3 years following termination of Cd applications.

4. Other Soil Factors

The oxidation–reduction potential of soil also has a marked influence on the concentration of Cd absorbed from soil by plants. This is so because under reducing
conditions Cd is substantially less soluble in soil solutions than it is under oxidizing conditions. Although the redox potential in soil influences Cd bioavailability,
it is only important in the culture of rice because all other agricultural crops fail
to grow under reducing conditions. BINGHAM et al. (1976a) has shown that the
concentration of Cd in rice grown under reducing conditions (flooded) is less than
that of rice grown under oxidizing conditions (nonflooded). Similar observations
have been made by TAKIJIMA et al. (1973).

Although other soil factors have been reported to influence the absorption of
Cd by terrestrial plants, their effects are not nearly as consistent and clear-cut as
those of soil pH and Cd content of soil. HAGHIRI (1974) reported a decrease in
the amount of Cd absorbed by oat shoots as the cation exchange capacity (CEC)
of the soil was increased by adding organic matter. However, MAHLER et al.
(1978) showed no consistent pattern in Cd absorption by either lettuce or chard
in relation to soil CEC. Data in STENSTROM and LONSJO (1974) also show no
change in the absorption of Cd by wheat grain in relation to changes in the CEC
of soil. It is quite possible that adjusting the CEC of a soil by introducing foreign
substances may have caused a decrease in Cd absorption by plants because the
introduced substances reacted preferentially with Cd. But over a broad range of
soils with varying CEC, other soil chemical properties tend to overshadow the influence of soil CEC on the absorption of Cd.

Several investigators suggested that oxides of iron and manganese exhibit
highly specific adsorption affinity for trace metals, including Cd (FORBES et al.
1976; COREY et al. 1981). There is limited information to support the thesis that
the quantity of Cd absorbed by plants can be influenced by the content of iron
and manganese oxides in soil (CHANEY and HORNICK 1978).

The synergistic and antagonistic effects of other trace metals in the soil substrate on the absorption of Cd by plants has been examined by a number of investigators. Studies on the interactive effects of Cd, Zn, Cu, and Ni by MITCHELL
et al. (1978) showed that increasing concentrations of both Cu and Ni in soil consistently reduced concentrations of Cd in the leaves of lettuce plants. However,
the effect of Zn depended upon the Cd concentration in soil. At low Cd levels
(~ 0.1 µg/g), increasing levels of Zn reduced the concentration of Cd in lettuce

leaves, but at higher Cd levels the added Zn either showed no effect or increased the Cd concentration in lettuce leaves. In solution culture experiments, LAGER-WERFF and BIERSDORF (1971) observed a similar Cd absorption pattern for radish. However, HAGHIRI (1974) presented data which showed an increased uptake of Cd by soybean plants with Zn additions to soil up to approximately 100 μg/g, followed by a progressive decrease in Cd uptake at concentrations of Zn added to soil greater than 100 μg/g. Other investigators (IWAI et al. 1975; JOHN 1973; CUN-NINGHAM et al. 1975; MCLEAN 1976), however, have observed that Zn added to substrates has little or no effect on the concentration of Cd in plants. An examination of data on interactive effects of Zn and Cd suggests that other soil chemical properties may be operative and in certain situations may tend to offset any possible synergistic or antagonistic effects of Zn on the absorption of Cd by plants.

In addition to Zn, Cu, and Ni, other elements in soils which have been reported to reduce Cd uptake by plants include Se (FRANCIS and RUSH 1974), Mn (CHANEY and HORNICK 1978), and P (WILLIAMS and DAVID 1977; STREET et al. 1978). Phosphorus additions to noncalcareous soils may reduce the solubility of Cd in the soil solution and thereby decrease Cd available to plants (SANTILLAN-MEDRANO and JURINAK 1975).

The absorption of Cd by plants may also be influenced by temperature of the substrate in which the plants are grown. GIORDANO et al. (1979) reported significant increases in the concentration of Cd in broccoli and potato plants with increased temperature of the soil. HAGHIRI (1974) made similar observations for soybean seedlings. Although increased temperatures of the soil tend to increase the absorption of Cd by some plants, the effect has not been consistently observed for all plants (GIORDANO et al. 1979).

F. Phytotoxic Effects of Cadmium

Excessive trace metal absorption may injure a plant. Although trace metal-induced crop damage has been reported in several instances where trace metals were allowed to accumulate in soils (LEE and PAGE 1967; LEE and CRADDOCK 1969), phytotoxic effects caused by cadmium contamination of soils in field situations were not found in the literature. However, numerous solution culture and pot experiments illustrate the potential adverse effects of cadmium on plant growth (JOHN et al. 1972; PAGE et al. 1972; BINGHAM and PAGE 1975; BINGHAM et al. 1975, 1976 b; BECKETT and DAVIS 1977). Plant species and even varieties within a species exhibited wide variation of tolerance to levels of cadmium in soil (JOHN 1973; JOHN and VAN LAERHOVEN 1976). Table 12 summarizes cadmium addition to a calcareous soil that will result in 50% yield reduction of various field and vegetable crops grown in containers in a greenhouse. In general, vegetable plants are less tolerant to cadmium than field crops. Leafy vegetables such as spinach and lettuce are especially susceptible to damage by cadmium. In acid soils, more acute crop damage is experienced than in calcareous soils containing equal levels of cadmium (CHANEY et al. 1979; CHANG et al. 1981). But Cd levels in soils that may result in phytotoxicity far exceed those that are associated with accelerated Cd

Table 12. Amounts of Cd addition to a calcareous soil resulting in 50% reduction of yield of container-grown field and vegetable crops[a]

Crop	Cd addition rate reducing yields 50% (µg/g)	Crop	Cd addition rate reducing yields 50% (µg/g)
Spinach	10	White clover	120
Soybean	11	Table beet	133
Curly cress	15	Alfalfa	145
Romaine lettuce	35	Radish	160
Sweet corn	35	Zucchini squash	200
Upland rice	36	Swiss chard	320
Sudan grass	58	Tall fescue	320
Carrot	65	Cabbage	350
Field bean	65	Bermuda grass	400
Wheat	80	Tomato	415
Turnip	100	Paddy rice	>640

[a] From Bingham and Page (1975)

uptake by plants. Unless the hazard of cadmium contamination of soils in terms of its effect on the accumulation of Cd by food chain crops is totally neglected, Cd phytotoxicity is not likely to become a problem.

G. Concentrations of Cadmium in Food Chain Crops

Cadmium is a naturally occurring element present in all soils in at least trace quantities. For this reason, all food chain crops contain at least trace amounts of Cd. The concentrations of Cd in plants vary among species and cultivars. Different plant parts (leaves, stems, fruit, roots) accumulate different amounts of Cd. The concentration of cadmium in the leaves and seeds of pea, wheat, and corn (Table 13) are representative of results reported in the literature. The concentration of Cd in a particular plant part is also influenced by its physiologic state of development (Chang et al. 1984).

Cadmium uptake is characterized by an initial rapid phase followed by a slower phase (Girling and Peterson 1981). Accumulation of cadmium generally is highest in roots, intermediate in leaves, and lowest in grains. About 20% of cadmium taken up by corn was translocated to parts above ground (Dupont et al. 1980). Only 5% or less of the Cd absorbed by rice plants was found in the polished grains (Biglicocca et al. 1979). In tobacco, most Cd is translocated to the tops and accumulated in leaves (Frank et al. 1977). Grasses, in general, tend to have high Cd concentration in tops.

Weigel and Jaer (1980) reported that the subcellular distribution and chemical form of Cd in bean plants is as follows: more than 70% localized in the cytoplasmic fraction in roots and leaves; 8%–14% bound either to the cell wall or organelles. In roots, cadmium is associated with compounds of molecular weight 5,000–10,000, whereas in leaves it is associated with compounds of molecular weight 700–5,000 and small amounts are found in high molecular weight proteins (Weigel and Jaer 1980).

Table 13. Cadmium concentrations of vegetative and reproductive tissues from plants grown on sewage sludge-supplemented soils in relation to species, application rate, and soil pH

Cd added from sludge	Soil pH	Cadmium (μg/g)[a]					
		Pea		Wheat		Corn	
(kg/ha)		Leaves	Seeds	Leaves	Grain	Leaves	Grain
0	4.4	0.94	0.20	0.19	0.06	0.11	0.03
2.2	4.6	4.40	0.64	0.82	0.25	1.44	0.06
4.5	5.0	3.80	1.11	1.10	0.32	1.83	0.08
9.0	5.2	6.05	1.45	0.89	0.58	3.37	0.09
0	7.8	0.43	0.14	0.14	0.04	0.07	0.01
2.2	7.6	0.43	0.17	0.18	0.12	0.14	0.02
4.5	7.4	0.42	0.18	0.25	0.23	0.41	0.03
9.0	7.3	0.48	0.30	0.33	0.34	0.92	0.03

[a] Dry weight basis

In the past decade, background concentrations for a wide variety of food chain crops have been published (FORSTNER 1980; PAGE et al. 1981). A summary of the data compiled by PAGE et al. (1981) is presented in Table 14. These data pertain to situations where the soils on which the crops were grown were not known to be subject to Cd contamination, and therefore should be representative of natural background levels of Cd in the crops listed. The data clearly demonstrate that background levels of Cd in crops vary substantially. Data of a national survey of the main production areas in the United States show Cd concentrations of lettuce, spinach, carrot, potato, onion, and wheat, of the same order of magnitude (Table 15). The data presented in Table 15 were obtained from a cooperative study jointly conducted by the US Department of Agriculture, the Food and Drug Administration, and the Environmental Protection Agency. Special care was taken to insure that all sites selected were remote from sources of contamination, and in the handling, packaging, and shipping of samples. All samples were analyzed in a specially equipped Food and Drug Administration laboratory. The senior author of this chapter served on the advisory committee for the study, and in his opinion the data are among the most reliable in existence.

Although only limited data are available, it appears that crops grown on soil naturally elevated in Cd show higher concentrations of Cd than those grown on similar soils, but not naturally elevated. FEENEY et al. (1984) recently reported results from a national survey of metal content of vegetable species. In the region where soils were naturally elevated in Cd (Salinas Valley, California), mean concentrations of Cd for lettuce, spinach, carrot, and tomato were, without exception, greater than mean concentrations for the same crops grown on soils with more or less normal Cd concentrations (Table 16). The Cd concentrations for the soils in the region designated as naturally elevated are not uniformly high throughout, and vary quite substantially from what would be considered normal (Table 16). This natural variation among the soils within the region accounts for

Table 14. Cadmium concentrations of various food chain crops[a]

Food class/crop	No. of observations	Cd (mg/kg)[b]		
		Minimum	Maximum	Range of reported means
Leafy vegetables				
Spinach	13	0.03	0.31	0.045–0.11
Lettuce	59	<0.001	0.198	0.012–0.093
Cabbage	43	0.002	0.15	0.006–0.04
Root vegetables				
Carrot	83	0.001	0.22	0.005–0.13
Potato	112	0.005	0.18	<0.05 –0.18
Onion	58	<0.002	0.09	0.006–0.08
Radish	12	0.008	0.027	0.016
Beet	28	0.01	0.069	0.016–0.041
Other vegetables				
Brussels sprout	20	0.01	0.11	0.027–0.03
Cauliflower	15	0.003	0.021	0.01
Tomato	65	<0.001	0.08	0.01 –0.03
Pepper	8	0.015	0.05	0.029–0.043
Bean	20	0.02	0.08	0.04 –0.042
Rutabaga	15	0.01	0.026	0.016
Cucumber	32	<0.001	0.014	0.003–0.01
Stone fruits				
Cherry	18	<0.001	0.076	<0.001–0.04
Plum	7	0.014	0.067	0.036
Peach	10	<0.001	0.006	0.002
Citrus fruits				
Orange	15	<0.001	0.007	0.002
Grapefruit	3	<0.01	0.01	<0.01
Lemon	5	0.01	0.04	0.01
Pomaceous fruits				
Apple	43	<0.001	0.027	0.005–0.027
Pear	9	0.01	0.09	0.011–0.03
Grains				
Wheat	250	<0.005	0.23	0.035–0.10
Barley	133	0.01	0.75	0.05 –0.37
Oats	101	0.01	0.28	0.01 –0.09
Rice	69	<0.001	0.31	0.11 –0.13

[a] Derived from information reviewed by PAGE et al. (1981)
[b] Wet weight basis

the wide range of Cd concentrations observed for the vegetable species sampled. More limited studies by LUND et al. (1981) and from our laboratory (A. L. PAGE 1982, unpublished work) for native vegetation and crops grown on similarly naturally elevated Cd soils also show elevated Cd concentrations in plants when compared with the same plants grown on soils with normal levels of Cd. The data demonstrate the background levels for crops will vary with the natural level of Cd in soil in addition to pH and possibly other soil properties.

Table 15. Background concentrations of cadmium for various food crops grown in the major producing regions of the United States[a]

Crop	No. of obser- vations	Cadmium (mg/kg)[b]			
		Minimum	Maximum	Mean	Median
Leafy vegetables					
Lettuce	150	0.001	0.160	0.026	0.017
Spinach	104	0.012	0.195	0.065	0.061
Root crops					
Peanuts	320	0.010	0.588	0.078	0.060
Carrots	207	<0.002	0.132	0.028	0.017
Onion	228	<0.002	0.054	0.011	0.009
Potatoes	297	0.002	0.182	0.031	0.028
Grain crops					
Soybeans	322	0.002	0.11	0.059	0.041
Sweet corn	268	<0.001	0.039	0.003	0.002
Field corn	277	<0.001	0.317	0.012	0.004
Wheat	288	<0.002	0.207	0.043	0.030
Rice	166	<0.001	0.226	0.012	0.004
Other vegetables					
Tomatoes	231	<0.003	0.048	0.017	0.014

[a] Derived from WOLNIK et al. (1983, 1985)
[b] Wet weight basis

Table 16. Cadmium concentrations of vegetable crops grown in a region naturally elevated in Cd and other regions[a]

Crop/region	No. of samples	Cd in soil (mg/kg)[b] Range	Cd in crop (mg/kg)[c]	
			Range	Mean
Lettuce				
Naturally elevated	13	0.33–5.98	0.52–24	4.63
Other	12	<0.33–1.38	0.48–1.54	0.88
Spinach				
Naturally elevated	5	0.26–1.26	2.38–3.8	3.09
Other	12	<0.33	0.38–1.98	0.85
Carrot				
Naturally elevated	8	0.16–5.97	0.39–2.79	0.98
Other	15	0.5 –1.10	0.04–0.39	0.25
Tomato				
Naturally elevated	10	0.6 –8.42	0.46–4.12	2.57
Other	8		0.09–0.78	0.35

[a] Derived from FEENEY et al. (1984)
[b] 0.1 M HCl soluble Cd, dry weight basis
[c] Dry weight basis

Table 17. Cadmium concentrations of various food classes[a]

Food class	No. of samples	Cadmium (mg/kg)[b]			
		Minimum	Maximum	Mean	Median
Leafy vegetables	266	0.001	0.388	0.044	0.028
Sprouting vegetables	38	0.0005	0.09	0.019	0.01
Fruity vegetables	92	0.0005	0.166	0.020	0.020
Root vegetables	79	0.001	0.104	0.023	0.020
Kernel fruit	150	0.0005	0.116	0.010	0.005
Stoned fruit	62	0.0005	0.076	0.014	0.005
Berries	82	0.0001	0.101	0.018	0.007
Grains	574	0.004	0.80[c]	0.035[c]	
Potatoes	188	0.001	0.202	0.05	0.042

[a] Derived from KAFERSTEIN et al. (1979)
[b] Total element content for the food
c For wheat only

A rather extensive data base for Cd concentrations of various food classes in the Federal Republic of Germany has also been published (KAFERSTEIN et al. 1979). These data, however, are considered to be conditional by the authors of the report because sampling was not done according to statistical criteria; the data were supplied from various sources and based on different methods of processing. Aside from the limitations stated by those who prepared the Federal Republic of Germany report, where comparisons are possible the data appear to fall within the range reported in the United States survey. Data from the Federal Republic of Germany survey (Table 17) show minimum, maximum, mean, and median Cd concentration for potatoes of 0.001, 0.202, 0.05, and 0.042 mg/kg, respectively. These values compare reasonably well with minimum, maximum, mean, and median Cd concentrations of 0.002, 0.182, 0.031, and 0.028 mg/kg, respectively, for potatoes grown in the United States. Comparisons for Cd concentrations of leafy vegetables, wheat, as well as potatoes are presented in Table 18. The maximum value for the Cd concentration of wheat reported in the Federal Republic of Germany survey (0.80 mg/kg) is considerably greater than maximum values reported from the United States and other areas. In a Finnish survey, VARO et al. (1980) reported a range of 0.026–0.112 mg/kg (dry weight) for 85 samples of winter and spring wheat. Likewise, TILLER et al. (1975) reported that 110 samples of wheat from Australia contained from <0.006 to 0.051 mg/kg, KJELLSTROM et al. (1975) that 79 samples of spring and fall wheat from Sweden contained 0.006–0.154 mg/kg, and ANDERSSON and PETTERSSON (1981) that 107 samples of winter wheat contained 0.028–0.171 mg/kg.

These data again demonstrate that Cd concentrations of food crops vary considerably within species and among species. Additionally, varieties within plant species also show substantial differences in their Cd absorption characteristics. JOHN and VAN LAERHOVEN (1976) showed substantial differences in the Cd concentrations of nine varieties of lettuce when they were grown under identical conditions. Likewise, HINESLY et al. (1978, 1982), PETTERSSON (1977), CHANG et al.

Table 18. Comparison of cadmium concentrations of three food chain crops[a]

Crop	Cd (mg/kg)[b]		
	United States	Federal Republic of Germany	Many countries
Potatoes			
Minimum	0.002	0.001	0.005
Maximum	0.182	0.202	0.18
Mean	0.031	0.05	
Median	0.028	0.042	
Leafy vegetables[c]			
Minimum	0.001	0.001	<0.001
Maximum	0.195	0.388	0.31
Mean	0.042	0.044	
Median	0.043	0.028	
Wheat			
Minimum	0.0017	0.004	<0.005
Maximum	0.207	0.80	0.23
Mean	0.043	0.035	
Median	0.030		

[a] Derived from data presented in tables 14, 15, and 17
[b] Wet weight basis
[c] Data from United States are for lettuce and spinach only

(1982a), and ANDERSSON and PETTERSSON (1981) observed that different varieties of corn (HINESLY et al. 1978, 1982), wheat and barley (PETTERSSON 1977), barley (CHANG et al. 1982a), and wheat (ANDERSSON and PETTERSSON 1981) absorbed different amounts of Cd. These observations have prompted attempts to breed plants with low Cd absorption characteristics.

In terms of comparing the concentrations of Cd in various food crops it is important to recognize the weight basis on which the data are expressed. In the literature, Cd concentrations in food are frequently expressed in terms of fresh (wet) or dry (freeze-dried or oven-dried, usually at 70 °C in a forced draft oven) weight, and less commonly on the basis of the weight of the ash (550 °C for 2–4 h). A comparison of the Cd concentration of various crops, expressed on a wet and dry weight basis and derived from data contained in WOLNIK et al. (1983, 1985), is presented in Table 19. The data demonstrate that the order of diminishing concentrations of Cd in crops depends on the weight basis upon which the concentrations are expressed. For example, when expressed on a wet weight basis, spinach, peanuts, soybeans, wheat, and potatoes have higher concentrations of Cd than lettuce, but when expressed on a dry weight basis, only spinach has a higher concentration than lettuce. Also, since the moisture content of a crop may vary considerably, depending upon its maturity, the length of time the sample is stored, and the relative humidity during storage, the concentrations in a specific food crop expressed on a fresh weight basis change as the water content changes. For example, WOLNIK et al. (1983) present data which show that the water content of 288 samples of wheat grain collected in the major producing regions of the United States varied from 1.2% to 27.8%. For comparative purposes and to

Table 19. Comparison of the concentration of Cd in various crops expressed on a wet (fresh) and dry weight basis[a]

Crop	Cd (mg/kg)	
	Wet weight basis	Dry weight basis
Spinach	0.061	0.80
Peanuts	0.060	0.068
Soybeans	0.041	0.045
Wheat	0.030	0.036
Potatoes	0.028	0.14
Lettuce	0.017	0.435
Carrots	0.017	0.16
Tomatoes	0.014	0.22
Onion	0.009	0.09
Field corn	0.004	0.004
Rice	0.004	0.005
Sweet corn	0.002	0.008

[a] Derived from WOLNIK et al. (1983, 1985)

avoid confusion associated with differences in moisture content among the same food crop, it would be desirable if all results were expressed on a dry weight basis.

H. Human Intake of Cadmium

Chapter 3 on Cd absorption reviews additional details on this topic. The daily intake of Cd from foods depends upon the caloric intake and dietary habits of individuals, the source of the raw food crops, and the methods by which the foods are processed prior to consumption. Because diets of individuals vary within and among ethnic groups the ingestion of cadmium in the general population will also vary. Since intake is a function of the amount of food consumed, those individuals consuming the largest amount of food (frequently teenage males) will have the highest daily Cd intake.

ELINDER (1985) recently compiled data for the average daily intake of Cd from all food sources from a number of countries throughout the world. The data show widespread variations in average daily intake among the various countries. The range of average daily intake from reports published after 1976 showed values of 10–51 µg/day for the United States, 10–20 µg/day for the United Kingdom, 11–18 µg/day for Sweden, and 20–70 µg/day for Japan. The more recent measurements of the average daily intake (after 1976) tend to show levels less than the earlier measurements (before 1976). This difference is generally attributed to the availability of more accurate and sensitive methodology to measure Cd intake in recent times. The consistently higher levels of intake for the Japanese population can be attributed to the relatively high per capita consumption of rice in Japan (average of 300 g per capita per day). In nonpolluted areas of Japan, the mean concentrations of Cd for rice is reported to be 0.09 µg/g (YAMAGATA 1978). As-

Table 20. Daily intake of cadmium from terrestrial food chain crops which directly enter the diet for the average individual in the United States and the Federal Republic of Germany

Food class	Cd (µg/kg)[a]	Consumption (g/day)	Cd intake (µg/day)
United States[b]			
Grain and cereal products	23.2	331	7.7
Potatoes	48.0	138	6.6
Leafy vegetables	40.5	42	1.7
Legume vegetables	6.2	51	0.3
Root vegetables	32.3	25	0.8
Garden fruits	14.7	69	1.0
Fruits	3.0	173	0.5
Federal Republic of Germany[c]			
Grains	35	276	9.7
Potatoes	42	242	10.2
Leafy vegetables	28	28.5	0.8
Sprouting vegetables	10	21.6	0.2
Fruity vegetables	20	28.4	0.6
Root vegetables	20	13.7	0.3
Berries	7	15.7	0.1
Kernel fruit	5	50.2	0.3
Stone fruit	5	16.7	0.1

[a] Wet weight basis
[b] Derived from RYAN et al. (1982)
[c] Derived from data presented by KAFERSTEIN et al. (1979)

suming this concentration is representative of the rice actually consumed, the consumption of rice in Japan on the average would contribute 27 µg Cd to the daily intake. Based upon an average intake of cadmium of 50 µg/day for the Japanese population, rice alone may contribute about 54% of the average daily intake of cadmium.

Available information suggests that for most populations any substantial increase in the average daily intake of Cd will come from terrestrially produced crops which directly enter the human food chain. Except for the liver and kidney of animals and poultry, the food products derived from warm-blooded animals do not appear to accumulate Cd. In the case of seafoods, although many tend to accumulate Cd in a polluted environment, the amount consumed by an average North American is relatively small, and therefore, should cause only a slight increase in average daily intake.

Average daily intake of Cd from terrestrially produced foods which directly enter the human food chain estimated for the population of the United States (RYAN et al. 1982) and for the Federal Republic of Germany (derived from KAFERSTEIN et al. 1979) are presented in Table 20. The data show that two food classes: grains and potatoes, account for about 76% and 90% of the daily intake "from terrestrial foods which directly enter the food chain" for populations in the United States and the Federal Republic of Germany, respectively. DAVIS et al.

(1982), from a more limited data set based upon the content of Cd in food crops grown on one soil, also conclude that grains/grain products and potatoes account for more than 90% of the Cd intake from foods of plant origin for individuals in the United Kingdom. In terms of minimizing the intake of Cd the analyses presented suggest that crops which contribute a substantial percentage to the daily intake of Cd should not be cultivated on Cd-contaminated soils. Since these considerations are only applicable to persons with diets comparable to the average adult population in the United States and the Federal Republic of Germany, caution should be excercised in their application to all individuals.

J. Methods to Control the Entry of Cadmium into Food Chain Crops

The information presented in the previous sections suggests a number of procedures to control the entry of Cd into food chain crops. In terms of soil properties, control of the soil pH at levels near neutral or greater, and controls on the amounts of Cd added to soils from extraneous sources should serve to minimize the entry of Cd into food chain crops. In situations where soils are naturally high in Cd, use of these soils for crops which tend to exclude Cd or crops which are used exclusively as animal feed are measures which can be taken to minimize the amounts of Cd which enter the human food chain. When warm-blooded animals (swine, cattle, goats, lambs) were fed diets elevated in Cd, only the liver and kidney of these animals was significantly elevated in Cd (SHARMA et al. 1979; FITZGERALD 1980; DOWDY et al. 1985). Since Cd tends not to accumulate in the animal muscle tissue, there is probably little concern about nonvisceral meats in the marketplace, even though the animal may have been fed a diet elevated in cadmium (KOWAL 1984). A discussion of bioavailability of Cd along with possible control measures is presented by CHANEY (1982) and LOGAN and CHANEY (1984).

In response to concern over possible increased levels of Cd in human diets resulting from environmental pollution, governmental agencies and others in various countries have suggested limits for amounts of Cd added to agricultural soils as well as limits for amounts of Cd in food crops. Limits on the amounts of trace elements added to agricultural soils from sewage sludge have been proposed by the Council of European Communities (OFFICIAL JOURNAL OF EUROPEAN COMMUNITIES 1982). With respect to cadmium, the Council recommends that the average annual applications of cadmium over a 10-year period not exceed 100 g Cd per hectare per year and sets a mandatory limit of 150 g Cd per hectare per year, again based upon a 10-year average. Earlier, Denmark and Sweden proposed that the maximum permissible annual application of Cd be 15 g/ha and Finland and Norway proposed 20 and 30 g/ha, respectively (cited by PURVES 1981). In the United States, the current annual application is based on the crop grown and the soil pH (U.S. ENVIRONMENTAL PROTECTION AGENCY 1979; NAYLOR and LOEHR 1981). For root crops, leafy vegetables, and tobacco, and for all crops grown on soils with a pH less than 6.5, the annual limit is established at 500 g/ha. For other crops grown on soils where the pH is maintained at levels greater than 6.5, the annual limit effective after 30 June 1984 is 1,250 g/ha and this level is scheduled to be reduced to 500 g/ha on 1 July 1987. The Federal Republic of Germany, United Kingdom, and Japan have not established guidelines which limit annual applications of Cd, but specify the permissible total cumulative addition of Cd. In the Federal Republic of Germany and the United Kingdom, guidelines state that the amount of Cd applied over any period of time should not result in a soil concentration in excess of 3 and 3.5 mg Cd per kilogram soil, respectively (KLOKE 1982; DEPARTMENT OF THE ENVIRONMENT 1981). If this limit applies to the surface 15 cm of a silt loam soil, it is approximately the equivalent of a surface application of 6,000–7,000 g/ha. In England, guidelines governing metal additions to agricultural land propose that additions be made gradually over a period of 30 years or more. On this basis, the annual suggested limit in England would be approximately 230 g/ha. Guidelines for the application of Cd to soils in Japan do not specify any absolute amount, but state that the amount added should not exceed an amount which will produce rice grain with a Cd content greater than 0.4 mg/kg (ASAMI 1981a). Total amounts of Cd permissible on agricultural land in the United States are also specified in the US Environmental Protection Agency Interim Criteria (U.S. ENVIRONMENTAL PROTECTION AGENCY 1979). These are based upon the pH and the CEC of the soil. For soils of pH less than 6.5, the criteria limit the total quantity of Cd applied to 5,000 g/ha. For soils maintained at pH greater than 6.5 and CEC less than 5, 5–15, and greater than 15 mequiv. per 100 g soil, the total cumulative limits are 5,000, 10,000, and 20,000 g/ha, respectively.

It is obvious that differences of opinion occur among the various countries regarding a safe level of Cd in soil utilized for the production of crops. In terms of annual applications, the Scandinavian countries limit annual applications to levels of 30 g/ha or less, the Council of European Communities proposes a mandatory limit of 150 g/ha and in the United States, in the most restrictive case, the annual application is limited to 500 g/ha. In terms of the maximum amount of Cd permitted on agricultural land, the Federal Republic of Germany and the United Kingdom permit about 5,000 g/ha while in the United States as much as 20,000 g/ha is permitted. Finally, it should be pointed out that soils may have background levels much in excess of the limits specified for the total permissible Cd addition (see Table 5).

Except for rice in Japan and for certain food classes in the Federal Republic of Germany, there are few suggested limits for Cd in food chain crops. The reason for the reluctance on the part of regulatory agencies to establish limits for food crops is probably related to the dependence of Cd intake on the nature of the diet. For example, in the Federal Republic of Germany and in the United States, potatoes and grains and cereals represent the largest single contribution to dietary intake of Cd from foodstuffs of plant origin (see Table 20). In terms of minimizing Cd daily intake, therefore, it would seem that stricter controls on the amounts of Cd in foods which make up a high percentage of the diet would be the most effective. In Japan, rice makes up a substantial percentage of the food consumed, and limits are established for this crop. The maximum allowable Cd concentration for rice is set at 1.0 mg/kg for unpolished rice, but the suggested limit is 0.4 mg/kg (ASAMI 1981b). KAFERSTEIN (1980) (also cited by KLOKE et al. 1984) has suggested guidelines for Cd concentrations of green vegetables, sprout vegetables, fruity vegetables, cereals, and potatoes of 0.1 mg/kg on a fresh weight basis, and

0.05 mg/kg (fresh weight basis) for root vegetables, pomaceous fruits, stone fruits, and berries. Where the content of foodstuffs of plant origin is twice as high as the guidelines suggested, the Ministry of Nutrition, Agriculture, Environment and Forestry of Baden-Württemberg, Federal Republic of Germany, suggests that the products be removed from commercial circulation (Anonymous 1980, cited by Kloke et al. 1984). Mean and median background concentrations of crops grown in the United States are less than the Federal Republic of Germany limit specified for commercial distribution; however, maximum background levels observed for some root crops (peanuts, carrots) and grain crops (soybeans, field corn, and rice) exceed the limit (see Table 15). Although the crop concentration as obtained from the field may exceed limits for the food class specified, the processing of the crop for human consumption may reduce the concentration in the refined product. When many grains (e.g., rice, wheat, corn) are processed into flour products, the refined product is substantially lower than the whole grain products (Hinesly et al. 1979 b; Kitageshi and Obata 1981). Oat groats, soybean cotyledons, and soy protein products, on the other hand, are as high in Cd as the whole grain (Kirleis et al. 1981; Braude et al. 1980). In examining human dietary intake of Cd, it is essential that the Cd content of the foodstuff as consumed be determined.

In polluted soils, the Cd is usually concentrated in the surface few centimeters of soil. One obvious means to correct the situation is to remove the contaminated layer of soil or to place a soil cover over the contaminated layer. This procedure has been practiced in Japan with some success. Asami (1981 b) presents data which show a substantial reduction in the Cd concentration of rice grain following covering of a polluted rice paddy soil with a 30-cm layer of nonpolluted soil.

K. Summary

Cadmium is a relatively rare metal not found in the pure state in nature. It is recovered as a by-product from the smelting and refining of zinc ore at rates equivalent to 0.02%–1.4% of Zn. Approximately 65% of the total world production took place in the past 20 years. Since 1970, the concern regarding the health effects of cadmium has resulted in a downward trend in its production. Six countries, France, Germany, Belgium, Japan, the United Kingdom, and the United States accounted for over 70% of the cadmium consumed during the last decade. Almost all of the cadmium produced went into electroplating, plastic stabilizing, pigments, and batteries. Other uses include fungicides, phosphorescent dials, and various miscellaneous uses.

In the environment, cadmium is regarded by many as one of the most toxic trace elements to humans. Although acute cadmium toxicity caused by consumption of food is rare, chronic exposure to high Cd levels in food may significantly increase the Cd accumulation in certain body organs. Concentrations of Cd in foods of plant origin are controlled by its concentration in the soil substrate as well as the chemical properties of the substrate. Typical noncontaminated soils will contain 0.05–1.0 µg/g with a median concentration of a few tenths of a microgram Cd per gram. Soils derived from igneous rocks are usually lowest in total cadmium, those derived from metamorphic rocks are intermediate, and those derived from sedimentary rocks contain the largest quantities of Cd. Soils may be contaminated with cadmium by fallout from aerial sources, by application of waters, fertilizers, or pesticides which contain Cd, or by the discharge of cadmium-containing waste materials. Cadmium added to soils, regardless of the chemical form, tends to remain at or near the depth of incorporation.

Two most important factors governing the absorption and accumulation of Cd by a crop are soil pH and the Cd level of the soil. If other conditions remain unchanged, the plant tissue Cd concentration would decrease as pH of the soil increases. Amounts of Cd absorbed by plants tend to increase as the concentration of Cd in the soil increases. However, the increased concentration in plants may or may not be proportional to the increased Cd concentration in the soil. The amount absorbed by plants is also influenced by source and form of Cd, and the synergistic and antagonistic effects of other trace elements such as Zn, Cu, and Ni.

All food chain crops contain at least trace concentrations of Cd. When concentrations are expressed on a dry weight basis, plant tissue accumulation of Cd is generally highest in roots, intermediate in leaves, and lowest in grains. Grasses often exhibit higher Cd concentrations in tops than roots. Cadmium levels in food crops vary quite substantially within species and among species.

The entry of Cd into food chain crops may be minimized by controlling the soil pH at levels near neutral or greater, and the amounts of Cd added to soils from anthropogenic sources. Amounts of Cd in foods which make up a higher percentage of the diet such as rice, potato, and wheat products have the most significant impact on the dietary intake of Cd. Guidelines for the maximum concentrations of Cd in food crops of plant origin and for maximum amounts of Cd added to and/or present in soils used for the production of crops as proposed by various countries are presented and discussed.

References

Alkezweeny AJ, Laulainen NS, Thorp JM (1982) Physical, chemical and optical characteristics of a clean air mass over northern Michigan. Atmos Environ 16:2421–2430

Allen RO, Steinnes E (1979) Contribution from long range atmospheric transport to the heavy metal pollution of surface soil. In: Proc International Conference Management and Control of Heavy Metals in the Environment. CEP Consultants, Edinburgh, p 271

Andersson A (1972) Enrichment of trace elements from sewage sludge fertilizer in soils and plants. Ambio 1:176–179

Andersson A, Hahlin M (1981) Cadmium effects from phosphorus fertilization in field experiments. Swed J Agric Res 11:3–10

Andersson A, Nilsson KO (1974) Influence of lime and soil pH on cadmium availability to plants. Ambio 3:198–200

Andersson A, Nilsson KO (1977) Heavy metals in Swedish soils: on their retention, distribution and amounts. Swed J Agric Res 7:7–20

Andersson A, Pettersson O (1981) Cadmium in Swedish winter wheat. Swed J Agric Res 11:49–55

Anonymous (1980) Erlaß des Ministeriums für Ernährung, Landwirtschaft, Umwelt und Forsten des Landes Baden-Württemberg der Schwermetallbelastung vom Boden. Gemeinsames Amtsblatt 28B:1186–1189

Asami T (1981a) Maximum allowable limit of heavy metals in rice and soil. In: Kitageshi K, Yamani I (eds) Heavy metal pollution in soils of Japan. Japan Scientific Societies Press, Tokyo, p 257

Asami T (1981b) The Ichi and Maruyama River basins: soil pollution by cadmium, zinc, lead, and copper discharged from Ikuno mine. In: Kitageshi K, Yamani I (eds) Heavy metal pollution in soils of Japan. Japan Scientific Societies Press, Tokyo, p 125

Auer C (1977) Cadmium in phosphate fertilizer production. US Environmental Protection Agency, Midwest Research Institute Report, Washington DC

Bates TE, Haig A, Soon YK, Moyer JA (1975) Uptake of metals from sludge amended soils. In: Hutchinson TC et al. (eds) Proc International Conference on Heavy Metals in the Environment, University of Toronto, Toronto, Canada, p 413

Beamish RJ (1976) Acidification of lakes in Canada by acid precipitation and the resulting effects on fishes. Water Air Soil Pollut 6:501–514

Beckett PHT, Davis RD (1977) Upper critical levels of toxic elements in plants. New Phytol 79:95–106

Bigliocca C, Giradi F, Orthmann E, Reiniger P (1979) The balance of Cd, Pb, Cr, and Cu in an experimental rice field for one growing season. Riso 28:23–35

Bingham FT, Page AL (1975) Cadmium accumulation by economic crops. In: Hutchinson TC (ed) Proc International Conference on Heavy Metals in the Environment. University of Toronto, Toronto, Canada, p 433

Bingham FT, Page AL, Mahler RJ, Ganje TJ (1975) Growth and cadmium accumulation of plants grown on a soil treated with a cadmium-enriched sewage sludge. J Environ Qual 4:207–211

Bingham FT, Page AL, Mahler RJ, Ganje TJ (1976a) Cadmium availability to rice in sludge-amended soil under "flood" and "nonflood" culture. Soil Sci Soc Am J 40:715–719

Bingham FT, Page AL, Mahler RJ, Ganje TJ (1976b) Yield and cadmium accumulation of forage species in relation to cadmium content of sludge-amended soils. J Environ Qual 5:57–60

Bingham FT, Page AL, Strong JE (1980) Yield and Cd content of rice grain in relation to addition rates of cadmium, copper, nickel, and zinc with sewage sludge and liming. Soil Sci 130:32–38

Bingham FT, Strong JE, Sposito G (1983) Influence of chloride salinity on cadmium uptake by swiss chard. Soil Sci 135:160–165

Bingham FT, Sposito G, Strong JE (1984) The effect of chloride on the availability of cadmium. J Environ Qual 13:71–74

Bitton G, Damron BL, Edds GT, Davidson JM (eds) (1980) Sludge – health risks of land application. Ann Arbor Science Publishers/The Butterworth Group, Ann Arbor, MI

Bowen JHM (1979) Environmental chemistry of the elements. Academic, London

Boyle EA, Schalter F, Edmond JM (1976) On the marine geochemistry of cadmium. Nature 263:42–44

Braude GL, Nash AM, Wolf WJ, Carr RL, Chaney RL (1980) Cadmium and lead content of soybean products. J Food Sci 45:1187–1189

Bruland KW, Knauer GA, Martin JH (1978) Cadmium in northeast Pacific waters. Limnol Oceanogr 23:618–625

Buchauer MJ (1973) Contamination of soil and vegetation near a zinc smelter by zinc, cadmium, copper and lead. Environ Sci Technol 7:131–135

Burau RG, Kaita KY, Inouye TS, Miller M (1973) Chemical analysis of soil samples from the Salinas Valley, California for cadmium, zinc and phosphate. Report to State Water Resources Control Board, University of Calif. Davis

Cartwright B, Merry RH, Tiller KG (1976) Heavy metal contamination of soils around a lead smelter at Port Pirie, South Australia. Aust J Soil Res 15:69–81

CEP Consultants Ltd (1979) International Conference Management and Control of Heavy Metals in the Environment. CEP Consultants Ltd, Edinburgh, UK

CEP Consultants Ltd (1981) International Conference Heavy Metals in the Environment. CEP Consultants Ltd, Edinburgh, UK

CEP Consultants Ltd (1983) International Conference Heavy Metals in the Environment. CEP Consultants Ltd, Edinburgh, UK

Chaney RL (1982) Fate of toxic substances in sludge applied to cropland. In: Proc International Symposium on Land Application of Sewage Sludge, Association for the Utilization of Sewage Sludge. Tokyo, Japan, p 259

Chaney RL, Hornick SB (1978) Accumulation and effects of cadmium on crops. In: Proceedings 1st International Cadmium Conference, San Francisco. Metal Bulletin, London, p 125

Chaney RL, White MC, Simon PW (1975) Plant uptake of heavy metals from sewage sludge applied to land. In: Proc. 2nd National Conf. Municipal Sludge Management. Information Transfer. Rockville MD, p 169

Chaney RL, Hornick SB, Simon PW (1977) Heavy metal relationships during land utilization of sludge in the northeast. In: Loehr RC (ed) Land as a waste management alternative, Ann Arbor Science, Ann Arbor, p 283

Chaney RL, Hundemann PT, Palmer WT, Small RJ, White MC, Decker AM (1979) Plant accumulation of heavy metals and phytotoxicity resulting from utilization of sewage sludge and sludge compost on cropland. In: Proc National Conference Composting Municipal Residues and Sludges. Information Transfer, Rockville MD, p 86

Chang AC, Page AL, Bingham FT (1981) Re-utilization of municipal wastewater sludges – metals and nitrates. J Water Pollut Contr Fed 53:237–245

Chang AC, Page AL, Foster KW, Jones TE (1982a) A comparison of cadmium and zinc accumulation by four cultivars of barley grown in sludge-amended soils. J Environ Qual 11:409–412

Chang AC, Page AL, Bingham FT (1982b) Heavy metal absorption by winter wheat following termination of cropland sludge application. J Environ Qual 11:705–708

Chang AC, Page AL, Warneke JE, Johanson JB (1982c) Effects of sludge application on the Cd, Pb and Zn levels of selected vegetable plants. Hilgardia 50:1–14

Chang AC, Page AL, Warneke JE, Resketo MR, Jones TE (1983) Accumulation of cadmium and zinc in barley grown in sludge-treated soils: a long-term field study. J Environ Qual 12:391–397

Chang AC, Warneke JE, Page AL, Lund LJ (1984) Accumulation of heavy metals in sewage sludge-treated soils. J Environ Qual 13:87–91

Chizhikov DM (1966) Cadmium. Pergamon, London

Coker EG, Davis RD, Hall JE, Carlton-Smith CH (1982) Field experiments on the use of consolidated sewage sludge for land reclamation. Water Research Centre-Technical Report-TR183, Stevenage UK

Corey RB, Fujii R, Hendrickson LL (1981) Bioavailability of heavy metals in soil-sludge. Conference on Application Research Practices of Municipal and Industrial Waste, University of Wisconsin-Extension, Madison, p 449

Council for Agricultural Science and Technology (1976) Application of sewage to plants and animals. CAST Report No. 64, US Environmental Protection Agency EPA-430/9-76-013

Council for Agricultural Science and Technology (1980) Effects of sewage sludge on cadmium and zinc content of crops. CAST Report No. 80, Ames IA

Cunningham JD, Kenney DR, Ryan JA (1975) Yield and metal composition of rye grown on sewage sludge-amended soil. J Environ Qual 4:448–454

Davis RD, Stark JH, Carlton-Smith CH (1982) Cadmium in sludge-treated soil in relation to potential human dietary intake of cadmium. Paper presented at the Commission of the European Communities Working Party – Concerted action on the characterization, treatment and use of sewage sludge. Water Research Centre, Stevenage UK

Davis WE and associates (1970) National inventory of sources and emissions of cadmium, nickel and asbestos. Cadmium Section 1 Report PB 192250, U.S. Department of Commerce, National Technology Transfer Services, Springfield VA

Department of the Environment/National Water Council (1981) Report of the sub-committee on the disposal of sewage sludge to land. DOE/NWC Standing Technical Committee Report 20, NWC, London

DeVries MPC, Tiller KG (1978) Sewage sludge as a soil amendment with special reference to Cd, Mn, Ni, Pb, and Zn – comparisons of results from experiments conducted inside and outside a glasshouse. Environ Pollut 16:231–240

D'Itri FM, Martinez JA, Lambarri MA (eds) (1981) Municipal wastewater in agriculture. Academic, New York

Dowdy RH, Larson WE, Titrud JM, Latterell JJ (1978) Growth and metal uptake of snap beans grown on sewage sludge-amended soil: a four year field study. J Environ Qual 7:252–257

Dowdy RH, Bray BJ, Goodrich RD (1985) Trace metal composition of organs of goats and lambs fed silage produced on sludge-amended soil. J Environ Qual (in press)

Dudas MG, Pawluk S (1977) Heavy metals in cultivated soils and in cereal crops in Alberta. Can J Soil Sci 57:329–339

Dupont JC, Casak G, Kirchmann R (1980) Cadmium contamination of *Zea mays* by root absorption. Int J Environ Studies 15:33–40

Elinder CG (1985) In: Friberg L (ed) Cadmium in the environment. 3rd ed, CRC Press, Boca Raton, FL (in press)

Elliott CF, Stevenson FJ (eds) (1977) Soils for management and utilization of organic waste waters. Soil Science Society of America, Madison WI

Feeney S, Peterson JR, Zenz DR, Lue-Hing C (1984) National survey of the metals content of seven vegetable species. Dept of Research and Development – Report No. 84-4 Metropolitan Sanitary Dist of Greater Chicago, Chicago IL

Fitzgerald PR (1980) Observations on the health of some animals exposed to anaerobically digested sludge originating in the Metropolitan Sanitary District of Greater Chicago System. In: Bitton G, Damron BL, Edds GT, Davidson JM (eds) Sludge – health risks of land application. Ann Arbor Science/The Butterworth Group, Ann Arbor MI, p 267

Fleischer M, Sarofim AF, Fassett DW, Hammond P, Shacklette HT, Nisbet IC, Epstein S (1974) Environmental impact of cadmium: a review by the panel on hazardous trace substances. Environ Health Persp 7:253–323

Forbes EA, Posner AM, Quirk JP (1976) The specific adsorption of divalent Cd, Co, Cu, Pb, and Zn on geothite. Soil Sci 27:154–160

Forstner U (1980) Cadmium. In: Hutzinger O (ed) Handbook of environmental chemistry, vol 3, part A. Anthropogenic compounds. Springer, Berlin Heidelberg New York, p 59

Francis CW, Rush SG (1974) Factors affecting uptake and distribution of cadmium in plants. In: Hemphill DD (ed) Trace substances in environmental health VII. University of Missouri Press, Columbia, p 75

Frank R, Braun HE, Holdrinet M, Stonefield KI, Elliot JM, Vickery B, Cheng HH (1977) Metal contents of insecticide residues in tobacco soils, and cured tobacco leaves collected in Southern Ontario. Tob Sci 21:417–428

Friberg L, Piscator M, Nordberg G, Kjellstrom T (1974) Cadmium in the environment. 2nd edn. CRC Press, Cleveland OH

Fulkerson W, Goeller HE (eds) (1973) Cadmium, the dissipated element. Oak Ridge National Laboratory, Oak Ridge Tennessee ORNL/NSF/EP-21

Gabby JL (1950) Toxicity of cadmium sulfide and cadmium sulfoselinide pigments. Arch Ind Hyg Occup Med 1:677

Giordano PM, Mays DA, Behel AD Jr (1979) Soil temperature effects on the uptake of cadmium and zinc by vegetables grown on sludge-amended soil. J Environ Qual 8:232–236

Girling CH, Peterson PJ (1981) The significance of the cadmium species in uptake and metabolism of cadmium in crop plants. J Plant Nutri 3:707–720

Goldschmidt VM (1958) Geochemistry. Oxford University Press, Oxford

Gong H, Rose AW, Suhr NH (1977) The geochemistry of cadmium in some sedimentary rocks. Geochim Cosmochim Acta 41:1687

Gunnarsson O (1980) The relative role of fertilizer for the cadmium levels in the food chain under Swedish circumstances. In: Gunnarsson O (ed) TFI-Cadmium Seminar, The Fertilizer Institute, Washington DC, p 115

Haghiri F (1974) Plant uptake of cadmium as influenced by cation exchange capacity, organic matter, zinc and soil temperature. J Environ Qual 3:180–183

Harler DNH, Barber J (1979) Relationships between vegetation and heavy metals in the atmosphere. In: International Conference on heavy metals in the environment. CEP Consultants, Edinburgh, p 275

Harrison RM, Williams CR (1982) Airborne cadmium, lead, and zinc at rural and urban sites in north-west England. Atmos Environ 16:2669–2681

Heinrichs H, Schulz-Dobrick B, Wedepohl KH (1980) Terrestrial geochemistry of Cd, Bi, Ti, Pb, Zn, and Rb. Geochim Cosmochim Acta 44:1519–1532

Hinesly TD, Alexander DE, Ziegler EL, Barrett GL (1978) Zinc and Cd accumulation by corn inbreds grown on sludge-amended soils. Agron J 70:425–458

Hinesly TD, Ziegler EL, Barrett GL (1979 a) Residual effects of irrigating corn with digested sewage sludge. J Environ Qual 8:35–38

Hinesly TD, Sudarski-Hack V, Alexander DE, Barrett GL (1979 b) Effect of sewage sludge applications on phosphorus and metal concentrations in fractions of corn and wheat kernels. Cereal Chem 56:238–287

Hinesly TD, Alexander DE, Redborg KE, Ziegler EL (1982) Differential accumulations of cadmium and zinc by corn hybrids grown on soil amended with sewage sludge. Agron J 74:469–474

Holmgren GGS, Meyer MW, Daniels RB, Kubota J, Chaney RL (1985) Cadmium, lead, zinc, copper, and nickel in agricultural soils in the United States. J Environ Qual 16 (in press)

Horn MK, Adams JAS (1966) Computer-derived geochemical balances and element abundances. Geochim Cosmochim Acta 30:279

Hunt WF, Pinkerton C, McNulty O, Creason JA (1971) A study of trace element pollution of air in 77 midwestern cities. In: Hemphill DD (ed) Trace substances in environmental health IV. University of Missouri, Columbia, MO, p 56

Hutton M (ed) (1982) Cadmium in the European community: a prospective assessment of sources, human exposure and environmental impact. MARC Report No. 26, Chelsea College, London

Hyde HC, Page AL, Bingham FT, Mahler RJ (1979) Effect of heavy metals in sludge on agricultural crops. J Water Pollut Control Fed 51:2475–2486

Iwai I, Hara T, Sonoda Y (1975) Factors affecting cadmium uptake by corn plant. Soil Sci Plant Nutr 21:37–46

John MK (1973) Cadmium uptake by eight food crops as influenced by various soil levels of cadmium. Environ Pollut 4:7–15

John MK (1976) Interrelationships between plants and cadmium and uptake of some other elements from culture solutions by oats and lettuce. Environ Pollut 11:85–95

John MK, Van Laerhoven CJ (1976) Differential effects of cadmium on lettuce varieties. Environ Pollut 10:163–173

John MK, Van Laerhoven CJ, Chuah HH (1972) Factors affecting plant uptake and phytotoxicity of cadmium added to soils. Environ Sci Technol 6:1005–1009

Johnson RD, Miller RJ, Williams RE, Wai CM, Wiese AC, Mitchell JE (1975) The heavy metal problem of Silver Valley, Northern Idaho. In: Hutchinson TC (ed) Proc International Conference on Heavy Metals In the Environment, vol II, part 2, University of Toronto, Toronto, p 465

Kaferstein FK (1980) Toxische Schwermetalle in Lebensmitteln. Zentralbl Bakteriol (B)171:352–358

Kaferstein FK, Altmann H-J, Kallischnig G, Klein H, Kossen M-T, Lorenz H, Muller J, Schmidt E, Zufeld KP (1979) Lead, cadmium, and mercury in and on foodstuffs, causes, consequences, requirements – a model study. Dietrich Reimer, Berlin (in german)

Kennedy UC, Sebetich MJ (1976) Trace elements in Northern California streams. Geological Survey Research, Washington DC, p 208

Kirleis AW, Sommers LE, Nelson DW (1981) Heavy metal content of grouts and hulls of oats grown on soil treated with sewage sludges. Cereal Chem 58:530–533

Kitageshi K, Obata H (1981) Accumulation of heavy metals in rice grains. In: Kitageshi K, Yamani I (eds) Heavy metal pollution in soils of Japan. Japan Scientific, Tokyo, p 95

Kjellstrom T, Nordberg GF (1978) A kinetic model of cadmium metabolism in human beings. Environ Res 16:248–269

Kjellstrom T, Lind B, Linnman L, Elinder CG (1975) Variation of cadmium concentration in Swedish wheat and barley: An indicator of changes in daily cadmium intake during the 20th century. Arch Environ Health 30:321–328

Klein DH (1972) Mercury and other metals in urban soils. Environ Sci Technol 6:558–559

Kloke A (1982) Reuse of sludges and treated wastewater in agriculture. Water Sci Technol 14:61–72

Kloke A, Sauerbeck DR, Vetter H (1984) The contamination of plants and soils with heavy metals and the transport of metals in terrestrial food chains. In: Nriagu JO (ed) Changing metal cycles and human health. Dahlem Conference. Springer, Berlin, p 113

Korcak RF, Fanning DS (1978) Extractability of cadmium, copper, nickel, and zinc by double acid vs. DTPA and plant content at excessive soil levels. J Environ Qual 7:506–512

Kowal NE (1984) An overview of public health effects. In: Page AL, Gleason TL, Smith JE, Iskandar IK, Sommers LE (eds) Utilization of municipal wastewater and sludge on land. University of California Press, Riverside, p 329

Lagerwerff JV, Biersdorf GT (1971) Interactions of zinc with uptake and translocation of cadmium in radish. In: Hemphill DD (ed) Trace substances in environmental health V. University of Missouri Press, Columbia, p 515

Lagerwerff JV, Brower DL (1975) Source determination of heavy metal contaminants in the soil of a mine and smelter area. In: Hemphill DD (ed) Trace substances in environmental health IX. University of Missouri Press, Columbia, p 207

Lannefors H, Hanssan HC (1983) Background aerosol composition in southern Sweden – Fourteen micro and macro constituents measured in seven particle size intervals at one site during one year. Atmos Environ 17:87–101

Lansche AM (1958) Cadmium. In: Minerals Year Book 1955, vol 1. U.S. Bureau of Mines US Government Printing Office, Washington DC, p 259

Lee CR, Cradelock GR (1969) Factors affecting plant growth in high-zinc medium: II. Influence of soil treatment on growth of soybean on strongly acid soil containing zinc from peach sprays. Agron J 61:565–569

Lee CR, Page NR (1967) Soil factors influencing the growth of cotton following peach orchards. Agron J 59:237–240

Leeper GW (1978) Managing the heavy metals on the land. Dekker, New York

Lepp NW (ed) (1981) Effects of heavy metal pollution on plants. Applied Science, London

Lieber M, Welsh WF (1954) Contamination of groundwater by cadmium. J Am Water Works 46:541

Lindberg SE, Turner RR, Shriner DS, Huff DD (1981) Atmospheric deposition of heavy metals and their interaction with acid precipitation in a North American deciduous forest. In: Proc Inter Conf on heavy metals in the environment. CEP Consultants Ltd, Edinburgh, p 306

Linnman L, Andersson A, Nilsson K, Lind B, Kjellstrom T, Friberg L (1973) Cadmium uptake by wheat from sewage sludge used as a plant nutrient source. Arch Environ Health 27:45–47

Loehr RC (ed) (1977) Land as a waste management alternative. Ann Arbor Science, Ann Arbor, MI

Logan TJ, Chaney R (1984) Metals. In: Page AL, Gleason TL, Smith JE, Iskandar IK, Sommers LE (eds) Utilization of municipal wastewater and sludge on land. University of California Press, Riverside, p 235

Logan TJ, Miller RH (1983) Background levels of heavy metals in Ohio farm soils. Research Circular 275 The Ohio State University Agricultural Research and Development, Wooster OH

Lund LJ, Betty EE, Page AL, Elliott RA (1981) Occurrence of naturally high Cd levels in soil and its accumulation by vegetation. J Environ Qual 10:551–556

Mahaffey KR, Corneliussen PE, Jelinek CF, Fiorino JA (1975) Heavy metal exposure from foods. Environ Health Perspec 12:63–69

Mahler RJ, Bingham FT, Page AL (1978) Cadmium-enriched sewage sludge application to acid and calcareous soils: I. Effect on yield and cadmium uptake by lettuce and Swiss chard. J Environ Qual 7:274–281

Marowsky G, Wedepohl KH (1971) General trends in the behavior of Cd, Hg, Ti, and Bi in some major rock forming processes. Geochim Cosmochim Acta 35:1255

Marples AE, Thornton I (1980) The distribution of cadmium derived from geochemical and industrial sources in agricultural soils and pasture herbage in parts of Britain. In: Cadmium 79, Proc 2nd Intern Cadmium Conf, Metal Bulletin, London, p 135

Martin JH, Bruland KW, Broenkow WW (1976) Cadmium transport in the California current. In: Windom HL, Duce RA (eds) Marine pollutant transfer. Heath, Lexington, p 159

McKee JE, Wolf HW (eds) (1971) Water quality criteria. 2nd ed. California State Water Quality Control Board Publ. 3A, p 149

McKim HL (ed) (1978) State of knowledge in land treatment of wastewater. U.S. Army Corps of Engineers Cold Regions Research and Engineering Laboratory, Hanover NH

McLean AJ (1976) Cadmium in different plant species and its availability in soils as influenced by organic matter and additions of lime, P, Cd, and Zn. Can J Soil Sci 56:129–138

Merry RH, Tiller KG (1978) The contamination of pasture by a lead smelter in a semi-arid environment. Aust J Exp Agric Animal Husb 18:89–96

Mitchell GA, Bingham FT, Page AL, Nash P (1978) Yield and metal composition of lettuce and wheat grown on soils amended with sewage sludge enriched with Cd, Cu, Ni, and Zn. J Environ Qual 7:165–171

Moorcroft S, Watt J, Thornton I, Wells J, Stehlow CD, Barltrop D (1982) Composition of dusts and soils in an apparently uncontaminated rural village in southwest England – Implications to human health. In: Hemphill DD (ed) Trace substances in environmental health XVI, University of Missouri, Columbia, p 155

Mulla DJ, Page AL, Ganje TJ (1980) Cadmium accumulation and bioavailability in soils from long-term phosphorus fertilization. J Environ Qual 9:408–412

Mullin JB, Riley JP (1956) The occurrence of cadmium in sea water and in marine organisms and sediments. J Marine Res 15:103

Munshower FF (1977) Cadmium accumulation in plants and animals of polluted and non-polluted grasslands. J Environ Qual 6:411–413

Naylor LM, Loehr RC (1981) Increase in dietary cadmium as a result of sewage sludge to agricultural land. Environ Sci Technol 15:881–886

Nriagu JO (ed) (1980) Cadmium in the environment. Part I. Ecological cycling. Wiley, New York

Nwankwo JN, Elinder CG (1979) Cadmium, lead, and zinc concentrations in soils and in food grown near a zinc and lead smelter in Zambia. Bull Environ Contam Toxicol 22:625

Official Journal of European Communities (1982) Proposal for a council directive on the use of sewage sludge in agriculture. No. C, 264/3–264/7

Oreshkin VN, Belyayev YI, Vnukovskaya GL, Tatsiy YG (1979) Determination of cadmium in soils by direct nonflame atomic-absorption analysis. Pochvovediniye 5:109–116 (in Soviet Soil Sci 1980:358–364)

Page AL (1974) Fate and effects of trace elements in sewage sludge when applied to agricultural lands. US Environmental Protection Agency Special Publication EPA 670/2-74-005

Page AL (1981) Cadmium in soils and its accumulation by food crops. In: International conference heavy metals in the environment. CEP Consultants LTD, Edinburgh, p 206

Page AL, Bingham FT (1973) Cadmium residues in the environment. Residue Rev 48:1–44

Page AL, Chang AC (1978) Trace elements impact on plants during cropland disposal of sewage sludges. In: Proc. 5th Nat. Conf. on Acceptable Sludge Disposal Techniques. Information Transfer, Rockville, MD, p 91

Page AL, Chang AC (1979) Contamination of soil and vegetation by atmospheric deposition of trace elements. Phytopath 69:1007–1011

Page AL, Bingham FT, Nelson CO (1972) Cadmium absorption and growth of various plant species as influenced by solution cadmium concentration. J Environ Qual 1:288–291

Page AL, Bingham FT, Chang AC (1981) Cadmium in terrestrial plants. In: Lepp NW (ed) Effect of heavy metal pollution on plants, vol 1. Effects of trace metals on plant function. Applied Science, London, p 77

Page AL, Gleason III TL, Smith JE Jr, Iskandar IK, Sommers LE (1984) Proceedings of the 1983 workshop on utilization of municipal wastewater and sludge on land. University of California, Riverside, CA

Pahren HR, Lucas JB, Ryan JA, Dotson GR (1979) Health risks associated with land application of municipal sludge. J Water Pollut Control Fed 51:2588–2601

Pettersson O (1977) Differences in cadmium uptake between plant species and cultivars. Swed J Agric Res 7:21–24

Pierce FJ, Dowdy RH, Grigal DF (1982) Concentrations of six trace metals in some major Minnesota soil series. J Environ Qual 11:416–422

Purves D (1981) National standards for metal addition to soil in sewage sludge. In: Proc International Conference Heavy Metals in the Environment. CEP Consultants, Edinburgh, p 176

Ragaini RC, Ralston HR, Roberts N (1977) Environmental trace metal contamination in Kellogg, Idaho near a lead smelting complex. Environ Sci Technol 11:773–781

Rohbock E, Georgii HW, Perseke C, Kins L (1981) Wet and dry deposition of heavy metal aerosols in the Federal Republic of Germany. In: Proc. Intern. Conf. on Heavy Metals in the Environment. CEP Consultants, Edinburgh, p 310

Rupp EM, Parzyck DC, Walsh PJ, Booth RS, Raridon RJ, Whitfield BL (1978) Composite hazard index for assessing limiting exposures to environmental pollutants: application through a case study. Environ Sci Technol 12:802–807

Ryan JA, Pahren HR, Lucas JB (1982) Controlling cadmium in the human food chain: a review and rationale based on health effects. Environ Res 28:251–302

Santillan-Medrano J, Jurinak JJ (1975) The chemistry of lead and cadmium in soil: Solid phase formation. Soil Sci Soc Am Proc 39:851–856

Schell WR, Nevissi A (1977) Heavy metals from waste disposal in central Puget Sound. Environ Sci Technol 11:887–893

Sharma RP, Street JC, Verma MP, Shupe JL (1979) Cadmium uptake from feed and its distribution to food products of livestock. Environ Health Perspect 28:59–66

Sikora LJ, Chaney RL, Frankos NH, Murray CM (1980) Metal uptake by crops grown over entrenched sewage sludge. J Agric Food Chem 28:1281–1285

Singh BR, Steinnes E (1976) Uptake of trace elements by barley in zinc-polluted soils 2. Lead, cadmium, mercury, selenium, arsenic, chromium, and vanadium in barley. Soil Sci 121:38–43

Sommers LE (1977) Chemical composition of sewage sludge and analysis of their potential use as fertilizers. J Environ Qual 6:225–232

Sommers LE (1982) Toxic metals in agricultural crops. In: Bitton G, Damron BL, Edds GT, Davidson JM (eds) Sludge-health risks of land application. Ann Arbor Science/The Butterworth Group, Ann Arbor, MI, p 105

Sopper WE, Seaker EM, Bastian RK (eds) (1982) Land reclamation and biomass production with municipal sludge. The Pennsylvania State University Press, University Park

Sposito G, Page AL (1985) Cycling of metal ions in the soil environment. In: Sigel H (ed) Metal ions in biological systems V. 18 Metal cycling in the environment (in press)

Stenstrom T, Lonsjo H (1974) Cadmium availability to wheat: a study with radioactive tracers under field conditions. Ambio 3:87–90

Street JJ, Sabey BR, Lindsay WL (1978) Influence of pH, phosphorus, cadmium, sewage sludge, and incubation time on the solubility and plant uptake of cadmium. J Environ Qual 7:286–290

Stubbs RL (1978) Cadmium – the metal of benign neglect. In: Cadmium 77: Proc 1st Intern Cadmium Conf Metal Bulletin, London, p 7

Thornton I (1983) Geochemistry applied to agriculture. In: Thornton I (ed) Applied environmental geochemistry. Academic, New York, p 231

Thornton I, John S, Moorcroft S, Watt J, Stehlow CD, Barltrop D, Wells J (1980) Cadmium at Shipham – A unique example of environmental geochemistry and health. In: Hemphill DD (ed) Trace substances in environmental health XIV. University of Missouri Press, Columbia MO, p 27

Takijima Y, Katsumi F, Takezawa K (1973) Cadmium contamination of soils and rice plants caused by zinc mining. II. Soil conditions of contaminated paddy fields which influence heavy metal contents of rice. Soil Sci Plant Nutri 19:173–182

Tiller KG, Cartwright B, deVries MPC, Merry RH, Spouncer LR (1975) Environmental pollution of the Port Pirie region: I. Accumulation of metals in wheat grain and vegetables grown on the coastal plain. Div of Soil Rept No 6. Commonwealth Scientific and Industrial Research Organization, Australia

Tjell JC, Hovmand MF (1978) Metal concentrations in Danish soils. Acta Agric Scand 28:81–89

Trefry JH, Presley BJ (1976) Heavy metals in sediments from San Antonio Bay and the northwest Gulf of Mexico. Environ Geol 1:283–294

Tsuchiya K (ed) (1978) Cadmium studies in Japan – a review. Elsevier/North-Holland Biomedical, Amsterdam

U.S. Bureau of Mines (1965–1980) Minerals Yearbooks. Government Printing Office, Washington DC

U.S. Environmental Protection Agency (1972) Helena Valley, Montana area environmental pollution study. EPA Office of Air Programs Publ AP-91 Research Triangle Park, North Carolina

U.S. Environmental Protection Agency (1978) Cadmium additions to agricultural lands via commercial phosphate fertilizers – A preliminary assessment. Office of Water and Waste Management, Washington DC. Soil Waste Management Series No SW-718, p 35

U.S. Environmental Protection Agency (1979) Criteria for classification of solid waste disposal facilities and practices. Federal Register 44:53438–53464

Valadares JMAS, Gal M, Mingelgrin U, Page AL (1983) Some heavy metals in soils treated with sewage sludge, their effects on yield, and their uptake by plants. J Environ Qual 12:49–57

Varo P, Muurtano M, Saari E, Koivistoinen P (1980) Mineral element composition of Finnish foods. III. Annual variations in the mineral element composition of cereal grains. Acta Agric Scand [Suppl] 22:27–35

Viitasalo I (1973) Heavy metals in soil and cereals fertilized with sewage sludge. Program Water Technol 10:309–316

Waketa H, Schmitt RA (1970) Cadmium. In: Wedepohl KH (ed) Handbook of geochemistry. Springer, New York, chap 48

Wedepohl KH (1968) Origin and distribution of elements. Ahrens LH (ed). Pergamon, London, p 999

Weigel HJ, Jaer HJ (1980) Subcellular distribution and chemical form of Cd in bean plants. Plant Physiol 65:480–482

Williams CH, David DJ (1973) The effect of superphosphates on the cadmium content of soils and plants. Aust J Soil Res 11:43–56

Williams CH, David DJ (1976) The accumulation in soil of cadmium residues from phosphate fertilizers and their effects on the cadmium content of plants. Soil Sci 121:86–93

Williams CH, David DJ (1977) Some effects of the distribution of cadmium and phosphate in the root zone on the cadmium content of plants. Aust J Soil Res 15:59–68

Williams DE, Vlamis J, Pukite AH, Corey JE (1980) Trace element accumulation, movement and distribution in the soil profile from massive applications of sewage sludge. Soil Sci 129:119–132

Wolnik KA, Fricke FL, Capar SG, Braude GL, Meyer MW, Satzger RD, Bonnin E (1983) Elements in major raw agricultural crops in the United States. I. Cadmium and lead in lettuce, peanuts, potatoes, soybeans, sweet corn and wheat. J Agric Food Chem 31:1240–1244

Wolnik KA, Fricke FL, Capar SG, Meyer MW, Satzger RD, Bonnin E, Gaston CM (1985) Elements in major raw agricultural crops in the United States. 3. Cadmium and lead and eleven other elements in carrots, field corn, onion, rice, spinach, and tomatoes. J Agric Food Chem 33 (in press)

Yamagata N (1978) Cadmium in the environment and in humans. In: Tsuchiya K (ed) Cadmium studies in Japan – a review. Elsevier/North-Holland Biomedical, Amsterdam, p 19

Yamagata N, Shigematsu I (1970) Cadmium pollution in perspective. Inst Public Health 19:1–27

CHAPTER 3

Absorption of Cadmium

E. C. FOULKES

A. Introduction

Even outside occupational settings, the human environment contains measurable concentrations of cadmium compounds. These may be derived from natural sources, or be contributed to the environment by mining, smelting, or other industrial activities. As further discussed in Chap. 2, cadmium enters the human food chain in a variety of ways, such as by application of Cd-containing fertilizer to agricultural lands, or through bioaccumulation in marine organisms. In addition, significant amounts of Cd may be present in polluted water, or may be inhaled in ambient air (BUCHET et al. 1980). Another significant source of Cd exposure is tobacco smoke. As a net result of overall exposure of the general population, the average body burden of the metal in a North American adult male amounts to perhaps 30 mg (SCHROEDER and BALASSA 1961); higher values have been reported in more polluted areas, such as Japan (TSUCHIYA et al. 1976).

Cadmium is excreted from the body primarily through the kidneys (see Chap. 6). Fecal loss of body Cd, reflecting both biliary excretion and possible secretion across the intestinal wall, is normally small, but may become more significant in the presence of chelating agents (KIYOZUMI and KOJIMA 1978; CHERIAN and RODGERS 1982). However, total excretion of body Cd, at least in the early stages of Cd exposure, is generally low. Accordingly, the biologic half-life of Cd is long, with values reported for humans in the range of 10–30 years (FRIBERG et al. 1974). As a result, the major determinant of the body burden of Cd is the absorption of the metal, and this forms the subject of the present chapter. In this connection absorption will be defined as systemic uptake; this does not include accumulation of Cd in the intestinal mucosa.

B. Routes of Exposure

I. Lungs

Significant pulmonary exposure to Cd most frequently is associated with occupational settings (see Chap. 5). Industrial contamination, however, may spread beyond the immediate workplace, and BUCHET et al. (1980) observed significantly increased blood Cd levels in children living close to a nonferrous smelter operation in Belgium. They attributed about 30% of the rise in blood Cd to pulmonary uptake. Another well-documented source of Cd exposure is cigarette smoke (LEWIS et al. 1972). Approximately 0.1 µg Cd may be inhaled per cigarette smoked (Menden et al. 1972). Even though such a value appears small compared with an average oral Cd intake of 50 µg/day (Friberg et al. 1974), it assumes greater significance in light of the finding that fractional absorption of inhaled Cd (25%–50%, see Friberg et al. 1974 for a detailed review) greatly exceeds that of ingested Cd (around 2%, see, e.g., Moore et al. 1973).

When humans or experimental animals are exposed to high levels of Cd in ambient air, the lungs can become a primary target organ. Thus, acute exposure causes massive pulmonary edema (see, e.g., Barret et al. 1947). After chronic exposure to lower levels of Cd compounds, pulmonary damage (emphysema) may be accompanied by renal lesions (Friberg 1959). Further details of the pulmonary effects of Cd are found in Chap. 5.

Little is known of the mechanism of pulmonary Cd absorption. In any case, except for heavy smokers, and away from close proximity to certain industrial operations, the pulmonary route of absorption contributes relatively little to the total Cd content of the body.

II. Skin

Small amounts of Cd may be absorbed through the skin (Wahlberg 1965), but the dermal route does not normally account for a significant fraction of total Cd absorption.

III. Intestine

The major fraction of the body burden of Cd in the general population is derived from food. This holds in spite of the fact that only a small portion of the ingested metal is normally absorbed in the intestine. Values for fractional absorption, as reviewed by Friberg et al. (1974), usually amount to only a few percent; the precise fraction is influenced by many factors, including the chemical form of the metal, the age of the organism, and a variety of dietary and endogenous factors, as further discussed in Sect. D.

In general, the evidence for low fractional absorption of Cd from the intestine is not based on direct measurement of unidirectional movement of the metal across the intestinal barrier. Instead, absorption is equated to the difference between ingestion and fecal excretion, measured over a period of several days, long enough to justify the assumption that the intestinal lumen is essentially free of Cd. For retention values to serve in this manner as basis for evaluating true absorption, several conditions must be met: (a) allowance must be made for any Cd trapped in the intestinal wall (see also Sect. C.III); (b) biliary excretion of Cd must remain low – actually, excretion through the bile is variable and depends on pretreatment of the animal with metals, or on the presence of certain chelating agents (Kiyozumi and Kojima 1978; Cherian and Rodgers 1982); (c) the assumption must be made that no Cd is secreted into the intestinal lumen – occurrence of secretion was reported by Kiyozumi and Kojima (1978), and influx of Cd into the lumen is influenced by treatment with chelating agents (Kiyozumi and Kojima 1978; Foulkes 1980). Schafer and Forth (1983) described the excretion of Cd and other metals down their concentration gradient into the intestinal lumen of the rat.

It is often not clear to what extent these three conditions are met in work on Cd absorption in whole animals. Thus, assumptions (b) and (c) are thrown into doubt by the repeated observation of fecal excretion of Cd following its systemic administration. A good example is the work of SHAIKH and LUCIS (1972) in which 5% of a subcutaneous dose was thus excreted in 4 days. MCLELLAN et al. (1978) reported that after oral administration of ^{115m}Cd to human volunteers, together with a fecal marker (^{51}CrCl$_3$), fecal Cd excretion continued after complete elimination of Cr. Mean Cd retention (4.6%) in this study clearly cannot serve as a measure of unidirectional absorption.

Cadmium absorption has been studied in different segments of the small intestine (FOULKES 1980 and unpublished work). Duodenum, jejunum, and ileum were each found capable of removing Cd from a luminal perfusate in situ; a pronounced activity gradient was observed along the jejunum. The question of which segment is primarily responsible for Cd absorption under physiologic conditions has not been clearly answered. The difficulty here arises, in part, from the fact that absorption can be influenced by age, by changes in diet, by the rate of intestinal transit, and by secretion of endogenous modulators (see Sect. D). As a result, the analysis of Cd transport in isolated segments can provide information of only limited quantitative significance to evaluation of absorption in the intact animal.

What is clear, however, is that absorption of Cd in the adult is normally slow. This fact is particularly well illustrated in the work of SMITH et al. (1978) who studied transfer of Zn and Cd across the intestinal barrier in a doubly perfused segment of the rat intestine in situ. Appearance of Zn in the vascular perfusate was readily demonstrated, but no Cd could be recovered from this perfusate. Nevertheless, constant absorption of Cd at even a very slow rate, coupled with its very low excretion, does lead to gradual Cd accumulation in the body. Because of its very long biologic half-life, Cd in essence acts as a cumulative poison (see Sect. A), whose body burden is primarily controlled by intestinal absorption.

A detailed discussion of Cd uptake by humans on various diets will be found in Chap. 2. The joint FAO/WHO Expert Committee on Food Additives (WORLD HEALTH ORGANIZATION 1972) provisionally established tolerable intakes of Cd from food at around 60–70 µg/day in adults. This value must be compared with the estimate that, assuming 5% fractional absorption of Cd, and a daily Cd excretion of less than 0.01% of the body burden, Cd intake of around 300 µg/day would permit toxic levels of Cd to accumulate in human kidneys by age 50 years (FRIBERG et al. 1974). Average daily intake on a North American diet may reach as high as 60 µg/day (MAHAFFEY et al. 1975). In other words, the safety margin between actual and toxic levels of Cd is not large.

C. Mechanism of Intestinal Absorption

I. General

A fairly extensive literature has accumulated dealing with intestinal Cd transport, as studied both in vivo and in vitro. In either situation, the metal is rapidly re-

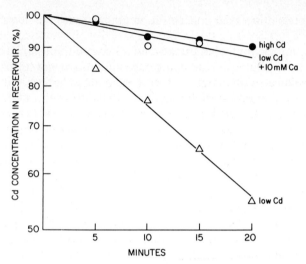

Fig. 1. Apparent saturation and inhibition of step 1 of jejunal Cd absorption in the rat. Rat jejunum was perfused in situ with 5 mM glucose in saline, containing 20 μM (low) or 200 μM (high) CdCl$_2$. (FOULKES 1980)

moved from the intestinal lumen, as illustrated in Fig. 1 by results of an experiment in which 5 mM glucose in saline containing 20 μM CdCl$_2$ was recirculated through the rat jejunum (FOULKES 1980). Autoradiography showed that the Cd thus removed from the lumen readily penetrates the mucosa (E. F. FOULKES and K. STEMMER 1980, unpublished work), so that the steady exponential rate of Cd uptake clearly represents more than absorption of the metal on the cell membranes. This conclusion is further supported by the fact (see Sect. C.IV) that reaction of Cd with brush border membrane is very rapid, while the exponential uptake proceeds at a constant rate for 20 min or longer.

Two further points emerge from Fig. 1. First, at higher concentrations, fractional uptake of Cd decreases. This effect was found to be at least in part reversible (FOULKES 1980), and was attributed to saturation of an uptake mechanism. The second point to be noted in Fig. 1 is that the uptake mechanism is inhibited by Ca ions, a finding whose significance will be further considered.

Formally, Fig. 1 depicts the first step in Cd absorption, as described in the following scheme

$$\text{Luminal Cd} \xrightarrow[\text{step 1}]{} \text{mucosal Cd} \xrightarrow[\text{step 2}]{} \text{systemic Cd.}$$

Transfer of Cd out of the lumen into the mucosa is labeled step 1; step 2 stands for the further transfer of Cd from mucosa into the body. Although under certain conditions movement of Cd in the opposite direction, from mucosa to lumen, can be demonstrated, it is normally very slow (FOULKES 1980), and the two steps are shown as irreversible. Note further that they are represented in series, not in parallel as implied in the work of SAHAGIAN et al. (1967). Justification for the series model is provided by the finding that the rate of step 2 limits overall Cd absorption. The dissipation of mucosal Cd into the body proceeds about 100 times more slowly than does its original uptake into the mucosa from glucose–saline solution (see Sects. C.II, C.III). The rapidity of step 1 seen in Fig. 1 therefore does not contradict the earlier conclusion (see Sect. B.III) that absorption of Cd from the intestine is slow. Comparison between Cd transport in the intact animal and in isolated segments in situ is complicated by the fact that conditions in the segment are quite unphysiologic. This follows from the absence of normal luminal contents, including digestion products and endogenous factors known to alter step 1 (see Sect. D), and represents a serious limitation of such studies. Advantages and disadvantages of various experimental techniques used in the analysis of intestinal metal absorption are discussed further in Sect. C.II.

The apparent saturability of step 1 shown in Fig. 1, and its sensitivity to inhibition (in this case by Ca), suggest that movement of Cd is facilitated under these conditions; in that case, passive diffusion would not contribute significantly to the process. More recent results may require reconsideration of those conclusions (see Sect. C.V.6), but in any case the first event in step 1 appears to be an interaction between cadmium and brush border cell membranes; Sect. C.IV focuses on this interaction.

If Cd transport reflects facilitation by a saturable mechanism, presumably involving reaction sites on the brush border membrane, a conceptual problem arises. It seems unlikely, indeed, that a specific mechanism should have evolved for absorption of a metal which acts as a cumulative poison, and for which no essential biologic role has been described. The observation that Cd can activate certain enzymes, or the report that Cd increases the growth rate of rats on a low-Cd diet (SCHWARTZ and SPALLHOLZ 1976) cannot be equated to an essential role of the metal. Another indication that Cd does not play an essential role in the body is furnished by the fact that, at least in the mouse, absorption of Cd is independent of its total body burden (COTZIAS et al. 1961). This observation may be contrasted with the homeostatic control of intestinal absorption of a variety of essential metals such as Ca, Zn, and Fe.

The conceptual difficulty considered here could be resolved if movement of Cd were facilitated by mechanisms whose primary role lies in the absorption of essential metals such as those just referred to. In other words, the hypothesis could be formulated that Cd absorption results from a less than complete specificity of other carrier systems. This possibility is discussed in Sect. C.V. An alternative hypothesis, also obviating the assumption of the existence of Cd carriers, is presented in Sect. C.V.6.

II. Methods of Study

Much of the information on Cd absorption is derived from feeding studies in intact animals and humans. As already pointed out in Sect. B.III, the problem here arises of distinguishing between retention of the metal and the magnitude of its actual absorption, i.e., of its movement across the intestinal barrier. This may be illustrated by the work of KOSTIAL et al. (1978) on Cd absorption in rats of different ages and on various diets. The specific influence of these variables will be further discussed in Sect. D; here we are concerned with the methodological aspects. Cadmium isotope was administered orally 6 days before the animals were

Table 1. Cd retention in rats as a function of age (modified from Kello and Kostial 1977; Kostial et al. 1978)[a]

Age (weeks)	Diet	Retention (%) (SD)	
1	Milk	25.6	(2.0)
6	Milk	6.9	(0.2)
6	Rat diet	0.5	(<0.1)
52	Milk	5.6	(0.4)
52	Rat diet	0.3	(<0.1)

[a] Measurements were made by whole body counting 6 days after an oral load of 40–60 µCi ^{115m}Cd, specific activity 0.5–1 mCi/mg. Results are expressed as percentages of oral dose

killed. Retention of Cd was then determined by scintillation counting, and the percentage of the oral dose retained was equated to absorption. Results are shown in Table 1. Clearly, retention under these conditions can at best provide an approximation to absorption. Need for some correction, as indicated in Sect. B.III, might have arisen because of retention of Cd in the intestinal wall. Further uncertainties are introduced by the unknown contribution of enterohepatic circulation or enteric secretion to cadmium turnover under these conditions, and possibly by significant effects of diet on passage times of food through the intestinal lumen of intact animals. In any case, no discrepancy necessarily arises between the conclusion that a milk diet increases Cd absorption in older rats (Kello and Kostial 1977; Kostial et al. 1978), and the observation of Foulkes (1980) that step 1 of Cd absorption in the isolated rat jejunum in situ is severely depressed by milk. The work with intact rats had compared retention of Cd in presence and absence of the constituents of normal rat diet, whereas the baseline in studies with isolated segments in situ was a perfusate containing only 5 mM glucose and 0.15 M NaCl; milk appears to slow down Cd uptake, but less so than does rat diet. Influence of diet on Cd uptake is further discussed in Sect. D.III.

A better estimate of fractional absorption in the intact organism can theoretically be obtained under steady state conditions. Long-term balance studies have been performed in humans (e.g., Tipton et al. 1969), but analytic difficulties make the results difficult to interpret (Friberg et al. 1974).

The advantage of the intact organism for the study of metal absorption rests largely on the presence of normal gastric and intestinal secretions as well as digestion products in the lumen; normal intestinal transit times are probably also important. All these advantages may be lost in work with isolated segments, in vivo or in vitro. However, a segment in situ with uninterrupted blood supply will serve as a much more valid system for the study of Cd absorption than can the same segment in vitro. Indeed, the high reactivity of heavy metals in general, and of Cd in particular, leads to extensive binding and consequent trapping of the metal in the tissue. It is unlikely, therefore, that significant values for step 2 in Cd absorption can be obtained in the absence of vascular perfusion. Not only will a major portion of the Cd taken up under those conditions be retained in the mucosa, but the long diffusion path from mucosa into serosal fluid will encourage further trapping of Cd in submucosal tissue. The problem of measuring step 2 for Cd is exacerbated by the fact that it is very much slower than step 1. Even in the doubly perfused intestine described by SMITH et al. (1978) (see also Sect. B.III), where step 1 of both Cd and Zn absorption is readily observed, step 2 can be demonstrated only for Zn.

A different approach to the problem of measuring step 2 was employed by HAMILTON and VALBERG (1974) in their work on uptake and absorption of ^{59}Fe and ^{109}Cd from the mouse duodenum in situ. Open duodenal loops were perfused for 30 min. The sum of Cd retained in the intestinal wall, and that counted in the carcass after removal of the perfused segment, was equated to uptake, i.e., step 1 of Cd absorption. The equivalent of the transfer from mucosa into the body (step 2) was defined by the ^{109}Cd content of the carcass. This definition implicitly assumes absence of significant urinary or biliary Cd excretion or Cd secretion. In any case, step 2 amounted to only around 1% of step 1 at Cd concentrations in the perfusate below 0.2 mM.

Another technique for overcoming the difficulties of measuring step 2 of Cd absorption was described by KELLO et al. (1979 b) as illustrated in Fig. 2. In these experiments, the intestine was first perfused through the lumen in situ for 20 min, and step 1 was computed by subtracting the amount of Cd remaining in the perfusate from that present at zero time. Essentially all Cd thus transported could be recovered from the intestinal wall immediately after the perfusion, indicating

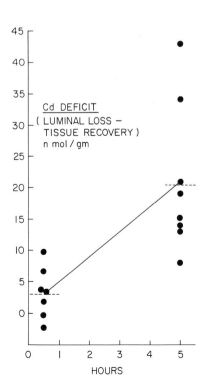

Fig. 2. Step 2 of jejunal Cd absorption in the rat. Step 2 is equated to the difference between the Cd removed from the luminal perfusate (initial Cd concentration 20 μM), and that recovered in the intestinal wall, immediately at the end of perfusion, and again 5 h after beginning of infusion. (KELLO et al. 1979 b)

again that step 2 proceeds much more slowly than step 1. However, 5 h later, only a portion of that Cd remained in the intestine. The difference between the amount of Cd transported by step 1, and that recovered from the intestine, must represent Cd which has moved beyond the intestine and can therefore be defined as step 2.

III. Kinetics

Kinetic analysis of Cd absorption requires accurate control over concentration and speciation of Cd compounds in the intestinal lumen. Such control cannot readily be achieved in the presence of food digests. As a result, kinetic studies have mostly been carried out under artificial conditions, largely in the absence of the many potential exogenous and endogenous modulators of Cd transport which may normally be present (see further, Sect. D).

Another difficulty encountered in these studies arises from the toxicity of Cd at higher concentrations. Exposure of rat duodenum in situ for 120 min to a Cd concentration as low as 0.1 mM was observed by Toraason (1983) to increase release of lactate dehydrogenase into the lumen; this finding may be attributed to cell damage. The apparent inability to saturate the rate of Cd removal from mucosal fluid in vitro (Chertok et al. 1979) may therefore reflect use of toxic Cd concentrations, as well as the limitations of the everted sac (see Sect. C.II). It is unlikely that studies with Cd concentrations higher than 0.2 mM possess much biologic significance. At lower concentrations, step 1 of Cd absorption follows first-order kinetics (see Fig. 1). The process approaches apparent saturation at concentrations of the order of 0.2 mM (Foulkes 1980).

Depression of fractional uptake of luminal Cd at higher Cd concentrations is, at least in part, reversible upon dilution (Foulkes 1980). Such dilution does not, however, cause any appreciable washout of Cd from the tissue. It follows that it is the Cd concentration at the membrane rather than in the cell which determines the apparent saturation of step 1. This conclusion implies that absorption of Cd is presumably initiated by its reaction with sites on the brush border membranes. Binding of Cd to such membranes can indeed readily be demonstrated in vitro (see Sect. C.IV). Section C.VI further considers the nature of the binding sites and of their role in step 1.

Little is known about step 2 in Cd absorption. Over a range of Cd concentrations in the lumen from 2 to 200 µM, step 2, as measured by the technique of Kello et al. (1979b), remains more or less constant below 2% of step 1 (E.C. Foulkes and C. Voner 1982, unpublished work). This finding confirms the observation of Hamilton and Valberg (1974) of a constant ratio of Cd transfer to Cd uptake in the mouse intestine in vivo. The dependence under many conditions of step 2 on step 1 provides additional support for the series model of absorption presented in Sect. C.I. The constant ratio of the two steps in these experiments may reflect the strong binding of Cd to mucosal binding sites; depending on the dissociation constant of such Cd complexes, only a small, constant fraction of the Cd transported by step 1 would remain in diffusible form. On this view one may predict that the ratio of step 2 to step 1 will be increased by presence of diffusible ligands which may compete with intracellular macromolecular metal ligands.

Table 2. Lack of correlation between Cd absorption and mucosal metallothionein in rats. (Modified from KELLO et al. 1979b)[a]

	Controls	Pretreated
Step 1 (nmol g^{-1}/min^{-1})	1.9 ± 0.8	1.3 ± 0.4
Step 2 (nmol g^{-1}/min^{-1})	0.023 ± 0.010	0.015 ± 0.009
Step 2/step 1 (%)	1.3 ± 0.7	1.3 ± 0.8
	(10)	(13)
Metallothionein	40 ± 6	144 ± 36
(µg per gram mucosa)	(6)	(6)
Absorbed Cd in metallothionein	2.3 ± 0.9	9.2 ± 1.7
fraction (nmol per gram mucosa)	(5)	(5)

[a] Means $\pm$ SD for (n) animals. Pretreatment consisted of 9 days exposure to Cd (50 ppm) in drinking water

This prediction is confirmed by results of several investigators (see Sect. D.III). The ratio of step 2 to step 1 should rise also if saturation on such binding sites could be achieved at nontoxic Cd concentrations.

The nature of the postulated intracellular metal ligands is not known. The metal-binding protein metallothionein has been considered as a possible sink of metals in the mucosa, especially for Zn (RICHARDS and COUSINS 1975). The results of KELLO et al. (1979 b) offer no support for such a role of metallothionein in Cd absorption. As shown in Table 2, step 2 of Cd absorption as a fraction of step 1 was not affected by an almost fourfold increase in the tissue metallothionein level and in the amount of Cd trapped in the metallothionein fraction. However, the ratio of step 2 to step 1 in these studies was measured at relatively low Cd concentrations in the perfusate. Subsequent studies at higher Cd levels (E. C. FOULKES and D. MCMULLEN 1984, unpublished work) have shown, as predicted, that metallothionein may contribute to the mucosal trapping of Cd. Reference is here made to endogenous metallothionein only, as exogenous Cd–metallothionein may slowly cross the intestinal epithelium (CHERIAN et al. 1978; VALBERG et al. 1977).

Whatever the reasons for the normally small extent of step 2 of Cd absorption, it causes the metal to accumulate in the intestinal mucosa, from which it may be lost upon sloughing of epithelial cells (VALBERG et al. 1976). Such an explanation, similar to the suggestion of RICHARDS and COUSINS (1975) on regulation of Zn absorption, could account for the low overall fractional absorption of Cd. An additional important mechanism for depressing intestinal uptake of Cd undoubtedly is the normal presence in the lumen of substances interfering with step 1, as further considered in Sect. D.

IV. Role of the Brush Border

As discussed in Sect. C.III, the first event in the uptake of Cd from the intestinal lumen appears to be a reaction of the metal with the brush border membranes.

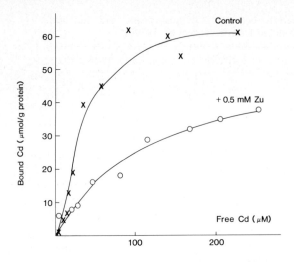

Fig. 3. Cd binding to jejunal brush border membrane vesicles. Vesicles were incubated for 5 min at 37 °C in the presence of $CdCl_2$ in HEPES-mannitol buffer, pH 7.0 (E. C. FOULKES and C. VONER 1983, unpublished work)

While details of this interaction have not been reported, it can readily be demonstrated in vitro with brush border membrane vesicles (E. C. FOULKES and C. VONER 1983, unpublished work). Significant amounts of the metal are rapidly taken up by such vesicles and the process reaches completion in less than 30 s. Because uptake is not altered by osmotically shocking the membrane preparation, the process presumably reflects Cd binding rather than intravesicular accumulation. This binding reaches apparent saturation at values above 100 μM Cd, and is depressed upon addition of relatively large amounts of Zn (Fig. 3). The possible nature of this Zn effect is further discussed in the next section.

V. Interaction Between Cd and Other Metals

1. Introduction

The extensive literature on trace metal interaction, and on effects of trace metal nutrition on Cd toxicity (see, e.g., NORDBERG et al. 1978) does not always conclusively indicate metal–metal interaction at the level of intestinal absorption. Indeed, in many instances no clear distinction is drawn between absorption of metals and their retention. However, effects of one trace metal on tissue levels of other trace metals (BREMNER 1978), or on step 1 in their absorption (see for instance SAHAGIAN et al. 1967) are well documented. Questions do remain on how one metal influences absorption of another; the expectation that the interaction would turn out to represent competition for common transport sites has not been fully confirmed.

To the extent that interaction between Cd and some essential metal like Zn does not result from competition, we may conclude that Cd absorption is not facilitated by the system transporting this essential metal. The problem then arises of how to reconcile the a priori improbability of the existence of specific Cd carriers with the apparent facilitation of Cd movement across brush border membranes.

2. Cd–Zn Interaction

Cadmium and zinc interact at many sites in the body, as might indeed be predicted from their similar chemical properties. In some cases such interactions have been attributed to competition for cofactor sites in Zn-requiring enzymes (VALLEE and ULLMER 1972). However, the common usage of referring to Cd–Zn antagonism as competitive in nature (e.g., BREMNER and CAMPBELL 1978) may not always be justified. This is true, in particular, in reference to intestinal Cd absorption.

The intestinal transport of Cd is inhibited by Zn (FOULKES 1980); a relatively high concentration of Zn is required for this effect (FOULKES 1985). This finding is hard to reconcile with the hypothesis that Cd competes with Zn for a Zn carrier system. Indeed, it would necessitate the assumption that such a system possesses a much higher affinity for Cd than for its natural substrate. Actually, when Zn uptake is measured as in the work of BONEWITZ et al. (1983), its inhibition by Cd can readily be demonstrated, but only in the presence of a large excess of Cd (Fig. 4). A similar discrepancy between the apparent half-saturating Cd or Zn concentrations (K_M) and K_i, the concentration of the inhibiting metal reducing Cd and Zn uptake by 50% in a line of hamster ovary cells, was attributed by COR-RIGAN and HUANG (1981) to the involvement of more than one carrier system in series.

The action of Zn on step 1 of Cd uptake is readily demonstrated, but no effect on step 2 has been established. Cadmium–zinc interactions have also been studied

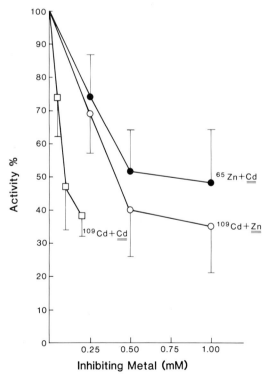

Fig. 4. Interaction between Cd and Zn. Jejunal segments were perfused with 20 μM ^{109}Cd or ^{65}Zn, as indicated, in the presence of various concentrations of inhibiting metal. Each point represents mean ± SD for six or more rats. (FOULKES 1985)

in vitro, as in the work of SAHAGIAN et al. (1967). The latter authors reported that addition of Zn to the mucosal fluid increased transmural movement of Cd. However, the significance of step 2 in such a preparation is open to question (see Sect. C.II), and the concentration of Cd used in these studies was relatively high (0.3 mM), exceeding acutely toxic (TORAASON 1983) and apparent saturation (FOULKES 1980) levels. It must also be noted that steps 1 and 2 in this case were considered to be in parallel, not in series (cf. Sect. C.I).

Also in vitro, the binding of Cd to brush border cell membranes, presumably the necessary event in initiation of step 1 of Cd uptake, is depressed by Zn (see Fig. 3). Attempts to quantify this effect by use of conventional Scatchard plots were unsuccessful, possibly because of the aggregation of membrane vesicles in the presence of polyvalent metal cations (KIRSCHBAUM 1982).

While interaction between Cd and Zn in the intestine has thus frequently been observed, the suggestion that the two metals might be competing for common carrier sites remains unproven. Evidence against competition is based on several studies, including experiments with Zn-deficient rats. The rationale here was the observation that Zn deficiency stimulates Zn absorption (EVANS et al. 1973); if the two metals were transported by the same system, this should be accompanied by increased Cd absorption. HAHN and EVANS (1975) could not demonstrate such stimulation of Cd transport in Zn-deficient rats, although they speculated about possible competition for cytoplasmic binding sites in the mucosa.

Table 3. Cd absorption in the jejunum of Zn-deficient rats. (Modified from FOULKES and VONER 1981)[a]

	Zn replete	Zn deficient	P
Plasma Zn (µg/ml)	1.9 ± 0.1	0.4 ± 0.1	<0.01
Step 1 (nmol g^{-1} min^{-1})	2.9 ± 0.8	2.5 ± 0.6	NS
Step 2 (nmol g^{-1} min^{-1})	0.025 ± 0.011	0.021 ± 0.012	NS
Step 2 step 1 (%)	0.7 ± 0.2	0.8 ± 0.4	NS

[a] Values shown are means $\pm$ SD for 3–6 animals

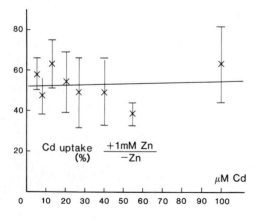

Fig. 5. Influence of Cd concentration on fractional inhibition of Cd uptake by Zn. Means $\pm$ SD are shown for groups of 5–12 rats studied at the Cd concentration shown. Each animal served as its own control, and was studied before and after addition of 1 mM Zn to the perfusate; no significant difference was observed between any groups by analysis of variance. (Modified from FOULKES 1985)

A more detailed analysis of steps 1 and 2 of Cd absorption in Zn-deficient rats was reported by FOULKES and VONER (1981), and is summarized in Table 3. Neither step 1 nor step 2 of Cd absorption was significantly altered by Zn deficiency, and the ratio of the two steps remained constant.

If Cd were transported by a rate-limiting and saturable one-step system, and if Zn shared common carrier sites with Cd, then the fractional inhibition of Cd uptake by Zn should be reversed at high Cd concentrations. Test of this hypothesis over the range of Cd concentrations approaching apparent saturation showed that Zn inhibition is independent of Cd concentration (Fig. 5). Together with the observation that Zn deficiency does not stimulate Cd transport, this finding thus argues against the hypothesis that the two metals compete for common transport sites, and makes it unlikely that Cd transport is facilitated by the system responsible for Zn absorption.

3. Cd–Ca Interaction

Many reports have dealt with the relationship between metabolism of Ca and Cd. This interaction became specially important because of the suggested role of Cd in the osteomalacia of itai-itai disease ((TSUCHIYA 1969a, b). According to MURATA et al. (1970) the primary lesion in this disease is produced by an enteric effect of Cd, leading to inhibition of intestinal Ca absorption. Although this view has not been generally accepted, Cd inhibition of Ca absorption and distribution is well documented (see, e.g., ANDO et al. 1978). It is worth recalling that the duodenum is a site of significant retention of orally administered Cd and it is also that segment of intestine which is primarily responsible for Ca absorption (PHILPOTTS 1980).

The reverse reaction, i.e., Ca interference with Cd absorption, has also been observed repeatedly. Such an inhibition could help explain the protection which a high Ca diet offers against Cd toxicity. LARSSON and PISCATOR (1971), for instance, observed that retention of Cd in rats increased on Ca-deficient diets and suggested that effects of Ca on Cd absorption could explain such an effect. The contrary finding by KELLO and KOSTIAL (1977), that a milk diet (high in Ca) favors Cd absorption, was discussed in Sect. C.II; it may be restated as suggesting that milk contains less substances interfering with Cd absorption than does normal rat food. What is clearly established is that Cd and Ca do interact, and that they can inhibit each other's absorption from the intestine.

The possibility that Cd and Ca actually compete with one another for common transport sites has been raised repeatedly. Thus, TSURUKI et al. (1978) explored the effect of Cd on vitamin D-stimulated Ca transport in rat duodenum in vitro. Limitations of the in vitro technique for the quantitative analysis of transmural metal transport have been discussed in Sect. C.II. In any case, appearance of Ca in serosal fluid as a function of mucosal Ca concentrations could be described by Michaelis–Menten kinetics, with apparent K_M and V_{max} values of 1.0 mM and 2.86 mmol ml^{-1} h^{-1}, respectively. In the presence of Cd, there was seen an apparently competitive inhibition of Ca transport, with an apparent K_i of 0.02 mM.

In the work of Koo et al. (1978) absorption of Cd in chicks was increased by vitamin D, or Ca and P deficiency, conditions known to stimulate Ca absorption. Such a finding is compatible with the view that Ca and Cd are transported by, and therefore presumably compete for, the same carrier system. Interpretation of these findings is made somewhat difficult by the complex kinetics of Cd absorption in that system. An observed increase in fractional Cd absorption at higher Cd concentrations may indicate toxic effects of Cd; alternatively, one might assume saturation of a mucosal trapping mechanism for Cd which normally prevents significant transmural movement of the metal.

One such binding site for Cd in the mucosa might be the calcium-binding protein (CBP) whose concentration is known to be raised by vitamin D treatment, or by Ca deficiency. This was the explanation offered by WASHKO and COUSINS (1977) for the acceleration of Cd absorption in rats on a low-Ca diet. Treatment with vitamin D had been observed by WORKER and MIGICOVSKY (1961) to stimulate Cd absorption in rachitic chicks. Cadmium also inhibits the vitamin D stimulation of Ca transport in vitro (ANDO et al. 1981). Along similar lines, SUGAWARA (1974) reported that administration of Cd decreases the Ca-binding activity of the duodenal mucosa in the rat. In the chick also, cadmium reduces the concentration of CBP in the duodenal mucosa (FULLMER et al. 1980).

CBP possesses significant affinity for Cd (INGERSOLL and WASSERMAN 1971). If there were competition between Cd and Ca for common transport mechanisms, the site of this competition might therefore well be on CBP. However, the role of CBP in Cd transport remains uncertain. Thus, HAMILTON and SMITH (1977) found the uptake of Cd in vitro to be unaffected by Ca deficiency in rats, a treatment expected to increase the concentration of CBP in the mucosa. Koo et al. (1978) found no correlation between CBP concentration and Cd absorption in the chick.

In the studies of FOULKES (1980), a concentration of 10 mM Ca was required to inhibit step 1 of Cd absorption in the rat jejunum perfused with 20 μM Cd. It must be pointed out that the primary site of active Ca absorption is the duodenum, not the jejunum. If, however, Cd and Ca shared a common transport system in the jejunum, this large excess of Ca would, as in the results of TSURUKI et al. (1978), lead to the surprising conclusion that Cd possesses an affinity for the Ca carriers several orders of magnitude higher than does Ca itself. Competition between Ca and Cd in the jejunum is also thrown into question by a kinetic analysis which yielded results for Ca inhibition of Cd movement similar to those shown for Zn in Fig. 5 (FOULKES 1985).

Further evidence against the view that the Ca–Cd interaction consists of competition for common binding sites may also be quoted. Thus, HAMILTON and SMITH (1978) measured what may be referred to as step 1 of Ca absorption in rat duodenum in vitro and reported a noncompetitive inhibition by Cd with a K_i of 0.8 mM. In an analysis of Cd and Ca transport by rat duodenum in situ, TORAASON (1983) and TORAASON and FOULKES (1984) observed that 10 mM Ca inhibits step 1 of Cd absorption independently of the Cd concentration over a range of 0.05–0.2 mM. Further, the effect of Cd was not abolished by removal of Cd from the perfusate, showing that Cd in this case could not have acted as a reversible competitive inhibitor. As in the work of ANDO et al. (1977), the toxic effect of Cd included a stimulation of Ca secretion into the lumen. In summary, Cd–Ca interaction during intestinal absorption, like that of Cd and Zn, is not likely to result from simple competition between the metals.

4. Cd–Fe Interaction

The ability of Cd to interfere with Fe metabolism is well documented (BREMNER 1978), and the possibility has repeatedly been raised that this effect of Cd results from interaction of the two metals in the intestine. An alternative explanation invokes disturbances in copper metabolism as the primary cause for the anemia of Cd intoxication; this will not be further discussed here.

Quite apart from the intrinsic interest in the question of how Cd affects Fe absorption, demonstration that Cd and Fe react at a common transport site would imply that Cd might be absorbed by the mechanism evolved for Fe absorption. It is important to define, therefore, the effects of the two metals on each other's absorption. In this connection, the observation that parenteral administration of Fe overcomes Cd-induced anemia in rats (POND and WALKER 1972) and pigs (POND et al. 1973) suggests that the action of Cd here is related to Fe absorption rather than to systemic inhibition of Fe metabolism. HAMILTON and VALBERG (1974) concluded that in Fe-deficient mice, duodenal uptake of Cd (i.e., step 1 of duodenal Cd absorption) is increased under conditions where Fe uptake is enhanced (see also VALBERG et al. 1976). When the capacity to absorb Fe was reduced by parenteral Fe loading and feeding of a diet supplemented with Fe, both uptake of Cd from the duodenal lumen (step 1) and further transfer into the body (step 2) were decreased.

The further conclusion that Cd increases the apparent Michaelis constant of Fe absorption without altering its maximum velocity (HAMILTON and VALBERG 1974) also supports the hypothesis that a common transport system may be shared by Fe and Cd. It must be pointed out, however, that the concentration of Cd used as inhibitor in these studies was relatively high and presumably toxic. In the neonatal rat, addition of 1.7 mM FeSO$_4$ (100 ppm Fe) to milk exerted no influence on retention of a tracer dose of Cd (RABAR and KOSTIAL 1981 b). However, uptake of Cd from 20 μM Cd in glucose saline in the jejunum of young rats was depressed by 0.4 mM FeSO$_4$ (LEON 1983). In summary, involvement of the Fe transport system in Cd absorption is possible, but remains unproven.

5. Other Metals

Exposure to Cd significantly affects metabolism of a variety of trace metals. For instance, as reviewed by PETERING (1978), Cd alters distribution of Cu, Zn, and Fe, but there is little evidence to suggest that these and other instances of metal–metal interaction primarily involve intestinal absorption. VAN CAMPEN (1966) reported that a large molar excess of Cd over Cu depresses absorption of Cu in the rat; more precisely, the results showed only a reduced total ^{64}Cu content in the tissues sampled, rather than a direct effect on absorption. EVANS et al. (1970) attributed the presumed Cd inhibition of Cu absorption to competition for a metallothionein-like protein in the mucosa. DAVIES and CAMPBELL (1977) found that

Table 4. Cation inhibition of Cd uptake from rat jejunum. (Modified from FOULKES 1985)[a]

Metal	Concentration (mM)	n	Inhibition (%)
Ca^{2+}	10	5	45 ± 6
Cr^{3+}	2	8	30 ± 17
La^{3+}	5	5	80 ± 4
Mg^{2+}	10	4	63 ± 15
Pb^{2+}	3	8	67 ± 19
Sr^{2+}	10	2	69
Zn^{2+}	1	6	50 ± 13
Polylysine	10	8	48 ± 18

[a] The percentage inhibition was calculated from n animals, each serving as its own control; values are presented as mean $\pm$ SD. Concentration of Cd in perfusate 0.02 mM. Concentration of polylysine (molecular weight 4,000–15,000) was calculated on the basis of lysine moieties

addition of Cd to the diet of rats, in a much smaller ratio to Cu than had been used by VAN CAMPEN (1966), increased rather than decreased uptake of ^{64}Cu from the lumen into the low molecular weight, metal-binding fraction. It is possible of course that this increase simply results from the raised concentration of metallothionein induced by chronic exposure to Cd in the diet. The significance of these results to the question whether the low molecular weight Cd-binding protein is involved in the effect of Cd on Cu absorption is therefore not clear. In summary, competition between Cu and Cd absorption has not been established.

A similar conclusion can be derived from other reports on metal–metal interactions in the intestine. Thus, SAHAGIAN et al. (1966, 1967) studied effects of Zn, Mn, and Hg on translocation of Cd by the rat small intestine in vitro. For reasons discussed in Sect. C.I and C.II, the bearing of these results on the mechanism of Cd absorption is not clear.

Step 1 of Cd absorption in the perfused jejunum can be depressed by relatively high concentrations not only of all polyvalent metal cations tested, but also by the organic polycation, poly(L-lysine). This is illustrated in Table 4, and leads to a simple explanation of how Cd may be taken up in the intestine, as discussed in Sect. C.VI.

VI. Conclusions

In spite of the extensive interaction between cadmium and other metals at the level of Cd uptake from the intestine, the evidence that these effects result from competition for common transport sites remains incomplete. It would be premature, therefore, to conclude that Cd absorption is facilitated by mechanisms responsible for absorption of essential metals like Ca and Zn. A simpler hypothesis is suggested by the finding that relatively high concentrations of all polyvalent metal cations tested, as well as the organic polycation polylysine, depress uptake of Cd. Conceivably, this interaction could result from nonspecific changes in electrostatic charges on the membrane (FOULKES 1985), similar to those observed by KIRSCHBAUM (1982) in a study of the aggregation of renal brush border membrane vesicles by different heavy metals. The neutralizing effect of La^{3+} on the net negative charge of vesicles prepared from intestinal brush border was demonstrated by STIEGER et al. (1983). Polycations (La^{3+}, ruthenium red) also inhibit Ca uptake by intestinal brush border membrane vesicles (MILLER and BRONNER 1981).

The hypothesis that a nonspecific polycation effect can explain the inhibitory action of various metals on Cd uptake suggests further that the depression of ^{109}Cd uptake by 0.2 mM Cd illustrated in Fig. 1 might also result from this general polycation effect. In that case there is no need to assume the existence of saturable Cd carriers in the membrane. Instead, the hypothesis implies that Cd uptake results from nonspecific binding to brush border membranes, followed by internalization due to pinocytosis. Presumably, other nonessential and toxic metals may gain access to the body in the same way. Once inside the cell, only a small fraction of mucosal Cd will remain in diffusible form, depending on the dissociation constants of intracellular Cd complexes. In agreement with this conclusion, the ratio of step 2 to step 1 of Cd absorption remains relatively constant over a fairly wide range of Cd concentrations in the perfusate, provided the binding capacity for Cd is not exceeded. How the diffusible Cd leaves the cells across the basolateral membranes (step 2) is not known.

D. Control of Cd Absorption

I. Introduction

As already discussed in Sect. C.I, there is no adequate reason to suspect that Cd is an essential trace element, or that its uptake from the intestine is under homeostatic control. Nevertheless, a variety of endogenous physiologic variables help determine fractional Cd absorption. These include in particular the age of the organism, its dietary status, and the composition and concentration of bile and possibly other secretions. In addition, exogenous factors also influence Cd absorption. These consist primarily of dietary constituents, among which the metals have already been considered (see Sect. C.V).

II. Endogenous Factors

1. Age and Sex

The ability of organisms to absorb metals varies at different stages in life. Although the source of these variations is not fully understood, they might well involve the endogenous factors considered in Sect. D.II.2. Whatever the mechanism, it is well recognized that neonates absorb or retain greater fractions of ingested metals than do adult organisms (see, e.g., FORBES and REINA 1972; KOSTIAL et al. 1978). Among these metals is Cd (see, e.g., SASSER and JARBOE 1977); this puts the immature organism at special risk of Cd intoxication.

One of the technical problems in this field is that of defining a basis for comparing function at different stages of growth. Weight of intestine per unit length, the diameter of the intestinal lumen and therefore the nominal surface area involved in absorption per unit length, as well as the density of microvilli and therefore the actual absorbing surface area per unit nominal surface area, all change with age. Neither absorption per unit weight of intestine, nor per unit length, nor per unit nominal surface area can therefore provide a useful basis for computing intrinsic functional changes of the intestine during maturation.

JUGO (1977) suggested that high pinocytotic activity in the neonatal intestine might explain the relatively efficient metal absorption at that age. SASSER and JARBOE (1977) observed major changes in Cd absorption occurring during the first day of life in rat pups; weaning further reduced whole body retention of Cd. On the other hand, feeding a milk diet to older rats increases Cd retention as compared with that seen in animals on normal rat diet. Both age and diet (see Sect. D.III) are important determinants of Cd retention (KELLO and KOSTIAL 1977). It is not known whether the effects of weaning result from changes in concentrations of specific dietary constituents, or whether the changed diet affects Cd absorption indirectly, perhaps by altering intrinsic properties of the intestine or the nature of gastrointestinal secretions.

One suggested example of how diet might alter those intrinsic properties of the intestine controlling Cd absorption is the influence of dietary iron (Sect. C.V.4). Milk is low in iron, so that pups before weaning are relatively Fe deficient. Iron deficiency, by increasing Fe absorption, should also increase absorption of Cd provided the two metals utilize the same carrier system (HAMILTON and VALBERG 1974). While KOSTIAL et al. (1980) could confirm an effect of Fe supplementation on Cd retention in 6-week-old rats on a milk diet, no such action was seen in 6-day-old pups (see also RABAR and KOSTIAL 1981 b). Other factors besides the low iron level in milk need therefore to be invoked to explain the high Cd retention in newborns (see Sect. C.V.4). Further physiologic variables known to increase fractional retention of ingested Cd include gestation and lactation. In the mouse, retention of Cd in the duodenum, for instance, is increased fivefold during gestation, and three- to fourfold during lactation. Such changes in the intestinal handling of Cd may be related to alterations in Ca metabolism in these conditions (BHATTACHARYYA et al. 1982).

An indication that Cd may be more toxic to females than to males arose from the analysis of itai-itai disease, a condition seen in elderly, poorly nourished Japanese women exposed to Cd in the diet (FRIBERG et al. 1974). Women have also been shown to accumulate more Cd than do men (SUMINO et al. 1975). Support for the view that these findings might reflect increased Cd absorption in the female was provided by KELLO et al. (1979a) who observed that whole body retention of Cd by rats 6 days following an oral load was $0.47 \pm 0.05\%$ (SE) of the dose in females, compared with $0.23 \pm 0.06\%$ in normal and $0.40 \pm 0.02\%$ in castrated males.

2. Constituents of Gastrointestinal Secretions

It has been suggested that absorption of heavy metals from the intestine requires the presence of low molecular weight ligands secreted into the intestinal lumen. Thus, EVANS et al. (1975) proposed that such a role is played by picolinic acid in Zn absorption. Evidence for an equivalent function of low molecular weight compounds in Cd absorption is lacking. The same arguments, indeed, can be adduced against the need of a low molecular weight ligand for Cd absorption as have previously been marshalled against the obligatory role of diffusible ligands in Zn absorption (BONEWITZ et al. 1982). In particular, it has often been observed that Cd is readily removed from the intestinal lumen perfused with saline solutions; the rate of removal is the same whether measured from a recirculating perfusate or from a perfusate passed through the lumen only once (FOULKES and VONER 1981). It seems unlikely therefore that accumulation of a secreted ligand in the lumen must precede Cd absorption. This conclusion does not of course deny the possibility that in competition with nonabsorbed macromolecules under physiologic conditions, low molecular weight ligands might render Cd more diffusible and more absorbable than would otherwise be the case.

Effects of Ca, Zn, and other metals on Cd absorption have been described in Sect. C.V. Whether compounds of these metals are present in sufficient concentrations in gastrointestinal secretions to inhibit Cd uptake is doubtful. There is at least one instance, however, of normal constituents of gastrointestinal secretions affecting Cd transport; this is the action of bile salts in the rat jejunum (FOULKES and VONER 1981). At a level corresponding to the critical micellar concentration range of 4–8 mg/ml, glycocholate inhibits step 1 of Cd absorption, as illustrated in Fig. 6. Similar results were obtained with taurocholate. The inhibition is fully reversible, and is not a function of the detergent properties of the compounds. The non-micelle-forming bile salt taurodehydrocholate is inactive. It seems likely that interaction between Cd and micellar bile salts in bulk solution is responsible for the observed inhibition.

The ability of mucus to influence Cd movement has not been explored, although binding of metals to mucus has been described (COLEMAN 1979). RI-

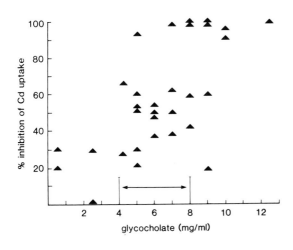

Fig. 6. Inhibition of Cd uptake by glycocholic acid. Each point was calculated for the rate of removal of Cd from a 20 μM Cd perfusate in rat jejunum in situ, before and after addition of glycocholate. The *arrow* indicates the critical micellar range. (FOULKES and VONER 1981)

CHARDSON and Fox (1974) observed that chronic ingestion of rather high amounts of Cd by Japanese quail led to a syndrome resembling tropical sprue, with marked goblet cell hyperplasia and large amounts of mucus in the intestinal lumen. The slow degradation of mucus, and its capacity to bind metals thus indicate that mucus secretion may represent another endogenous determinant of Cd absorption.

III. Influence of Diet

The influence of diet on metal absorption has been studied extensively in many laboratories. Mechanisms responsible for the action of diet could involve direct effects on Cd transport mechanisms, changes in the availability of Cd for diffusion and absorption, or indirect effects on the intestine. An example of direct interference with Cd absorption would be the inhibitory metals discussed in Sect. C.V, if present in sufficiently high concentration; acute inhibition of Cd absorption from the rat jejunum by Ca in milk illustrates such an effect (FOULKES 1980).

Constituents of digested food may stimulate transport of Cd if their reaction with the metal renders it more diffusible, or better able to penetrate cell membranes. The stimulation of calcium absorption by phosphopeptides provides an illustration (LEE et al. 1983). Low molecular weight metal ligands could thus readily increase uptake of Cd in competition with nonabsorbed macromolecules capable of binding the metal in nonavailable form. Such a binding reaction of macromolecules is illustrated by the finding that zeolites (3% in the diet) protect growing swine against the toxic effects of Cd, and more particularly against Cd-induced anemia (POND and YEN 1983).

Formation of stable, low molecular weight complexes could further prevent or diminish Cd trapping by mucosal macromolecules and thus increase the rate of step 2 of Cd absorption, the transfer of the metal from the mucosa into the body. One such compound may be exogenous Cd–metallothionein, which is slowly absorbed from the intestinal lumen, either as such or as partial breakdown product (CHERIAN et al. 1978). If the metal remains in dissociable form, the nature of the administered anion does not affect retention (MOORE et al. 1973).

Different diffusible Cd complexes may be transported to a varying extent, depending presumably on stability, lipid solubility, and other factors. For instance, KOJIMA and KIYOZUMI (1974) reported that in rat intestine perfused in vitro with solutions containing relatively high concentrations of Cd, step 1 of Cd absorption, i.e., the sum of Cd accumulated in the tissue plus that recovered from serosal fluid, was greatly depressed by several chelating agents, including EDTA and citric acid. Citrate has been suspected of playing a role in Zn absorption (LÖNNER-DAL et al. 1980).

An influence of diet on both steps 1 and 2 of Cd absorption may be deduced from the results of RABAR and KOSTIAL (1981 a), as shown in Table 5. Assuming that the rats in these experiments excreted little Cd in urine or bile during the 6 days following its oral administration, whole body Cd here may be equated to the net amount of Cd transported by step 1, while that transported by step 2 is given by the amount recovered from the gut-free carcasses. Note that milk, meat, or

Table 5. Influence of diet on Cd retention in rats (based on results of RABAR and KOSTIAL 1981a)[a]

Diet	n	Percentage of oral dose			
		Whole body (step 1)	Gut	Gut-free carcass (Step 2)	Step 2/step 1
Rat diet	18	1.75 ± 0.23	0.23 ± 0.04	1.52 ± 0.21	0.9
Meat	10	8.26 ± 0.45	3.12 ± 0.39	5.14 ± 0.20	0.6
Bread	10	7.30 ± 0.34	2.25 ± 0.22	5.05 ± 0.20	0.7
Milk	18	7.80 ± 0.27	2.63 ± 0.23	5.17 ± 0.33	0.7

[a] Results are expressed as means $\pm$ SE for n rats; 6-week-old animals were maintained on the respective diets for 3 days before, and 6 days after oral administration of Cd 0.5 mg/kg, at which time they were killed for analysis

bread permitted significantly greater transport of Cd by both steps than was seen in control animals. However, the ratio of step 2 to step 1 was not significantly altered by these diets, i.e., they did not change the likelihood of Cd taken up by step 1 being further transported by step 2. The low step 1 seen in control animals presumably reflects the presence in commercial rat food of one or more substances interfering with Cd movement.

Under different conditions, a high protein diet may reduce absorption or retention of Cd (SUZUKI et al. 1969). Within 24 h of being placed on such a diet, mice retained significantly less of an oral Cd load than did control animals. The subsequent report that levels of bovine serum albumin as high as 30% are required in a jejunal perfusate before a significant depression of step 1 of Cd absorption can be observed (FOULKES and VONER 1981) not only provides some indication of the relative affinity of the protein and of brush border receptors for Cd, but also makes it unlikely that the observation of SUZUKI et al. (1969) can be explained by assuming binding of Cd to nonabsorbable macromolecules. Other factors, such as mucosal changes, or luminal passage times, might be involved here.

Other apparent effects of diet may not be directly related to changes in Cd absorption. Thus, the beneficial action of ascorbic acid in Cd-poisoned animals may be related to stimulation of Fe absorption (FOX et al. 1980). A useful review by Fox (1983) further considers the influence of diet on metal absorption.

E. Summary

Cadmium is a toxic, nonessential metal which possesses a very long biologic half-life and as a consequence acts as a cumulative poison in humans and higher animals. Outside of the industrial environment, most of the body burden of the metal is derived from food, and the WORLD HEALTH ORGANIZATION (1972) recommends that the level of Cd in food should not exceed around 0.1 ppm. This recommendation is based on a mathematical model (FRIBERG et al. 1974) which, among other assumptions, states that potentially irreversible renal damage may be expected to occur in a significant fraction of a chronically exposed population when the concentration of Cd in renal cortex approaches 200 µg/g (KJELLSTROM et al. 1984) (see Chap. 6), and that fractional absorption of ingested Cd amounts to 5%. Full consensus on the critical level has not yet been reached; it may vary with the nature of Cd exposure and with other factors, including the distribution of the metal between different chemical species, e.g., metallothionein-bound and non-metallothionein-bound Cd (NOMIYAMA and NOMIYAMA 1982).

The low fractional absorption of an oral load of Cd has been well established. However, the 5% value commonly assumed also represents no more than a convenient approximation, as a multitude of endogenous and exogenous variables determine actual uptake under various conditions. It is conceivable therefore that changes in the composition of the diet could reduce absorption sufficiently to permit some increase in the acceptable Cd concentration in food.

An earlier observation that Cd uptake at low concentrations obeys saturation kinetics suggested the involvement of a carrier system in Cd transport. A priori it seems unlikely, however, that a specific mechanism should have evolved in higher species for uptake of a nonessential toxic metal with a very long half-life in the body. If Cd uptake were the result of its reaction with other systems primarily responsible for absorption of essential metals like Zn, Fe, or Ca, then competition between these metals and Cd for common binding sites would be predicted. Although Cd does interact with these metals during absorption from the intestine, competition between them has not been established. In the case of Zn and Cd, in particular, interaction with Cd is clearly not competitive in nature.

In relatively high concentrations, a variety of polyvalent metal cations other than Zn also inhibit Cd uptake (see Table 4). They include La^{3+}, Cr^{3+}, Sr^{2+}, Mg^{2+}, Fe^{2+}, and Pb^{2+}; the organic polycation polylysine exerts the same effect. The one common factor in each case is the electric charge, and this leads to the conclusion that the effect of these cations may be mediated by charge redistribution on the brush border membrane. If the ability of high concentrations of Cd to depress fractional uptake of ^{109}Cd is also the consequence of such a nonspecific cation effect, the need to postulate the existence of a saturable Cd transport mechanism in the membrane disappears. Step 1 of Cd uptake, and presumably of that of other toxic metals like Pb, may then be visualized as a process initiated by their nonspecific binding to the brush border membranes, followed by pinocytotic internalization of the bound metals.

In intestinal segments isolated in situ and perfused with glucose–saline, the rate of Cd uptake by the mucosal cells (step 1 of Cd absorption) greatly exceeds that of its further movement from mucosa into the body (step 2). The avid retention of Cd in the mucosa plays an important role in minimizing Cd absorption and presumably results from binding of Cd to macromolecular ligands. The fact that under a given set of conditions the ratio of step 1 to step 2 remains constant and independent of Cd concentration suggests that step 2 may be determined by the small diffusible fraction of cellular Cd in equilibrium with bound Cd. Whatever the nature of step 2, there is no indication of a facilitating mechanism involved at that level.

References

Ando M, Sayato Y, Tonomura M, Osawa T (1977) Studies on excretion and uptake of calcium by rats after continuous oral administration of cadmium. Toxicol Appl Pharmacol 39:321–327

Ando M, Sayato Y, Osawa T (1978) Studies of the disposition of calcium in bones of rats after continuous oral administration of cadmium. Toxicol Appl Pharmacol 46:625–632

Ando M, Shimuzu M, Sayato Y, Tanimura A, Tobe M (1981) The inhibition of vitamin D-stimulated intestinal calcium transport in rats after continuous oral administration of cadmium. Toxicol Appl Pharmacol 61:297–301

Barret HM, Irwin DA, Semmons E (1947) Studies on the toxicity of inhaled cadmium. J Ind Hyg Toxicol 29:279–301

Bhattacharyya MH, Whelton BD, Peterson DP (1982) Gastrointestinal absorption of cadmium in mice during gestation and lactation. Toxicol Appl Pharmacol 66:368–375

Bonewitz RF, Voner C, Foulkes EC (1982) Uptake and absorption of zinc in perfused rat jejunum: the role of endogenous factors in the lumen. Nutr Res 2:301–307

Bonewitz RF, Foulkes EC, O'Flaherty EJ, Hertzberg VS (1983) Kinetics of Zn absorption by the rat jejunum: effects of adrenalectomy and dexamethasone. Am J Physiol 244:G314–G320

Bremner I (1978) Cadmium toxicity. Nutritional influences and the role of metallothionein. World Rev Nutr Diet 32:165–197

Bremner I, Campbell JK (1978) Effects of Cu and Zn status on susceptibility to Cd intoxication. Environ Health Persp 25:125–128

Buchet JP, Roels H, Lauwerys R, Bruaux P, Claeys-Thoreau F, Lafontaine A, Verduyn G (1980) Repeated surveillance of exposure to cadmium, manganese and arsenic in school-age children living in rural, urban and non-ferrous smelter areas in Belgium. Environ Res 22:95–108

Cherian MG, Rodgers K (1982) Chelation of cadmium from metallothionein in vivo and its excretion in rats repeatedly injected with cadmium chloride. J Pharmacol Exp Ther 222:699–704

Cherian MG, Goyer RA, Valberg LS (1978) Gastrointestinal absorption and organ distribution of oral $CdCl_2$ and Cd-metallothionein in mice. J Toxicol Environ Health 4:861–868

Chertok RJ, Sadder LB, Callahan MF, Jarboe GE (1979) Intestinal absorption of Cd in vitro. Environ Res 20:125–132

Coleman JR (1979) Electron probe microanalysis and the cellular basis of transepithelial Ca transport. In: Lechene CP, Warner RR (eds) Proceedings Workshop Biol. X-ray microanalysis and electron beam excitation. Academic, New York, pp 509–515

Corrigan AJ, Huang PC (1981) Cellular uptake of cadmium and zinc. Biol Trace Elem Res 3:197–216

Cotzias GC, Borg DC, Selleck B (1961) Virtual absence of turnover in cadmium metabolism: [109]Cd studies in the mouse. Am J Physiol 201:927–930

Davies NT, Campbell JK (1977) The effect of cadmium on intestinal copper absorption and binding in the rat. Life Sci 20:955–960

Evans GW, Majors PF, Cornatzer WE (1970) Mechanism for cadmium and zinc antagonism of copper metabolism. Biochem Biophys Res Commun 40:1142–1148

Evans GW, Grace CI, Hahn CJ (1973) Homeostatic regulation of Zn absorption in the rat. Proc Soc Exp Biol Med 143:723–725

Evans GW, Grace CI, Votava HJ (1975) A proposed mechanism for zinc absorption in the rat. Am J Physiol 228:501–505

Forbes GB, Reina JC (1972) Effect of age on gastrointestinal absorption (Fe, Sr, Pb) in the rat. J Nutr 102:647–652

Foulkes EC (1980) Some determinants of intestinal cadmium transport in the rat. J Environ Pathol Toxicol 3:471–481

Foulkes EC (1985) Interactions between metals in rat jejunum: implications on the nature of cadmium uptake. Toxicology 37:117–125

Foulkes EC, Voner C (1981) Effects of Zn status, bile and other endogenous factors on jejunal Cd absorption. Toxicology 22:115–122

Fox MRS (1983) Cadmium bioavailability. Fed Proc 42:1726–1729

Fox MRS, Jacobs RM, Lee-Jones AO, Fry BE, Stone CL (1980) Effects of vitamin C and iron on cadmium metabolism. Ann NY Acad Sci 355:249–261

Friberg L (1959) Chronic cadmium poisoning. Arch Ind Health 20:401–407

Friberg L, Piscator M, Nordberg GF, Kjellstrom T (1974) Cadmium in the environment, 2nd edn. Chemical Rubber, Cleveland

Fullmer CS, Oku T, Wasserman RH (1980) Effect of cadmium administration on intestinal calcium absorption and vitamin D-dependent calcium-binding protein. Environ Res 22:386–399

Hahn CJ, Evans GW (1975) Absorption of trace metals in the zinc-deficient rat. Am J Physiol 228:1020–1023

Hamilton DL, Smith MW (1977) Cadmium inhibits calcium absorption by rat intestine. J Physiol 265:54P–55P

Hamilton DL, Smith MW (1978) Inhibition of intestinal calcium uptake by cadmium and the effect of a low calcium diet on cadmium retention. Environ Res 15:175–184

Hamilton DL, Valberg LS (1974) Relationship between cadmium and iron absorption. Am J Physiol 227:1033–1037

Ingersoll RJ, Wasserman RH (1971) Vitamin D_3-induced calcium-binding protein. J Biol Chem 246:2808–2814

Jugo S (1977) Metabolism of toxic heavy metals in growing organisms. Environ Res 13:36–46

Kello D, Kostial K (1977) Influence of age and milk diet on cadmium absorption from the gut. Toxicol Appl Pharmacol 40:277–282

Kello D, Dekanic D, Kostial K (1979a) Influence of sex and dietary calcium on intestinal cadmium absorption in rats. Arch Environ Health 34:30–33

Kello D, Sugawara N, Voner C, Foulkes EC (1979b) On the role of metallothionein in cadmium absorption by rat jejunum in situ. Toxicology 14:199–208

Kirschbaum BB (1982) Aggregation of renal brush border membranes by concanavalin A and heavy metals. Toxicol Appl Pharmacol 64:10–19

Kiyozumi M, Kojima S (1978) Studies on poisonous metals. V. Excretion of cadmium through bile and gastrointestinal mucosa and effect of chelating agents on its excretion in cadmium-pretreated rats. Chem Pharm Bull 26:3410–3415

Kjellstrom T, Elinder CG, Friberg L (1984) Conceptual problems in establishing the critical concentration of cadmium in human kidney cortex. Environ Res 33:284–295

Kojima S, Kiyozumi M (1974) Studies on poisonous metals. I. Transfer of cadmium chloride across rat small intestine in vitro and effect of chelating agents on its transfer. Yakugaku Zasshi 94:695–701

Koo SI, Fullmer CS, Wasserman RH (1978) Intestinal absorption and retention of ^{109}Cd: effects of cholecalciferol, calcium status and other variables. J Nutr 108:1812–1822

Kostial K, Kello D, Jugo S, Rabar I, Maljkovic T (1978) Influence of age on metal metabolism and toxicity. Environ Health Perspect 25:81–86

Kostial K, Rabar I, Blanusa M, Simonovic I (1980) The effect of iron additive to milk on cadmium, mercury, and manganese absorption in rats. Environ Res 22:40–45

Larsson S, Piscator M (1971) Effect of cadmium on skeletal tissue in normal and calcium-deficient rats. Israel J Med Sci 7:495–498

Lee YS, Noguchi T, Naito H (1983) Intestinal absorption of calcium in rats given diets containing casein or amino acid mixture: the role of casein phosphopeptides. Br J Nutr 49:67–76

Leon L (1983) The role of iron in the intestinal uptake of cadmium in the newborn rat. PhD thesis, University of Cincinnati

Lewis GP, Coughlin L, Jusko W, Hartz S (1972) Contribution of cigarette smoking to cadmium accumulation in man. Lancet 1:291–292

Lönnerdal B, Stanislowski AG, Hurley LS (1980) Isolation of a low molecular weight Zn-binding ligand from human milk. J Inorg Biochem 12:71–78

Mahaffey KR, Corneiussen PE, Jellinek CF, Fiorino JA (1975) Heavy metal exposure from foods. Environ Health Perspec 12:63–69

McLellan JS, Flanigan PR, Chamberlain MJ, Valberg LS (1978) Measurement of dietary cadmium absorption in humans. J Toxicol Environ Health 4:131–138

Menden EE, Elia VJ, Michael LM, Petering HG (1972) Distribution of cadmium and nickel of tobacco during cigarette smoking. Environ Sci Technol 6:830–832

Miller A, Bronner F (1981) Calcium uptake in isolated brush-border vesicles from rat small intestine. Biochem J 196:391–401

Moore W Jr, Stara JF, Crocker WC (1973) Gastrointestinal absorption of different compounds of [115m]cadmium and the effect of different concentrations in the rat. Environ Res 6:159–164

Murata I, Hirono T, Soeki Y (1970) Cadmium enteropathy, renal osteomalacia (Itai-Itai disease) in Japan. Bull Soc Int Chir 1:34–42

Nomiyama K, Nomiyama H (1982) Tissue metallothioneins in rabbits chronically exposed to cadmium, with special reference to the critical concentration of cadmium in the renal cortex. In: Foulkes EC (ed) Biological roles of metallothionein. Elsevier/North-Holland, Amsterdam, pp 47–67

Nordberg GF, Fowler BA, Friberg L, Jeruelöv A, Nelson N, Piscator M, Sandstead HH, Vostal J, Vouk VB (1978) Factors influencing metabolism and toxicity of metals: a consensus report. Environ Health Perspect 25:31–41

Petering HG (1978) Some observations on the interaction of zinc, copper and iron metabolism in lead and cadmium toxicity. Environ Health Perspect 25:141–145

Phillpotts CJ (1980) Retention of cadmium in the duodenum of the rat following oral administration. Toxicology 14:245–253

Pond WG, Walker EF (1972) Cadmium induced anemia in growing rats: prevention by oral or parenteral iron. Nutr Rep Int 5:365–370

Pond WG, Yen JT (1983) Protection by Clinoptilite or Zeolite NaA against cadmium-induced anemia in growing swine. Proc Soc Exp Biol Med 173:332–337

Pond WG, Walker EF, Kirtland D (1973) Cadmium induced anemia in growing pigs: protective effect of oral and parenteral iron. J Animal Sci 36:1122–1128

Rabar I, Kostial K (1981a) Bioavailability of cadmium in rats fed various diet. Arch Toxicol 47:63–66

Rabar I, Kostial K (1981b) Failure of trace element additives to decrease cadmium, mercury and manganese absorption in suckling rats. In: Gut I, Cikrt M, Plaa GL (eds) Industrial and environmental xenobiotics. Springer, Berlin Heidelberg New York, pp 45–47

Richards MP, Cousins RJ (1975) Mammalian zinc homeostatis: requirement for RNA and metallothionein synthesis. Biochem Biophys Res Commun 64:1215–1223

Richardson ME, Fox MRS (1974) Dietary Cd and enteropathy in the Japanese quail. Lab Invest 31:722–731

Sasser LB, Jarboe GE (1977) Intestinal absorption and retention of cadmium in neonatal rat. Toxicol Appl Pharmacol 41:423–431

Sahagian BM, Harding-Barlow I, Perry HM (1966) Uptakes of zinc, manganese, cadmium and mercury by intact strips of rat intestine. J Nutr 90:259–267

Sahagian BM, Harding-Barlow I, Perry HM (1967) Transmural movements of zinc, manganese, cadmium, and mercury by rat small intestine. J Nutr 93:291–300

Schafer SG, Forth W (1983) Excretion of metals into the rat intestine. Biol Trace Element Res 5:205–217

Schroeder HA, Balassa JJ (1961) Abnormal trace metals in man: cadmium. J Chronic Dis 14:236–258

Schwartz K, Spallholz J (1976) Growth effects of small cadmium supplements in rats maintained under trace-element controlled conditions. Fed Proc 35:255 (abstract)

Shaikh ZA, Lucis OJ (1972) Biological differences in cadmium and zinc turnover. Arch Environ Health 24:410–425

Smith KT, Cousins RJ, Silbon BL, Failla ML (1978) Zinc absorption and metabolism by isolated vascularly perfused rat intestine. J Nutr 108:1849–1857

Stieger B, Burckhardt G, Murer H (1983) Application of a potential-sensitive cyanine dye to rat small intestine brush border membrane vesicles. Biochem Biophys Acta 732:324–326

Sugawara N (1974) Calcium-binding activity of duodenal mucosa, renal cortex and medulla in cadmium poisoning in rats. Jpn J Hyg 29:399–402

Sumino K, Hayakawa K, Shibata T, Kitamura S (1975) Heavy metals in normal Japanese tissues. Arch Environ Health 30:487–494

Suzuki S, Taguchi T, Yokohashi G (1969) Dietary factors influencing upon the retention rate of orally administered ^{115m}CdCl$_2$ in mice, with special reference to calcium and protein concentrations in diet. Ind Health 7:155–162

Tipton IH, Stewart PL, Dickson J (1969) Patterns of elemental excretion in long-term balance studies. Health Physics 16:455–462

Toraason M (1983) Interaction between calcium and cadmium during absorption in the duodenum of the rat. PhD Thesis, University of Cincinnati

Toraason M, Foulkes EC (1984) Interaction between calcium and cadmium in the 1,25 dihydroxy vitamin D$_3$ stimulated rat duodenum. Toxicol Appl Pharmacol 75:98–104

Tsuchiya K (1969a) Causation of ouch-ouch disease (Itai-Itai Byo). An introductory review. I. Nature of the disease. Keio J Med 18:181–194

Tsuchiya K (1969b) Causation of ouch-ouch disease (Itai-Itai Byo). II. Epidemiology and evaluation. Keio J Med 18:195–211

Tsuchiya K, Seki Y, Sugita M (1976) Cadmium concentrations in the organs and tissues of cadavers from accidental deaths. Keio J Med 25:83–90

Tsuruki F, Otawara Y, Wung HL, Moriuchi S, Hosoya N (1978) Inhibitory effect of cadmium on vitamin-D stimulated calcium transport in rat duodenum in vitro. J Nutr Sci Vitaminol 24:237–242

Valberg LS, Sorbe J, Hamilton DL (1976) Gastrointestinal metabolism of cadmium in experimental iron deficiency. Am J Physiol 231:462–467

Valberg LS, Haist J, Cherian MG, Delaquerriere-Richardson L, Goyer RA (1977) Cadmium-induced enteropathy: comparative toxicity of cadmium chloride and cadmium-thionein. J Toxicol Environ Health 2:963–975

Vallee BL, Ulmer DD (1972) Biochemical effects of Hg, Cd, and Pb. Ann Rev Biochem 41:91–128

Van Campen DR (1966) Effects of zinc, cadmium, silver and mercury on the absorption and distribution of copper-64 in rats. J Nutr 88:125–130

Wahlberg JE (1965) Percutaneous toxicity of metal compounds. Arch Environ Health 11:201–204

Washko PW, Cousins RJ (1977) Role of dietary calcium and calcium binding protein in cadmium toxicity in rats. J Nutr 107:920–928

Worker NA, Migicovsky BB (1961) Effect of vitamin D on the utilization of zinc, cadmium and mercury in the chick. J Nutr 75:222–224

World Health Organization (1972) Evaluation of certain food additives and the contaminants mercury, lead and cadmium. WHO Tech Rep Ser No 505

CHAPTER 4

The Chronic Toxicity of Cadmium: Influence of Environmental and Other Variables

K. Nomiyama

A. Introduction

As referred to elsewhere in this volume (see especially Chaps. 5 and 6), a series of episodes of chronic human exposure to apparently toxic levels of cadmium have been reported. These will be reviewed in some detail here, followed by the specific health effects seen. The major emphasis in this chapter is placed on the variability of the response to cadmium, and on the factors determining this response.

B. Environmental Pollution with Cadmium and Health Effects

The public health effects of cadmium pollution have been reviewed previously (Nomiyama 1981a). The major episodes of cadmium pollution in Japan and Europe are discussed in the following sections.

I. Itai-Itai Disease

Itai-itai disease was endemic among elderly women in the Zinzu river basin after the Second World War. The patients suffered from intolerable pain, especially on movement. Even slight movements could result in pathologic fractures. X-ray films of the bones showed bending, deformation, decalcification, fracture, and signs of healing suggestive of osteomalacia in combination with osteoporosis (Fig. 1). Proteinuria, glycosuria, low molecular weight proteinuria, and aminoaciduria were also observed. Tissue cadmium was found to be high. The administration of a high protein diet and vitamin D were effective in treating the disease.

The total number of patients was estimated in 1955 by the Toyama prefecture as being 41 of a total of 1,666 residents (849 women). In 1961, the disease was thought to be associated with heavy metal pollution, presumably derived from mine tailings. In 1963, a health survey was conducted on villagers in the Zinzu river basin, and the results pointed to cadmium as the most likely metal to be the etiologic agent of itai-itai disease. However, a low protein and calcium diet was also thought to contribute to the onset of the disease. In May 1968, itai-itai disease was officially recognized as a pollution-related disease by the Japan Ministry of Health and Welfare. By March 1983, a total of 116 cases of itai-itai disease had been officially recognized, as well as 52 patients suspected of suffering from the disease. The onset of the disease occurred most frequently between the ages of 50

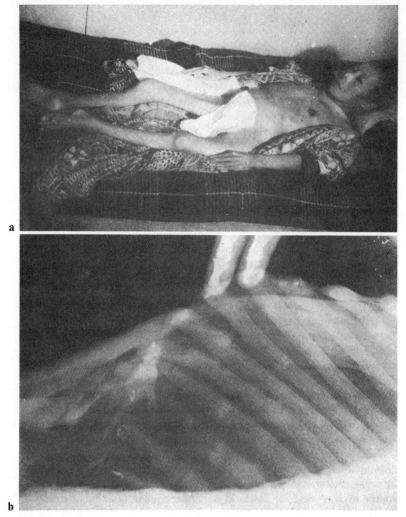

Fig. 1 a, b. Itai-itai disease patient and her roentgenogram. **a** A severe case of itai-itai disease, 55-year-old female, **b** roentgenogram of multiple Milkman's pseudofracture of ribs (osteomalacia). (Murata et al. 1970)

and 55 years. Since 1968, patients have been given free medical care by the government, and since 1971, the disease has been subject to the Pollution-Related Health Damage Compensation Law.

II. An Episode in Annaka District, Japan

The Toho Zinc Corporation began to smelt zinc in the town of Annaka (Gunma Prefecture; Fig. 2) in June 1937. With the initiation of smelting, bamboo leaves near the factory became white and this change was attributed to sulfur dioxide gas leaking from the factory. The topsoil of 20 ha of rice-growing land was contaminated with slag from the factory in 1938. In 1949, the Toho Zinc Corporation intended to add a smelting plant and sulfuric acid factory, in spite of local opposition to the plan. In 1960, local inhabitants requested that the company should pay compensation for the agricultural damage, and appealed to the Diet and Prime Minister. With the initiation of the operation of the new zinc and sulfuric acid factories in 1961, 10 ha of farms were affected. In 1961, dead fish were found in the river and liquid waste from the factories was once more suspected of causing the pollution; crop yields were reduced for several years, in spite of the fact that a large reservoir and concentrating equipment had come into use in the factory in 1956. By the end of 1963, the completion of the sewage work from the factory at Takasaki helped to reduce pollution entering the Yanase river. In 1964–1965, the company installed a highly efficient scrubber and Cottrell precipitator to clean the exhaust gas. In order to neutralize exhaust gases from the sulfuric acid factory, an absorber was also installed in 1967. In early 1967, the company promised to pay compensation for damage caused to the community. The company expanded its electrolysis factory in March 1967. In May 1969, silk production near the factory was seriously decreased by damage to mulberry leaves by a leak of sulfur dioxide gas from the factory after its electric power supply was stopped by lightning.

In October 1968, the Takasaki Central Hospital performed a cadmium health effects survey on some local residents and the results of this survey caused serious concern. On 27 March 1969, the Committee on Cadmium Health Effects, for the Ministry of Health and Welfare, concluded that there was no case of itai-itai disease in the Annaka district. However, the possibility of the existence of itai-itai disease was discussed at the House of Councilors on 9 April 1969. On 23 June the company gained permission from the Ministry of International Trade and Industry to enlarge the factory. This decision triggered more local protests to the Ministry of International Trade and Industry. The Ministry of Health and Welfare took tentative measures for reducing environmental pollution with cadmium, and settled safe guidelines for rice contamination with cadmium: 1.0 ppm for unpolished rice and 0.9 ppm for polished rice in 1970. In late July, cadmium was detected at a high concentration in grasses from a farm close to the factory, and cows' milk was suspected of being highly polluted with cadmium. In the same month, Takasaki Central Hospital announced that eight farmers in the Annaka district were suffering from cadmium-induced deformity of the fingers. However, the Committee on Cadmium Health Effects for the Ministry of Health and Welfare later concluded that this particular incidence was not caused by cadmium intoxication. On 1 February 1971, cadmium was detected by Professor J. Kobayashi in a concentration as high as 20,000 µg per gram ash in the kidneys of a deceased woman who had been employed as a cadmium foil worker in the Annaka factory. Nevertheless, after examining the detailed history, signs, and symptoms, the Committee concluded that she had not suffered from cadmium poisoning. At the end of June 1971, itai-itai disease patients won their case in court, and on 1 April 1972, neighbors of the Annaka factory sued the Toho Zinc Corporation for compensation. Gunma Prefecture had exchanged the soil of cadmium-polluted rice fields with soil from areas not exposed to cadmium, and demanded

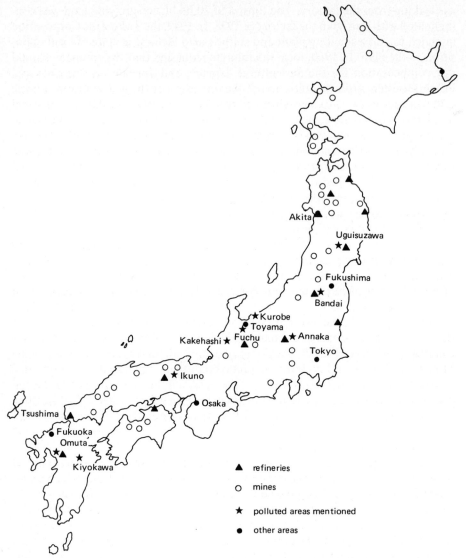

Fig. 2. Location of sulfide ore mines and refineries and cadmium-polluted areas in Japan. (Yamamoto 1972)

that the company should pay 470 million yen for the cost. Cadmium health effects surveys have been conducted every year, but no itai-itai disease patients have been found in the Annaka district.

III. Other Episodes in Japan

By the analysis of cadmium in rice samples from each km² of rice fields, cadmium-polluted areas were found in most prefectures. Health surveys have been performed on residents in cadmium-polluted areas by the local health authorities to discover itai-itai disease patients. Since 1976, the Japan Environment Agency has conducted an epidemiologic health survey on 8,800 residents of above 50 years of age in eight cadmium-polluted areas. However, no itai-itai disease patients have been found outside the Zinzu river basin. An increased prevalence of β_2-microglobulinuria was found in some cadmium-polluted areas. However, it is still difficult to establish an association of cadmium exposure with the occurrence of β_2-microglobulinuria, because the association with polluted areas could not always be observed. The Japanese government, in any event, has withheld distribution of rice of more than 0.4 ppm cadmium concentration in order to safeguard public health.

IV. Episodes in Europe

In late January 1979, newspapers that a very high concentration of cadmium had been detected from soil of the village of Shipham, 30 km south-west of Bristol. The soil of Shipham was contaminated by wastes from old mining operations; the village was built on these wastes. It had been well known locally that soil in the village was contaminated by metals and adverse effects on plant growth had been observed. A pilot study was carried out on 31 volunteers from among 1,000 Shipham villagers. Raised blood cadmium and abnormal clinical and biochemical findings suggesting renal tubular dysfunction and hypertension were observed, and the average cadmium level in the liver of 21 volunteer villagers (11.0 µg/g) was higher than the normal level of 2.2 µg/g. Later, the Department of the Environment conducted a health survey of all Shipham villagers, but no medical history nor any signs of cadmium health effects were found. Because of high cadmium levels in vegetables grown in the village, inhabitants were advised not to use these as food (THOMAS 1984).

The Liège area, Belgium, is known to be highly polluted by cadmium owing to the presence of nonferrous metal smelters, in activity since the end of the nineteenth century. Health surveys in 1980 revealed that elderly women from the Liège area have a higher cadmium body burden than women of the same age in other areas. A mortality study also indicated excess death from glomerulonephritis in the Liège area (LAUWERYS et al. 1980).

The town of Freiberg, between Karl-Marx-Stadt and Dresden, German Democratic Republic, has been known to be polluted with cadmium emitted from a nonferrous metal smelting factory. The first report of land contamination of this district occurred in 1975 after the deaths of cattle grazing in the vicinity of the smelter (SCHNEIDER et al. 1979). Health effects on residents in Freiberg have not been reported so far.

Stadskanaal, a canal in the town of Sangster (North-East Netherlands), was reported to be contaminated with cadmium emitted from a television screen factory over a period of 17 years. Cadmium concentrations of vegetables in large vegetable gardens along the canal appeared to be increased. However, a health survey revealed nothing of clinical significance among the residents in the polluted area (SANGSTER and DE GROOT 1984).

C. Renal Effects

I. Renal Effects Among Residents in Cadmium-Polluted Areas in Japan

Since cadmium was announced officially as the etiologic agent probably responsible for itai-itai disease in 1968, administrative health surveys have been carried out on residents in recognized cadmium-polluted areas in Japan (Table 1; SHIGE-MATSU et al. 1981 b). Emphasis was placed on discovery of itai-itai disease (osteomalacia). As indicated before, no itai-itai disease has been found in areas with cadmium pollution other than Fuchu, Toyama Prefecture. Thus, the procedure

Table 1. Environmental pollution with cadmium and health effects in Japan (compiled from TSUCHIYA 1978)

Area	History of exposure	Cadmium in rice (μg/g)	Daily intake (μg/day)	Effects
Kosaka (Akita)	91 years (Cu mine and refinery)	0.16–0.58	139–177	β_2-Microglobulinuria, glycosuria (male, dose-related)
Uguisuzawa (Miyagi)	250 years (As, Pb, Zn mine)	0.6 –0.7		No proteinuria, nor glycosuria
Bandai (Fukushima)	50 years (Zn refinery)	0.16–0.38	180–309	No proteinuria, nor glycosuria
Yoshino (Yamagata)	400 years (Au, Ag, Cu, Zn refinery)	0.58		Glycosuria (female)
Annaka (Gunma)	40 years (Zn refinery)	0.40–0.54	180–380	No proteinuria, nor glycosuria
Izu (Shizuoka)	250 years (Au, Cu mine)	0.40		No proteinuria, nor glycosuria
Kurobe (Toyama)	40 years (Cu mine)	0.6		
Fuchu (Toyama)	370 years (Zn, Pb, Cd mine and refinery)	0.5 –2		Proteinuria, glycosuria, β_2-microgloburinuria (dose-related)
Kakehashi (Ishikawa)	40 years (Cu mine)	0.2 –0.8	160–190	β_2-Globulinuria, retinol-binding proteinuria (dose-related), glycosuria (dose-related)
Ikuno (Hyogo)	440 years (Ag, Cu mine)	0.24–1.0		Proteinuria (male), glycosuria, β_2-microglobulinuria
Tsushima (Nagasaki)	30 years (Pb, Zn mine)	0.0.45–0.75	210–255	Glycosuria (female, dose-related), β_2-microglobulinuria
Okutake (Oita)	40 years (Au, Cu, Pb, Zn, As mine)	0.16–0.46	222–391	No proteinuria, nor glycosuria
Ohmuta (Fukuoka)	55 years (Zn refinery)			No proteinuria, nor glycosuria

for detecting health effects of cadmium was revised in 1976 to detect renal tubular dysfunction among residents in cadmium-polluted areas. Administrative and epidemiologic surveys on cadmium-induced renal dysfunction were carried out with the use of the revised procedure in the fiscal year 1976–1978 in seven prefectures (Akita, Ishikawa, Nagasaki, Fukushima, Hyogo, and Oita). Subjects over 50 years old numbered 4,658 (2,067 and 2,591 females) from polluted areas and 4,200 (1,820 males and 2,380 females) from areas believed to be free of pollution. In some prefectures (Ishikawa, Akita, and Nagasaki) cadmium pollution could be correlated with urinary sugar and low molecular weight protein, symptoms of depressed proximal tubular function, while in other prefectures (Fukushima, Hyogo, and Oita) such was not the case. Elevated urinary excretion of low molecular weight protein, believed to result from the action of cadmium, was found to have very little relationship to cadmium pollution. A total of 57 persons with depressed proximal tubular function were found in cadmium-polluted areas. Cadmium concentrations of rice in these areas were recorded as 0.16–0.58 µg/g in Akita, 0.5–2.0 µg/g in Toyama, 0.2–0.7 µg/g in Ishikawa, and 0.45–0.75 µg/g in Nagasaki Prefectures. The levels of cadmium also were relatively high in Fukushima (0.16–0.38 µg/g), in Hyogo (0.24–1.0 µg/g), and in Oita Prefectures (0.16–0.46 µg/g), but no relationships were found between cadmium exposure and the incidence of renal dysfunction. Daily intake of cadmium was 139–177 µg in Akita, 160–190 µg in Ishikawa, 210–250 µg in Nagasaki, 180–309 µg in Fukushima, and 222–391 µg in Oita Prefectures. No high incidence of renal dysfunction was observed in Annaka (Gunma Prefecture), where the cadmium level in rice was 0.40–0.54 µg/g and daily intake of cadmium was 180–380 µg. These data indicate that no significant difference exists between cadmium level in rice or in daily Cd intake between areas with and without elevated incidence of renal dysfunction. This conclusion raises some questions about a definite critical level of cadmium in rice, required to induce renal dysfunction among residents in cadmium-polluted areas. Annaka in Gunma Prefecture and Bandai in Miyagi Prefecture have been polluted with cadmium, but also with zinc in the air, because zinc refineries have operated in these areas. It is quite possible that the simultaneous exposure to cadmium and zinc does not readily induce renal dysfunction. On the other hand, areas with elevated incidence of cadmium-induced renal dysfunction, such as Fuchu (Toyama Prefecture), Kakehashi (Ishikawa Prefecture), and Tsushima (Nagasaki Prefecture) have been polluted with cadmium through river water, primarily emitted from copper mines and refineres. In addition, the pollution in Kosaka (Akita Prefecture) was caused by atmospheric emissions from a copper mine and refinery. Clearly, it is necessary to study the possible involvement of metals other than cadmium.

The incidence of renal dysfunction has been claimed to be related to the degree of cadmium pollution in Akita, Toyama, Ishikawa, and Nagasaki Prefectures, where renal dysfunction was already acknowledged by the administrative survey, as discussed previously. A measure frequently used for quantifying exposure to cadmium pollution is the product of the cadmium concentration in rice and the duration of residence in the cadmium-polluted areas. However, the duration of residence is usually a function of age, and susceptibility to cadmium varies with age, as discussed later. In addition, cadmium in rice varies greatly from year to year, even among crops grown in the same cadmium-polluted rice paddy field, presumably because cadmium accumulation in rice is known to depend upon the oxygen content of the soil. It is, therefore, not correct to use the product of cadmium concentration in rice and duration of residence in the cadmium-polluted areas for estimation of Cd exposure. The following alternate exposure indexes are suggested: the average cadmium level in rice in the area for several years, or the urinary excretion of cadmium of individual persons. The mechanism of urinary excretion of cadmium is described later.

II. Mortality Study on Residents in Cadmium-Polluted Areas

The past mortality data involving 333,000 inhabitants of both cadmium-polluted and control areas in Akita, Miyagi, Toyama, and Nagasaki Prefectures were collected retrospectively for a period of 6–30 years, based on vital statistics or death certificates (Fig. 3). The standardized mortality ratios (SMR) from all causes and

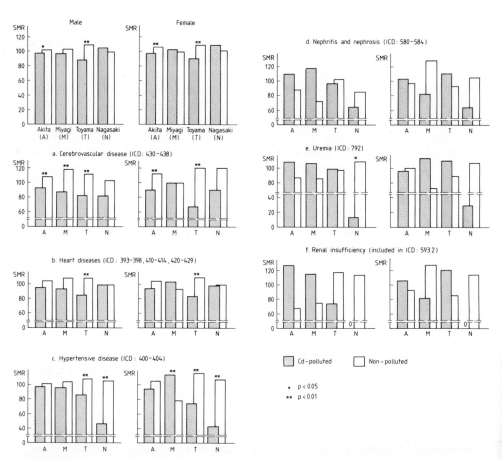

Fig. 3. Sex specified standard mortality ratios (SMR) in areas with or without cadmium pollution in Japan. (SHIGEMATSU et al. 1981 c)

from cardiovascular diseases such as cerebrovascular and hypertensive disease were even lower in cadmium-polluted than in control areas, while no distinct difference in SMR from renal diseases was found (SHIGEMATSU et al. 1982).

These findings agree well with a British report on cadmium workers where no excess death due to renal disease was observed (ARMSTRONG and KAZANTZIS 1983; SORAHAN 1982). Furthermore, even cadmium workers who showed cadmium-induced proteinura did not show excess deaths due to renal disease (HOLDEN 1980).

D. Skeletal Effects of Cadmium

I. Itai-Itai Disease

Itai-itai disease, as indicated already, was officially recognized as a cadmium-induced osteopathy in May 1968. The development of itai-itai disease begins after chronic cadmium poisoning has induced renal disturbance leading to renal osteomalacia. Apparently, factors such as pregnancy, nursing, changes in endocrine secretion, senility, and nutritional calcium deficiency were thought to contribute to the development of the disease (JAPAN MINISTRY OF HEALTH AND WELFARE 1968). Up to now the number of officially recognized itai-itai disease patients is 129.

However, no conclusive agreement has been reached on whether renal dysfunction precedes osteomalacia. Autopsy data on two cases of itai-itai disease prior to 1960 showed typical osteomalacia on histologic examination, but no renal tubular changes. After 1960, in six other itai-itai disease cases, osteomalacia accompanied by renal tubular changes was observed (KAJIKAWA et al. 1974). In addition, some clinical data before 1960 did not directly indicate the existence of significant renal dysfunction in itai-itai disease patients, even though patients suffered from osteomalacia (NAKAGAWA 1960).

II. Epidemiologic Studies on Residents in Cadmium-Polluted Areas

To follow up the clinical symptoms, 53 patients were admitted to hospitals for detailed health checks in 1975–1976. They were characterized by small physique and deformed spinal column and thorax, high incidence of peripheral nervous disturbance, normochromic anemia and granulocytosis with a tendency toward lymphocytopenia, moderate glomerular dysfunction as well as tubular dysfunction, and relatively low blood pressure; urinalysis indicated proteinuria, glycosuria, low molecular weight proteinuria, and a high amino acid level of over 280 mg/l. There was a fairly large urinary excretion of proline, related to bone metabolism. The average cadmium level in urine was low: 9.5 µg/l (24-h urine) and 11.3 µg/l (early morning urine) (SHINODA et al. 1977).

Because cadmium was thought to cause the osteomalacia of itai-itai disease, health examinations were performed on about 52,000 residents in cadmium-polluted areas: 4,900 (Gunma), 1,400 (Oita), 12,000 (Hyogo), 2,300 (Sizuoka), 440 (Nagasaki), 400 (Akita), 11,600 (Yamagata), 1,800 (Fukushima), 1,100 (Miyagi), 2,800 (Ishikawa), 6,700 (Fuchu, Toyama), 10,600 (Kurobe, Toyama), and 2,500

(Fukuoka). However, no itai-itai disease could be found in other than the Fuchu area. Some researchers reported that they succeeded in finding itai-itai disease in the Ichikawa river basin (Hyogo Prefecture), downstream from a copper mine and refinery (NOGAWA et al. 1975) and on Tsushima Island (Nagasaki Prefecture) close to a zinc mine (TAKEBAYASHI 1979). These cases indicated biochemical findings similar to those in recognized itai-itai disease cases. However, osteomalacia was not clinically observed in these residents (TSUCHIYA 1978).

III. Animal Experiments

The Japan Environment Agency sponsored long-term cadmium feeding experiments on monkeys. In the first study, 10 monkeys were fed for 1 year with pelleted food with a cadmium content of 0–300 µg/g as $CdCl_2$. Monkeys receiving 300 µg/g developed typical tubular dysfunction in 4 months, but showed no osseous changes after 1 year (NOMIYAMA et al. 1979 a). In the second experiment, 35 monkeys were fed pelleted food containing $CdCl_2$ at cadmium dose levels of 0–100 µg/g over a period of 7 years. Monkeys in the 100 µg/g group developed proximal tubular dysfunction 1 year after the cadmium feeding started. However, no osseous changes were detected in the following 6 years (AKAHORI et al. 1983). In the third experiment, 40 monkeys were fed with a synthetic diet deficient in calcium, phosphate, vitamin D, and protein, but with cadmium at a dose level of 30 µg/g. However, cadmium-induced renal dysfunction did not precede osteomalacia in these monkeys in 6 years of experiment (YOSHIKI et al. 1983).

IV. Discussion at the International Conference on Cadmium-Induced Osteopathy

In 1979, an International Conference on Cadmium-Induced Osteopathy considered the question whether cadmium induces osteomalacia or not. It was clearly demonstrated that renal tubular dysfunction was followed by osteomalacia in cadmium workers (SHIGEMATSU and NOMIYAMA 1979; KAZANTZIS 1979; ADAMS 1979; MAROUBY 1979). However, it was also pointed out that only a few workers with severe renal tubular dysfunction developed osteomalacia. Furthermore, it is quite difficult to induce renal tubular osteomalacia in animals by cadmium administration (KAWAI and KIMURA 1979; KAJIKAWA 1979; NOMIYAMA et al. 1979 b). Some researchers reported success in inducing renal osteomalacia (ITOKAWA 1979; NOGAWA 1979), but the interpretation of their results by other pathologists did not generally agree with this conclusion. The definition and diagnosis of renal osteomalacia was clearly a subject of controversy.

Vitamin D_3 is converted in the body to 25-OH-D_3 in the liver, and then to 1,25-$(OH)_2$-D_3 in mitochondria of renal proximal tubular cells. This 1,25-$(OH)_2$-D_3 is the biologically active vitamin D. Cadmium has been thought to bring on renal osteomalacia as follows: cadmium accumulates in the proximal tubular cells, depressing cellular function; this is followed by the depressed conversion of 25-OH-D_3 to 1,25-$(OH)_2$-D_3. Therefore, cadmium induces vitamin D deficiency, and subsequently osteomalacia. However, there are findings which contradict this

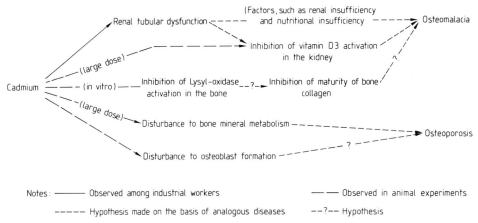

Fig. 4. Mechanism of skeletal effects of cadmium. (Japan Public Health Association 1976)

hypothesis: decreased nephron mass depresses vitamin D activation in the kidneys, but not so severely as to induce vitamin D deficiency. In addition, it has not been proven that acidosis, hypophosphatemia, and bicarbonate wasting in proximal tubular dysfunction induce osteomalacia. The etiology of osteomalacia cannot be elucidated without taking into consideration nutritional factors such as low calcium and vitamin D deficiency.

Recently, an animal experiment was reported which suggests that cadmium might disturb bone mineral metabolism directly, without the involvement of the kidneys; this may represent an effect on maturation of bone collagen (Japan Public Health Association 1976). The relationship between cadmium and bone changes is illustrated in Fig. 4. It must be emphasized that the interaction between the various factors may depend on the levels of exposure to cadmium, and these must always be considered.

E. Blood Pressure, Cerebrovascular Disease, and Heart Disease

I. Depressed Blood Pressure

Epidemiologic surveys have been performed on about 50,000 residents in cadmium-polluted areas in Japan. The incidence of hypertension among residents in cadmium-polluted areas such as Ishikawa, Nagasaki, and Oita Prefectures was lower than that among residents in nonpolluted areas (Fig. 5; Shigematsu et al. 1981 a). Systolic blood pressure of itai-itai disease patients has been reported to be depressed (Nogawa and Kohno 1969).

A monkey experiment (Akahori et al. 1984) supported the conclusions of the epidemiologic surveys. Monkeys fed cadmium at dose levels of 0–100 µg Cd per gram food over a period of 7 years showed no increased blood pressure at the higher dose levels, while it increased with age on a normal diet or with lower doses

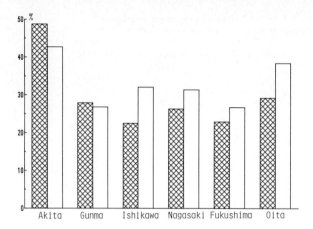

Fig. 5. Incidence of hypertension in areas with or without cadmium pollution in Japan. *Hatched* and *open bars* indicate cadmium-polluted and nonpolluted areas, respectively. (SHIGEMATSU et al. 1981 b)

of Cd. Plasma cholesterol and triglyceride were also lower in monkeys fed cadmium at higher dose levels than in monkeys at lower dose levels. This finding is contrary to those of many investigators, but agrees with the report of KOPP et al. (1982). However, such experiments have usually been performed over relatively short periods and with relatively high dose levels. Monkey data suggest that long-term and low-level exposure to cadmium may decrease blood pressure owing to depressed lipid metabolism. Long-term exposure experiments appear to be required to stimulate the effects of cadmium on blood pressure in humans.

II. Epidemiologic Studies on Mortality from Cerebrovascular Disease and Heart Disease

A retrospective mortality study in Japan revealed that the SMR from heart disease, hypertensive disease, and cerebrovascular disease among residents of cadmium-polluted areas were, in general, lower than in residents of nonpolluted areas (SHIGEMATSU et al. 1981 c). LEMEN et al. (1976) also clearly demonstrated the depressive effects of cadmium on mortality from heart disease among cadmium workers, but provided no further comment. The data of SORAHAN (1982) and HOLDEN (1980) also showed a depressed SMR from circulatory disease in nickel–cadmium battery workers heavily exposed to cadmium.

F. Recovery from Cadmium-Induced Health Effects

Cadmium taken up into the human body accumulates in the kidneys, the critical organ, and induces renal dysfunction. The biologic half-life of cadmium has been reported as 16–38 years in humans not specifically exposed to cadmium (TSU-CHIYA and SUGITA 1971; HAMMER and FINKLEA 1972), but the cadmium level in the kidneys decreased very little. Therefore, once cadmium-induced renal dysfunction occurs, it was believed to be essentially irreversible. PISCATOR (1966) reported that cadmium-induced proteinura could not be reversed and even appeared to be progressive.

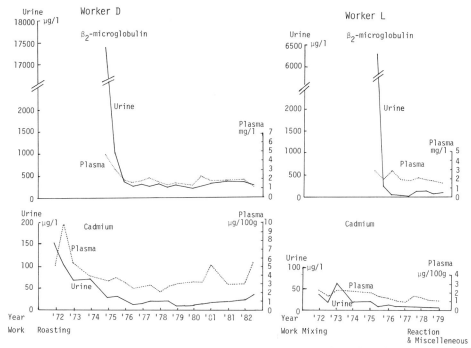

Fig. 6. Examples of dramatic recoveries from cadmium health effects in cadmium pigment workers by improving the working environment; worker D (46 years old) worked for 22 years, and worker L (38 years old) for 17 years. (SHIBUYA et al. 1984)

TSUCHIYA (1976) observed that proteinuria seen among cadmium workers decreased after cadmium exposure had ceased. Two other Japanese reports mentioned that cadmium-induced proteinuria was reversible (Fig. 6; OHMORI et al. 1984; SHIBUYA et al. 1984). The difference between the Swedish and Japanese findings may relate to the severity of cadmium health effects. When cadmium workers were exposed to cadmium at extremely high levels for a long period, even though they were suffering from cadmium-induced proteinuria, the cadmium effects might be irreversible. On the contrary, occupational health regulations in Japan demand that cadmium workers should be removed from cadmium exposure as soon as cadmium-induced proteinura is detected. As a result, the severity of cadmium health effects might have been quite different in Sweden and Japan. There is some support for this hypothesis from animal experiments. One group of rabbits was given cadmium only until slight proteinuria appeared, while another group of rabbits was given cadmium until renal effects became dominant. Cadmium-induced renal effects disappeared quickly in the first group of rabbits, while they were not reversed in the second group (NOMIYAMA and NOMIYAMA 1984a).

Low molecular weight proteinuria, such as β_2-microglobulinuria, in cadmium workers has been thought to be a precursor of severe renal disease. However, SHI-BUYA et al. (1984) clearly demonstrated that low molecular weight proteinuria did not develop into general proteinuria, but was readily reversed. HOLDEN (1980) also indicated in his mortality study that cadmium workers with proteinuria died of diseases other than renal diseases.

G. Chemical Forms of Cadmium in Food and Health Effects

Most cadmium taken up by humans is derived from food. However, the chemical forms of cadmium in food remain to be fully clarified. The cadmium concentration in vegetables is generally lower than that in animal products. Thus, cadmium in crops may amount to 0.1 ppm, while cadmium in liver of octopus or shellfish is 100–200 µg/g (ISHIZAKI et al. 1970).

Cadmium in contaminated rice is reported to bind with phytic acid and protein mainly located in the aleurone layer (SUZUKI et al. 1977), or with glutelin, and also to some extent with globulin (MINAGAWA 1978). Cadmium in soybean seems to bind with proteins of molecular weight 10,000, and also with compounds of molecular weight below 500 (CATALDO et al. 1981). Cadmium in mushrooms binds with mucoprotein of molecular weight 8,000 (MEISCH et al. 1983).

The chemical form of cadmium in oysters has not been fully elucidated. Binding does not apparently involve metallothionein, but proteins of molecular weight 40,000–50,000 containing relatively few sulfhydryl groups, but a high concentration of dicarboxylic amino acids (RIDLINGTON and FOWLER 1979). According to SHARMA (1983), 60% of cadmium in oysters bound to proteins of molecular weight 20,000, 34% to metallothionein, and 4% to low molecular weight substance (less than 2,000). Cadmium in other shellfish differs from that in oyster: it binds with glycoproteins of molecular weight of 8,000 and 13,000 (DOHI et al. 1983).

Intestinal absorption rates differ according to the chemical form of cadmium in food. Cadmium bound with glutelin is reported to be very little absorbed compared with cadmium chloride (KOHASHI 1978), while cadmium bound with glutenin is absorbed at almost the same rate as cadmium chloride (NOMIYAMA et al. 1979 c). Cadmium–metallothionein readily crosses the intestinal wall without breakdown and reaches the kidneys (CHERIAN et al. 1978).

New Zealand fishermen were reported to eat a large amount of oysters, which contained the highest level of cadmium observed in normal food, but they did not suffer from overt renal dysfunction (MCKENZIE et al. 1982). Perhaps the high level of zinc in oysters prevents cadmium-induced renal dysfunction; alternately, the intestinal absorption of oyster cadmium might be very slow.

H. Elevated Sensitivity to Cadmium

I. Aging

The incidence of renal dysfunction among residents in cadmium-polluted areas was higher in aged people than in younger people; this could be related to greater accumulation of cadmium in the kidneys, the critical organ, following the longer exposure to Cd. However, experiments revealed that old animals were more sus-

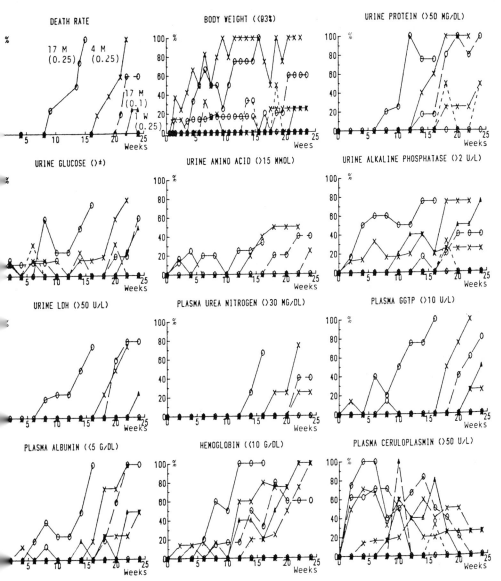

Fig. 7. Aging, an aggravating factor for chronic toxicity of cadmium. Rabbits of 1 week, 4 months, and 17 months old were given subcutaneous injections of cadmium chloride at cadmium dose levels of 0, 0.1, and 0.25 mg/kg six times a week over a period of 24 weeks. (Nomiyama et al. 1984b)

ceptible to cadmium intoxication and accumulated cadmium in the renal cortex more rapidly than younger animals (Fig. 7; Nomiyama et al. 1980a, 1984b). A depressed ability to synthesize metallothionein interfered with cadmium detoxification in the kidneys when aged animals were heavily exposed to cadmium (Nomiyama et al. 1984c).

II. Protein–Calorie Malnutrition

Environmental pollution with cadmium is likely to become a social concern in developing countries. In such countries, malnutrition often prevails among residents. However, acute toxicity of cadmium in rats was reported not to be aggravated, but possibly even reduced by protein malnutrition (Nomiyama and Nomiyama 1984 b).

III. Environmental Temperature

Environmental temperature was found to modify acute toxicity of cadmium: mice were acclimatized to 8 °, 22 °, and 38 °C for 3 weeks, and then they were given cadmium intraperitoneally or orally. Toxicity of cadmium was enhanced in both cold and hot environments, but more so in the cold (Nomiyama et al. 1980 b).

Exposure to cadmium for 8 months at various dose levels in mice acclimatized to 8 °, 22 °, and 38 °C revealed that at higher environmental temperature less cadmium accumulated in the kidneys and the critical concentration of cadmium was lower. In the hot environment, there was also greater loss of body weight and proteinuria was more readily produced than at lower temperatures (Nomiyama et al. 1978).

IV. Combination of Hot Environment and Protein–Calorie Malnutrition

Rats were acclimatized to a hot environment as well as to protein–calorie malnutrition, and then they were administered organic solvents or heavy metals. The

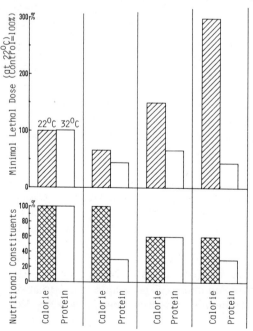

Fig. 8. Combined effects of high temperature and malnutrition on minimal lethal dose of cadmium chloride intraperitoneally given to rats. (Nomiyama and Nomiyama 1984 c)

combination of hot environment and protein–calorie malnutrition enhanced acute toxicity of cadmium, regardless of the fact that protein–calorie malnutrition per se decreases toxicity of cadmium (Fig. 8; NOMIYAMA and NOMIYAMA 1984c). It follows that inhabitants of tropical underdeveloped countries may be at special risk with regard to cadmium pollution.

J. Metal Shift in Cadmium Intoxication

Cadmium from the environment enters the body through the lungs and intestines. Then cadmium is transported into the blood and first accumulates in the liver where it induces synthesis of metallothionein (Fig. 9). The induced metallothionein detoxifies cadmium by binding it (KAGI and NORDBERG 1979). However, when excessive cadmium enters the body, metallothionein induction is insufficient to detoxify it all, and liver dysfunction is produced by cadmium not bound to metallothionein (non-MT-Cd). Cadmium–metallothionein may leak from damaged hepatic cells into the blood (TANAKA et al. 1981). Cadmium in the blood, mostly cadmium–metallothionein, does not enter erythrocytes, but is directly distributed to the kidneys (NOMIYAMA 1977b), where it is freely filtered at the glomeruli. Filtered Cd–metallothionein is reabsorbed by proximal tubule cells by an easily saturable and another nonsaturable transport mechanism (NOMIYAMA and FOULKES 1977). In the tubular cells, cadmium–metallothionein is catabolized to cadmium and protein. The cadmium set free induces metallothionein production and this induced metallothionein again detoxifies the Cd.

This represents the generally accepted view of Cd–metallothionein. It implies that renal dysfunction is caused by non-MT-Cd. The critical concentration of non-MT-Cd in the renal cortex was estimated at 35 µg Cd per gram wet weight in rabbits and monkeys given cadmium for long periods (NOMIYAMA and NOMIYAMA 1982; NOMIYAMA et al. 1982b). Because the biologic half-life of cadmium-induced metallothionein is only 3 days, depressed induction of metallothionein synthesis in cadmium-damaged kidneys results in the release of cadmium from the kidneys. In addition, the decreased reabsorption of metallothionein at the tubuli may result in the elevated urinary excretion of cadmium–metallothionein.

On the other hand, cadmium taken into the human body elevates plasma and tissue zinc and copper (SUZUKI 1981; NOMIYAMA and NOMIYAMA 1982; NOMIYAMA and NOMIYAMA 1983b). These heavy metals also induce production of metal enzymes and metallothionein in tissues (NOMIYAMA and NOMIYAMA 1983a, b). Excess cadmium in liver depresses hepatic function (NOMIYAMA and NOMIYAMA 1982, 1983a, 1984a; NOMIYAMA et al. 1980a, 1982b) and results in decreased production of metal enzymes and metallothionein. In advanced stage of cadmium intoxication, intestinal absorption of zinc and copper may be depressed owing to cadmium-induced enteropathy (MURATA et al. 1970), and hepatic and renal zinc and copper decrease rapidly (NOMIYAMA and NOMIYAMA 1982, 1983b; NOMIYAMA et al. 1981a, 1982b) to result in copper deficiency anemia (NOMIYAMA and NOMIYAMA 1983b). Intravenous administration of copper prevented or delayed cadmium-induced renal and hepatic dysfunction as well as anemia (Fig. 10; NOMIYAMA and NOMIYAMA 1983c).

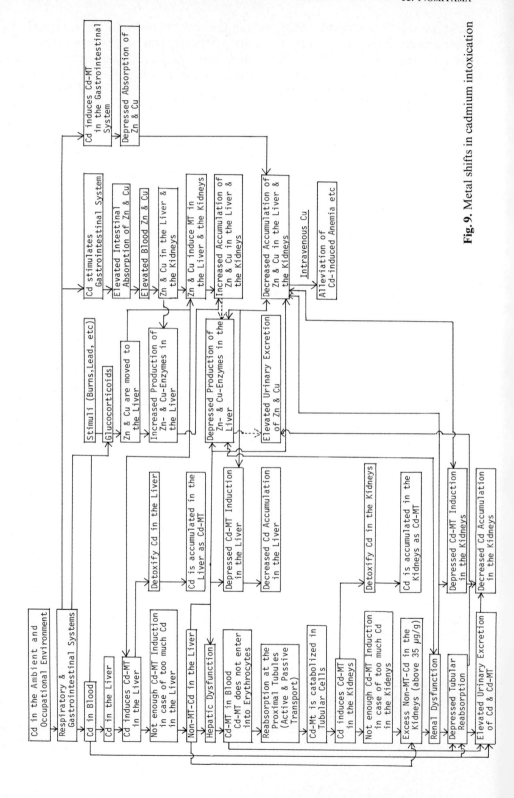

Fig. 9. Metal shifts in cadmium intoxication

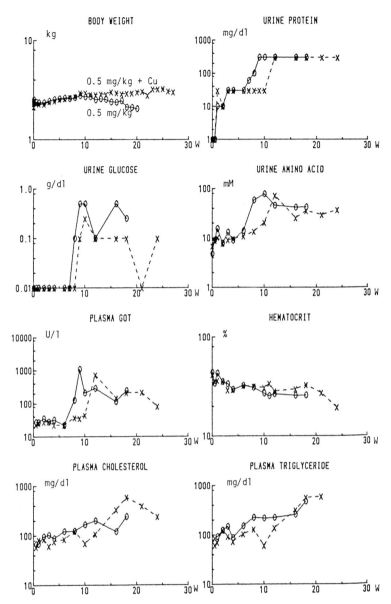

Fig. 10. Preventive effect of intravenous injections of copper acetate on cadmium health effects in rabbits. (NOMIYAMA and NOMIYAMA 1983c)

K. Biologic Monitoring of Cadmium Exposure

I. Urinary Cadmium

FRIBERG et al. (1972) stated in their review that urinary excretion of cadmium is only 1% of the daily absorbed dose, and that there will be a gradual but pronounced increase in urinary excretion when renal dysfunction occurs. It follows that determination of urinary cadmium could not serve as a biologic monitor of cadmium exposure, but would rather reflect renal dysfunction resulting from exposure. After renal dysfunction occurs, a sharp increase in urinary excretion of cadmium has been observed in mice (NORDBERG 1972), rats (FUKUSHIMA and KO-BAYASHI 1974; GOYER et al. 1978; SUZUKI 1980), and rabbits (FRIBERG 1952). After the appearance of renal damage, no further elevation in urinary excretion of cadmium was reported (AXELSSON and PISCATOR 1966; SUZUKI 1980).

However, some questions have been raised about the model of FRIBERG et al. (1972). Thus, cadmium clearance is proportional to cadmium concentration in the renal cortex, and no elevated cadmium clearance was observed in rabbits with uranium-induced renal dysfunction (Fig. 11; NOMIYAMA and NOMIYAMA 1976 a); the latter resembles cadmium nephropathy (NOMIYAMA et al. 1982 a). In addition, uranium-induced nephropathy did not elevate urinary excretion of cadmium in rabbits previously fully loaded with cadmium, nor reduce cadmium in the renal cortex (Fig. 12; NOMIYAMA and NOMIYAMA 1976 a). These results suggest that a significantly elevated urinary excretion of cadmium is not solely related to renal dysfunction.

NORDBERG (1972) found that urinary excretion of cadmium was correlated with the dose of cadmium in repeated injection experiments on mice. Similar re-

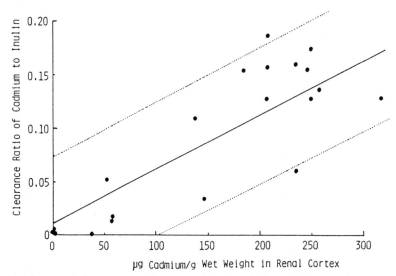

Fig. 11. Relationship between the clearance ratio of cadmium to inulin and the renal cadmium level in 20 rabbits given successive subcutaneous injections of cadmium. *Full* and *broken lines* represent the correlation line and the confidence limits at 95% level, respectively. (NOMIYAMA and NOMIYAMA 1976 a)

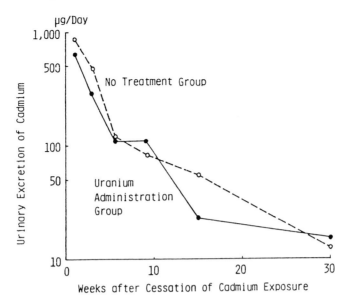

Fig. 12. Effect of uranium administration on urinary excretion of cadmium. Uranium was given intravenously at certain intervals after cessation of subcutaneous cadmium injection of 1.5 mg/kg^{-1} day^{-1} for 21 days. (NOMIYAMA and NOMIYAMA 1976 a)

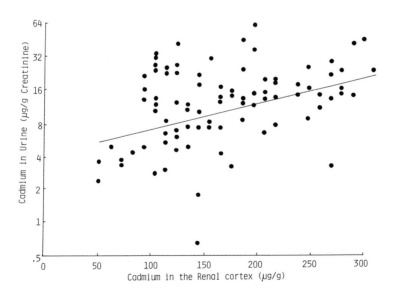

Fig. 13. Relationship between cadmium in urine and the renal cortex of cadmium workers. Cadmium in the renal cortex was determined by prompt gamma-ray neutron activation analysis. (ROELS et al. 1981)

sults have been reported with rabbits given cadmium by subcutaneous injections (Nomiyama 1973; Nomiyama and Nomiyama 1976 b), oral administration (No- miyama and Nomiyama 1974, 1976 c), and with monkeys fed cadmium (No- miyama et al. 1979 a, 1981 a). The increase in urinary excretion of cadmium paral- lels that of cadmium in the renal cortex (Nomiyama and Nomiyama 1976 a; Su- zuki 1980). Some reports indicated no increase in urinary excretion of cadmium in animals chronically exposed to cadmium prior to the appearance of renal dys- function. This may be due to a poor detection limit for cadmium in urine. Roels et al. (1981) and Ellis et al. (1984) later correlated the cadmium in the renal cor- tex, liver, blood, and urine in cadmium workers by γ-ray activation analysis, and proved that urine cadmium correlated quite well with renal and hepatic cadmium (Fig. 13). Urinary excretion of cadmium is, therefore, now believed to be a good biologic monitoring parameter for the body burden of cadmium, at least before significant renal dysfunction appears.

II. In Vivo Determination of Organ Cadmium

In the last 10 years, estimation of body or organ burden in vivo has become pos- sible with the aid of neutron activation analysis. Details of this technique are dis- cussed in Chap. 1. This technique is very useful for the biologic monitoring of cad- mium in humans. Its detection limit is around 5 mg, and it has now also been ap- plied to animals given cadmium (Nomiyama et al. 1984 a). An important variable may be the depth of the kidneys (Fletcher et al. 1982); care must therefore be taken when discussing the critical concentration of cadmium in the renal cortex on the basis of neutron activation analysis. The alternate use of X-ray fluores- cence analysis to determine cadmium in vivo (Alhlgren and Mattsson 1981; Christoffersson and Mattsson 1983) is also not yet fully reliable because of the deep location of the liver and kidneys in the body.

L. Estimation of Allowable Intake of Cadmium

The body burden of metal is related to its health effects. Therefore, it is important to estimate the metals at early stages of exposure. The body burden of metals is, in general, calculated as follows

$$q = \frac{I \cdot a \cdot t_{1/2}}{\log 2},$$

where, q, I, a, and $t_{1/2}$ stand for body burden, daily intake of metal, fractional absorption, and biologic half-life. With this equation, the allowable intake of cad- mium might be estimated, given values for critical body burden (or critical con- centration of cadmium in the renal cortex, the critical organ), absorption rate, and biologic half-life of cadmium (in the renal cortex). The following discussion considers whether and how parameters for the critical concentration and the bio- logic half-life of cadmium in the renal cortex can be estimated.

I. Biologic Half-Life of Cadmium in the Renal Cortex

Most metals exhibit a characteristic biologic half-life. For cadmium a biologic half-life of 16–38 years was deduced from analysis of cadavers from accidental death (Tsuchiya and Sugita 1971; Hammer and Finklee 1972). Estimates of the biologic half-life available to date vary greatly according to animal species. Estimates range from several weeks in mice to 22 years in monkeys (Nomiyama and Nomiyama 1979; Nomiyama et al. 1979 a). However, the biologic half-life of cadmium in the renal cortex was found to be shorter in animals given cadmium in large doses, even before renal dysfunction appeared. This was observed in mice (Nomiyama et al. 1977), rabbits (Nomiyama 1976; Nomiyama and Nomiyama 1976 d), and monkeys (Nomiyama et al. 1979 a, 1981 b). The biologic half-life of cadmium in the liver of cadmium workers is also shorter in the case of heavy exposure to cadmium (Fig. 14; Fletcher et al. 1982). Data of Ellis et al. (1984) also suggest that the biologic half-life in cadmium workers is around 5 years, which is far shorter than in individuals not excessively exposed to cadmium. There is only one report in which increased half-life of cadmium was found with increased dose (Engstrom and Nordberg 1979). The biologic half-life of cadmium also differs with sex and age (Taguchi and Suzuki 1981).

A single exposure to cadmium, furthermore, led to a steady increase in cadmium in the renal cortex, the critical organ, over a period of 24 months (Kawai and Kimura 1975). It is difficult to assign a fixed biologic half-life to cadmium; the large variations may be related to differences in the production of metallothionein.

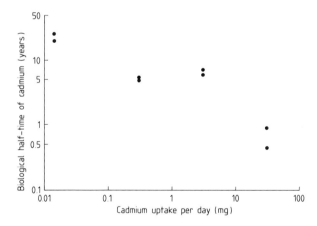

Fig. 14. Shortened biologic half-life of cadmium in the renal cortex by increasing the dose of cadmium, even before renal dysfunction appeared in monkeys fed cadmium over a period of 1 year. (Nomiyama and Nomiyama 1979)

II. Critical Concentration of Cadmium in the Renal Cortex

After a long-term exposure to cadmium, cadmium taken into the human body accumulates in the liver and the kidneys. When cadmium in the renal cortex exceeds a certain concentration, renal tubular dysfunction such as proteinuria, glycosuria, and aminoaciduria appear. This cadmium concentration is referred to as the critical concentration in the renal cortex (Task Group on Metal Toxicology 1976). Knowledge of the critical concentration is required to permit estimation of the allowable concentration of cadmium in the environment or in the diet. Efforts have therefore been focused on determination of the critical concentration of cadmium in the renal cortex of humans and animals.

The critical concentration of cadmium in human renal cortex was discussed officially by the TASK GROUP ON METAL TOXICOLOGY (1976) and by the WHO TASK GROUP (1977). It was estimated as being about 200 μg Cd per gram wet weight (ranging from 100 to 300 μg/g), based on 20 autopsy and biopsy cases of cadmium workers and 8 autopsy cases of inhabitants of cadmium-polluted areas in Japan (WHO TASK GROUP 1977). However, NOMIYAMA (1977a) criticized this estimate, because the proposed value of 200 μg/g was arbitrarily chosen on the basis of a limited number of cases and in spite of large variation of the data.

Recently, prompt gamma-ray neutron activation analysis has made it possible to determine in vivo cadmium in the human renal cortex (HARVEY et al. 1975; VARTESKY et al. 1977). ROELS et al. (1981) and ELLIS et al. (1981) thus measured in vivo cadmium in the kidneys of cadmium workers and claimed that the critical concentrations of this element were 210 and 260 μg/g using β_2-microglobulinuria, respectively. As end point, values of 300–400 μg/g were proposed. This estimate was subsequently corrected to 210 μg/g (ROELS et al. 1981) and 350 μg/g (FLETCHER et al. 1982) on the basis of proper allowance for the depth of the kidneys.

In addition, ROELS et al. (1981) and ELLIS et al. (1981) dealt with the critical concentration of cadmium by correlating liver with kidney cadmium, and then with renal dysfunction parameters, based on a single cross-sectional determination of organ cadmium in cadmium workers. The criticism of these estimates has been raised that the critical concentration should be primarily estimated on the basis of time-dependent dose–response data from many workers or inhabitants in cadmium-polluted areas, rather than on a single cross-sectional dose–response analysis. Probably because of this, a considerable variation is seen in these data, and it is difficult to arrive at a firm estimate of the critical concentration of cadmium in the renal cortex in this manner.

Although renal cadmium did not correlate with hepatic cadmium, a correlation line was drawn. The authors discriminated between workers with and without renal dysfunction on the graphs, and estimated the critical concentration of cadmium in liver and kidney. The age of the workers was not considered. ELLIS et al. (1984) clearly demonstrated, as shown in Table 2, that cadmium in the kidneys and the liver reached a maximum after 5–15 years of exposure, but that slight renal dysfunction appeared only at a later stage; significant renal dysfunction was seen only after 20 years. It follows that cadmium can reach its maximum concentration in the renal cortex without any immediate signs of renal dysfunction. In addition, cadmium workers with longer duration of cadmium exposure were older than cadmium workers with shorter duration of exposure. Therefore, a major factor in the production of these renal signs might have been aging. This hypothesis is supported by the data on noncadmium production workers in whom kidney cadmium exceeded 32 mg without concomitant renal dysfunction. On the other hand, retired workers who had not been exposed to cadmium (probably older men) had less cadmium in kidneys and liver, but showed significant renal dysfunction. As was discussed in Sect. H.I, aging elevates the susceptibility to cad-

Table 2. Mean values for kidney cadmium, liver cadmium, urinary β_2-microglobulin, and urinary total protein for industrial workers and controls. (ELLIS et al. 1984)

Exposure group	Expo-sure (years)[c]	No. of sub-jects	Kidney Cd (mg)	Liver Cd (ppm)	Urinary excretion β_2 (µg/liter)	Protein (mg/24 h)
Cadmium production						
Active workers	< 1	8	5.0 (1.7)[a]	3.5 (2.8)[a]	93 ± 78[b]	275 ± 50[b]
	1– 5	2	16.7 (1.1)	10.7 (1.2)	123 ± 51	150 ± 71
	5–10	2	30.2 (1.2)	34.2 (1.3)	31 ± 24	238 ± 88
	10–15	9	24.9 (1.9)	38.5 2.0)	70 ± 36	271 ± 138
	15–20	8	24.5 (1.7)	39.6 (2.1)	376 ± 369	417 ± 240
	> 20	11	23.9 (1.7)	35.1 (2.2)	5,192 ± 11,015	500 ± 237
Retired workers[c]	< 5	12	25.8 (1.6)	43.8 (3.1)	9,078 ± 21,675	1,457 ± 1,377
	5–10	7	13.7 (1.7)	29.4 (2.5)	43,192 ± 40,749	1,280 ± 1,228
	> 10	2	10.6 (5.2)	13.5 (1.5)	5,156 ± 6,466	567 ± 345
Noncadmium production						
Active workers	15	3	32.5 (2.0)	46.4 (1.4)	62 ± 42	300 ± 100
Retired workers	20	6	14.4 (1.5)	34.4 (1.5)	10,940 ± 9,064	233 ± 58
Office, managements, labs						
Active workers	1–25	8	5.2 (1.5)	7.5 (1.7)	182 ± 207	200 ± 89
Retired workers	1–20	4	6.9 (1.5)	5.7 (1.5)	180 ± 150	350 ± 129
Controls						
Smokers		30	4.4 (2.2)	2.8 (2.2)	92 ± 105	178 ± 109
Nonsmokers		17	6.7 (1.5)	3.8 (1.7)	99 ± 119	
		13	2.6 (2.3)	1.9 (2.5)	85 ± 91	

[a] Geometric mean (geometric standard deviation) values for log-normal distribution
[b] Arithmetic mean ± arithmetic standard deviation for normal distribution
[c] All retired workers had been employed at least 15 years. The values given in the table for the retired workers are the number of years of retirement

mium. Therefore, age must be considered when the critical concentration of cadmium is discussed.

ROELS et al. (1981) estimated the critical concentration of the saturation value of renal cadmium. However, renal cadmium can reach a maximum at different levels, depending on the age of the host and the dose level of cadmium. Therefore, the saturation value is not a good basis upon which to estimate the critical concentration at which cadmium-induced renal dysfunction appears. Finally, the critical concentrations of cadmium calculated by ROELS et al. (1981) and ELLIS et al. (1981, 1984) cannot easily be compared because different levels of urinary β_2-microglobulin were used as end point.

Animal experimentation provides another approach to the question of the critical concentration of cadmium. Cadmium was given to experimental animals such as mice, rats, rabbits, or monkeys at various dose levels for long periods. Data so far available (Table 3) indicate that the critical concentration lies between 200 and 300 µg/g in mice, rats, and rabbits, while it is much higher in monkeys (NOMIYAMA and NOMIYAMA 1979).

Table 3. Critical concentrations of cadmium in various animals. (NOMIYAMA 1981b and references therein)

Animal species	Index medium	Cadmium (µg/g)	Animal species	Index medium	Cadmium (µg/g)
Mouse	Proteinuria	250	Rabbit	Aminoaciduria	200
		225			230
	Glycosuria	225			300
Rat	Proteinuria	225		Enzymuria	117
		234			200
		255		Decreased tubular	250
	Enzymuria	135		function	238
		300		Pathologic change	250
	Pathologic change	400			250
		300			200
		56	Monkey	Proteinuria	450
Rabbit	Proteinuria	450–1,050			610
		142		Low molecular	380
		300		weihgt proteinuria	
		230		Glycosuria	450
		300			610
	Low molecular	300		Aminoaciduria	450
	weight proteinuria				610
	Glycosuria	117		Pathologic change	300–465
		300			
		300			

The difficulty of determining critical levels of Cd may be illustrated by recent findings of NOMIYAMA et al. (1984d): 35 male rhesus monkeys were given pelleted food containing cadmium chloride at cadmium dose levels of 0, 3, 10, 30, and 100 µg/g over a period of 5 years (Fig. 15). In the 100 µg/g group, cadmium in the renal cortex increased rapidly, reaching the maximum at the 79th week, and then decreased. Slight and occasional proteinuria and glycosuria appeared in the 16th week; persistent proteinuria, glycosuria, decreased creatinine clearance, and tubular reabsorption of phosphorus in the 49th week; aminoaciduria appeared after the 161st week. From this data, the critical concentration of cadmium in the renal cortex of the 100 µg/g group was estimated at 680 µg/g (NOMIYAMA et al. 1982b). However, cadmium in the renal cortex of the 10 and 30 µg/g groups increased to 1,200 µg/g without any renal dysfunction. This suggests that no unique critical concentration of cadmium in the renal cortex may exist. Furthermore, it is known that the critical concentration varies with environmental temperature (NOMIYAMA and NOMIYAMA 1979) or the dose level of cadmium (NOMIYAMA et al. 1979a, 1981b).

Because metallothionein detoxifies tissue cadmium, only cadmium not bound to metallothionein (non-MT-Cd) may cause nephropathy in animals and humans exposed to cadmium (NOMIYAMA and NOMIYAMA 1984d). Renal dysfunction appeared in rabbits and monkeys exposed to cadmium for a long period when non-MT-Cd in the renal cortex was elevated to reach a cadmium concentration of 35–60 µg/g (NOMIYAMA and NOMIYAMA 1982; NOMIYAMA et al. 1982b, 1984d). Fur-

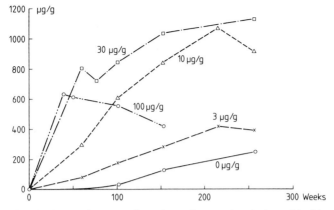

Fig. 15. Cadmium in the renal cortex of monkeys given oral cadmium chloride at dose levels of 0, 3, 10, 30, and 100 µg Cd per gram food over a period of 5 years. (NOMIYAMA et al. 1984 d)

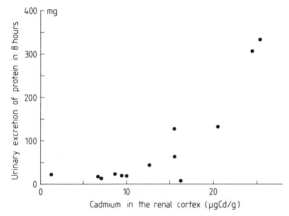

Fig. 16. Relationship of urinary excretion of protein and cadmium in the renal cortex of 13 rabbits given a single intravenous injection of cadmium chloride at various dose levels simultaneously with excess mercaptoethanol, 8 h after cadmium injection. (NOMIYAMA and NOMIYAMA 1984 d)

thermore, the critical concentration of non-MT-Cd in rabbit renal cortex was studied by exposing renal tubular cells to non-MT-Cd in vivo (Fig. 16; NOMIYAMA and NOMIYAMA 1984 d). Rabbits were given cadmium chloride at various dose levels with excessive mercaptoethanol to prevent cadmium from binding to plasma proteins and to enable cadmium to be freely filtered at the glomeruli. Urinary excretion of protein in 8 h after cadmium administration was slightly elevated when the renal cadmium level exceeded 10 µg/g and became significantly elevated when cadmium exceeded 20 µg/g. This result suggests a possible critical concentration of non-MT-Cd in the renal cortex of around 10 µg/g for subclinical intoxication and 20 µg/g for overt renal dysfunction. Non-MT-Cd levels in human renal cortex have not been determined.

In conclusion, the maximum permissible daily intake of cadmium needs to be determined on the basis of epidemiologic data on cadmium workers and residents in cadmium-polluted areas, rather than being estimated with the aid of a mathematical model such as that of KJELLSTRÖM(1974), using uncertain data on intestinal absorption of cadmium, its critical concentration, and its biologic half-life in the renal cortex.

References

Adams RG (1979) Osteopathy associated with tubular nephropathy in employees in an alkaline battery factory. In: Shigematsu I, Nomiyama K (eds) Cadmium-induced osteopathy. Japan Public Health Association, Tokyo, pp 66–73

Ahlgren L, Mattsson S (1981) Cadmium in man measured in vivo by x-ray fluorescence analysis. Phys Med Biol 26:19–26

Akahori F, Nomiyama K, Masaoka T, Nomiyama H, Nomura Y, Kobayashi K, Suzuki T (1983) Experimental studies on chronic effects of cadmium on monkeys. Kankyo Hoken Rep 49:1–27

Akahori F, Masaoka T, Nomiyama K, Nomiyama H, Nomura Y, Kobayashi K, Suzuki T (1984) Health effects of dietary cadmium on monkeys. Kankyo Hoken Rep 50: 1–26

Armstrong BG, Kazantzis G (1983) The mortality of cadmium workers. Lancet 1:1424–1427

Axelsson B, Piscator M (1966) Renal damage after prolonged exposure to cadmium, an experimental study. Arch Environ Health 12:360–373

Cataldo DA, Garland TR, Wildung RE (1981) Cadmium distribution and chemical fate in soybean plants. Plant Physiol 68:835–839

Cherian MG, Goyer RA, Valverg LS (1978) Gastrointestinal absorption and organ distribution of oral cadmium chloride and cadmium-metallothionein in mice. J Toxicol Environ Health 4:861–868

Christoffersson J-O, Mattsson S (1983) Polarised x-rays in XRF-analysis for improved in vivo detectability of cadmium in man. Phys Med Biol 28:1135–1144

Dohi Y, Ohba K, Yoneyama Y (1983) Purification and molecular properties of two cadmium-binding glycoproteins from the hepatopancreas of a whelk. *Buccinum tenuissimum*. Biochim Biophys Acta 745:50–60

Ellis KJ, Morgan WD, Zanzi I, Yasumura S, Vartesky D, Cohn SH (1981) Critical concentration of cadmium in human renal cortex: dose-effect studies in cadmium smelter workers. J Toxicol Environ Health 7:691–703

Ellis KJ, Yuen K, Yasumura S, Cohn SH (1984) Dose-response analysis of cadmium in man: body burden vs kidney dysfunction. Environ Res 33:216–226

Engstrom B, Nordberg GF (1979) Dose dependence of gastrointestinal absorption and biological half-time of cadmium in mice. Toxicology 13:215–222

Fletcher JG, Chettle DR, Al-Haddad IK, Harvey TC, Roels H, Buchet A, Berdnard A, Lauwerys R (1982) In vivo measurement of liver and kidney cadmium: estimate of critical levels. Cadmium 81. Proc 3rd Int Cadmium Conf. Miami, Cadmium Assoc, London, pp 157–160

Friberg L (1952) Further investigations on chronic cadmium poisoning; a study on rabbits with radioactive cadmium. AMA Arch Ind Hyg Occup Med 5:30–36

Friberg L, Piscator M, Nordberg GF, Kjellstrom T (1972) Cadmium in the environment. CRC Press, Cleveland

Fukushima M, Kobayashi E (1974) Urinary excretion of cadmium after its administration in female rats. Jpn J Ind Health 16:91–97

Goyer RG, Cherian MG, Richardson LD (1978) Renal effects of cadmium. Cadmium 77. Proc 1st Int Cadmium Conf San Francisco. Cadmium Assoc, London, pp 183–185

Hammer DI, Finklea JF (1972) Cadmium body burdens at autopsy in the United States. 17th Int Congress Occup Health

Harvey TC, McLellan JS, Thomas BJ, Fremlin JH (1975) Measurement of liver-cadmium concentrations in patients and industrial workers by neutron-activation analysis. Lancet 1:1269–1272

Holden H (1980) A mortality study of workers exposed to cadmium fumes. Cadmium 79. Edited Proc Int Cadmium Conference Miami. Cadmium Assoc, London, pp 211–215

Ishizaki A, Fukushima M, Sakamoto M (1970) Distribution of cadmium in biological materials. Part 2. Cadmium and zinc contents of foodstuffs. Jpn J Hyg 25:207–222

Itokawa I (1979) Histological and biochemical studies on bone changes in cadmium poisoned rats. In: Shigematsu I, Nomiyama K (eds) Cadmium-induced osteopathy. Japan Public Health Association, Tokyo, pp 21–29

Japan Ministry of Health and Welfare (1968) Etiology of Itai-Itai disease. May 8, 1968

Japan Public Health Association (1976) Effects of cadmium on human, a review study mainly performed in Japan. Japan Public Health Association, Tokyo

Kagi JHR, Nordberg M (eds) (1979) Metallothionein. Birkhäuser, Basel

Kajikawa K (1979) The effects of cadmium on the kidney and bone of rats. In: Shigematsu I, Nomiyama K (eds) Cadmium-induced osteopathy. Japan Public Health Association, Tokyo, pp 48–50

Kajikawa K, Kitagawa M, Nakanishi I (1974) A pathological study of "Itai-Itai disease". Med J Kanazawa Univ 83:309–347

Kawai K, Kimura M (1975) Renal lesion after single injection of cadmium. Ind Health 13:261–265

Kawai K, Kimura M (1979) A note on bone changes due to cadmium – comparison of two long-term oral administrations –. In: Shigematsu I, Nomiyama K (eds) Cadmium-induced osteopathy. Japan Public Health Association, Tokyo, pp 43–47

Kazantzis G (1979) Renal tubular dysfunction and osteopathy in cadmium workers. In: Shigematsu I, Nomiyama K (eds) Cadmium-induced osteopathy. Japan Public Health Association, Tokyo, pp 60–65

Kjellstrom Y (1974) Theoretical models of uptake and retention of cadmium in human beings. In: Friberg L et al. (eds) Cadmium in the environment. CRC Press, Cleveland, pp 79–86

Kohashi K (1978) Chemical forms of cadmium in rice. 1977 Report to Japan Environ Agency

Kopp SJ, Glonek T, Perry M Jr, Erlanger M, Perry EF (1982) Cardiovascular actions of cadmium at environmental exposure levels. Science 217:837–839

Lauwerys R, Roels H, Berdnard A, Buchet JP (1980) Renal response to cadmium in a nonferrous smelter area in Belgium. Int Arch Occup Environ Health 45:271–274

Lemen RA, Lee JS, Wagoner JK, Blejer HP (1976) Cancer mortality among cadmium production workers. Ann NY Acad Sci 271:273–279

Marouby J (1979) Osteopathy in cadmium workers in France. In: Shigematsu I, Nomiyama K (eds) Cadmium-induced osteopathy. Japan Public Health Association, Tokyo, pp 74–77

McKenzie JM, Kjellstrom T, Sharma RP (1982) Cadmium intake, metabolism and effects in people with a high intake of oyster in New Zealand. Report to US Enciron Protec Agency

Meisch HU, Beckman I, Schmitt JA (1983) A new cadmium-binding phosphoglycoprotein, cadmium-mycophosphophatin, from the mushroom, *Agaricus macroporus*. Biochim Biophys Acta 745:259–266

Minagawa K (1978) Chemical form of heavy metals in cadmium-polluted rice. Jpn J Public Health 25:97–102

Murata I, Hirono T, Saeki Y, Nakagawa S (1970) Cadmium enteropathy, renal osteomalacia ("Itai Itai" disease in Japan). Bull Soc Inter Chir 2:34–42

Nakagawa S (1960) A study of osteomalacia in Toyama prefecture (So-called Itai-Itai disease). Med J Kanazawa Univ 56:1–51

Nogawa K (1979) Comparison of bone lesions in chronic cadmium poisoning and vitamin D deficiency – an experimental study. In: Shigematsu I, Nomiyama K (eds) Cadmium-induced osteopathy. Japan Public Health Association, Tokyo, pp 30–42

Nogawa K, Kohno S (1969) A survey on the blood pressure of women suspected of "Itai-Itai" disease. Med J Kanazawa Univ 77:357–363

Nogawa K, Ishizaki A, Fukushima M, Shibata I, Hagino N (1975) Studies on the women with acquired Fanconi syndrome observed in the Ichi River basin polluted with cadmium. Environ Res 10:280–307

Nomiyama K (1973) Mechanism and diagnosis of cadmium poisoning. Kankyo Hoken Rep 24:11–15

Nomiyama K (1976) Critical concentration of cadmium in human renal cortex and biological half-time of cadmium. Kankyo Hoken 36:62–66

Nomiyama K (1977a) Does a critical concentration of cadmium in human renal cortex exist? J Toxicol Environ Health 3:607–609

Nomiyama K (1977b) Metallothionein dynamics in rabbits. Kankyo Hoken Rep 41:22–28

Nomiyama K (1981a) "Kogai", environmental pollution and the related public nuisance. Public Health. The Taniguchi Foundation, Tokyo, pp 82–98

Nomiyama K (1981b) Renal effects of cadmium. In: Nriagu JO (ed) Cadmium in the environment. Wiley, New York, pp 643–689

Nomiyama K, Foulkes EC (1977) Renal absorption of filtered cadmium-thionein in rabbits. Proc Exp Biol Med 156:97–99

Nomiyama K, Nomiyama H (1974) Urinary and fecal excretion of cadmium in rabbits. Kankyo Hoken Rep 31:53–59

Nomiyama K, Nomiyama H (1976a) Mechanism of urinary excretion of cadmium; experimental study. In: Nordberg G (ed) Effects and dose response relationships of toxic metals. Elsevier, Amsterdam, pp 371–379

Nomiyama K, Nomiyama H (1976b) Metabolism of cadmium and mechanism of cadmium poisoning. Kankyo Hoken Rep 31:53–59

Nomiyama K, Nomiyama H (1976c) Long-term feeding experiment on rabbits with 300 ppm cadmium – Intermediate report at 12th month. Kankyo Hoken Rep 38:161–163

Nomiyama K, Nomiyama H (1976d) Biological half time of cadmium in rabbits. Kankyo Hoken Rep 38:156–158

Nomiyama K, Nomiyama H (1979) Factors modifying critical concentration and biological half-time of cadmium. Arh Hig Rada Toksikol [Suppl] 30:191–200

Nomiyama K, Nomiyama H (1982) Tissue metallothionein in rabbits chronically exposed to cadmium, with special reference to the critical concentration of cadmium in the renal cortex. In: Foulkes EC (ed) Biological roles of metallothionein. Elsevier, New York, pp 47–67

Nomiyama K, Nomiyama H (1983a) Dose-effect relationship for cadmium in rabbits. Jpn J Hyg 38:250

Nomiyama H, Nomiyama K (1983b) Dose-effect relationship for plasma, urine and tissue cadmium, copper and zinc in rabbits given cadmium. Proc 56th Ann Meeting of Japan Industr Hyg Assoc, pp 522–523

Nomiyama K, Nomiyama H (1983c) Prevention and treatment of cadmium-induced health effects by intravenous administration of copper. Proc 56th Annual Meeting of Japan Assoc Industr Health, pp 524–525

Nomiyama K, Nomiyama H (1984a) Reversibility of cadmium-induced health effects in rabbits. Environ Health Perspect 54:201–211

Nomiyama K, Nomiyama H (1984b) Minimal lethal doses of heavy metals, organic solvents and agricultural chemicals in rats given low calorie-low protein diet. Jpn J Hyg 39:255

Nomiyama K, Nomiyama H (1984c) Hot environment and low calorie and/or low protein diet, factors modifying toxicity of organic solvents, heavy metals and agricultural chemicals. 21th Int Congr Occup Health

Nomiyama K, Nomiyama H (1984d) Critical concentration of "active cadmium" in the renal cortex. 21th Int Congr Occup Health

Nomiyama K, Nomiyama H, Taguchi T (1977) Effects of environmental temperatures on the chronic toxicity of cadmium in mice. Kankyo Hoken Rep 41:29–37

Nomiyama K, Nomiyama H, Taguchi T (1978) Effects of environmental temperatures on the toxicity of cadmium in mice. Proc 8th Asian Conf Occup Health. Jpn Ind Occup Safety Assoc, Tokyo, pp 221–225

Nomiyama K, Nomiyama H, Nomura Y, Taguchi T, Matsui K, Yotoriyama M, Akahori F, Iwao S, Koizumi N, Masaoka T, Kitamura K, Tsuchiya K, Suzuki T, Kobayashi K (1979a) Effects of dietary cadmium on rhesus monkeys. Environ Health Perspect 28:223–243

Nomiyama K, Nomiyama H, Taguchi T (1979b) No osteomalacia found in mice, rabbits and monkeys given cadmium for a prolonged period. In: Shigematsu I, Nomiyama K (eds) Cadmium-induced osteopathy. Japan Public Health Association, Tokyo, pp 51–53

Nomiyama K, Nomiyama H, Matsui K (1979c) Chemical form and intestinal absorption of cadmium in rice. Jpn J Hyg 34:103

Nomiyama K, Nomiyama H, Yotoriyama M (1980a) Ageing, a factor aggravating chronic toxicity of cadmium. Toxicol Lett 6:225–230

Nomiyama K, Matsui K, Nomiyama H (1980b) Environmental temperature, a factor modifying the acute toxicity of organic solvents, heavy metals, and agricultural chemicals. Toxicol Lett 6:67–70

Nomiyama K, Nomiyama H, Akahori F, Masaoka T (1981a) Further studies on effects of dietary cadmium on rhesus monkeys (9) Cadmium, zinc and copper in urine. Recent studies on health effects of cadmium in Japan. Japan Environ Agency, Tokyo, pp 139–153

Nomiyama K, Nomiyama H, Akahori F, Masaoka T (1981b) Further studies on dietary cadmium on rhesus monkeys (10) Tissue cadmium, zinc and copper. Recent studies on health effects of cadmium in Japan. Japan Environ Agency, Tokyo, pp 154–188

Nomiyama K, Nomiyama H, Yotoriyama M (1982a) Low-molecular-weight proteins in urine form rabbits given nephrotoxic compounds. Ind Health 20:1–10

Nomiyama K, Nomiyama H, Akahori F, Masaoka T (1982b) Cadmium health effects in monkeys with special reference to the critical concentration of cadmium in the renal cortex. Cadmium 81. Proc 3rd Int Cadmium Conf Miami, Cadmium Assoc, London, pp 151–156

Nomiyama K, Ohshiro H, Nomiyama H (1984a) In vivo determination of animal organ metals by the prompt gamma ray neutron activation analysis. Jpn J Hyg 39:464

Nomiyama K, Nomiyama H, Kamal A-AM, Ohshiro H (1984b) Ageing, a factor aggravating chronic toxicity of cadmium in rabbits. Jpn J Hyg 39:466

Nomiyama K, Nomiyama K, Ohshiro H, Kamal A-AM (1984c) Effects of ageing on metallothionein induction in rabbits given cadmium. Jpn J Hyg 39:467

Nomiyama K, Nomiyama H, Akahori F, Masaoka T (1984d) Some comments and proposals on dose and effect for estimating critical concentration of cadmium in the renal cortex. Cadmium 83. Proc 4th Int Cadmium Conf Munich. Cadmium Assoc, London, pp 161–171

Nordberg GF (1972) Cadmium metabolism and toxicity. Environ Physiol Biochem 2:7–36

Ohmori K, Ikemi Y, Tozawa T, Abe K, Yamaga K (1984) Urinary excretion of cadmium workers. Proc Jpn Assoc Ind Health 510–511

Piscator M (1966) Proteinuria in chronic cadmium poisoning III. Electrophoretic and immunoelectrophoretic studies on urinary proteins from cadmium workers with special reference to the excretion of low molecular weight protein. Arch Environ Health 12:335–344

Ridlington JW, Fowler BA (1979) Isolation and partial characterization of a cadmium-binding protein from the American oyster (Crassostrea virginica). Chem Biol Interact 25:127–138

Roels HA, Lauwerys RR, Buchet J-P, Berdnard A, Chettle DR, Harvey TC, Al-Haddak IK (1981) In vivo measurement of liver and kidney cadmium in workers exposed to this metal: its significance with respect to cadmium in blood and urine. Environ Res 26:217–240

Sangster B, de Groot G (1984) Cadmium pollution in Stadskanaal: screening of the inhabitants of a polluted quarter. Cadmium 83. 4th Int Cadmium Conference Munich, Cadmium Assoc, London, pp 110–112

Schneider H-J, Anke M, Grun M, Partschefeld M (1979) The Cd-, Zn-, Cu-, and Mn-level of different organs of human beings from an area exposed to Cd in comparison with standard values. In: Anke M, Schneider H-J (eds) Kadmium-Symposium. Friedrich-Schiller-Universität, Jena, pp 282–289

Sharma RP (1983) Ligands binding cadmium, zinc, and copper in a species of New Zealand oyster (Ostrea Lutaria). Bull Environ Contam Toxicol 30:428–434

Shibuya Y, Hirota M, Taniguchi M, Takayama T, Harada A, Sakagami Y (1984) Eleven years follow-up study on the health effects of cadmium pigment production. Proc Jpn Assoc Ind Health 514–515

Shigematsu I, Nomiyama K (eds) (1979) Cadmium-induced osteopathy. Japan Public Health Association, Tokyo

Shigematsu I, Tsuchiya K, Nomiyama K, Kitamura S, Kimura M, Harada A, Ishimoto F, Kato T, Nogawa K, Kajikawa K, Takebayashi S (1981a) General research report and summary reports of research team. In: Recent studies on health effects of cadmium in Japan. Jpn Environ Agency, Tokyo, pp 381–398

Shigematsu I, Tsuchiya K, Kitamura S, Takeuchi J, Kajikawa K, Kato T, Nomiyama K, Ishimoto F, Ogata H, Saito H, Minowa M (1981b) Analysis and report of the results on the health survey on the inhabitants in environmentally contaminated areas by cadmium. In: Recent studies on health effects of cadmium in Japan. Jpn Environ Agency, Tokyo, pp 319–380

Shigematsu I, Kitamura S, Takeuchi J, Minowa M, Nagai M, Usui T, Fukushima M (1981c) A retrospective mortality study on cadmium exposed population in Japan. In: Recent studies on health effects of cadmium in Japan. Jpn Environ Agency, Tokyo, pp 303–317

Shigematsu I, Kitamura S, Takeuchi J, Minowa M, Nagai M, Usui T, Fukushima M (1982) A retrospective mortality study on cadmium exposed populations in Japan. Cadmium 81. Edited Proc 3rd Int Cadmium Conference Miami. Cadmium Assoc, London, pp 115–118

Shinoda S, Yuri T, Nakagawa S (1977) Present medical findings of Itai-Itai disease patients. Kankyo Hoken Rep 41:44–52

Sorahan Y (1982) A mortality study of nickel-cadmium battery workers. Cadmium 81. Edited Proc 3rd Int Cadmium Conference Miami. Cadmium Assoc, London, pp 138–141

Suzuki T, Takeda M, Uchiyama M (1977) Chemical form of cadmium in foodstuff I. Investigation of chemical form in rice grain. J Hyg Chem 23:345–351

Suzuki Y (1980) Cadmium metabolism and toxicity in rats after long-term subcutaneous administration. J Toxicol Environ Health 6:469–482

Suzuki Y (1981) Cadmium, copper, and zinc distribution in blood of rats after long-term cadmium administration. J Toxicol Environ Health 7:251–262

Taguchi T, Suzuki S (1981) Influence of sex and age on the biological half-life of cadmium in mice. J Toxicol Environ Health 7:239–249

Takebayashi S (1979) First autopsy case, suspicious of cadmium intoxication, from the cadmium-polluted area in Tsushima, Nagasaki Prefecture. In: Shigematsu I, Nomiyama K (eds) Cadmium-induced nephropathy. Japan Public Health Association, Tokyo, pp 124–138

Tanaka K, Nomura H, Onosaka S, Min K-S (1981) Release of hepatic cadmium by carbon tetrachloride treatment. Toxicol Appl Pharmacol 59:535–539

Task Group on Metal Toxicology (1976) Effects and dose-response relationships of toxic metals. In: Nordberg GF (ed) Effects and dose-response relationships of toxic metals. Elsevier, Amsterdam, pp 1–111

Thomas JFA (1984) Some conclusions of the Shipham survey and implications for general UK policy on cadmium, Cadmium 83. 4th Int Cadmium Conference Munich, Cadmium Association, London, pp 104–106

Tsuchiya K (1976) Proteinuria of cadmium workers. J Occup Med 18:463–466

Tsuchiya K (ed) (1978) Cadmium studies in Japan, a review. Kodansha, Tokyo, pp 159–
160

Tsuchiya K, Sugita M (1971) A mathematical model for deriving the biological half-life of
a chemical. Nord Hyg Tidskr 53:105–110

Vartesky D, Ellis KJ, Chen NS, Cohn SH (1977) A facility for in vivo measurement of kidney and liver cadmium by neutron capture prompt gamma ray analysis. Phys Med Biol
22:1085–1096

WHO Task Group (1977) Environmental health criteria for cadmium (summary). WHO,
Geneva

Yamamoto Y (1972) Present status of cadmium pollution in Japan. Kankyo Hoken Rep
11:7–12

Yoshiki S, Tachikawa T, Yamaguchi R, Yamazaki T, Yamana H, Sakai K (1983) Effects
of nutritional factors on cadmium-administered monkeys 6. Bone change. Kankyo
Hoken Rep 49:68–75

CHAPTER 5

Effects of Cadmium Exposure in Humans

A. Bernard and R. Lauwerys

A. Introduction

Cadmium is an occupational and environmental contaminant which has received
a great deal of attention in the last few years. This concern about the potential
hazards of cadmium for human health appears justified in view of the biologic
properties of this element. An important toxicologic feature of cadmium is its exceptionally long biologic half-life in the human organism (10–30 years). Evolution has not provided humans with a metabolic pathway for the elimination of
this metal. Once absorbed, cadmium is efficiently retained in the organism in
which it accumulates throughout life. In the newborn, cadmium is nearly absent,
but at the age of 50 years, the cadmium body burden may increase up to 20–30 mg
and in people occupationally exposed, it may reach values as high as 200–300 mg.
Furthermore, cadmium concentrates in vital organs, particularly in the kidneys.
Under low levels of exposure, such as occur in the general environment, 30%–
50% of the cadmium body burden is found in the kidneys alone.

In addition to this cumulative property, cadmium is a toxic element which
may interfere with a large number of biologic systems. In humans, excessive exposure to cadmium has been linked to the development of lung insufficiency, renal disturbances, and osteomalacia. Cadmium has also been implicated in the development of hypertension and of various types of cancer. The industrial production of cadmium began in the early part of this century and many aspects of its
toxicity for humans are still obscure or matters of controversy. In particular, the
potential health effects of the current environmental pollution by cadmium in industrialized countries remain to be clarified.

This chapter reviews the toxic effects of cadmium on organ systems in humans, focusing mainly on the most recent observations. The available data on the
dose–response relationships for the two main target organs, the kidney and the
lung, are also discussed.

B. Human Exposure to Cadmium

I. Environmental Exposure

Food and cigarettes constitute the two main sources of cadmium for the general
population. Cadmium is present in all foodstuffs. The lowest concentrations are
found in milk (around 1 ppm). In meat, fish, and fruit, the concentration of cadmium ranges from 1 to 50 ppm and in staple foods such as wheat, rice, and po-

tatoes, concentrations are often between 10 and 150 ppm. The highest cadmium levels (100–1,000 ppm) are found in internal organs of adult mammals (kidneys and liver) and in certain species of mussels, scallops, and oysters (LAUWERYS 1978).

When grown on a cadmium-polluted soil, some vegetables, such as rice, can accumulate considerable amounts of cadmium. For instance, the JAPAN ENVIRONMENT AGENCY (1972) made a survey of cadmium concentration in rice from areas where cadmium pollution was suspected. A total of 4,477 rice samples was collected in fields covering an area of 11,700 ha. Rice samples containing 1,000 ppm or more of cadmium were detected in 24% of the fields surveyed; 292 samples (6.5%) had a cadmium content of 1,000 ppm or more.

It is very likely that the concentration of cadmium in some basic foodstuffs (e.g., wheat and rice) grown in industrialized countries has progressively increased during the twentieth century (KJELLSTRÖM et al. 1975; ELINDER and

Table 1. Dietary cadmium intake in various countries

Country	Cd intake (µg/day)	Methods of estimation	References
Belgium	18	B	BUCHET et al. (1983)
	45	A	FOUASSIN and Fondu (1980)
United Kingdom	< 20	A	HUBBARD and LINDSAY (1979)
	15–30		TOLAN and ELTON (1973)
Federal Republic	32	C	ESSING et al. (1969)
of Germany	48	A	ESSING et al. (1969)
United States	< 26–61	A	FDA (1977)
	13–16	C	KOWAL et al. (1979)
	17	C	KJELLSTRÖM (1979a)
Denmark	< 30	A	MILJOMINISTERIET (1980)
The Netherlands	29	A	MINISTRY OF HEALTH DEN HAAG (1980)
	32		DE VOOGT and VAN HATTOM (1981)
Sweden	17	C	KJELLSTRÖM (1979a)
New Zealand	21		GUTHRIE and ROBINSON (1977)
Japan	600–2,000	A	FRIBERG et al. (1974)
(polluted areas)	211–245	A	Japan Public Health Association (1980) (cited by TSUCHIYA, 1978)
	180–281	B	
(control areas)	59–113	A	
	57–108	B	
(various areas)	31 (3–149)	B	YAMAGATA and IWASHIMA (1975) (cited by TSUCHIYA, 1978)
Japan (Tokyo)	36	C	IWAO (1977) (cited by TSUCHIYA, 1978)
	34	C	
Japan	47	A	FUKUSHIMA (1972) (cited by TSUCHIYA, 1978)
	17–43	B	YAMAGATA et al. (1971) (cited by TSUCHIYA, 1978)

A, market basket survey; B, duplicate meal study; C, fecal analysis

KJELLSTRÖM 1977). However, the impact of this increase on the cadmium intake of the general population may vary, depending on the dietary habits. In the United States, it has been recently estimated that, even assuming an increase of cadmium levels in food (namely wheat) between 1945 and 1975, the intake of cadmium has remained fairly constant as a result of profound changes in eating habits (TRAVIS and ETNIER 1982). By contrast, in Japan where rice has remained a staple food, the cadmium intake has increased in parallel with the environmental pollution by this metal.

Three methods have usually been used to estimate the dietary intake of cadmium: the market basket survey, the duplicate meal study, and the analysis of fecal cadmium (the gastrointestinal absorption of cadmium is assumed to be 5%). Table 1 summarizes the values obtained in several countries. The estimates based on market basket survey are generally higher than those derived from duplicate meal or fecal analysis. For example, with the first method, FOUASSIN and FONDU (1980) have reported that in Belgium the weekly cadmium intake was 315–330 µg. This value is three times higher than that recently found during a duplicate meal study (BUCHET et al. 1983).

Estimates of the cadmium intake in Japan, even in areas regarded as nonpolluted, are constantly higher than anywhere else in the world. The highest values ever reported for the general population (600–2,000 µg/day) were observed in the Fuchu area where itai-itai disease broke out (FRIBERG et al. 1974).

Cadmium levels in drinking water are usually less than 1 µg/l so that the contribution of water to the cadmium intake is very small. The concentration of cadmium in ambient air is of the order of 0.001–0.005 $\mu g/m^3$ in rural areas, 0.003–0.05 $\mu g/m^3$ in urban areas, and up to 0.6 $\mu g/m^3$ near cadmium-emitting sources. It can be calculated (see Sect. C) that, the latter situation excepted, the cadmium intake from air is negligible compared with that from food. In the case of children, it should be mentioned that, as for lead, they may ingest relatively large amounts of cadmium-containing dust when playing on areas contaminated by cadmium (e.g., around cadmium smelters) (BUCHET et al. 1980a).

II. Industrial Exposure

Exposure to cadmium may occur during several industrial processes: production of cadmium and its compounds, fabrication of alloys and solders, plating of metals, use of cadmium in pigments and stabilizers for plastics, fabrication of Cd–Ni batteries, etc. In industry, the exposure is mainly due to inhalation of cadmium fumes and dusts. Cadmium has a relatively high vapor pressure. Hence, the hazard is particularly high during thermal treatment of cadmium or cadmium-containing materials. Significant oral intake of cadmium may also occur (e.g., eating or smoking with contaminated hands). It has also been shown that cigarettes may be contaminated by cadmium when kept in work clothes (PISCATOR et al. 1976). The total airborne cadmium concentrations vary according to the type of industry and the efforts made to control the emissions. In the past (Table 2), cadmium concentrations around 100 $\mu g/m^3$ were frequent. In some factories where no precaution was taken to minimize exposure, values as high as 10,000 $\mu g/m^3$ were reported. Working conditions are currently being improved and in modern fac-

Table 2. Clinical studies on lung changes in workers chronically exposed to cadmium

Number and sex of exposed workers	Conditions of exposure[a]	Observations	References
20 Males	0.2–22 years exposure (mean 8 years) in cadmium smelters; 40–1,440 $\mu g/m^3$	No chest X-ray change	PRINCI (1947)
5 Males	4–8 years exposure in the production of cadmium-faced bearings; 0.1 mg/m^3 on average	No chest X-ray change	HARDY and SKINNER (1947)
43 Males	9–34 years exposure (20 years on average) in an alkaline accumulator factory; 3–15 mg/m^3	Disturbance of lung function tests in 14 subjects	FRIBERG (1948a, b, 1950)
15 Males	Less than 4 years in the above alkaline accumulator	No disturbance of lung function tests	
8 Males	9–19 years exposure in an alkaline accumulator factory	Chest X-ray suggestive of emphysema in 6 subjects	BAADER (1951)
Females	Alkaline accumulator factory	Diffuse pulmonary fibrosis	VOROBJEVA (1957a)
100 Males	More than 5 years of exposure in the production of copper-cadmium alloys; 13–89 $\mu g/m^3$ (mean 40–50 $\mu g/m^3$) in the 1st factory and 1–270 $\mu g/m^3$ (mean 132 $\mu g/m^3$) in the 2nd factory	Disturbance of lung function tests and chest X-ray suggestive of emphysema in 21 subjects	BONNELL (1955), KAZANTZIS (1956), BUXTON (1956), BONNELL et al. (1959)
12 Males	0.5–31 years exposure in a cadmium pigment factory	3 Subjects with disturbance of lung function and 1 with emphysema	KAZANTZIS et al. (1963)
70 Males	10–40 years exposure in an alkaline accumulator factory; 0.6–23.6 $\mu g/m^3$ to 1949 and later below 0.5 mg/m^3	Emphysema and chronic bronchitis in 4 subjects	POTTS (1965)
19 Males	On average 3.3 years exposure to cadmium oxide dust; 30–690 $\mu g/m^3$	No disturbance of lung function	SUZUKI et al. (1965)
26 Males		Diffuse interstitial fibrosis	HORSTOWA et al. (1966)
13 Males	0.75–12 years exposure in smelting alloys of silver and cadmium; 68–241 $\mu g/m^3$ (mean 126 $\mu g/m^3$)	No chest X-ray change	TSUCHIYA (1967)
27 Males	5–44 years exposure in an alkaline accumulator factory; 0.3–5 mg/m^3	Disturbance of lung function tests in 5 subjects	ADAMS et al. (1969)
11 Males	7–11 years exposure in a cadmium refinery; 1.2–2.7 mg/m^3	No disturbance of lung function tests	TECULESCU and STANESCU (1970)

Table 2 (contiued)

Number and sex of exposed workers	Conditions of exposure[a]	Observations	References
72 Males		Diffuse interstitial fibrosis observed by chest X-ray in 17 subjects	TARASENKO and VOROBJEVA (1973)
32 Females	On average 4.4 years exposure in an electronic workshop; 6.8–18.6 µg/m³	No disturbance of lung function tests	LAUWERYS et al. (1974),
90 Males	Less than 20 years exposure in a cadmium-producing plant (mean 8 years); 36–256 µg/m³	Mild obstructive syndrome	MATERNA et al. (1975)
25 Males	More than 20 years exposure in a cadmium-producing plant (mean 24.5 years; 3.7–556 µg/m³	Mild obstructive syndrome	
17 Males	On average 26.4 years exposure in a cadmium-producing plant	5 Subjects with lung fibrosis on chest X-ray; slight disturbance of lung function tests	SMITH et al. (1976)
18 Males	More than 22 years exposure (average 32 years) in a cadmium-producing plant	Slight disturbance of lung function tests suggestive of a mild obstructive syndrome; no chest X-ray change	STANESCU et al. (1977)
34 Males	3–7 years exposure in a cadmium-producing plant; 0.15–31 µg/m³	Increased prevalence of exertional dyspnea and of respiratory infection	GILL (1978)
42 Males	1–33 years (average 13 years) exposure in a nonferrous metal plant	Emphysema in 3 subjects; disturbance of lung function tests in about 50% of the subjects	KOSSMAN et al. (1969)
10 Males	1–17 years exposure in a pigment-manufacturing plant; 0.4–2.31 mg/m³ (in 1977)	2 Workers with dyspnea, severe airways obstruction and emphysema (7 and 13 years exposure); 1 worker with mild airway obstruction	DE SILVA and DONNAN (1981)

[a] Cadmium concentration in total dust

tories using or producing cadmium, the concentration of cadmium in air can be maintained at rather low levels (below 20 µg/m³) (ADAMSSON 1979).

III. Tobacco Smoke

Smoking may be an important additional source of cadmium. One cigarette contains approximately 1–2 µg cadmium, of which about 10% may be absorbed by the lungs (SCHROEDER and BALASSA 1961; SZADKOWSKY et al. 1969; NANDI et al. 1969; MENDEN et al. 1972; FRIBERG et al. 1974). The cadmium content of cigarettes depends on the country of origin (ELINDER et al. 1983); for instance, it is rather low in cigarettes produced in India, Zambia, and Argentina (0.1–0.5 µg per cigarette).

C. Metabolism

I. Absorption

1. Inhalation

In the general environment, 20%–30% of the inhaled cadmium is probably deposited in the lungs. As about 64% of the cadmium deposited can be absorbed, this means that 13%–19% of the total amount of cadmium inhaled is effectively absorbed (LAUWERYS 1982). If we except special circumstances, like living close to a cadmium emission source, the amount of cadmium absorbed by the pulmonary route in nonsmokers does not exceed 0.2 µg/day. In smokers, cigarettes represent an additional source of cadmium which may equal or exceed that from food. The US ENVIRONMENTAL PROTECTION AGENCY (1979) has estimated that smoking 20 cigarettes per day results in the absorption of 1.4 µg cadmium. In industry, the absorption of inhaled cadmium may be quite variable, depending on the size of cadmium particles and on their chemical form. Animal experiments indicate that whereas cadmium oxide is rapidly translocated from the respiratory surface to the general circulation, cadmium pigments are much less easily absorbed (LAUWERYS 1982).

2. Ingestion

In humans, the average oral absorption of cadmium has been estimated at 5% (RAHOLA et al. 1972; MCLELLAN et al. 1978). Physiologic and nutritional factors may modify this absorption rate. The study of FLANAGAN et al. (1978) has demonstrated that subjects with low iron stores (low ferritin levels in serum) absorb significantly more cadmium (up to 15% of the ingested amount) than persons with normal iron stores. Oral absorption of cadmium is therefore higher in females than in males. Furthermore, animal experiments have shown that a low intake of calcium and protein may considerably increase the intestinal absorption of cadmium (LARSSON and PISCATOR 1971; SUZUKI et al. 1969). It is likely that the low calcium, protein, and iron intake in Japan at the end of World War II has contributed to the exceptional accumulation of cadmium in itai-itai disease patients. Depending on the dietary intake and on the iron status, it has been estimated that a European adult absorbs cadmium orally at an average rate of 1.4–8 µg/day (LAUWERYS 1982).

II. Distribution

In blood, more than 90% of cadmium is found in cells. In vitro experiments have shown that red blood cells accumulate little cadmium whereas lymphocytes, which synthesize metallothionein, can concentrate cadmium to a level 3,000-fold greater than in the culture medium (HILDEBRAND and CRAM 1979). In adults not exposed to cadmium at work, the level of cadmium in blood is usually below 0.5 µg per 100 ml. The concentration of cadmium in blood is usually higher in smokers than in nonsmokers.

Cadmium is efficiently retained in the organism in which it accumulates throughout life. The cadmium body burden of European and American adults not exposed to cadmium at work has been estimated to range from 5 to 40 mg (LAUWERYS 1978). A partial body neutron activation technique was used by ELLIS et al. (1979) to measure the absolute amounts of cadmium present in the left kidney and in the liver of 20 adult male Americans. By assuming that kidney and liver contain 50% of the total cadmium body burden, they estimated that the average body burden at the age of 50 years is 19.3 mg for nonsmokers and 35.5 mg for smokers.

The two main sites of storage of cadmium are the liver and kidneys. In normal subjects, about 40%–80% of the body burden is found in these two organs and in the case of low level exposures, such as those occurring in the general environment, about 30%–50% is stored in the kidneys alone. The concentration of cadmium in the renal cortex is about 1.5 times higher than that in the whole organ (LIVINGSTONE 1972), but according to a recent estimate, the true cortex : whole kidney cadmium concentration ratio might be 1.15 : 1 (KJELLSTRÖM et al. 1983). In the United States and Europe, the mean cadmium concentration in the renal cortex at age 40–50 years has been shown to range from 15 to 50 ppm (SCHROEDER et al. 1967; PISCATOR and LIND 1972; HAMMER et al. 1973; KJELLSTRÖM 1979 a). Higher values have been found in some population groups in Japan (60–120 ppm) and in cadmium-exposed workers (up to 300 ppm) (TSUCHIYA 1978; KJELLSTRÖM 1979 a; FRIBERG et al. 1974; ROELS et al 1981 a).

Recently, a study was carried out to assess the human exposure to cadmium in different areas of the world. The concentration of cadmium was measured in samples of kidney cortex obtained at autopsy of deceased teachers (VAHTER 1982). The highest values were observed in Japan in the age group 40–49 years (geometric mean 67 ppm). Values obtained in other countries for the same age group were 2–4 times lower, with geometric means ranging from 15.7 ppm (India) to 39.3 ppm (Belgium). Since these values are average estimates, it can be assumed that in certain countries such as Japan and Belgium, a small fraction of the population has already reached the critical level (around 200 ppm, see Sect. E.VII.2). The zinc concentration in the renal cortex tends to increase with increasing cadmium concentration at least up to a cadmium level of 60 ppm (PISCATOR and LIND 1972; ELINDER et al. 1977). When renal dysfunction occurs, the cadmium level in the renal cortex decreases because of increased urinary excretion (Adams et al. 1969; Lauwerys et al. 1974, 1976). The decrease of renal cadmium is very likely due to a release of cadmium stored in the kidney combined with a depressed tubular reabsorption of circulating cadmium (Bernard and Lauwerys 1981 a). This phenomenon explains why in most severely poisoned workers and also in patients with itai-itai disease, the concentration of cadmium in the renal cortex may be relatively low and sometimes not markedly different from that observed in normal subjects. In these persons, however, the concentration of cadmium in liver remains elevated. The levels of cadmium in the liver are generally much lower than those in the renal cortex. Nevertheless, because of its weight, the liver contains a significant fraction of the total body burden. In adults not exposed to cadmium at work, the concentration of cadmium in liver ranges approximately from 0.5 to 5 ppm (Nriagu 1981). In cadmium-exposed workers, hepatic cadmium levels may exceed 150 ppm (Roels et al. 1981 a). The ratio between the cadmium concentration in the liver and that in the kidney increases with the intensity of exposure (Friberg et al. 1974); it is for instance much higher for occupationally exposed persons than in the general population (Kjellström 1979 a). The thyroid, the pancreas, and the salivary glands can also accumulate significant amounts of cadmium. In humans, placental transfer of cadmium seems to be limited. An investigation of more than 500 pregnant women living in different areas of Belgium has shown that in comparison with maternal blood, the placenta concentrates cadmium about tenfold (Roels et al. 1978). The barrier role of the placenta explains why the cadmium concentration in newborn blood is on average 50% lower than that in maternal blood (Lauwerys et al. 1978). Cadmium levels in the placenta are significantly higher in smokers than in nonsmokers (Roels et al. 1978; Copius Pereboom et al. 1979).

In tissues, the majority of cadmium is bound to metallothionein, a low molecular weight protein (molecular weight 6,600) rich in cysteine residues, but deficient in aromatic amino acids. At the cellular level, the synthesis of this protein may represent a defense mechanism against the toxic cadmium ion. However, when administered intravenously or intraperitoneally, the cadmium–metallothionein complex is highly nephrotoxic, causing extensive necrosis to the proximal tubules (Nordberg et al. 1975). According to Webb and Etienne (1977), this toxic action is due to the ion released intracellularly during the lysosomal degradation of the reabsorbed cadmium–metallothionein complex. For Cherian (1978), however, the cadmium–metallothionein complex would be toxic by itself, inducing membrane damage during the process of pinocytosis. Metallothionein is probably also involved in the transport of cadmium from the liver to the kidneys. Because of its small size, the cadmium–protein complex released from the liver is freely filtered through the glomeruli to be reabsorbed by the tubular cells. Such a mechanism could explain the selective accumulation of cadmium in the renal cortex during long-term exposure. For a more detailed discussion of metallothionein, see Chap. 8.

III. Excretion

Cadmium is eliminated from the organism mainly via urine. The amount of cadmium excreted daily in urine is, however, very small; it represents about 0.005%–0.01% of the total body burden, which corresponds to a biologic half-life of about 20–40 years (FRIBERG et al. 1974). On a group basis, the urinary excretion of cadmium is proportional to the body burden (LAUWERYS et al. 1974; ROELS et al. 1981a) and thus increases with age, at least up to 50–60 years (ELINDER et al. 1978). When renal damage occurs, cadmium excretion in urine usually increases sharply and the relationship to body burden disappears. In persons not exposed to cadmium at work, the urinary excretion of cadmium is normally below 2 µg/day, even in smokers. A fraction of urinary cadmium is probably bound to metallothionein, as suggested by the close relationship between the two parameters (CHANG et al. 1980; ROELS et al. 1983b). Cadmium can also be excreted by other routes (bile, gastrointestinal tract, saliva, hair, nails), but to a lesser extent than in urine. Secretion into milk is also very limited.

IV. Evaluation of Cadmium Exposure

In view of the cumulative property of cadmium, any biologic monitoring program of population groups chronically exposed to cadmium should attempt to evaluate both the current and the integrated exposure. The determination of cadmium concentration in liver and kidney samples collected at autopsy or by biopsy provides a direct assessment of the cadmium body burden of population groups. Another approach, more directly useful on an individual basis consists in measuring in vivo by a neutron capture γ-ray analysis technique the amounts of cadmium accumulated in tissues (BIGGIN et al. 1974). Initially, the method used neutrons produced by a cyclotron (HARVEY et al. 1975) but recently, a portable system has been developed (THOMAS et al. 1979; AL-HADDAD et al. 1981; VARTSKY et al. 1977). This system which can measure both hepatic and renal stores of cadmium, has been applied to occupationally exposed workers (ROELS et al. 1979, 1981a, 1983a; ELLIS et al. 1980, 1981) and to the general population (ELLIS et al. 1979). A method based on X-ray fluorescence has recently been proposed by AHLGREN and MATTSON (1980) as an alternative to the neutron activation technique. Compared with the latter, the X-ray fluorescence technique presents the advantage of lower irradiation. Unfortunately, the present detection limit for the determination of cadmium in kidney is higher than that obtained by neutron activation. It amounts to 20 ppm when the kidney surface is 3 cm below the skin, but reaches 100 ppm when the distance is 5 cm.

So far, in the health surveillance of workers in industry or in large-scale studies on the general population, the exposure to cadmium has usually been evaluated indirectly by measuring the metal in urine and blood. The detailed kinetics of cadmium in humans is not yet fully elucidated, but in practice, the following conclusions can be formulated regarding the significance of cadmium in blood and urine. In persons currently exposed to cadmium, the concentration of cadmium in the blood reflects mainly the average intake during recent months (KJELLSTRÖM and NORDBERG 1978; LAUWERYS et al. 1979a). The relative influence of the cadmium body burden on the cadmium level in the blood may be more important in persons who have accumulated a large amount of cadmium and have been removed from exposure. Several studies on humans and animals have indicated that the level of cadmium in urine can be interpreted as follows (LAUWERYS et al. 1979 a). In the absence of acute overexposure to cadmium and as long as the storage capability of the kidney cortex is not exceeded or cadmium-induced nephropathy has not yet occurred, the level of cadmium in urine increases progressively with the amount of cadmium stored in the kidneys. Under such conditions, which prevail mainly in the general population and in workers moderately exposed to cadmium, there is a significant correlation between urinary cadmium and cadmium in the kidneys (ROELS et al. 1981 a). If exposure to cadmium has been excessive, the cadmium-binding sites in the organism become progressively saturated and, despite continuous exposure, the cadmium concentration in the renal cortex levels off. From this stage on, the absorbed cadmium cannot be further retained in that organ and it is rapidly excreted in the urine. At this stage, urinary cadmium is influenced by both the boby burden and the recent intake. If exposure is continued, some subjects may develop renal damage, which gives rise to a further increase of urinary cadmium (release of cadmium stored in the kidney and depressed reabsorption of circulating cadmium). Recent studies indicate that metallothionein in urine has the same biologic significance. Good correlations $(0.6 < r < 0.8, P < 0.001)$ have been observed between the urinary concentration of metallothionein and that of cadmium, independent of the intensity of exposure and the status of renal function (ROELS et al. 1983 b; CHANG et al. 1980). Contrary to the suggestion made by TOHYAMA et al. (1981, 1982), there is so far no reason to regard metallothionein levels in urine as of better predictive significance with regard to the risk of renal dysfunction than urinary cadmium levels.

D. Acute Toxicity

The principal acute manifestations observed in humans are gastrointestinal disturbances following ingestion and chemical pneumonitis following inhalation of cadmium oxide fumes.

I. Acute Toxicity by Inhalation

The first known cases of acute cadmium poisoning were reported in Belgium by SOVET (1858). The poisoning occurred in three persons who were polishing silverware with cadmium carbonate and were exposed to a cloud of cadmium dust. In industry, intoxication results from acute inhalation of cadmium fumes, generated by welding cadmium-containing materials or by smelting or soldering such materials. Maintenance workers who have not been properly instructed about the risk have usually been the victims of such intoxications. Acute exposure to a moderately high concentration of freshly generated cadmium fumes $(200–500 \ \mu g/m^3)$ may cause symptoms similar to those of metal fume fever. The prognosis is usually favorable with complete recovery within a few days. More intense exposure may lead, after a latent interval of several hours, to more serious manifestations resulting from severe bronchial and pulmonary irritation. Symptoms include irritation and dryness of the nose and throat, cough, headache, dizziness, weakness, chills, fever, chest pain, and breathlessness. Nausea and vomiting may also occur. A fatal outcome several days after exposure is frequently due to pulmonary edema. There is no apparent relationship between the latency period and the severity of symptoms. The persons who survive the acute episode may recover without permanent damage, but it is also possible that repeated or even a single episode of acute or subacute pneumonitis may result in delayed development of lung impairment. Recently, TOWNSHEND (1982) reported the case of a welder who developed acute cadmium pneumonitis after a single day's exposure to cadmium fumes. Follow-up of the patient for 4 years did not reveal any permanent pulmonary damage, but 17 years later, the man developed a progressive pulmonary fibrosis which, according to the author, is undoubtedly the late result of the acute poisoning. As indicated, the initial symptoms after exposure to cadmium fumes are very similar to those of metal fume fever. The treatment and prognosis of the two diseases are, however, quite different and confusion between them may have dramatic consequences. Acute cadmium inhalation constitutes a medical emergency whereas metal fume fever (welder's fever) is a relatively benign and self-limiting condition occurring after exposure to freshly generated fumes of metals, most frequently zinc oxide fumes.

The lethal concentration of cadmium oxide fumes for human beings has been estimated to be around 5 mg/m^3 (as Cd) for an 8-h exposure (FRIBERG et al. 1974). For an 8-h exposure period, the threshold effect levels in the lung for cadmium oxide fumes and "respirable" dust are approximately 0.5 and 3 mg/m^3, respectively (WORLD HEALTH ORGANIZATION 1980).

II. Acute Toxicity by Ingestion

Ingestion of food or beverages which have been contaminated with cadmium can cause gastrointestinal disturbances. In the past, the use of cadmium-plated cooking utensils and the storage of acid juice in cadmium-containing earthenware has been responsible for several episodes of such intoxications. Acute oral intoxications have also been observed in workers exposed to cadmium dust who ate their meals with dirty hands.

The main symptoms are nausea, vomiting, diarrhea, abdominal cramps, headache, and salivation. In the case of fatal intoxication, these symptoms have been followed either by shock due to the loss of fluid and death within 24 h, or by acute renal failure with cardiopulmonary depression and death within 7–14 days. Liver damage may also be observed. The no-effect level of cadmium administered as a single oral dose to humans is estimated at 3 mg and the letal dose 350–8,900 mg. The concentration of cadmium in water that induces vomiting is about 15 mg/l.

E. Chronic Toxicity

The first known case of chronic cadmium poisoning was reported by STEPHENS (1920). This author cited the case of a man employed in a zinc smelter for many

years. When he died at the age of 67 years, the autopsy revealed chronic interstitial nephritis and cardiac hypertrophy. Stephens was able to differentiate this case
from saturnism because the liver contained no lead, but high amounts of cadmium.

Later, in a paper entitled "The possibility of chronic cadmium poisoning,"
HARDY and SKINNER (1947) reported observations made on five men exposed
chronically to cadmium dusts and fumes. Signs of fatigue, loss of appetite, and
coughing were common to all. However, these earlier reports lack supporting
data, and chronic cadmium poisoning was not recognized as a clinical entity until
the early 1950s. At that time, in Sweden, FRIBERG (1948a, b, 1950) started his extensive studies on chronic cadmium poisoning in a factory manufacturing alkaline accumulators. Clinical examinations were conducted on 58 workers, 43 of
whom had been employed on average for 20 years and 15 for about 2 years. The
main findings were pulmonary emphysema, anosmia, yellowing of teeth, impaired renal function with proteinuria, and low physical working capacity. Since
Friberg's report, a number of studies have documented the chronic toxicity of
cadmium in humans. The two main toxic effects resulting from long-term exposure to cadmium in industry are renal dysfunction and lung impairment. Other
reported toxic changes include osteomalacia, slight anemia, and anosmia. The
epidemiologic data on the carcinogenic risk of cadmium are not yet conclusive.
Conflicting results have also been reported regarding the occurrence of chromosomal anomalies in cultured lymphocytes of workers exposed to cadmium and on
the role of cadmium as an etiologic agent in the development of cardiovascular
diseases, particularly hypertension (see Chap. 7).

I. Effects on the Bones

At the end of World War II, an unusual endemic bone disease broke out in Japan,
confined to the Fuchu area in the Zinzu river basin. The disease was called itai-itai
disease, because the patients complained of severe pain in the bones, and *itai-itai*
is the Japanese term for a cry of pain. The main features of itai-itai disease are
pseudofractures of the bones, osteomalacia with eventual osteoporosis, and renal
dysfunction. High concentrations of cadmium, and also zinc and lead, were found
in tissues of autopsied cases as well as in the daily foods in the area (HAGINO and
YOSHIOKA 1961). The patients had been exposed to cadmium as a result of contamination of water and rice by discharges from a zinc mine located 50 km upstream from the endemic area. Clinically apparent cases of the disease were
limited to women over 40 years of age who had given birth to many children and
who had lived in the area for more than 30 years. Up to 1966, nearly 100 deaths
from this disease had been reported and between 1967 and 1982, 132 cases including 90 deaths were officially notified.

The role of cadmium in the occurrence of itai-itai disease has been questioned,
a few authors suggesting that it was not related to cadmium pollution, but caused
by vitamin D deficiency. However, in 1977, a World Health Organization Task
Group concluded that the close epidemiologic association between cadmium exposure and the disease, the accumulation of cadmium in tissues, and the finding
of osteomalacia in cadmium-exposed workers indicate that cadmium was a nec-

essary factor in the development of itai-itai disease. As the disease mainly affected aged women who have had several children and had suffered from calcium and phosphorus deficiency, it is now believed that this severe bone disease resulted from the combination of various nutritional deficiencies with an exceptionally high intake of cadmium.

Bone lesions have also been found in cadmium-exposed workers, but usually as a late manifestation of severe chronic cadmium poisoning. NICAUD et al. (1942) investigated workers in a French alkaline accumulator factory. They observed impairment of the general health with loss of weight, iron deficiency anemia, and severe osteoporosis with pseudofractures of the bones such as are seen in osteomalacia. A few cases of cadmium workers with pseudofractures of the bones suggestive of osteomalacia were also reported from the USSR (TARASENKO and VOROBJEVA 1973) and Poland (HORSTOWA et al. 1966). ADAMS et al. (1969) described the case of a worker in the alkaline battery industry, who developed osteomalacia with multiple spontaneous fractures after 36 years of exposure to cadmium. PUJOL et al. (1970) also found signs of osteomalacia in a subject with 16 years exposure to cadmium. KAZANTZIS (1978) reported the case of a cadmium-exposed worker who developed osteomalacia 12 years after a renal tubular defect was diagnosed.

Several mechanisms are probably involved in the demineralization of the bones induced by cadmium. First, it may be secondary to the increased urinary excretion of calcium and phosphate observed in workers with renal tubular dysfunction (see Sect. E.III.1). Animal experiments suggest that bone changes are associated with a disturbance in vitamin D metabolism. It has been shown that the activation of vitamin D in chicken kidney is inhibited by cadmium, which leads to decreased synthesis of calcium-binding protein in the intestinal mucosa and hence to reduced calcium absorption (FELDMAN and COUSINS 1973). Cadmium may also inhibit directly both the calcium-dependent ATPase and the calcium-binding protein which are implicated in the intestinal absorption of calcium (SAMARAWICKRAMA 1979). Finally, it has also been hypothesized that the bone lesion could result from a direct action of the metal on the bone tissue (KAWAMURA et al. 1978).

II. Effects on the Lung

Impairment of lung function has been described only in workers exposed to cadmium by inhalation. The main clinical studies on the chronic effects of cadmium on the lungs are summarized in Table 2. FRIBERG (1948a, b, 1950) was the first to draw attention to the risk of lung impairment in workers chronically exposed to cadmium. Shortness of breath was among the main complaints of 43 workers exposed on the average for 20 years to cadmium oxide dust in an alkaline accumulator factory. In one-third of the subjects, the residual volume : total lung capacity ratio was decreased, which led Friberg to suggest that emphysema was present. The Swedish report was then supported by observations made in Germany by BAADER (1951) and in the United Kingdom by BONNELL (1955), BONNELL et al. (1959), KAZANTZIS (1956), KAZANTZIS et al. (1963), BUXTON (1956), and ADAMS et al. (1969). The symptoms and findings in these studies were also suggestive of emphysema. In the USSR, lung changes suggestive of diffuse interstitial fibrosis were observed by several authors (VOROBJEVA 1957a; HORSTOWA et al. 1966; TARASENKO and VOROBJEVA 1973). In these early investigations, however, the influence of smoking was not always considered, and it is not likely that all the effects reported were caused by cadmium alone.

In Belgium, LAUWERYS et al. (1974) did take smoking habits into account when matching control and cadmium workers. The workers examined were from different factories: an electronics workshop, a nickel–cadmium battery factory, and a cadmium-producing plant. In each factory, a control group was selected to match the exposed group according to the sex, age, height, weight, smoking habits, and socioeconomic status. The authors observed signs of a mild obstructive syndrome in a group of workers exposed for more than 20 years. Of these workers, the 18 most exposed were carefully examined later by STANESCU et al. (1977) who confirmed the existence of a mild form of obstructive lung disease. The functional impairment was, however, rather slight by comparison with that caused by smoking. Chest X-ray examination of these workers gave no indication of pulmonary emphysema. SMITH et al. (1976) have also examined workers from a cadmium-producing plant. Of 17 male workers exposed on the average for 26.4 years to cadmium, 5 had evidence of mild to moderate lung fibrosis by chest X-ray examination. No such findings were observed in a low-exposure control group, selected from the same plant and matched with the exposed group according to age and smoking habits. In these workers, a significant decrease of the forced vital capacity was found, correlated with the urinary excretion of cadmium. SMITH et al. (1976) suggested that exposure to cadmium fumes may give rise to mild fibrotic reactions in the lung.

GILL (1978) reported a study on 34 men who had worked for 3–37 years in a cadmium plant. By comparison with a control group of office workers, the exposed group exhibited an increased prevalence of exertional dyspnea, but no differences in chest X-ray and ventilatory function were found between the exposed and control workers. In Poland, KOSSMAN et al. (1979) examined the respiratory function of 42 workers exposed to cadmium for periods ranging from 1 to 3 years. Chest X-ray examination revealed emphysema in three workers. Signs of obstructive lung disease were observed in about 50% of the workers examined. Unfortunately, this study cannot be conclusive as smoking habits were not taken into account and no control group was examined. In Australia, DE SILVA and DONNAN (1981) performed respiratory function tests on ten workers employed in a cadmium pigment plant for periods ranging from less than 1 year to 19 years. Two workers with 7 and 13 years exposure suffered from dyspnea and had respiratory function tests indicating severe airway obstruction and emphysema. A third worker, after 3 years exposure, had signs of mild airway obstruction. However, nine of the ten workers were smokers, including the two with emphysema. The authors concluded that the respiratory function was more severely affected than could be explained by the smoking habits alone. A few retrospective studies have shown a slightly increased mortality from respiratory diseases in workers who had been exposed to cadmium (KJELLSTRÖM et al. 1979; HOLDEN 1980). These studies were based on a comparison of the mortality of the cadmium workers with that expected from the mortality of the general population. Since manual workers usually have a higher tobacco consumption than the general population, the exact role of cadmium in this excess mortality from lung disease is difficult to assess.

Recently, ARMSTRONG and KAZANTZIS (1983) reported the results of a mortality study on a cohort of 6,995 workers born before 1940 and exposed to cadmium for at least 1 year between 1942 and 1970. By 1979, a total of 1,902 men aged under 85 years had died, compared with 1968 expected. No excess of deaths due to prostatic cancer, cerebrovascular disease, or renal disease was observed. There were marginally more deaths from lung cancer than expected, but this excess was not related to exposure levels. However, a statistically significant excess of deaths due to bronchitis showed a strong correlation to duration and intensity of exposure, being predominant in the group of men with heavy past exposure to cadmium. According to the authors, the clear relationship with intensity of exposure, the discrepancy between mortality from bronchitis and that from lung cancer, and the implausibility that the high-exposure group smoked much more than the other group, make it unlikely that the excess mortality observed in the high-exposure group can be accounted for by cigarette smoking.

The association between familial α_1-antitrypsin deficiency and pulmonary emphysema is well known (MITTMAN 1972). CHOWDHURY and LOURIA (1976) have reported that in contrast to other metals (Fe^{2+}, Hg^{2+}, Ni^{2+}, Pb^{2+}, and Zn^{2+}), cadmium in vitro causes a dose-related reduction in α_1-antitrypsin content of human plasma and its trypsin inhibitory capacity. They suggested that these in vitro effects of cadmium on α_1-antitrypsin offer a potential explanation for the emphysema reported in some workers exposed to cadmium. However, this specific action of cadmium on the immunologic and biologic activity of α_1-antitrypsin could not be reproduced by GLASER et al. (1976). These authors demonstrated that the decrease of plasma α_1-antitrypsin as reported by CHOWDHURY and LOURIA (1976) was in fact due to a lack of pH control in their experimental protocol. This conclusion was confirmed by BERNARD et al. (1977) who also failed to show any in vitro effect of cadmium on α_1-antitrypsin activity and concentration. Furthermore, these authors measured the concentration and the trypsin inhibitory activity of α_1-antitrypsin in the plasma of 19 cadmium workers and in a similar group of matched controls. No difference between the two groups was found, although the workers had been exposed to cadmium for more than 20 years and 50% of them presented signs of kidney damage. Recently, MARCK et al. (1980) reported a slight reduction of α_1-antitrypsin concentration in serum obtained from cadmium-exposed workers by comparison with controls not occupationally exposed. The difference was however small, about 10% on average, and may have been related to factors other than cadmium.

Several autopsy studies have indicated that persons who died of emphysema and/or chronic bronchitis have high levels of cadmium in lung, liver, and kidneys (MORGAN 1969, 1970; MORGAN et al. 1971; HIRST et al. 1973). It was suggested that cadmium may play a role in the development of these diseases. However, smoking is associated with cadmium exposure and increases the cadmium body burden (see Sect. C). In view of the well-known causal relationship between smoking and chronic bronchitis or emphysema, the accumulation of cadmium in these patients is probably more a secondary effect than a causal factor.

In summary, the following conclusions can be drawn from the various clinical studies on the chronic effects of cadmium on the lung:

1. In the absence of acute episodes of overexposure, the changes induced by cadmium in the lung are usually mild. This conclusion must be tempered by the fact that most investigations have been performed on active workers. This may have introduced a bias in the sense that only "resistant" workers have been examined.

2. The type of function and morphological disturbances induced by cadmium do not agree. Emphysema as reported by the early investigators has not always been found in recent studies in which smoking habits have been taken into account. However, the possibility remains that lung damage develops after several episodes of acute pneumonitis, or even a single episode (see Sect. D.I). In this regard, it should be remembered that exposure levels were much higher in the past.

III. Effects on the Kidney

It is commonly accepted that the kidney is the most important target organ in long-term exposure to cadmium. Cadmium nephropathy has been described in both occupationally exposed workers and in population groups living in a cadmium-polluted environment (e.g., some parts of Japan). Further details on renal effects of Cd will be found in Chap. 6.

1. Observations in Cadmium-Exposed Workers

The nephrotoxic effects of cadmium were first described by Friberg (1948a, b, 1950) who studied a group of alkaline battery workers in Sweden during the late 1940s. The most prominent feature and probably the earliest sign of cadmium nephropathy is an increased proteinuria. Further studies performed in Sweden and the United Kingdom (the main studies on renal function of workers exposed to cadmium are summarized in Table 3) showed that the proteinuria of cadmium

Table 3. Main studies on kidney function in workers exposed to cadmium

Number of workers and conditions of exposure	Observations	References
38 Workers in a cadmium battery factory; 0.4–15 mg/m^3	In 19 subjects exposed for more than 8 years, 18 exhibited a proteinuria of tubular type and 14 had abnormal kidney function tests	Friberg (1948a, b)
58 Workers in the same factory as above	As above, with in addition, 25% of nephrolithiasis	Friberg (1950)
9 Workers exposed more than 9 years in the same factory as above	Deterioration of renal function after removal from exposure; proteinuria may occur after less than 2 years of exposure	Friberg and Nyström (1952), Friberg (1957)

Table 3 (continued)

Number of workers and conditions of exposure	Observations	References
100 Workers in 2 factories producing copper-cadmium alloys; 4–118 µg/m³ (factory 1) and 1–270 µg/m³ (factory 2); higher concentrations in the past	16 Workers with a tubular type proteinuria	BONNELL (1955), KEKWICK (1955)
12 Workers in a cadmium battery factory	Aminoaciduria	CLARKSON and KENCH (1956)
8–30 years exposure in a cadmium battery factory	Proteinuria in 60% of subjects exposed to CdO fumes, in 20% of subjects exposed to CdO dust and in 5% control workers	SMITH and KENCH (1957)
Follow-up study of 83 workers examined in 1955	Proteinuria may appear after cessation of exposure; glucosuria	BONNELL et al. (1959)
40 Workers examined previously by FRIBERG	Proteinuria related to exposure time; electrophoresis of urinary proteins: tubular type pattern	PISCATOR (1962)
As above	Urinary proteins derived from plasma; 50% of low molecular weight proteins constituted by β_2-microglobulin; moderate glucosuria; enzymuria (lysozyme, ribonuclease)	PISCATOR (1966a, b)
12 Workers in a cadmium pigment factory	Clinical tubular type proteinuria in 5 workers exposed for more than 25 years; in 3 workers with 12–14 years of exposure, tubular type pattern on electrophoresis with signs of impaired tubular function (aminoaciduria, glucosuria, hypercalciuria, decreased concentration capacity of the kidneys, impaired acid excretion)	KAZANTZIS et al. (1963)
70 Workers in a cadmium battery factory	44% of subjects with proteinuria	POTTS (1965)
3 Workers in a Swedish cadmium battery factory	30%–35% of urinary proteins constituted by light chains of immunoglobulin	VIGLIANI et al. (1966)
13 Workers producing alloys of silver and cadmium; 68–250 µg/m³	Proteinuria in 7 subjects with more than 1 year exposure	TSUCHIYA (1967)
27 Workers in a cadmium battery factory; 0.5–5 mg/m³	Proteinuria in 19 workers after 4–24 years exposure; tubular type pattern on electrophoresis; decreased creatinine clearance; increased urinary excretion of uric acid, calcium, phosphate, glucose, and amino acids; nephrolithiasis	ADAMS et al. (1969)

Table 3 (continued)

Number of workers and conditions of exposure	Observations	References
21 Workers in a cadmium battery factory; 91 workers in a cadmium-producing plant; 31–134 µg/m³	23 Subjects with proteinuria; electrophoresis of urinary proteins: increased urinary excretion of both low and high molecular weight proteins	LAUWERYS et al. (1974), MATERNE et al. (1975)
Workers in a cadmium-producing plant	Increased urinary excretion of low (lysozyme, β_2-microglobulin) and high molecular weight proteins (albumin, transferrin, IgG, orosomucoid)	ROELS et al. (1975), BERNARD et al. (1976)
55 Workers in a cadmium battery factory	Increased urinary excretion of both low and high molecular weight proteins; larger relative increase of β_2-microglobulin	HANSEN et al. (1977)
240 Workers in a cadmium battery factory; 50 µg/m³	19% of workers exposed for 6–12 years have an increased β_2-microglobulinuria; 10 years exposure to 25 µg Cd/m³ may have increased the β_2-microglobulinuria	KJELLSTRÖM et al. (1977a)
11 Workers in a cadmium pigment factory (median level of exposure 50 µg/m³)	3 Workers with proteinuria (1 glomerular, 1 tubular and 1 mixed type proteinuria) after 3–4 years of exposure	LAUWERYS et al. (1979)
42 Workers in a cadmium-producing plant	Increased renal clearance of β_2-microglobulin, orosomucoid, albumin, transferrin, and IgG; increased plasma creatinine and β_2-microglobulin; β-galactosiduria; independent occurrence of signs of tubular and glomerular dysfunction	BERNARD et al. (1979a)
148 Workers in a cadmium-producing plant	13% of workers with increased β_2-microglobulinuria and 15% with increased albuminuria	BUCHET et al. (1980b)
27 Workers in a cadmium-producing plant	Decreased creatinine clearance; increased urinary excretion of β_2-microglobulin and uric acid	SMITH et al. (1980)
11 Workers in a cadmium pigment plant; 0.4–2.31 mg/m³ (in 1977)	6 Workers exposed for 7 years or more exhibited signs of renal tubular damage	DE SILVA and DONNAN (1981)
21 Workers exposed to cadmium and copper fumes and/or dust for 2–25 years	Increased β_2-microglobulinuria (higher than 200 µ/g creatinine) in 6 workers	DI COSTANZO et al. (1982)
37 Workers exposed for a few months to 28 years in a cadmium-producing plant	Signs of renal dysfunction in workers exposed for more than 10 years; increased urinary excretion of albumin, β_2-microglobulin, alkaline phosphatase, and β-N-acetyl-D-glucosaminidase	GOMPERTZ et al. (1983)

workers was similar to the tubular proteinuria described by BUTLER and FLYNN (1958) in patients with renal tubular disorders (BUTLER et al. 1962; KAZANTZIS et al. 1963; PISCATOR 1962). The electrophoretic patterns (paper electrophoresis) of urinary proteins were characterized by the presence of a relatively small albumin fraction with larger α_2, β, and γ protein fractions. In some cases, a post-γ-globulin band was also present. By ultracentrifugation and gel filtration techniques, it was shown that the components of cadmium proteinuria were mainly low molecular weight proteins, chiefly derived from the plasma (PISCATOR 1966a, b). According to PISCATOR (1966b), more than 50% of the proteins had molecular weights less than that of albumin. The low molecular weight proteins so far identified in cadmium proteinuria are β_2-microglobulin, retinol-binding protein, lysozyme, ribonuclease, immunoglobulin light chains, and carbonic anhydrase C.

From 1972, we have performed several studies in which cadmium proteinuria was characterized not only by electrophoresis (on agarose and SDS–polyacrylamide gel), but also by a quantitative determination of specific proteins with molecular weight ranging from 10,000 to 400,000 (LAUWERYS et al. 1974, 1984; ROELS et al. 1975; BERNARD et al. 1976, 1979a, b; BUCHET et al. 1980b). These investigations revealed that cadmium can induce an increased urinary excretion not only of low molecular weight proteins (β_2-microglobulin and lysozyme), but also of high molecular weight proteins such as albumin, transferrin, and IgG. Both types of proteins were often associated in a mixed type of proteinuria, but in some cases an increased urinary excretion of low molecular weight proteins only (tubular proteinuria) or of high molecular weight proteins only (glomerular proteinuria) was observed. Quantitatively, high molecular weight proteins, namely albumin, are the most important components of cadmium-induced proteinuria. Nevertheless, the excretion of low molecular weight proteins, namely β_2-microglobulin, is proportionally much more increased than that of high molecular weight proteins. For instance, in a group of 42 cadmium-exposed workers, a 30-fold increase in the mean relative clearance of β_2-microglobulin was observed against a 5-fold increase only for that of albumin, transferrin, and IgG (BERNARD et al. 1979a). These observations were confirmed by HANSEN et al. (1977) who studied the urinary proteins from cadmium workers by isoelectric focusing on polyacrylamide gel. These authors concluded: "the most pronounced relative increases in average concentrations in relation to years of cadmium exposure were seen in some zones, e.g. those containing albumin and β_2-microglobulin, respectively. The largest quantitative increase was observed for the zone containing albumin." Although many investigators claim that tubular proteinuria is the first event in cadmium proteinuria and that glomerular dysfunction arises secondarily to tubular damage (FRIBERG et al. 1974), no evidence was found in our studies that one component (tubular or glomerular proteinuria) occurs systematically before the other. Even though extensive literature has been published on cadmium proteinuria, little is known about the mechanisms of cadmium nephrotoxicity. Increased urinary excretion of β_2-microglobulin, which passes freely through the glomerulus, indicates a defect in protein reabsorption by the proximal tubules, at least when there is no marked increased in serum β_2-microglobulin. Serum β_2-microglobulin is indeed inversely correlated with the glomerular filtration rate (GFR) (WIBELL et al. 1973; KULT et al. 1974). A semilogarithmic plot of urine versus serum concentration of β_2-microglobulin in patients with various degrees of renal failure has suggested a renal threshold for the tubular reabsorption of β_2-microglobulin at a serum level of about 4.5 mg/l (Wibell 1978). As long as this serum level is not reached, the urinary excretion of β_2-microglobulin may be used as an index of tubular dysfunction. Serum levels of β_2-microglobulin around 4 mg/l have been observed in some cadmium workers (Kjellström and Piscator 1977; Piscator 1978; Bernard et al. 1979a). In these subjects, the increased urinary excretion of β_2-microglobulin may not be related to the extent of tubular dysfunction.

An increased urinary excretion of high molecular weight proteins only (e.g., albumin and γ-globulin), as observed in a few cases of cadmium-exposed workers (Roels et al. 1975; Bernard et al. 1976, 1979a), is generally associated with a change in glomerular filtration. However, when the increased urinary excretion of high molecular weight proteins is accompanied by a concomitant increase in the excretion of low molecular weight proteins, its origin is much more difficult to assess. First, it can result from an incomplete reabsorption by the proximal tubule of high molecular weight proteins which have filtered through the glomerulus. This implies that cadmium affects the reabsorption mechanisms for both low and high molecular weight proteins. Another explanation is that high molecular weight proteins present in urine of cadmium workers are released from the kidneys. Among the various high molecular weight proteins we have so far detected in excessive amounts in the urine from cadmium workers (albumin, transferrin, IgG, and ferritin), this possibility applies mainly to ferritin (Lauwerys et al. 1984). Albumin and transferrin are not synthesized by the kidney. Since IgG excretion is highly related to that of the latter proteins, it is likely that its increased urinary excretion results from a similar mechanism, i.e., an increased glomerular permeability. Ferritin is a large anionic protein, efficiently retained by the glomerular barrier, and present only in trace amounts in plasma. Even assuming that in cadmium-exposed workers ferritin is cleared from the plasma at the same rate as albumin and that no tubular reabsorption takes place, the amount of ferritin which originates from plasma, could account for only a minute fraction of the total amount found in urine(100–200 µg/day in some cadmium workers compared with 5–10 µg/day in control subjects).

Finally, cadmium might also directly lead to increased glomerular permeability. The metal could bind to the negatively charged components of the glomerular capillary wall and reduce the electrostatic restriction to polyanionic proteins such as albumin. An immunologic reaction, as described for inorganic mercury, might also be involved. The recent finding of circulating anti-laminin antibodies (laminin is a glycoprotein of the glomerular basement membrane) in rats chronically exposed to cadmium offers some support to the latter hypothesis (Bernard et al. 1984). That cadmium can affect the glomerular function was already suggested by the studies of Friberg (1950), Ahlmark et al. (1961), and Adams et al. (1969) who reported a decreased GFR in cadmium-exposed workers. For these authors, however, glomerular dysfunction is an advanced feature of cadmium intoxication, occurring only after other signs of tubular damage. Increased serum levels of creatinine and β_2-microglobulin have been observed in recent surveys on cadmium workers (Kjellström and Piscator 1977; Piscator 1978; Bernard et al. 1979a; Smith et al. 1980). The correlations observed between serum β_2-microglobulin, serum creatinine, and creatinine clearance indicate that the increased plasma levels of these components result from a reduction in GFR (KJELLSTRÖM and PISCATOR 1977; BERNARD et al. 1979 a).

A group of Japanese authors has suggested that cadmium could stimulate the synthesis of β_2-microglobulin, and that the increased urinary excretion of β_2-microglobulin might be a consequence of increased serum levels (TSUCHIYA et al. 1979; IAWO et al. 1980; SAKURAI 1980). PISCATOR (1978) compared the concentration of β_2-microglobulin in serum between two groups of cadmium-exposed workers of the same age, but with different blood levels of cadmium. One group (12 workers) had a concentration of cadmium in blood below 10 µg/l and the other group (8 workers) had values between 10 and 20 µg/l. The concentration of creatinine in serum and that of β_2-microglobulin in urine, and also the creatinine clearance did not differ significantly between both groups, but the serum level of β_2-microglobulin was significantly higher in the group with high blood levels of cadmium. According to the authors, this tends to support the hypothesis of a stimulation of β_2-microglobulin synthesis by cadmium. However, this observation could also be explained by the fact that serum β_2-microglobulin is a more sensitive index of decreased GFR than serum creatinine (WIBELL et al. 1973; KULT et al. 1974). The slope of the regression line between inulin clearance and serum β_2-microglobulin is closer to -1 than that observed between inulin clearance and serum creatinine. PISCATOR et al. (1981) further studied the relationship between cadmium and serum β_2-microglobulin in rabbits chronically treated with cadmium, but they failed to show any effect of cadmium exposure on the serum level of β_2-microglobulin. PISCATOR and KJELLSTRÖM (1977) had already presented data on the relationship between β_2-microglobulin and creatinine in serum from cadmium-exposed workers. Among 33 workers exposed to CdO, 4 had increased β_2-microglobulinuria (>360 µg/l) with normal serum β_2-microglobulin (<2.5 mg/l), 5 had increased levels of both parameters, but 6 had high values of β_2-microglobulin in serum with a normal β_2-microglobulinuria. In the total population, a significant correlation was observed between creatinine and β_2-microglobulin in serum ($r=0.59$) which led the authors to conclude that "the etiology of high serum β_2-microglobulin is more likely to be caused by decreased GFR than increased production of β_2-microglobulin." If the increased β_2-microglobulin concentration in serum observed in the 6 workers mentioned is really due to a decreased GFR and not to an increased synthesis (which can not yet be totally excluded), this would support the hypothesis that cadmium may induce glomerular dysfunction before the occurrence of tubular damage.

The question whether cadmium may disturb glomerular function as early as tubular function remains thus a matter of controversy. In subjects with high concentrations of β_2-microglobulin in the urine, the decrease of GFR is probably the consequence of both interstitial and tubular changes, which is consistent with the concept of tubulointerstitial nephritis. However, it can not be excluded that another mechanism is involved, particularly in the cases of decreased GFR associated with normal β_2-microglobulinuria. Other signs of cadmium nephropathy are aminoaciduria, glucosuria, increased urinary excretion of calcium, phosphorus, and uric acid, and decreased concentrating ability of the kidneys (FRIBERG et al. 1974). An increased release in urine of lysosomal enzymes such as β-galactosidase

(Bernard et al. 1979a) or β-N-acetylglucosaminidase or of the brush border enzyme, alkaline phosphatase (Gompertz et al. 1983) may also be observed. These modifications are usually moderate. The disturbances in calcium and phosphorus metabolism may lead to a demineralization of the bones (see Sect. E.I) and also to the formation of kidney stones (Friberg 1950; Ahlmark et al. 1961; Axelsson 1963). In a group of coppersmiths exposed to cadmium, Scott et al. (1976, 1978) found an increased prevalence of urinary tract stones associated with a highly significant hypercalciuria and reduced serum inorganic phosphate. Scott et al. (1980) were also able to demonstrate by neutron activation analysis a significant deficit ($P < 0.01$) in whole body calcium in 15 coppersmiths as compared with two groups of control subjects. The deficit was significantly correlated with the duration of exposure.

2. Observations in the General Population

In cadmium-polluted areas of Japan, signs of renal dysfunction very similar to those observed in cadmium workers were commonly found. A higher incidence of proteinuria, glucosuria, aminoaciduria, and β_2-microglobulinuria has been observed in the Zinzu river basin in Toyama prefecture where itai-itai disease was first seen (Ishizaki and Fukushima 1968; Fukushima et al. 1974; Kjellström et al. 1977b; Shiroishi et al. 1977). Further investigations of renal function of the inhabitants in this area revealed a significant decrease in both creatinine clearance and renal phosphorus reabsorption. Renal dysfunction due to chronic cadmium poisoning was also found in other areas of Japan where the rice was contaminated by cadmium (Saito et al. 1977; Kojima et al. 1977). It seems, however, that Japan is not the only country where environmental exposure to cadmium may induce renal changes in the general population. Recently, a study was carried out in Belgium, suggesting that environmental exposure to cadmium in an industrialized area polluted by this metal may exacerbate the age-related decline of renal function in elderly residents (Lauwerys et al. 1980; Roels et al. 1981b). The renal function of a group of 60 women over 60 years of age who had spent the major part of their lives in the cadmium-polluted area around Liège, was compared with that of two groups of aged women from areas less polluted by this heavy metal (Brussels and Charleroi areas). The group of aged women from the contaminated area had on average a higher cadmium body burden (as reflected by a higher urinary excretion of cadmium) than the groups from the other areas. The parameters selected for evaluating renal function (total protein, amino acids, β_2-microglobulin, and albumin in urine) followed the same trend. Significant correlations were observed between the urinary excretion of cadmium and that of the four renal function parameters. Furthermore, a retrospective mortality study carried out shortly after these observations (Lauwerys and de Wals 1981) revealed that the standardized mortality ratio from nephritis and nephrosis was significantly higher in the cadmium-polluted area than in other areas. The increase was observed for both males and females, which tends to confirm the influence of an environmental factor. Soon after the publication of these results, Boelart et al. (1981) published a letter in *The Lancet,* claiming that the increased mortality by renal diseases in the Liège area was likely due to a greater consumption of nephrotoxic analgesics in Liège by comparison with reference areas. This suggestion is refuted by the results of a recent epidemiologic study on analgesic-induced nephropathy in Belgium (VANHERWEGHEM and EVEN-ADIN 1981). The number of patients with analgesic nephropathy treated by hemodialysis was not significantly different from that in the control areas. An autopsy study is still under way in our laboratory, comparing the cadmium body burden of inhabitants in the Liège area with that of persons living in other parts of Belgium. Preliminary results indicate that the cadmium concentration in the renal cortex in the age group 40–60 years is on average nearly twice as high in the Liège area (geometric mean 37 ppm) than in other areas of the country (LAUWERYS et al. 1983).

In Great Britain, a national geologic survey carried out in 1979 revealed a high degree of soil contamination by cadmium in Shipham, a village in Somerset. Cadmium originated from nearby extinct calamine workings. The cadmium level in the liver of inhabitants was found to be on average five times higher than in control subjects (on the average 11 ppm compared with 2.2 in control subjects; HARVEY et al. 1979). After examining 32 residents of the village, CARRUTHERS and SMITH (1979) concluded that some of the abnormal renal findings could be attributed to cadmium. However, no definitive conclusion can be drawn from this study, which was based on volunteers and did not even include a control group. A mortality study among Shipham residents with a 40-year follow-up was carried out by INSKIP and BERAL (1982). Slight increases in the standardized mortality ratios from nephritis, genitourinary disease, and hypertensive and cardiovascular diseases were found by comparison with a nearby control village. But again, it is difficult to draw a conclusion from this study because of the small size of the population examined and the low number of deaths from specific causes. More interesting is the epidemiologic study performed by BARLTROP and STREHLOW (1982) and by BARLTROP et al. (1983). The authors compared the health status of 548 inhabitants of Shipham with that of 543 inhabitants of a nearby control town (North Petherton). The average cadmium concentration in soil was 100 ppm in Shipham and less than 1 ppm in North Petherton. Cadmium and β_2-microglobulin concentrations were found to be greater in the urine of Shipham adults although values for both groups were within the accepted normal range. However, after correction for age, sex, and smoking history, no statistically significant correlation was found between urinary β_2-microglobulin and length of residence. Only a weak correlation was observed between length of residence and blood or urine cadmium. Little correlation was found between the biochemical parameters and cadmium in soil, dust, or diet. Average dietary intake of cadmium was found to be only moderately elevated in Shipham, rarely exceeding the WORLD HEALTH ORGANIZATION (1972) tolerable weekly intake (400–500 µg/week). Furthermore, a health inventory revealed few significant differences between the populations studied and none that could be related to cadmium. Thus, this study failed to reveal in Shipham residents any health effect which could be attributed to the contamination of soil by cadmium. It is possible that cadmium naturally present in soil is not as easily bioavailable as that contaminating the soil following surface deposition (dustfall, use of cadmium-containing fertilizers, etc.).

3. Diagnosis and Prognosis of Cadmium Nephropathy

Currently, the determination of β_2-microglobulin in urine is widely used as a sensitive test for the detection of cadmium-induced tubular dysfunction. The choice of β_2-microglobulin for this purpose has been questioned since this protein is unstable in acid urine. When the urinary pH is below about 5.5, a time- and temperature-dependent degradation of β_2-microglobulin occurs (EVRIN and WIBELL 1972). This degradation may start in the bladder so that neutralization immediately after urine collection is not always a satisfactory solution to the problem. The rate of degradation is higher in pathologic urine samples, very likely because of an increased release of proteolytic enzymes from damaged tubular cells (DAVEY and GOSLING 1982). It should be stressed that the urinary pH zone in which β_2-microglobulin is unstable is very close to the mean urinary pH in humans (around 5.7–5.8). This explains why usually 20%–30% of random urine samples can not be used for the β_2-microglobulin test (BERNARD et al. 1982; BASTABLE 1983; GOMPERTZ et al. 1983). For a reliable evaluation of urinary excretion of β_2-microglobulin, the urine specimen should be collected several hours after ingestion of sodium bicarbonate, an impracticable procedure during the routine monitoring of workers in industry. Recently, we have demonstrated that the practical difficulties of correct urine sampling encountered with the β_2-microglobulin test are obviated when measuring retinol-binding protein in urine. While being an index as sensitive and as specific as β_2-microglobulin for detecting tubular dysfunction, retinol-binding protein offers the advantage of being stable in acid urine (degradation occurs only at pH below 4.5) (BERNARD and LAUWERYS 1981 b; BERNARD et al. 1982). According to GOMPERTZ et al. (1983), β_2-microglobulinuria goes hand in hand with the excretion of albumin, total protein, and enzymuria (β-N-acetyl-β-D-glucosaminidase and alkaline phosphatase) and it can not be argued, on the basis of their results, that the urinary excretion of β_2-microglobulin is an early sign of renal damage. They suggest that monitoring strategies should be designed to obtain maximum information on both renal function and cadmium status of workers.

Several studies have shown that, once an increased proteinuria has been demonstrated, it is often irreversible (BONNELL et al. 1959; ADAMS et al. 1969; PISCATOR and PETERSON 1977; LAUWERYS et al. 1979 b; ROELS et al. 1982). However, according to TSUCHIYA (1976), the proteinuria may disappear after removal from cadmium exposure. It is possible, indeed, that a slight proteinuria detectable only by the determination of urinary β_2-microglobulin may be reversible, depending on the past exposure conditions and on the health status of the worker (especially age).

The progression of renal dysfunction after cessation of exposure is very slow (ROELS et al. 1982; PISCATOR and PETERSON 1977). Persistent proteinuria is frequently found in retired cadmium workers without any evidence of renal insufficiency. Similar observations were also made in inhabitants of cadmium-polluted areas in Japan. Follow-up of subjects with marked β_2-microglobulinuria did not reveal any evolution to renal insufficiency (uremia). The majority were active and did not require any special medical care.

KJELLSTRÖM (1982) however reported a significant excess of deaths from genitourinary disease (4 compared with 0.93 expected) (mainly nephritis) in a group of workers with more than 20 years exposure to cadmium and 20 years latency.

For this author "it is clear that cadmium exposure increases mortality from kidney diseases after high exposure intensity and long duration of exposure." By contrast, ARMSTRONG and KAZANTZIS (1983) and SORAHAN et al. (1983) did not find any significant increase of the mortality rate from nephritis and nephrosis in cadmium-exposed workers. In the study of SORAHAN et al. (1983), the observed number of deaths was nevertheless nearly twice as high as expected (10 compared with 5.49). More recently, ANDERSSON et al. (1983) reported a significant increase in deaths from nephritis and nephrosis (3 observed compared with 0.41 expected) in a group of 175 workers exposed to cadmium for more than 15 years. The health significance of an increased β_2-microglobulinuria is thus not clear and the question remains whether this renal disturbance must be considered as an adverse health effect. The subcommittee on cadmium of the British Occupational Hygiene Society Committee on Hygiene Standards does not consider as an adverse effect an increase in the excretion of proteins as far as it is undetectable by classical tests for proteinuria. Nevertheless, from the standpoint of preventive medicine, it is certainly advisable to prevent the occurrence of such an effect and therefore the permissible levels of exposure (cadmium in air, in dust, etc.) should be defined accordingly.

In their study on the renal function of inhabitants living in a cadmium-polluted area of Japan, NOGAWA et al. (1980) suggested that reduction in creatinine clearance may occur at the early stage of chronic cadmium poisoning and may be useful in early detection of renal dysfunction in chronic cadmium poisoning.

The various studies we have performed on cadmium-exposed workers in Belgium have shown that the most sensitive method for the early detection of cadmium nephropathy is the determination of specific proteins in urine. These studies stress also the usefulness of measuring at least two proteins, a low molecular weight protein (e.g., retinol-binding protein) and a higher molecular weight protein such as albumin, for the early detection of cadmium-induced renal disturbances (LAUWERYS and BERNARD 1982).

IV. Effects on the Cardiovascular System: Hypertension

SCHROEDER (1965) was the first to suggest that cadmium might contribute to the development of essential hypertension in humans. His hypothesis was based on both animal and human data. He demonstrated that long-term oral administration of cadmium to rats may induce a systolic hypertension persisting throughout their life. In humans, he observed that patients dying from hypertension and/or cardiovascular diseases had somewhat higher cadmium levels in liver and kidneys than people dying from other causes. The hypertensive action of cadmium in animals has been confirmed in subsequent studies (SAMARAWICKRAMA 1979). Its mechanism is however still obscure and in particular, the role of nutritional factors in the dose–effect and dose–response relationships remains to be clarified. Epidemiologic studies which have focused on the possible relationship between prevalence of cardiovascular diseases and exposure to cadmium have provided conflicting results. The association between arterial pressure and cadmium levels in tissues, initially reported by SCHROEDER (1965), has been found, depending on the study, to be positive, nonexistent, or even negative.

Similarly, the positive correlation between arterial pressure and blood or urinary cadmium observed in some studies has not been confirmed by others (STAESSEN et al. 1984). Part of this discrepancy may be due to confounding factors such as age, sex, nutritional status, and, mainly, smoking habits. Indeed, as smoking is a contributory factor in the development of cardiovascular diseases (including hypertension) and also a source of cadmium exposure, the relationship between cadmium and hypertension seen in some studies might be secondary. Recently, we have examined the relationship between urinary cadmium, β_2-microglobulin in urine, and blood pressure in a random 4% sample of the population of a small Belgian town (STAESSEN et al. 1984). After adjusting for age, body weight, and smoking habits, a weak but negative correlation became apparent between urinary cadmium and systolic pressure in women and between urinary cadmium and diastolic pressure in men. Of course, these correlations do not necessarily imply a causal relationship between urinary cadmium and blood pressure, since an unknown third factor might be the common link and produce the association. Nevertheless, they suggest that cadmium, even at the environmental level, might have some kind of biologic action and for unknown reasons reduce blood pressure. A striking and still unexplained observation was also made in this study: in women, the urinary excretion of β_2-microglobulin was negatively correlated with both systolic and diastolic pressure.

In the United States, CARROLL (1966) and later HICKEY et al. (1967) observed that the cadmium concentration in air of more than twenty cities was significantly correlated with death rate from cardiovascular diseases. However, HUNT et al. (1971) in a study involving 77 American cities, failed to show any correlation between cadmium fallout and mortality from cardiovascular diseases. Furthermore, reanalyzing Carroll's data, they were able to demonstrate a higher correlation between population density and hypertension than between hypertension and the cadmium level in air. A significant negative correlation between total water hardness and cardiovascular diseases has been frequently reported (MASIROMI 1974). Since hard water usually contains less heavy metals, in particular cadmium, than soft water, this explains why one may find a positive correlation between cadmium in water and the prevalence of hypertension. Furthermore, when considering the possible relationships between cadmium in air or in water and hypertension, it should be remembered that the cadmium intake of the general population from water and from air is very low in comparison with that from food.

So far, there is no serious evidence of increased morbidity or mortality due to cardiovascular diseases in workers exposed to cadmium. In a recent study, VOROBJEVA and EREMEEVA (1980) reported an increased prevalence of hypertension and several types of ECG abnormalities in cadmium-exposed workers. However, as no matched control group was examined, it is difficult to draw clear-cut conclusions from this study. In cadmium-polluted areas in Japan, blood pressure was monitored during several epidemiologic studies, but no association between blood pressure and the degree of cadmium pollution could be detected (JAPAN PUBLIC HEALTH ASSOCIATION 1976; SHIGEMATSU et al. 1981). The results of two mortality studies among cadmium-exposed populations in Japan have also been published. In one study, it was found that the cerebrovascular disease mortality rate was twice as high in people with proteinuria as in those without proteinuria

(NOGAWA et al. 1981). This was not confirmed in the second study which compared the cerebrovascular disease mortality rate between administrative units
with polluted areas and those without such areas (SHIGEMATSU et al. 1982). It is
however possible that, in the latter study, the effect has been masked because the
"exposed groups" included large numbers of people with low exposure to cadmium. These negative findings under conditions of relatively high exposure to
cadmium do not necessarily disprove that cadmium at a low environmental level
plays a role in the etiology of hypertension. As suggested by PERRY and ERLANGER
(1974), the relationship between cadmium and blood pressure may not be linear
and the potential action of cadmium on blood pressure may vary according to
the intensity of exposure. It is also possible that the hypertensive action of cadmium is determined by factors such as age, sex, smoking habits, genetic susceptibility, or mineral content of the diet.

In conclusion, the role of cadmium in the development of hypertension remains uncertain. The failure, after nearly 20 years of epidemiologic investigations, to show a clear relationship between cadmium and hypertension, suggests
that if cadmium really plays a role in the etiology of hypertension, it is in association with other factors involved in the pathogenesis of this disease (for further
discussion see Chap. 7).

V. Carcinogenicity

Cadmium metal or various cadmium salts can produce injection site sarcomas in
rats and interstitial cell testicular tumors in mice and rats after subcutaneous injections (INTERNATIONAL AGENCY for RESEARCH on CANCER 1976). In a lifetime
rat inhalation study, TANEKAKA et al. (1983) have found a dose-dependent induction of lung carcinoma by cadmium chloride aerosol.

So far, the available epidemiologic data (summarized in Table 4) provide
limited evidence that cadmium or certain cadmium compounds are carcinogenic
for humans. Of these studies, only three show a statistically significant association
between cadmium exposure and prostate cancer (KIPLING and WATERHOUSE
1967; LEMEN et al. 1976; HOLDEN 1980). The increase of death rate from prostatic
cancer found in the studies of McMICHAEL et al. (1976) and KJELLSTRÖM et al.
(1979) did not reach the level of significance whereas that reported initially by
POTTS (1965) cannot be evaluated statistically for lack of a comparison group.

In addition to the risk of prostate cancer, LEMEN et al. (1976) and HOLDEN
(1980) also found a significant excess of deaths from bronchogenic carcinoma in
cadmium-exposed workers. But these workers were simultaneously exposed to
low levels of lead, zinc, and arsenic. The latter is a well-known pulmonary carcinogen and according to HOLDEN (1980) probably responsible for the increased
death rate from lung cancer. The concomitant exposure to other known or suspected carcinogens (nickel, arsenic, tobacco smoke) may be the origin of the excess of renal carcinomas reported by KOLONEL (1976), which, so far, has been observed in no other epidemiologic study.

There is presently no clinical or experimental indication that exposure to cadmium via food favors the development of cancer. The lowest death rate for prostatic cancer is in Japan (1.4/100,000 in 1974–1975), where the daily intake of cad-

Table 4. Clinical studies on the carcinogenic effects of cadmium

Observations	Reference
5 Cancer cases (3 of the prostate) in 74 men exposed for more than 10 years to CdO dust (no comparison group)	Potts (1965)
Increased prevalence of prostate cancers (4 vs 0.58 expected, $p < 0.05$) among 248 cadmium workers exposed for at least 1 year. These cancer cases include the 3 cases by Potts (1965)	Kipling and Waterhouse (1967)
5 Cancer cases (2 of lung, 1 of liver, 1 of prostate, and 1 of heart) among 536 workers who between 1949 and 1966 had been in contact with cadmium (and also nickel hydroxide). The author concluded that the information was insufficient to establish an association between cadmium and cancer	Humperdinck (1968)
1 Prostate carcinoma and 1 bronchus carcinoma among 42 men exposed to cadmium for 2–40 years	Holden (1969)
Case history study (64 patients with renal tumor) revealing a significant association of renal cancer with exposure to cadmium (greater risk in smokers)	
Increased rate of total malignancies (27 vs 17.5 expected), lung cancer (12 vs 5.11 expected, $P < 0.05$), and prostate cancer (4 vs 1.15 expected, $P < 0.05$) among 292 workers who had been employed in a cadmium smelter for at least 2 years	Lemen et al. (1976)
Mortality study among rubber workers. An excess of death from prostate cancer associated with the use of metallic oxides (including cadmium oxide)	McMichael et al. (1976)
Case history study (176 prostate carcinoma cases). No association with occupational exposure to cadmium	Kolonel and Winkelstein (1977)
Among 269 workers in a cadmium-nickel battery factory, no increase in total cancer mortality (15 vs. 16.4 expected). The death rate from nasopharynx cancer was significantly increased, probably owing to nickel dust. Among 94 workers in a cadmium-copper alloy factory, 4 cases of prostate cancer vs 2.69 expected	Kjellström et al. (1979)
Significant excess of deaths from cancer (all causes), from lung cancer and prostate cancer in 624 cadmium factory workers	Holden (1980)
4 Prostate cancer deaths vs 3.1 expected in 619 workers employed in a cadmiun-nickel battery factory	Kjellström (1982)
No excess of deaths due to prostate cancer in a cohort of 6995 workers exposed to cadmium for more than 1 year. A slight increase in lung cancer, but not related to exposure levels	Armstrong and Kazantzis (1983)
No excess of deaths from cancer (all causes, prostate included) in a cohort of 3025	Sorahan et al. (1983)
No significant increases for cancer of the prostate (3 vs 1.58 expected), urinary bladder (2 vs 0.44 expected), and lung (3 vs 2.5 expected) in a group of 175 workers exposed to cadmium for more than 15 years	Andersson et al. (1983)

mium is the highest in the world (see Sect. B.I). On the other hand, Sweden has the highest age-adjusted death rate from prostate cancer in the world (21.9/ 100,000 in 1974–1975) with a low daily intake and low body burdens of cadmium (KJELLSTRÖM et al. 1979). Mortality studies of cadmium-polluted areas in Japan (NOGAWA et al. 1981; SHIGEMATSU et al. 1981, 1982) or in Europe (LAUWERYS and DE WALS 1981) have provided little or no evidence of an increased mortality rate from total malignancies or prostatic cancer. Additional information cannot be obtained from mutagenesis studies from which conflicting results have emerged (see Sect. E.VI).

In conclusion, although there is sufficient evidence that cadmium may be carcinogenic in animals under certain exposure conditions, the association between cadmium exposure and cancer in humans remains tenuous. Only the increased risk of prostatic cancer in workers exposed to cadmium by inhalation has been found to be significant, but the number of cases so far reported is very small. The INTERNATIONAL AGENCY for RESEARCH on CANCER (1976) has nevertheless classified cadmium among chemicals which are probably carcinogenic for humans (category 2A).

VI. Other Effects

Among other effects reported in persons chronically exposed to cadmium, one can mention: anosmia, ulceration of the nasal mucosa, yellowing of dental necks, mild anemia, and occasionally signs of liver damage. So far, no report on teratogenic effects of cadmium in humans has been published. In a study on cadmium-exposed women in the USSR, congenital malformations were not observed, but the birth weights of offspring were lower than those from control mothers (CVETKOVA 1970). Data on mutagenic effects of cadmium in humans are conflicting. SHIRAISHI (1975) reported the existence of chromosomal aberrations in itai-itai patients, but this was not confirmed by BUI et al. (1975). The latter authors also examined chromosomes from lymphocytes of five cadmium workers, but no abnormality was found. By contrast, DEKNUDT and LEONARD (1975) and BAUCHINGER et al. (1976) found a slight but significant increase of chromosomal anomalies in workers exposed to cadmium. In these two studies, however, the workers were also exposed to other metals, such as lead, zinc, or arsenic, so that the anomalies observed cannot be firmly attributed to cadmium. O'RIORDAN et al. (1978) found no increased frequency of aberration in blood lymphocytes of cadmium workers. They suggest that aberrations described previously result from a synergistic action of heavy metals with some environmental mutagens. Negative results were also recently reported by FLEIG et al. (1983). GASIOREK and BAUCHINGER (1981) have studied the in vivo effect of lead, cadmium, and zinc, separately and in combination, on the incidence of chromosomal aberrations in human lymphocytes. They observed a significantly increased incidence of anomalies exclusively with cadmium, an observation the authors relate to the accumulation of cadmium in lymphocytes (metallothionein synthesis). Functional disturbances in the nervous system of cadmium-exposed workers have been reported by VOROBJEVA (1957b) in the USSR. Physical examination revealed an increase in patellar reflex, tremor, dermatographia, and sweating. Changes were also observed in chronaxy. Cadmium sulfide is sometimes used as a yellow tattoo pigment. Local phototoxic reactions may occur when the tattooed skin is exposed to UV radiation. Of 24 subjects with yellow tattoos examined by BJORNBERG (1963), 18 complained of skin swelling when exposed to sunlight.

VII. Dose–Effect and Dose–Response Relationships

In occupational exposure to cadmium, the kidney and the lung are the two main target organs, but in the absence of episodes of subacute exposure, the kidney is usually the first affected and therefore constitutes the critical organ. For the general population, mainly exposed to cadmium present in food, the lung is not a target organ; damage is usually detected in the kidney first and much later in the bones.

1. Lung

Since lung disturbances induced by cadmium are most likely the result of a local toxic action, their occurrence and intensity must be related to external exposure factors such as concentration in air and duration of exposure. However, it is not yet clear from the literature whether lung impairment results from long-term exposure above a critical airborne cadmium concentration or from several episodes of subacute exposure leading to permanent changes. Various types of lung disturbances (e.g., emphysema, chronic obstructive lung disease, fibrosis) have been linked with cadmium exposure. Unfortunately, in many studies reporting lung impairment induced by cadmium, insufficient consideration was given to simultaneous exposure to other lung irritants such as tobacco smoke or industrial pollutants. Furthermore, the data on the concentration of cadmium in air are fragmentary and provide no information on the particle size or the chemical form of cadmium.

In view of these uncertainties, only a tentative proposal for a long-term no-effect level of cadmium in air can be formulated. The available epidemiologic data (see Table 2) suggest that to prevent any deleterious effect of cadmium on the respiratory system, the time-weighted average exposure to cadmium oxide fumes or to respirable cadmium dust should not exceed a Cd concentration of $20 \, \mu g/m^3$ (duration of exposure: 40 h per week over the whole working life) (WORLD HEALTH ORGANIZATION 1980).

2. Kidney

The chronic effects of cadmium in the kidney result from an excessive accumulation of the metal in the organ following long-term exposure by inhalation (occupational exposure) or by ingestion (environmental exposure). The risk of renal damage has been evaluated by studying the relationships between the effect (or the response) and: (a) the amount of cadmium stored in the kidney; (b) the concentration of cadmium in urine, which may be used as an indirect indicator of the renal cadmium store; or (c) the daily intake of cadmium. The latter method is only applicable to the general population exposed to cadmium essentially through food (smokers excepted).

As inhalation is the major route of cadmium exposure in the working environment, several authors have also examined the relationship between the prevalence of renal dysfunction and the integrated exposure to airborne cadmium ($\mu g/m^3 \times$ years) and, on this basis, have attempted to estimate a threshold effect level. MATERNE et al. (1975) and LAUWERYS et al. (1974) have reported that exposure to 20 $\mu g/m^3$ for 40 h a week over 20 years could be close to the threshold effect level. KJELLSTRÖM et al. (1977a) have found that 19% of workers with 6–12 years exposure to Cd dust at about 50 $\mu g/m^3$, equivalent to an exposure of 20 $\mu g/m^3$ for about 20 years, had tubular proteinuria as compared with 3% in the control group. A follow-up study on 27 workers with a median of 25 years exposure to airborne cadmium was recently published by SMITH et al. (1980). Comparing the time-weighted cumulative exposure for each worker with the β_2-microglobulin excretion, they confirmed that exposure to airborne cadmium should be kept below 50 $\mu g/m^3$ for a worker's lifetime to prevent increased β_2-microglobulin excretion. All these findings are in agreement with the calculation made by FRIBERG et al. (1974), indicating that after 10 years of occupational exposure to 25 $\mu g/m^3$, sensitive persons may have accumulated cadmium in the renal cortex up to the critical concentration. In practice, however, technical measures based on a threshold effect level of cadmium in air do not suffice for effective prevention of renal damage. We know from previous experience that measurements of airborne concentration, even with personal samplers, provide only a rough estimate of the amount of cadmium inhaled by the worker. Furthermore, only total cadmium concentration is generally measured and the physicochemical characteristics of the particles which influence the respiratory absorption are not taken into account.

a) Critical Concentration of Cadmium in the Renal Cortex

From a comparison of the cadmium concentrations in the renal cortex of cadmium-exposed persons with and without signs of kidney damage, FRIBERG et al. (1974) suggested that the critical level of cadmium in the renal cortex for the appearance of tubular proteinuria is around 200 ppm. In 1977, a World Health Organization Task Group, reviewing the available animal and human data, concluded that "the critical concentration is between 100 and 300 ppm in kidney cortex, but the most likely estimate is about 200 ppm" (WORLD HEALTH ORGANIZATION 1977).

As already pointed out by FRIBERG et al. (1974), a critical concentration of 200 ppm does not mean that 200 ppm cadmium in the renal cortex will give rise to renal tubular dysfunction in all persons exposed. The critical level must be regarded as the concentration of cadmium in the renal cortex at which a fraction of the population (the most susceptible group) may suffer from adverse renal effects. This concept has been recently clearly expressed by KJELLSTRÖM et al. (1984) who proposed the term "population critical concentration" with a defined response rate (generally 10%). With the development of neutron activation techniques allowing the in vivo determination of cadmium in tissues, the critical level of cadmium in human kidney has been more precisely assessed. By using this technique, we have measured the concentrations of cadmium in kidney and liver of

309 male workers employed in two Belgian zinc–cadmium plants (ROELS et al. 1979, 1981 a). Renal function was evaluated by determining the urinary excretion of β_2-microglobulin and albumin. The levels of cadmium in blood and urine were also measured. For computing the kidney cadmium content, we had assumed a kidney depth of 5 cm for all the workers. With this assumption, the critical concentration of cadmium in the renal cortex, corresponding to a 10% response rate of renal dysfunction, was estimated at 160 ppm. However, in a subsequent study, we had to reassess this estimate after the kidney depth of the examined workers was measured by echography (ROELS et al. 1983 a). The mean kidney depth was found to be 8.1 cm (range 5.1–12.4 cm). After correcting each individual value for the kidney depth, the critical level of cadmium in the renal cortex was estimated at 216 ppm, which corresponds to a mean concentration of cadmium in the liver of 30 ppm and to a mean total body burden of 182 mg. This critical level of cadmium in the renal cortex (216 ppm) protects probably more than 90% of male workers from cadmium-induced renal dysfunction.

ELLIS et al. (1980, 1981) also performed a study designed to estimate the critical level of cadmium in the renal cortex. Cadmium was measured in vivo in the left kidney and liver of 83 American cadmium workers. Evaluation of renal function was based on the determination of β_2-microglobulin and total protein in urine. Estimates of the critical level yielded values of 300–400 ppm, which are much higher than those obtained by ROELS et al. (1981 a). As suggested by KJELLSTRÖM et al. (1984), this could result from the fact that different approaches have been used for estimating the critical concentration. In fact, the critical concentration as estimated by ROELS et al. (1981 a) corresponds to a 10% response rate in the exposed population, whereas that calculated by ELLIS et al. (1981) is an average for exposed groups (50% response rate). Furthermore, according to KJELLSTRÖM et al. (1984), the estimates made by ROELS et al. (1981 a) and ELLIS et al. (1981) are too high by about 25% because the true cortex : whole kidney cadmium concentration ratio would be 1.15 : 1 instead of 1.5 : 1.

b) Critical Concentration of Cadmium in Urine

On the basis of the correlation between the urinary excretion of cadmium and that of total protein in occupationally exposed workers, LAUWERYS et al. (1974) suggested that "urinary cadmium concentration in workers currently exposed should be kept below 15 μg per gram creatinine, at which level the probability of detecting renal damage is low." This conclusion was corroborated by subsequent studies in which renal function was evaluated by more sensitive methods (e.g., renal clearance of β_2-microglobulin and of albumin) (BERNARD et al. 1979 a; LAUWERYS et al. 1979 a; BUCHET et al. 1980 b). Whatever the population examined and the intensity of exposure, renal dysfunction was found to be present when the concentration of urinary cadmium exceeded 10 μg per gram creatinine.

These observations led LAUWERYS et al. (1979 a) to propose a tentative biologic threshold for urinary cadmium of 10 μg per gram creatinine. The validity of this proposal was confirmed by the relationship between cadmium in urine and cadmium in the renal cortex in the 309 Belgian workers whose renal cadmium was measured by neutron activation analysis (ROELS et al. 1981 a, 1983 a). This relationship, established only in cadmium workers without signs of renal damage, shows that a concentration of cadmium in the renal cortex of 216 ppm (the critical level) corresponds to a urinary concentration of 10.8 µg per gram creatinine.

The relationship between urinary cadmium and prevalence of increased β_2-microglobulinuria was also examined by HUTTON (1982) in a group of 143 British cadmium workers. A urinary concentration of cadmium of 5 µg/l was found to be associated with elevated β_2-microglobulinuria in 10% of the population and at a urinary cadmium level of 15 µg/l, β_2-microglobulinuria was increased in 50% of the population. According to HUTTON (1982), these data would suggest that a 5 µg/l threshold should be required to protect 90% of occupationally exposed workers. In Japan, NOGAWA et al. (1979) studied the dose–response relationships between urinary cadmium and urinary β_2-microglobulin in inhabitants of the Zinzu river basin (itai-itai disease endemic area). In men, a urinary excretion of cadmium of 6.3 and 14 µg per gram creatinine was associated with increased β_2-microglobulinuria in 10% and 50% of the population, respectively. TSUCHIYA et al. (1979) also reported data on cadmium and β_2-microglobulin in urine from environmentally exposed people in Japan, but the dose–response analysis of these data yields surprising results. About 20% of the population exhibited excessive β_2-microglobulinuria for a level of cadmium in urine of only 2 µg per gram creatinine (a level generally considered as the upper normal limit for nonexposed people) (HUTTON 1982). Regarding these two Japanese studies, it should be stressed that the susceptibility of the general population to cadmium toxicity might be different from that of adult male workers. Some epidemiologic data suggest that the critical level of cadmium in urine (and thus in kidney) in old persons with declining renal function is much lower than that estimated in middle-aged male workers (LAUWERYS et al. 1980; ROELS et al. 1981 b).

c) Critical Intake of Cadmium

Two approaches have been used to estimate the critical intake of cadmium for the development of renal dysfunction: (a) study of the dose–response relationships in population groups exposed to cadmium mainly via food (Japan); (b) calculation with a mathematical model of the intake necessary to reach the critical level in the renal cortex. The few epidemiologic studies designed for dose–response analysis between oral intake and renal effects of cadmium originate from Japan (KJELLSTRÖM 1977; NOGAWA et al. 1978). These studies were critically reviewed by HUTTON (1982). Using KJELLSTRÖM's (1977) data, HUTTON (1982) calculated that a daily cadmium intake of 118 µg for a Japanese (53 kg) or of 156 µg for a European (70 kg) is required to increase β_2-microglobulin excretion in 10% of the population after 50 years of exposure. Hutton applied the same calculation to the data collected by NOGAWA et al. (1978), but in this case, the estimates of critical intake were twice as high as those derived from Kjellström's data: 269 µg for a Japanese and 355 µg for a European. This difference between the two studies results very likely from the fact that the authors used methods of different sensitivity to detect renal dysfunction. NOGAWA et al. (1978) measured the urinary excretion of retinol-binding protein by radial immunodiffusion, a method about 100-fold less sensitive than the β_2-microglobulin radioimmunoassay used by KJELLSTRÖM (1977).

FRIBERG et al. (1974) proposed a mathematical model to calculate the cadmium intake by different routes, which is necessary to reach the critical level in the renal cortex (200 ppm). Considering only the oral intake, they estimated that a daily cadmium intake of 248 µg is necessary to reach 200 ppm in the renal cortex at the age of 50 years. KJELLSTRÖM and NORDBERG (1978) published an eight-compartment kinetic model for the metabolism of cadmium. Assuming a 4.8% gastrointestinal absorption, KJELLSTRÖM (1979 b) calculated with this model that a daily oral intake of cadmium of 108 µg for a Japanese (53 kg) and of 142 µg for a European (70 kg) is necessary to increase the concentration of cadmium in the renal cortex to 200 ppm at the age of 45 years in 10% of the population (nonsmokers).

In 1972, a FAO/WHO Expert Committee proposed a value of 1 µg/kg (70 µg mean European body weight) as the provisional tolerable daily intake of cadmium through food (WORLD HEALTH ORGANIZATION 1972). The estimates of the critical oral intake of cadmium reviewed range from 2 to 4 µg/kg^{-1} day^{-1}. This suggests that adherence to the WHO guideline will protect a large majority of the exposed population (probably more than 95%). In Europe, the average current daily intake of cadmium is around 15 µg according to the most recent estimate (see Table 1) and is thus below the WHO guideline. Nevertheless, we have obtained preliminary data suggesting that environmental pollution by cadmium in an industrialized area of Belgium may exacerbate the age-related decline of renal function in the general population, and possibly may influence both the morbidity and mortality from renal diseases (LAUWERYS et al. 1980; ROELS et al. 1981 b; LAUWERYS and DE WALS 1981). The question arises whether the current estimate of the critical level of cadmium in the renal cortex, mainly based on observations in occupationally exposed persons, and the critical intake derived from it, are applicable to the general population, some groups of which may be specially susceptible to the toxic action of this environmental pollutant.

References

Adams RG, Harrison JG, Scott P (1969) The development of cadmium-induced proteinuria, impaired renal function and osteomalacia in alkaline battery workers. Quart J Med 38:442–443

Adamsson E (1979) Long-term sampling of airborne cadmium dust in an alkaline battery factory. Scand J Work Environ Health 5:178–187

Ahlgren L, Mattson S (1980) Cadmium in man measured in vivo by x-ray fluorescence analysis. Phys Med Biol 26:19–26

Ahlmark A, Axelsson B, Friberg L, Piscator M (1961) Further investigations into kidney function and proteinuria in chronic cadmium poisoning. Proc 13th Int Cong Occup Health, New York

Al-Haddad IK, Chettle DR, Fletcher JG, Fremlin JH (1981) A transportable system for measurement of kidney cadmium in vivo. Int J Appl Radiat Isot 32:109–112

Andersson K, Elinder CG, Kjellström T, Spang G (1983) Mortality among cadmium workers in a Swedish battery factory. In: Wilson D, Volpe RA (eds) Proceedings of Fourth International Cadmium Conference. Cadmium Association, Cadmium Council, ILZRO, London, pp 101–103

Armstrong BG, Kazantzis (1983) The mortality of cadmium workers. Lancet I:1425–1427

Axelsson B (1963) Urinary calculus in long-term exposure to cadmium. Proc XIV Int Cong Occup Health, pp 939–942

Baader EW (1951) Public health and occupational medicine: chronic cadmium poisoning. Dtsch Med Woch 76:484–487 (in German)

Barltrop D, Strehlow CD (1982) Cadmium and health in Shipham. Lancet II:1394

Barltrop D, Strehlow CD, Wells J (1983) Health implications of cadmium exposure in Shipham. In: Proc IV Int Cadmium Conf Munich. Wilson D, Cadmium Association; Volpe RA, Cadmium Council and ILZRO London (eds), pp 101–103

Bastable MD (1983) β_2-microglobulin in urine: not suitable for assessing renal tubular function. Clin Chem 29:996–997

Bauchinger M, Schmid E, Einbrodt HJ, Dresp J (1976) Chromosome aberrations in lymphocytes after occupational exposure to lead and cadmium. Mutat Res 40:57–62

Bernard A, Lauwerys R (1981 a) The effects of sodium chromate and carbon tetrachloride on the urinary excretion and tissue distribution of cadmium in cadmium-pretreated rats. Toxicol Appl Pharm 57:30–38

Bernard A, Lauwerys R (1981 b) Retinol-binding protein in urine: a more practical index than urinary β_2-microglobulin for the routine screening of renal tubular function. Clin Chem 27:1781–1782

Bernard A, Roels H, Hubermont G, Buchet JP, Masson PL, Lauwerys R (1976) Characterization of the proteinuria in cadmium-exposed workers. Int Arch Occup Environ Health 38:19–30

Bernard A, Roels H, Buchet JP, Lauwerys R, Masson P (1977) α_1-antitrypsin in cadmium toxicity: an evaluation of its suggested role. Toxicology 9:249–253

Bernard A, Buchet JP, Roels H, Masson P, Lauwerys R (1979 a) Renal excretion of proteins and enzymes in workers exposed to cadmium. Eur J Clin Invest 9:11–22

Bernard A, Goret A, Buchet JP, Roels H, Lauwerys R (1979 b) Comparison of sodium dodecyl sulfate polyacrylamide gel electrophoresis with quantitative methods for the analyses of cadmium-induced proteinuria. Int Arch Occup Environ Health 44:139–148

Bernard A, Moreau D, Lauwerys R (1982) Comparison of retinol-binding protein and β_2-microglobulin determination in urine for the early detection of tubular proteinuria. Clin Chim Acta 126:1–7

Bernard A, Lauwerys R, Gengoux P, Mahieu P, Foidart JM, Druet P, Weening JJ (1984) Anti-laminin and anti-type IV procollagen antibodies in Sprague-Dawley and Brown Norway rats chronically exposed to cadmium. Toxicology 31:307–313

Biggin CH, Chen NS, Ettinger KV, Fremlin JH, Morgan WD, Nowotny R, Chamberlain MG, Harvey TC (1974) Cadmium by in vivo neutron activation analysis. J Radioanal Chem 19:207–214

Bjornberg A (1963) Reactions to light in yellow tattoos from cadmium sulfide. Arch Dermatology 88:267–271

Boelaert J, Daneels R, Schurgers M (1981) Cadmium, kidneys and Belgian industry. Lancet I:672

Bonnell JA (1955) Emphysema and proteinuria in men casting copper-cadmium alloys. Br J Ind Med 12:181–197

Bonnell JA, Kazantzis G, King E (1959) A follow-up study of men exposed to cadmium oxide fume. Br J Ind Med 16:135–147

Buchet JP, Roels H, Lauwerys R, Bruaux P, Claeys-Thoreau F, Lafontaine A, Verduyn G (1980 a) Repeated surveillance of exposure to cadmium, manganese and arsenic in school-age children living in rural, urban and nonferrous smelter areas in Belgium. Environ Res 22:95–108

Buchet JP, Roels H, Bernard A, Lauwerys R (1980 b) Assessment of renal function of workers exposed to inorganic lead, cadmium or mercury vapor. J Occup Med 22:741–750

Buchet JP, Lauwerys R, Vandevoorde A, Pycke JM (1983) Oral daily intake of cadmium, lead, manganese, copper, chromium, mercury, calcium, zinc and arsenic in Belgium: a duplicate meal study. Food Chem Toxicol 21:19–24

Bui TH, Lindsten J, Nordberg GF (1975) Chromosome analysis of lymphocytes from cadmium workers and Itai-Itai patients. Environ Res 9:187–195

Butler EA, Flynn FV (1958) The proteinuria of renal tubular disorders. Lancet II:978–980

Butler EA, Flynn FV, Harris H, Robson EB (1962) A study of urine proteins by two dimensional electrophoresis with special reference to the proteinuria of renal tubular disorders. Clin Chim Acta 7:34–41

Buxton R (1956) Respiratory function in cadmium alloy casters. Part II: The estimation of the total lung volume, its subdivisions and the mixing coefficient. Br J Ind Med 13:36–40

Carrol RE (1966) The relationship of cadmium in the air to cardiovascular disease death rates. J Am Med Assoc 198:267–269

Carruthers M, Smith B (1979) Evidence of cadmium toxicity in a population living in a zinc-mining area. Pilot survey of Shipham residents. Lancet I:845–847

Chang CC, Lauwerys R, Bernard A, Roels H, Buchet JP, Garvey JS (1980) Metallothionein in cadmium-exposed workers. Environ Research 23:422–428

Cherian MG (1978) Induction of renal metallothionein synthesis by parenteral cadmiumthionein in rats. Biochem Pharmacol 27:1163–1166

Chowdhury P, Louria DB (1976) Influence of cadmium and other trace metals on human α_1-antitrypsin: an in vitro study. Science 191:480–481

Clarkson TW, Kench JE (1956) Urinary excretion of amino acids by men absorbing heavy metals. Biochem J 62:361–372

Copius Peereboom JW, de Voogt P, Van Hattum B, Velde WVD, Copius Peereboom-Stegeman JHJ (1979) The use of the human placenta as a biological indicator for cadmium exposure. Management and control of heavy metals in the environment. CEP Consultants LTD, Edinburgh

Cvetkova RP (1970) Materials on the study of the influence of the cadmium compounds on the generative function. Gi Tr Prof Zabol 14:31–33 (in Russian with English summary)

Davey PG, Gosling P (1982) β_2-microglobulin instability in pathological urine. Clin Chem 28:1330–1333

Deknudt GL, Leonard A (1975) Cytogenetic investigations on leucocytes of workers from a cadmium plant. Environ Physiol Biochem 5:319–327

Di Costanzo J, Mallet B, Romette J, Charrel M (1982) Explorations biologique et clinique dans l'exposition professionnelle aux poussières de cuivre et cadmium. Ann Biol Clin 40:173–179

Elinder CG, Kjellström T (1977) Cadmium concentration in samples of human kidney cortex from the 19th century. Ambio 6:270–272

Elinder CG, Piscator M, Linnman L (1977) Cadmium and zinc relationships in kidney cortex, liver and pancreas. Environ Research 13:432–440

Elinder CG, Kjellström T, Linnman L, Pershagen G (1978) Urinary excretion of cadmium and zinc among persons from Sweden. Environ Research 15:473–484

Elinder CG, Kjellström T, Lind B, Linnman L, Piscator M, Sundstedt K (1983) Cadmium exposure from smoking cigarettes. Variations with time and country where purchased. Environ Research 32:220–227

Ellis KJ, Vartsky D, Zanzi I, Cohn SH, Yasumura S (1979) Cadmium: in vivo measurement in smokers and nonsmokers. Science 205:323–335

Ellis KJ, Wynford D, Zanzi I, Yasumura S, Vartsky D (1980) In vivo measurement of critical level of kidney cadmium: dose-effect studies in cadmium smelter workers. Am J Ind Med 1:339–348

Ellis KJ, Morgan WD, Zanzi I, Yasumura S, Vartsky D, Cohn SH (1981) Critical concentration of cadmium in human renal cortex: dose-effect studies in cadmium smelter workers. J Toxicol Environ Health 7:691–703

Essing HB, Schaller KH, Szadkowski D, Lehnert G (1969) Normal cadmium load in man by food and beverages. Arch Hyg Bakt 153:490–494 (in German)

Evrin PE, Wibell L (1972) The serum level and urinary excretion of β_2-microglobulin in apparently healthy subjects. Scand J Clin Lab Invest 29:69–74

FDA (1977) Compliance program evaluation, total diet studies (7320.08) FDA Bureau of Foods, Washington DC

Feldman SL, Cousins RJ (1973) Influence of cadmium on the metabolism of 2,5-hydroxy-cholecalciferol in chicks. Nutr Rep Int 8:251–259

Flanagan PR, McLellan JS, Haist J, Cherian G, Chamberlain M, Valberg L (1978) Increased dietary cadmium absorption in mice and human subjects with iron deficiency. Gastroenterology 74:841–846

Fleig I, Rieth H, Stocker WG, Thiess AM (1983) Chromosome investigations of workers exposed to cadmium in the manufacturing of cadmium stabilizers and pigments. Ecotoxicol Environ Safety 7:106–110

Fouassin A, Fondu M (1980) Evaluation de la teneur moyenne en plomb et en cadmium de la ration alimentaire en Belgique. Arch Belg 38:453–467

Friberg L (1948 a) Proteinuria and kidney injury among workmen exposed to cadmium and nickel dust. J Ind Toxicol 30:32–36

Friberg L (1948 b) Proteinuria and emphysema among workers exposed to cadmium and nickel dust in a storage battery plant. Proc Int Congr Ind Med 9:641–644

Friberg L (1950) Health hazards in the manufacture of alkaline accumulators with special reference to chronic cadmium poisoning. Acta Med Scand 138 (Suppl 240) 1–124

Friberg L (1957) Proteinuria in chronic cadmium poisoning after comparatively short exposure to cadmium dust: a report of 2 cases. AMA Arch Ind Health 16:27–29

Friberg L, Nyström A (1952) Aspects of the prognosis in chronic cadmium poisoning. Läkartidningen 49:2629–2639 (in Swedish)

Friberg L, Piscator M, Nordberg GF, Kjellström T (1974) Cadmium in the environment, 2nd edn. Cleveland, CRC Press

Fukushima M, Ishizaki A, Nogawa K, Sakamoto M, Kobayashi E (1974) Epidemiological studies on renal failure of inhabitants in Itai-Itai disease endemic district. I. Some urinary findings of inhabitants living in and around the endemic district of the Jinzu River basin. Jpn J Pub Health 21:67–73

Gasiorek K, Bauchinger M (1981) Chromosome changes in human lymphocytes after separate and combined treatment with bivalent salts of lead, cadmium and zinc. Environ Mutagens 3:513–518

Gill PF (1978) Respiratory function in a group of workers exposed to cadmium in Hobart. Proc First Int Cadmium Conf. San Francisco. Metal Bulletin Survey, pp 207–210

Glaser CB, Karic L, Huffaker T, Fallat RJ (1976) Influence of cadmium on human α_1-antitrypsin: a reexamination. Science 196:556–557

Gompertz D, Fletcher JG, Perkins J, Smith NY, Chettle DR, Mason H, Scott MC, Topping MD, Blindt M (1983) Renal dysfunction in cadmium smelters: relation to in-vivo liver and kidney cadmium concentrations. Lancet I:1185–1187

Guthrie BE, Robinson MF (1977) Daily intakes of manganese, copper, zinc and cadmium by New Zealand women. Br J Nutr 38:55–63

Hagino N, Yoshioka Y (1961) A study of the etiology of Itai-Itai disease. J Jpn Orthop Assoc 35:812–815 (in Japanese)

Hammer DI, Calocci AV, Hasselblad V, Williams ME, Pinkerson C (1973) Cadmium and lead in autopsy tissue. J Occup Med 15:956–963

Hansen L, Kjellström T, Vesterberg O (1977) Evaluation of different urinary proteins excreted after occupational cadmium exposure. Int Arch Occup Environ Health 40:273–282

Hardy HL, Skinner JB (1947) The possibility of chronic cadmium poisoning. J Ind Hyg Toxicol 29:321–325

Harvey TC, McLellan JS, Thomas BJ, Fremlin JF (1975) Measurement of liver cadmium concentrations in patients and industrial workers by neutron activation analysis. Lancet I:1269–1272

Harvey TC, Chettle DR, Fremlin JH, Al-Haddad IK, Downey SPMJ (1979) Cadmium in Shipham. Lancet I:551

Hickey RJ, Schoff EP, Clelland RC (1967) Relationship between air pollution and certain chronic disease death rates. Arch Environ Health 15:728–738

Hildebrand CE, Cram LS (1979) Distribution of cadmium in human blood culture in low levels of $CdCl_2$. Accumulation in lymphocytes and preferential binding to metallothionein. Proc Soc Exp Biol Med 161:438–443

Hirst RN, Perry HM, Cruz MC (1973) Elevated cadmium concentration in emphysema-tous lungs. Am Rev Resp Dis 108:30–39

Holden H (1969) Cadmium toxicology. Lancet II:57

Holden H (1980) Further mortality studies in workers exposed to cadmium fume. In: Occupational exposure to cadmium, Cadmium Association, London, pp 23–24

Horstowa H, Sikorski M, Tyborski H (1966) Chronic cadmium poisoning in the clinical and radiological picture (in Polish). Med Pr 17:13–25

Hubbard AW, Lindsay DG (1979) Dietary intakes of heavy metals by consumers in the United-Kingdom. In: Management and control of heavy metals in the environment. London, September 1979. CEP Consultants, Edinburgh, pp 52–55

Humperdinck K (1968) Cadmium and lung cancer. Med Klin 63:948–951 (in German)

Hunt WF, Pinkerton C, McNulty O, Creason J (1971) A study in trace element pollution of air in 77 midwestern cities. In: Hemphill DD (ed) Trace substances in environmental health. University of Missouri Press, Columbia, pp 55–68

Hutton MC (1982) Evaluation of the dose-effect and dose-response relationships for cadmium-induced renal dysfunction. Monitoring and Assessment Research Center, MARC report no 29, Chelsea College, University of London

Inskip H, Beral V (1982) Mortality of Shipham residents: 40-year follow-up. Lancet I:896–899

International Agency for Research on Cancer (IARC) (1976) Monographs on the evaluation of carcinogenic risk of chemicals to man. Cadmium and cadmium compounds 11:39–75

Ishizaki A, Fukushima M (1968) Itai-Itai disease (review). Jpn J Hyg 23:271–285

Iwao S, Tsuchiya K, Sakurai H (1980) Serum and urinary β_2-microglobulin among cadmium-exposed workers. J Occup Med 22:399–402

Japan Environment Agency (1972) Results of soil pollution survey in 1971, soil and agricultural chemical division, Water Quality Bureau, Tokyo, pp 1–129

Japan Public Health Association (1976) Effects of cadmium on human health: a review on studies mainly performed in Japan, Tokyo

Kawamura J, Yoshida O, Nishino K, Itokawa Y (1978) Disturbances in kidney functions and calcium and phosphate metabolism in cadmium-poisoned rats. Nephron 20:101–110

Kazantzis G (1956) Respiratory function in men casting cadmium alloys. Part I: Assessment of ventilatory function. Br J Ind Med 13:30–36

Kazantzis G (1978) Some long term effects of cadmium on the human kidney. Metal Bulletin Survey. Proc First Int Cadmium Conf, San Francisco, pp 194–198

Kazantzis G, Flynn FV, Spowage JS, Trott DG (1963) Renal tubular malfunction and pulmonary emphysema in cadmium pigments workers. Q J Med 32:165–192

Kekwick RA (1955) Physico-chemical examination of the serum and urine proteins in some cases of cadmium poisoning. Br J Ind Med 12:196–197

Kipling MD, Waterhouse JAH (1967) Cadmium and prostatic carcinoma. Lancet I:730–731

Kjellström T (1977) Accumulation and renal effects of cadmium in man. A dose-response study. PhD thesis, Karolinska Institute, Stockholm

Kjellström T (1979a) Exposure and accumulation of cadmium in people from Japan, USA and Sweden. Report on a 3-year cooperative research project. Environ Health Perspect 28:169–197

Kjellström T (1979b) Epidemiological aspects of the dose-response relationship of cadmium-induced renal damage. Proc Sec Int Cadmium Conf Cannes, Metal Bulletin, Survey, pp 118–122

Kjellström T (1982) Mortality and cancer morbidity in people exposed to cadmium. Report prepared for health effects research laboratory, US Environmental Protection Agency, Research Triangle Park, NC

Kjellström T, Nordberg GF (1978) A kinetic model of cadmium metabolism in the human being. Environ Res 16:248–266

Kjellström T, Piscator M (1977) Quantitative analysis of β_2-microglobulin in urine as an indicator of renal tubular damage induced by cadmium. Pharmacia Diagnostics AB, Uppsala Sweden

Kjellström T, Lind B, Linnman L, Elinder CG (1975) Variation of cadmium concentration in Swedish wheat and barley. An indicator of changes in daily cadmium intake during the 20th century. Arch Environ Health 30:321–338

Kjellström T, Evrin PE, Rahnster B (1977a) Dose-response analysis of cadmium-induced tubular proteinuria. A study of urinary β_2-microglobulin excretion among workers in a battery factory. Environ Res 13:303–317

Kjellström T, Shiroishi K, Evrin P (1977b) Urinary β_2-microglobulin excretion among people exposed to cadmium in the general environment. An epidemiological study in cooperation between Japan and Sweden. Environ Res 13:318–344

Kjellström T, Friberg L, Rahnster D (1979) Mortality and cancer morbidity among cadmium-exposed workers. Environ Health Perspect 28:199–204

Kjellström T, Elinder CG, Friberg L (1984) Conceptual problems in establishing the critical concentration of cadmium in human kidney cortex. Environ Res 33:284–295

Kojima S, Haga Y, Kurihara T, Yamawaki T (1977) A comparison between fecal cadmium and urinary β_2-microglobulin, total protein and cadmium among Japanese farmers. Environ Res 14:436–451

Kolonel LN (1976) Association of cadmium with renal cancer. Cancer 37:1782–1787

Kolonel L, Winhelstein W (1977) Cadmium and prostatic carcinoma. Lancet II:566–567

Kossman S, Pierzchala W, Rusiecki Z, Scieska J, Andryjewski J, Tomaszczyk S (1979) Estimation of ventilation efficiency of lungs in workers of cadmium division of nonferrous foundry. Pneumonol Pol 9:627–633

Kowal NE, Johnson DE, Kraemer DF, Pahren HR (1979) Normal levels of cadmium in diet, urine, blood and tissues of inhabitants of the United States. J Toxicol Environ Health 5:995–1014

Kult J, Lammelein C, Röckel A, Heideland A (1974) β_2-microglobulin in serum – a parameter of glomerular filtrate. Dtsch Med Wochenschr 99:1686–1688

Larsson SE, Piscator M (1971) Effect of cadmium on skeletal tissue in normal and calcium deficient rats. Israel J Med Sc 7:495–498

Lauwerys R (1978) CEC Criteria (Dose/Effect Relationship) for cadmium. Pergamon, Oxford

Lauwerys R (1982) The toxicology of cadmium. Environment and quality of life, Report EUR 7649 EN, Commission of the European Communities, Luxembourg

Lauwerys R, Bernard A (1982) Diagnosis of metal-induced nephropathy in humans. In: Bach PH, Bonner FW, Bridges JW, Loch EA (eds) Nephrotoxicity-assessment and pathogenesis. Wiley, Chichester, pp 371–377

Lauwerys R, De Wals PH (1981) Environmental pollution by cadmium and mortality from renal diseases. Lancet I:383

Lauwerys R, Buchet JP, Roels H, Brouwers J, Stanescu D (1974) Epidemiological survey of workers exposed to cadmium. Arch Environ Health 28:145–148

Lauwerys R, Buchet JP, Roels H (1976) The relationship between cadmium exposure or body burden and the concentration of cadmium in blood and urine in man. Int Arch Occup Environ Health 36:275–285

Lauwerys R, Buchet JP, Roels H, Hubermont G (1978) Placental transfer of lead, mercury, cadmium and carbon monoxide in women. I. Comparison of the frequency distributions of the biological indices in maternal and umbilical cord blood. Environ Res 15:278–289

Lauwerys R, Roels H, Regniers M, Buchet JP, Bernard A, Goret A (1979a) Significance of cadmium concentration in blood and in urine in workers exposed to cadmium. Environ Res 20:375–391

Lauwerys R, Vos A, Roels H, Buchet JP, Bernard A (1979b) Surveillance d'un travailleur écarté de son poste de travail suite à la découverte de lésions rénales induites par le cadmium. Arch Belg 37:137–146

Lauwerys R, Roels H, Bernard A, Buchet JP (1980) Renal response to cadmium in a population living in a non-ferrous smelter area in Belgium. Int Arch Occup Environ Health 45:271–274

Lauwerys R, Buchet JP, Roels H, Viau C, Bernard A, Bruaux P, Claeys-Thoreau F, Rondia R (1983) Potential risk of cadmium for the general population. Update of Liège study. In: Proceedings Forth Int Cadmium Conference Munich. Wilson D, Cadmium Association; Volpe RA, Cadmium Council and ILZRO, London (eds), pp 113–114

Lauwerys R, Bernard A, Roels H, Buchet JP, Viau C (1984) Characterization of cadmium proteinuria in man and rat. Environ Health Perspect 54:147–152

Lemen RA, Lee JS, Wagoner JK, Blejer HP (1976) Cancer mortality among cadmium production workers. Ann NY Acad Sci 271:273–279

Livingson HD (1972) Measurement and distribution of zinc, cadmium and mercury in human kidney tissues. Clin Chem 18:67–72

Marck K, Wocka-Marell T, Marks J (1980) Effect of occupational exposure to cadmium on the activity of α_1-antitrypsin in the serum. Pol Arch Med Wewn 63:53–56

Masiromi R (1974) Trace elements in relation to cardiovascular diseases. WHO, Geneva

Materne D, Lauwerys R, Buchet JP, Roels H, Brouwers J, Stanescu D (1975) Investigations sur les risques résultant de l'exposition au cadmium dans deux entreprises de production et deux entreprises d'utilisation du cadmium. Cah Med Trav 12:1–76

McLellan JS, Flanagan PR, Chamberlain MJ, Valberg LS (1978) Measurement of dietary cadmium absorption in human. J Toxicol Environ Health 4:131–138

McMichael AJ, Andjelkovic DA, Tyroler HA (1976) Cancer mortality among rubber workers: an epidemiologic study. Ann NY Acad Sci 271:124–128

Menden EE, Elia VJ, Michael LW, Petering HG (1972) Distribution of cadmium and nickel of tobacco during cigarette smoking. Environ Sci Technol 6:830–832

Miljoministeriet (1980) Cadmiumforurening. En redegorelse om anvedelse, forekomst og skadevirkninger af cadmium i Danmark. Jensen, Kobenhavn

Ministry of Health (1980) Surveillance Programme. Man and Nutrition. State Supervisory Public Health Service, Den Haag

Mittman C (1972) Pulmonary emphysema and proteolysis. Academic, New York

Morgan JM (1969) Tissue cadmium concentrations in man. Arch Int Med 123:405–408

Morgan JM (1970) Cadmium and zinc abnormalities in bronchogenic carcinoma. Cancer 25:1394–1398

Morgan JM, Burch HB, Watkin JB (1971) Tissue cadmium and zinc content in emphysema and bronchogenic carcinoma. J Chron Dis 24:107–110

Nandi M, Slone D, Jick H, Shapiro S, Lewis GP (1969) Cadmium content of cigarettes. Lancet II:1329–1330

Nicaud P, Lafitte A, Gros A (1942) Les troubles de l'intoxication chronique par le cadmium. Arch Mal Prof 4:192–202

Nogawa K, Ishizaki A, Kawano S (1978) Statistical observations of the dose-response relationships for cadmium based on epidemiological studies in the Kakehashi River basin. Environ Res 15:185–198

Nogawa K, Kobayashi E, Honda R (1979) A study of the relationship between cadmium concentrations in urine and renal effects of cadmium. Environ Health Perspect 28:161–168

Nogawa K, Kobayashi E, Honda R, Ishizaki A, Kawano S, Matusda H (1980) Renal dysfunction of inhabitants in a cadmium-polluted area. Environ Res 23:13–23

Nogawa K, Kawano S, Nishi M (1981) Mortality study of inhabitants in a cadmium-polluted area with special reference to low molecular weight proteinuria. In: Heavy metals in the environment, CEP Consultants, Edinburgh, UK, pp 538–540

Nordberg GF, Goyer R, Nordberg M (1975) Comparative toxicity of cadmium-metallothionein and cadmium chloride on mouse kidney. Arch Pathol 99:192–197

Nriagu JO (1981) Cadmium in the environment. Part II: Health effects. Wiley, New York

O'Riordan ML, Hughes EG, Evans H (1978) Chromosomal studies on blood lymphocytes of men occupationally exposed to cadmium. Mutat Res 58:305–311

Perry HM, Erlanger MW (1974) Metal-induced hypertension following chronic finding of low doses of cadmium and mercury. J Lab Clin Med 83:541–547

Piscator M (1962) Proteinuria in chronic cadmium poisoning. I. an electrophoretic and chemical study of urinary and serum proteins from workers with chronic cadmium poisoning. Arch Environ Health 4:607–622

Piscator M (1966a) Proteinuria in chronic cadmium poisoning. III. Electrophoretic and immunoelectrophoretic studies on urinary proteins from cadmium workers, with special reference to the excretion of low molecular weight proteins. Arch Environ Health 12:335–344

Piscator M (1966 b) Proteinuria in chronic cadmium poisoning. IV. Gel filtration and ion exchange chromatography on urinary proteins from cadmium workers. Arch Environ Health 12:345–359

Piscator M (1978) Serum β_2-microglobulin in cadmium exposed workers. Pathol Biol 26:321–323

Piscator M, Lind B (1972) Cadmium, zinc, copper and lead in human renal cortex. Arch Environ Health 24:426–431

Piscator M, Peterson B (1977) Chronic cadmium poisoning: diagnosis and prevention. In: Brown SJ (ed) Clinical chemistry and chemical toxicology of metals. Elsevier/North-Holland Biomedical Press, Amsterdam, pp 143–155

Piscator M, Kjellström T, Lind B (1976) Contamination of cigarettes and pipe tobacco by cadmium-oxide dust. Lancet II:587

Piscator M, Björck L, Nordberg M (1981) β_2-microglobulin levels in serum and urine of cadmium-exposed rabbits. Acta Pharmacol Toxicol 49:1–7

Potts CL (1965) Cadmium proteinuria – the health of battery workers exposed to cadmium oxide dust. Ann Occup Hyg 8:55–61

Princi F (1947) A study of industrial exposure to cadmium. J Ind Hyg Toxicol 29:315–320

Pujol M, Arlet J, Bollinelli R, Carles P (1970) Tubulopathie des intoxications chroniques par le cadmium. Arch Mal Prof 31:637–648

Rahola T, Aaran RK, Miettinen JK (1972) Half-time studies of mercury and cadmium by whole body counting. In: Assessment of radioactive organ and body burdens. IAEA, Vienne

Roels HA, Lauwerys RR, Buchet JP, Materne D (1975) Study on cadmium proteinuria, glomerular dysfunction: an early sign of renal impairment. CEC-EPA-WHO Int Symposium, Paris

Roels H, Hubermont G, Buchet JP, Lauwerys R (1978) Placental transfer of lead, mercury, cadmium and carbon monoxide in women. III. Factors influencing the accumulation of heavy metals in the placenta and the relationship between the metal concentration in the placenta and in maternal and cord blood. Environ Res 6:236–247

Roels H, Bernard A, Buchet JP, Goret A, Lauwerys R, Chettle DR, Harvey TC, Al-Haddad IK (1979) The critical concentration of cadmium in the renal cortex and in urine in man. Lancet I:221

Roels H, Lauwerys R, Buchet JP, Bernard A, Chettle D, Harvey TC, Al-Haddad IK (1981 a) In vivo measurement of liver and kidney cadmium in workers exposed to this metal. Environ Res 26:217–240

Roels H, Lauwerys R, Buchet JP, Bernard A (1981 b) Environmental exposure to cadmium and renal function of aged women in three areas of Belgium. Environ Res 24:117–130

Roels H, Djubgang J, Buchet JP, Bernard A, Lauwerys R (1982) Evolution of cadmium-induced renal dysfunction in workers removed from exposure. Scand J Work Environ Health 8:191–200

Roels H, Lauwerys R, Dardenne AN (1983 a) The critical level of cadmium in human renal cortex: a reevaluation. Toxicology Lett 15:357–360

Roels H, Lauwerys R, Buchet JP, Bernard A, Garvey JS, Linton HJ (1983 b) Significance of urinary metallothionein in workers exposed to cadmium. Int Arch Occup Environ Health 52:159–166

Saito H, Shioji R, Hurukawa Y, Nagai K, Arikawa T, Saito T, Sasaki Y, Furuyama T, Yoshinaga K (1977) Cadmium-induced proximal tubular dysfunction in a cadmium polluted area. Contrib Nephrol 6:1–12

Sakurai H (1980) Epidemiological approach to subclinical effects of metals in long term occupational exposures. In: Homstedt B, Lauwerys R, Mercier M, Roberfroid M (eds) Mechanisms of toxicity and hazard evaluation, vol 8. Elsevier/North-Holland Biomedical, Amsterdam, pp 293–305

Samarawickrama GP (1979) Biological effects of cadmium in mammals. In: Webb M (ed) The chemistry, biochemistry and biology of cadmium. Elsevier/North-Holland Biomedical, Amsterdam., pp 357–361

Schroeder HA (1965) Cadmium as a factor of hypertension. J Chron Dis 18:647–656

Schroeder HA, Balassa JJ (1961) Abnormal trace metals in man: cadmium. J Chron Dis 14:236–258

Schroeder HA, Nason AP, Tipton IH, Balassa IJ (1967) Essential trace metals in man: zinc-relation to environmental cadmium. J Chron Dis 20:179–210

Scott R, Mills EA, Fell GS, Husain F, Yates A, Paterson PJ, McKirdy A, Ottoway J, Fitz-gerald-Finchi O, Lamont A (1976) Clinical and biochemical abnormalities in copper-smiths exposed to cadmium. Lancet II:396–389

Scott R, Patterson PJ, Burns R, Ottoway JM, Husain FE, Fell GS, Dumbuya S, Igbal M (1978) Hypercalciuria related to cadmium exposure. Urology 11:462–465

Scott R, Haywood JK, Boddy K, Williams ED, Harvey I, Paterson PJ (1980) Whole body calcium deficit in cadmium-exposed workers with hypercalciuria. Urology 15:356–359

Shigematsu I, Kitamura S, Takeuchi J, Minowa M, Nagai M, Usui T, Fukushima M (1981) A retrospective mortality study on cadmium-exposed populations in Japan. In: Recent studies on health effects of cadmium in Japan. The Japan Cadmium Research Commit-tee, Japan Public Health Association, Tokyo, p 303

Shigematsu I, Mitamura S, Takeuchi J, Minowa M, Nagai M, Fukushima M (1982) A retrospective mortality study on cadmium-exposed populations in Japan. In: Cadmium 81, Proc Third Int Cadmium Conf, Miami, Cadmium Association, London

Shiraishi Y (1975) Cytogenetic studies in 12 patients with Itai-Itai disease. Hum genet 27:31–44

Shiroishi K, Kjellström T, Kubota K, Evrin PE, Anayama M, Vesterberg O, Shimada T, Piscator M, Iwata T, Nishino H (1977) Urine analysis for detection of cadmium-in-duced renal changes, with special reference to β_2-microglobulin. Environ Res 13:407–424

Silva PE de, Donnan MB (1981) Chronic cadmium poisoning in a pigment manufacturing plant. Br J Ind Med 38:76–86

Smith JC, Kench JE (1957) Observations on urinary cadmium and protein excretion in men exposed to cadmium oxide dust and fume. Br J Ind Med 14:240–249

Smith TJ, Petty TL, Reading JC, Lakshminarayan S (1976) Pulmonary effects of chronic exposure to airborne cadmium. Am Rev Resp Dis 114:161–169

Smith TJ, Anderson RJ, Reading JC (1980) Chronic cadmium exposures associated with kidney function tests. Am J Ind Med 1:319–337

Sorahan T (1983) A further mortality study of nickel-cadmium battery workers. In: Proc Fourth Int Cadmium Conf Munich. Wilson D, Cadmium Association; Volpe RA, Cadmium Council and ILZRO, London (eds), pp 143–148

Sovet (1858) Empoisonnement par une poudre à récurer l'argenterie. Press Méd Belge 10:69–71

Staessen J, Bulpitt CJ, Roels H, Bernard A, Fagard R, Joossens JV, Lauwerys R, Lynen P, Amery A (1984) Urinary cadmium and lead and their relationship to blood pressure in a population with low average exposure. Br J Ind Med 4:241–248

Stanescu D, Veriter C, Frans A, Goncette L, Roels H, Lauwerys R, Brasseur L (1977) Ef-fects on lung of chronic occupational exposure to cadmium. Scand J Resp Dis 58:289–303

Stephens GA (1920) Cadmium poisoning. J Ind Hyg 2:129–138

Suzuki S, Suzuki T, Ashizawa M (1965) Proteinuria due to inhalation of cadmium stearate dust. Ind Health 3:73–85

Suzuki S, Tageuchi T, Yokohashi G (1969) Dietary factors influencing upon the retention rate of orally administered 115m $CdCl_2$ in mice with special reference to calcium and protein concentration in diet. Ind Health 7:155–162

Szadkowsky D, Schultze H, Schaller KH, Lehnert G (1969) On the ecological consequence of the heavy metal content in cigarettes. Arch Hyg Bakteriol 153:1–8 (in German)

Tanekaka S, Oldiges H, König H, Hchrainer D, Oberdörster G (1983) Carcinogenicity of cadmium chloride aerosols in W rats. J Natl Cancer Inst 70:367–373

Tarasenko N, Vorobjeva RS (1973) Hygienic problems connected with the use of cadmium (in Russian with English abstract). Vestn Akad Med Nauk SSSR 28:37–43

Teculescu DB, Stanescu DC (1970) Pulmonary function in workers with chronic exposure to cadmium oxide fumes. Int Arch Arbeitsmed 26:335–345

Thomas BJ, Harvey DR, Chettle D, McLellan JS, Fremlin JH (1979) A transportable system for the measurement of liver cadmium in vivo. Phys Med Biol 24:432–437

Tohyama C, Shaikh ZA, Nogawa K, Kobayashi E, Honda R (1981) Elevated urinary excretion of metallothionein due to environmental cadmium exposure. Toxicology 20:289–297

Tohyama C, Shaikh ZA, Nogawa K, Kobayashi E, Honda R (1982) Urinary metallothionein as a new index of renal dysfunction in "Itai-Itai" disease patients and other Japanese women environmentally exposed to cadmium. Toxicology 50:159–166

Townshend RH (1982) Acute cadmium pneumonitis: a 17-year follow-up. Br J Ind Med 39:411–412

Tolan A, Elton GA (1973) Total diet studies with special reference to mercury and cadmium. In: European colloquium: problems of the contamination of man and his environment by mercury and cadmium. Commission of the European Community, Luxembourg, pp 335–352

Travis CC, Etnier EL (1982) Dietary intake of cadmium in the United States: 1920–1975. Environ Res 27:1–9

Tsuchiya K (1967) Proteinuria of workers exposed to cadmium fume. The relationship to concentration in the working environment. Arch Environ Health 14:875–880

Tsuchiya K (1976) Proteinuria of cadmium workers. J Occup Med 18:463–466

Tsuchiya K (1978) Cadmium studies in Japan. A review. Elsevier/North-Holland Biomedical, Amsterdam

Tsuchiya K, Iwao S, Sugita M, Sakuria H (1979) Increased urinary β_2-microglobulin in cadmium exposure: dose-effect relationship and biological significance of β_2-microglobulin. Environ Health Perspect 28:147–153

US Environmental Protection Agency (1979) Health Assessment Document for cadmium, Office of Health and Environmental Assessment EPA 600/8-79-003, Washington DC

Vanherweghem JL, Even Adin D (1981) Epidemiology of analgesic nephropathy in Belgium. Clin Nephrology 17:129–133

Vahter M (1982) Assessment of human exposure to lead and cadmium through biological monitoring. National Swedish Institute of Environmental Medicine and Karolinska Institute, Stockholm

Vartsky D, Ellis KJ, Chen NS, Cohn SH (1977) A facility for in vivo measurement of kidney and liver cadmium by neutron capture prompt gamma ray analysis. Phys Med Biol 22:1085–1086

Vigliani EC, Pernis B, Amate L (1966) Etudes biochimiques et immunologiques sur la nature de la protéinurie cadmique. Med Lav 57:321–330

Voogt P de, Van Hattum B (1981) Cadmium: expositie and dagelijkse opname in Nederland. Tijdschr Soc Genesk 59:368–372

Vorobjeva RS (1957a) On occupational lung disease in prolonged action of aerosol of cadmium oxide (in Russian). Arch Pathologii 8:25–29

Vorobjeva RS (1957b) Investigations of the nervous system function in workers exposed to cadmium oxide (in Russian). Neuropath Psikhrat 57:385–388

Vorobjeva RS, Eremeeva EP (1980) Cardiovascular function in workers exposed to cadmium (in Russian). Gig Sanit 10:22–25

Webb M, Etienne AT (1977) Studies on the toxicity and metabolism of cadmium-thionein. Biochem Pharmacol 26:25–30

Wibell L (1978) The serum level and urinary excretion of β_2-microglobulin in health and renal disease. Path Biol 26:295–301

Wibell L, Evrin PE, Berggard I (1973) Serum β_2-microglobulin in renal disease. Nephron 10:320–331

World Health Organization (1972) Evaluation of certain food additives and the contaminants mercury, lead and cadmium. Technical report series no 505. WHO, Geneve

World Health Organization (1977) WHO environmental health criteria for cadmium. Ambio 6:287–290

World Health Organization (1980) Recommended health-based limits in occupational exposure to heavy metals. WHO, Geneva

CHAPTER 6

The Nephropathy
of Chronic Cadmium Poisoning

M. Piscator

A. Introduction

The fact that exposure to cadmium could cause severe acute poisoning was known in the last century, but that cadmium could cause chronic disease was not conclusively shown until the 1940s. In 1950 Friberg presented extensive data on investigations of workers exposed to cadmium oxide dust in an alkaline battery factory. The main findings were chronic lung disease (see Chap. 5 for further details) and chronic renal disease. A decrease in glomerular filtration rate was seen, but the unique feature was a high prevalence of proteinuria of a hitherto unknown type. Examination of urine proteins by electrophoresis and ultracentrifugation showed that the main component of the urine proteins had a molecular weight below that of albumin. Other findings were a decreased concentrating capacity of the kidneys, and a high incidence of nephrolithiasis among the exposed workers. To verify the findings in human beings, Friberg (1950) also performed animal experiments. It was found that cadmium exposure caused proteinuria which differed from the type of proteinuria induced by uranyl salts. Since the workers were also exposed to nickel hydroxide, animals were also exposed to nickel, but the nickel exposure did not produce the same changes as cadmium exposure.

The unique proteinuria, with α-globulins dominating the urine protein pattern, was intriguing, but the state of the art at that time did not allow any certain conclusions about its origin. The so-called Bence Jones proteinuria was the only type of low molecular weight proteinuria then known, and it was speculated that exposure to cadmium could cause the formation of a low molecular weight protein that could cause damage during its passage through the kidneys.

An important discovery was made by Butler and Flynn (1958) who found that the electrophoretic pattern of urine proteins in patients with renal tubular disease of varying etiology, e.g., Fanconi's syndrome and hypokalemia, had no similarities to the one seen in patients with classic renal disease, i.e., nephritis and nephrosis. The electrophoretic pattern was dominated by α- and β-globulins, and the percentage of albumin was low. The pattern was very similar to the one seen among Friberg's patients with chronic cadmium poisoning. Further studies in the United Kingdom and Sweden in the early 1960s by Butler et al. (1962), Kazantzis et al. (1963), and Piscator (1962 a) gave further evidence for the similarity between proteinuria of chronic cadmium poisoning and the tubular proteinuria described by Butler and Flynn (1958).

More detailed examinations showed that a variety of low molecular weight proteins constituted a large part of the urine proteins. Among these proteins were

β_2-microglobulin (β_2-m), lysozyme, ribonuclease, immunoglobulin chains, and retinol-binding proteins (PETERSON and BERGGÅRD 1971; PISCATOR 1966a, b). These proteins occur normally in serum in very small amounts and can all be filtered through the glomeruli. The proteinuria in chronic cadmium poisoning, as in other tubular disorders, was thought to be caused by decreased reabsorption in the tubuli of filtered proteins. Low molecular weight proteins, as well as proteins of higher molecular weight, e.g., albumin and transferrin, were also found in normal urine.

In more advanced cases, glucosuria, aminoaciduria, and phosphaturia were seen and the end result thus resembled a complete Fanconi's syndrome. The finding of osteomalacia in French cadmium workers (NICAUD et al. 1942) could thus be explained by severe renal dysfunction. Osteomalacia has otherwise only been reported in a few occupational cases, but in the Toyama Prefecture in Japan, there was an epidemic of osteomalacia in a population of women who had been exposed to cadmium via rice. The cases generally occurred among women above 40 years of age who had had several pregnancies and nutritional deficiencies, especially low intakes of calcium and vitamin D (FRIBERG et al. 1974). Proteinuria and other signs of tubular dysfunction were also seen among the males in the contaminated area, but osteomalacia has only occasionally been reported to occur in males. There are many areas in Japan where cadmium contamination occurs, and tubular proteinuria and other signs of tubular defects have been common findings in studies of these people exposed to cadmium via food, mainly rice (KJELLSTRÖM et al. 1977; KOJIMA et al. 1977; NOGAWA et al. 1980; SAITO et al. 1977a, b). Moderate decreases in glomerular filtration rate (GFR) have been noticed in many of these studies, but chronic cadmium poisoning generally does not lead to severe uremia requiring dialysis. It has, however, been claimed (BERNARD et al. 1976, 1979; BUCHET et al. 1980; LAUWERYS et al. 1974) that cadmium can also cause primary glomerular disease. The main evidence for this has been the finding of an increase in the excretion of albumin, but as mentioned, albumin occurs normally in the glomerular filtrate and a reabsorption defect will also influence the reabsorption of albumin. The determination of β_2-m or other low molecular weight proteins in urine is generally regarded as the most specific test for detecting early signs of cadmium exposure, but it has been claimed (IWAO et al. 1980) that cadmium can cause an increase in the synthesis of β_2-m which might influence the urinary excretion of that protein. However, experiments on rabbits did not show any major effect of cadmium on β_2-m levels in serum (PISCATOR et al. 1981). Information on the general effects of cadmium will be found in Chap. 5 and other chapters of this book, as well as in other major reviews (FRIBERG et al. 1974; TSU-CHIYA 1978).

B. Uptake, Storage, and Turnover of Cadmium in the Kidneys

Most of the cadmium absorbed from the lungs or from the gastrointestinal tract will initially be stored in the liver and then gradually transferred to other organs, mainly the kidney. In the liver, cadmium is stored in metallothionein (see also Chap. 8). This protein has a rapid turnover, but the liver has a very high capacity to synthesize metallothionein according to the degree of cadmium exposure, and thus cadmium is efficiently trapped in the liver. The liver slowly releases Cd–metallothionein, and metallothionein has been found in small amounts in plasma (CHANG et al. 1980; FALCK et al. 1983a). Since metallothionein has a low molecular weight which allows complete passage through the glomeruli, the reabsorption of cadmium–metallothionein can explain the renal accumulation of cadmium. Absorbed metallothionein will be rapidly catabolized, but the kidney also has the capacity to synthesize the protein. Thus, cadmium will be stored in the kidneys in metallothionein as an inert compound. However, the kidney seems to have a limited capacity to synthesize metallothionein (NORDBERG et al. 1979). At a certain total level of cadmium in the kidney, some cadmium will not be bound in metallothionein and can be bound to other structures, thus explaining the renal effects of cadmium. Both in liver and kidney, cadmium has a very long biologic half-life (5–10, 10–15 years, respectively). These long storage times are also related to the metabolism of metallothionein.

Many of the enzymes in the kidney are zinc–metalloenzymes or zinc-dependent enzymes, and it has been speculated that cadmium may interfere with such systems. The renal accumulation of cadmium is accompanied by an increase in renal zinc owing to the storage of cadmium and zinc in metallothionein (PISCATOR and LIND 1972; NORDBERG et al. 1979). At lower renal cadmium levels, increases in zinc and Cd are practically equimolar, but with increasing Cd uptake, there will be relatively more cadmium in the renal metallothionein. Studies on horses have revealed that when renal cadmium concentrations exceed 160 mg per kilogram renal cortex, there is no further increase of zinc. This concentration is close to the so-called critical concentration of cadmium in the renal cortex, i.e., the concentration that may cause low molecular weight proteinuria in the most sensitive members of the population (FRIBERG et al. 1974). It was earlier estimated, based on autopsy data and some biopsy data from human beings, that this concentration was around 200 mg Cd per kilogram wet weight renal cortex (FRIBERG et al. 1974). Recent studies by in vivo neutron activation analyses of the cadmium content of kidneys from Belgian cadmium workers have verified that this earlier estimate was relatively accurate (ROELS et al. 1981, 1983). There have been claims that the critical concentration is above 300 mg per kilogram wet weight renal cortex, but this estimate is to be regarded as an average critical concentration which does not agree with the original definition (ELLIS et al. 1981). Since urine cadmium is a good indicator of the body burden of cadmium, there is also a critical concentration for cadmium in urine which is about 10 µg Cd per gram creatinine (FRIBERG et al. 1974; LAUWERYS et al. 1979; ROELS et al. 1981, 1983). These data for critical concentrations in kidney and urine should be compared with the present levels of cadmium in kidney and urine of members of the general population. The average cadmium concentration in the renal cortex of adults in most European countries and in North America lies between 20 and 30 mg per kilogram wet weight and urinary excretion averages 0.5–1 µg Cd per gram creatinine. In Japan, even in areas which are not regarded as cadmium polluted, renal concentrations of cadmium are about three times higher (FRIBERG et al. 1974; KJELLSTRÖM 1979; FRIBERG and VAHTER 1983). Nonsmokers generally have about half the renal burden of smokers.

C. Effects on Tubular Function

I. Proteinuria

The proteinuria in chronic cadmium poisoning has been called tubular proteinuria caused by tubular dysfunction, to distinguish it from the classic type of proteinuria, glomerular proteinuria, seen in disorders such as nephritis and
nephrosis, where the main effect is exerted on the glomeruli, leading to increased
permeability to plasma proteins or further damage.

Normally, about 20–30 mg plasma proteins will be excreted in the urine in
24 h and about the same amount of proteins originates in the urinary tract. The
relatively small protein excretion results from very efficient reabsorption of 1–2 g
plasma proteins filtered through the glomeruli per day. However, the estimate for
the filtered daily amount of protein is based on very limited data. MOGENSEN and
SÖLLING (1977) found in human beings that injections of basic amino acids, especially lysine, caused almost complete inhibition of protein reabsorption. Based on
the amount of albumin found in the urine after lysine administration, the glomerular filtrate on average might contain a little more than 2.5 mg/l albumin.
This corresponds to a filtered amount of albumin up to 500 mg, and other plasma
proteins may contribute 500–1,000 mg/day. Other evidence supporting the calculation of protein filtration is provided by the finding that in cadmium workers
with tubular proteinuria the total excretion of protein, even in very advanced
cases, never exceeds 2 g/day (PISCATOR 1962a). Other proteins appearing in urine
and with relatively high molecular weight are transferrin and immunoglobulins.
Among the normal urine proteins, albumin constitutes about 20%–25%, and it
is easily recognized on electrophoresis in different media (PISCATOR 1962a). Owing to the mixture of proteins of different sizes from the urinary tract, the electrophoretic pattern is otherwise rather diffuse, with no distinct peaks as seen on electrophoresis of plasma proteins. A concentrate of normal urine proteins usually
has a deep brown color, which to a large extent is due to the presence of an α-
globulin-containing brown pigment (PISCATOR 1966a), identified as α_1-micro-
globulin (EKSTRÖM et al. 1975).

Among the low molecular weight proteins in urine, β_2-m is the one which has
been studied and best characterized. The concentration of β_2-m in plasma is
about 1.5 mg/l and since its molecular weight, 11,800, gives it a very high sieving
coefficient, the concentration in the glomerular filtrate will probably be very close
to that level. This means that about 200 mg β_2-m may be filtered daily. This also
corresponds to the amount of β_2-m synthesized daily in the body. The daily excretion in normal urine is only about 0.1 mg, which indicates that more than 99%
of the filtered amount has been reabsorbed. Since β_2-m might be degraded at low
urine pH, the determination of that protein in urine should be performed only on
urine samples with a pH above 5.5, preferably above 6.

The absorption site for β_2-m seems to be in an area of the proximal tubule,
where some other anionic or neutral proteins also may be reabsorbed. This reabsorption process for β_2-m, as for other proteins, depends on the isoelectric point
since reabsorption of β_2-m is not influenced by cationic proteins such as cytochrome c and lysozyme (SUMPIO and MAACK 1982), whereas the neutral myo-

globin can interfere with the reabsorption of β_2-m (PESCE et al. 1980). Also certain basic amino acids, especially lysine, can inhibit the reabsorption of β_2-m.

Myoglobin can also inhibit the reabsorption of metallothionein (FOULKES 1978, 1982). This indicates that metallothionein may be reabsorbed at the same site as β_2-m. This will result in cadmium accumulation at the site and this is consistent with the fact that an increased excretion of β_2-m is an early sign of the effects of cadmium on the kidney.

Even though use of β_2-m for studies on urinary excretion of low molecular weight proteins demands control of urine pH, it possesses definite advantages. The simultaneous determination of β_2-m in serum and urine and the determination of parameters such as creatinine clearance makes it easy to calculate the relative clearance of β_2-m, a direct estimate of the degree of reabsorption.

The processes for glomerular filtration, tubular transport, and reabsorption of proteins are very complex. For more details of these subjects reference is made to some recent papers (MAACK et al. 1979; SUMPIO and MAACK 1982; DEEN and SATVAT 1981; PESCE and FIRST 1979; RYAN 1981). From what has been stated it is quite clear that physiologic proteinuria is in fact a tubular proteinuria, since it is caused by incomplete reabsorption of filtered proteins.

Exposure to cadmium will result in accumulation of cadmium in the proximal tubule. It can be expected that the cadmium concentrations will vary along the tubule, being highest in the proximal part of the proximal tubule. Eventually the local concentration of cadmium will be too high, and the synthesis of metallothionein will not be able to keep up. This will depress tubular reabsorption of low molecular weight proteins normally reabsorbed by that tubule segment. Because this may be a very slow process in human beings, it takes some time before increased β_2-m excretion in the urine can be demonstrated. The accumulation of cadmium will go on, but the increase will be smaller owing to the decreased reabsorption of metallothionein. On the other hand, the accumulation will go on as before in adjacent sites and eventually other parts of the tubule will also reach the critical concentration.

Basic proteins will be affected late in the process, as indicated by data from PISCATOR (1966a), where it was found that lysozyme excretion was only markedly increased when the total protein excretion exceeded 1 g/day. There will also be an increase in the excretion of albumin. It is not known if this starts at the same time as the increase in excretion of β_2-m, or if it comes later. It may be added that there was no increase of the urinary tract proteins which normally constitute about 50% of urinary protein. Now, if the reabsorption processes for albumin and β_2-m were affected simultaneously, and to the same extent, one would expect the same percentage increases in excretion of both proteins, or an even higher increase for albumin in the case of glomerular damage. In fact, the percentage of urine albumins generally tends to decrease with increasing total protein (PISCATOR 1962a, 1966a).

Since an increase in urinary albumin has been found in cadmium-exposed workers, Lauwerys and co-workers suggested in a series of papers that the increased albumin in urine from cadmium workers is a sign primarily of glomerular dysfunction (BERNARD et al. 1976, 1979; BUCHET et al. 1980; LAUWERYS et al. 1974). A review of these papers has been presented elsewhere (PISCATOR 1983) and some of the comments made will only be summarized here. The hypothesis was based on a finding of "glomerular patterns" in electrophoresis of urine proteins from cadmium-exposed workers (Lauwerys et al. 1974). However, these patterns were obtained by electrophoresis in agarose, which permits very distinct staining of the albumin fraction, whereas other protein fractions are not so clearly marked, especially if the proteins are not sufficiently concentrated. The method had been used in two studies (Lauwerys et al. 1974; Bernard et al. 1976) before it was recognized that they may not be suitable; increased excretion of β_2-m was found in several workers who had been classified as normal based on the agarose patterns. In later studies (Bernard et al. 1979; Buchet et al. 1980) several proteins were examined by immunologic techniques, and in some cases only an increase in albumin and transferrin was found, but not in β_2-m. However, there is no report on the control of pH in these studies.

One of the conclusions drawn by Bernard et al. (1979) was that

> ... this study shows that the proteinuria after prolonged exposure to cadmium has two components, the tubular proteinuria characterized by enhanced excretion of β_2-m, and a glomerular proteinuria with an increased excretion of HMW proteins, such as albumin, transferrin and IgG. Also both components can appear independently. They are often associated giving rise to a mixed type proteinuria.

Glomerular proteinuria could be explained according to the authors by binding of cadmium to the glomerular membrane with a consequent change in electric charge.

The findings of the Belgian group are very interesting, but the evidence for a primarily glomerular dysfunction remains incomplete. Serious consideration needs to be given to increases in albumin which might result from decreased reabsorption. Furthermore, it may be inadvisable to base a diagnosis of glomerular damage solely on increased albumin excretion since factors including blood pressure, posture, exercise, and water loading can influence excretion of that protein.

The question raised by Lauwerys and co-workers is important and their conclusions are now quoted extensively in the literature (Chan and Rennert 1981; Murray et al. 1981; Sakurai 1980; Falck et al. 1983b). It should be noted that in people with chronic cadmium poisoning there is a decrease in GFR, but, as will be discussed in a later section, this could result indirectly from interstitial changes. Experiments on rats indicate that cadmium exposure can cause an immune complex nephritis (Joshi et al. 1981), but it is doubtful if the rat is a good model for the effects of cadmium. More reliance should be placed on the human data.

II. Glucosuria and Aminoaciduria

An increased excretion of glucose and amino acids occurs among cadmium workers, as shown in several studies (Clarkson and Kench 1956; Kazantzis et al. 1963; Piscator 1966a). In the studies by Piscator (1966a), a slight glucosuria existed among cadmium workers, but even in cases with very pronounced proteinuria the glucose excretion generally was only a few hundred milligrams per day. It was also found that it was not possible to detect the glucosuria by common qualitative tests, e.g., dipsticks. In some cases, a slight positive reaction was seen if the sticks were read after about 15 min. No relationship was found between protein excretion and glucose excretion. In another study (KAZANTZIS et al. 1963), glucosuria had been detected with qualitative tests, but these cases probably had more severe tubular dysfunction than the Swedish workers.

The increase in the excretion of endogenous amino acids also seems moderate. In the study by PISCATOR (1966a), most cases showed normal excretion even when there was heavy proteinuria, and no relationship was found between excretion of amino acids and glucose or protein excretion. More pronounced increases in amino acid excretion were reported by KAZANTZIS et al. (1963) and CLARKSON and KENCH (1956). In the study by CLARKSON and KENCH (1956), it was shown that there was a generalized aminoaciduria with a tendency for increased excretion of hydroxyamino acids.

The filtered load of proteins and its reabsorption do not vary much and are not influenced by factors such as diet. In contrast, the filtered load of glucose and amino acids may vary considerably owing to dietary and endogenous factors; these compounds should be studied under standardized metabolic conditions in order to obtain more quantitative information on their renal handling in cadmium-exposed workers. Urinary losses of these substances are very small, and since any significant increase only seems to occur when there is already a significant proteinuria, studies of these compounds for evaluating Cd nephropathy possesses little or no value.

In animal experiments, it was also shown that chronic cadmium exposure may affect excretion of glucose and amino acids (AXELSSON and PISCATOR 1966). Aminoaciduria was only studied by determination of total amino acids, and increased excretion only occurred after proteinuria. A considerable drop in the reabsorption capacity for glucose was seen at about the same time as heavy proteinuria in these rabbits, and cadmium levels in the kidney had already started to decrease, a sign of severe renal damage. However, in rabbits followed for half a year after cessation of exposure, the glucose-loading test showed that there must have been a considerable regression of the renal damage, since the reabsorption capacity was no different from that seen in controls. In these rabbits, there also seemed to have been a regression of the proteinuria (PISCATOR and AXELSSON 1970).

III. Disturbances in Mineral Metabolism

Since FRIBERG (1950) had found a high incidence of renal stones among Swedish battery workers, further studies were made (AHLMARK et al. 1961; AXELSSON 1963). The stones consisted mainly of calcium phosphate; this is relatively uncommon, only occurring in 5% of stone-formers (AXELSSON 1963). Renal stones were more common in cases with slight disturbances than among cases with heavy proteinuria, but excretion of calcium and phosphorus was found to be normal. KAZANTZIS et al. (1963) studied a group of cadmium-exposed workers and found several with severe tubular dysfunction who also had increased calcium excretion and acidosis. One of these patients later developed osteomalacia (KAZANTZIS 1980). Some of the workers had a history of renal stones. A high incidence of renal stone disease has also been reported among other groups of British cadmium workers (ADAMS et al. 1969; SCOTT et al. 1976). In one group, hypercalciuria was common (SCOTT et al. 1978). In studies in the United States, a disturbed renal handling of phosphorus and calcium has been noted, but there have been no reports on the occurrence of renal stones (SMITH et al. 1980).

There is thus plenty of evidence that in men exposed occupationally to cadmium, disturbances in mineral metabolism may occur and there is a tendency toward formation of renal stones. A large number of studies have been performed in Japan on tubular dysfunction in members of the general population exposed to cadmium and with proteinuria and other signs of renal dysfunction as severe as those seen among cadmium workers. However, no increased incidence of renal stones was reported from Japan. The reason for the difference between Japanese and Europeans may be dietary. Japanese generally produce a more alkaline urine owing to a high intake of vegetables, especially in the farming population, whereas on a Western diet the urine tends to be acid, presumably owing to a higher protein intake.

Stone-formation is known to be prevented by giving bicarbonate if the cause is a distal renal tubular acidosis (AGUS et al. 1981; BACKMAN et al. 1980; BATTLE and ARRUDA 1981). The bicarbonate is thought to increase the citrate concentration in tubular fluid, which will prevent calcium from being precipitated (CHAN 1981). The reabsorption of calcium as well as citrate is also partly dependent on sodium transport across the proximal tubules (COHEN and BARAC-NIETO 1973; SIMPSON 1983; SUTTON 1983). However, there is a lack of data on how such mechanisms function in cadmium-exposed persons who form calcium phosphate stones. Some animal studies indicate that renal handling of sodium is influenced by low doses of cadmium (FRIBERG et al. 1974).

The most severe effects of Cd on mineral metabolism were seen in Japan in Toyama Prefecture, where itai-itai disease occurred; this, as mentioned earlier, is characterized by osteomalacia. A low intake of calcium and vitamin D and calcium losses during pregnancy and lactation may have contributed to this condition. Combination of mineral deficiency and a severe tubular dysfunction will of course cause very severe effects on the bone tissue. Other factors may be that cadmium interferes with intestinal absorption of calcium or with the renal synthesis of vitamin D_3.

As mentioned earlier, renal stones did not appear when there was very pronounced renal damage, and in such cases proximal renal tubular acidosis may exist. This generally does not cause renal stone formation (BACKMAN et al. 1980; BATTLE and ARUDA 1981) and may explain the peculiar dose–response relationship with regard to renal stones. Acidosis may however cause an increased resorption of calcium from bone which will be a further cause for the severe osteomalacia seen among Japanese women.

There is a lack of hard data on the disturbances in renal handling of acids and bases in cadmium-exposed people. One reason for this lack is that it is difficult to carry out good studies under field conditions; obviously, more data would be of great interest.

D. Effects on Glomerular Function

The finding by FRIBERG (1950) of reduced GFR among heavily exposed workers has been verified in several studies on cadmium-exposed workers (AHLMARK et al. 1961; BERNARD et al. 1979; KAZANTZIS et al. 1963; PETERSON et al. 1969; SMITH et al. 1980), as well as in Japanese women exposed to cadmium via food (NOGAWA et al. 1979, 1980). In animal experiments, a slight reduction of GFR could also be seen, but 6 months after cessation of exposure, there was no difference compared with controls (AXELSSON and PISCATOR 1966; PISCATOR and AXELSSON 1970).

As mentioned in Sect. C.I, small changes in the tubular reabsorption of proteins can be detected, e.g., by the determination of the relative clearance of β_2-m, but it is much more difficult to detect changes in GFR. Whereas a 0.1% decrease in the tubular reabsorption of β_2-m may double its excretion, and thus can readily be detected, it is difficult except under rigidly controlled conditions to demonstrate a 10% reduction in GFR. It is thus impossible to decide whether minor decreases in GFR occur together with changes in protein excretion. As mentioned in Sect. C.I, increased excretion of albumin has been used as an argument for glomerular damage caused by cadmium, but since albumin excretion is both related to tubular reabsorption functions and varies with many physiologic factors and disease states, it is not a reliable indicator for small changes in glomerular function.

There have been a few renal biopsies on cadmium workers, but microscopic examination did not reveal abnormal glomerular changes (FRIBERG et al. 1974). Studies on exposed rabbits have shown that even heavy exposure to cadmium caused little or no change in the glomeruli, whereas tubular damage was pronounced (AXELSSON and PISCATOR 1966; AXELSSON et al. 1968; PISCATOR and AXELSSON 1970). The most logical explanation for the slow decrease in GFR is that it is the result of the tubular effects and interstitial changes in the kidney. If there is fibrosis and atrophy of the tubules, this means loss of nephrons which will cause the decrease in GFR. Some similarities exist between chronic cadmium poisoning and the early stages of another primary tubular lesion as seen in endemic Balkan nephropathy (HALL and DAMMIN 1978). In this disease, severe glomerular dysfunction may occur as the result of the interstitial renal changes. It is also known that there is a correlation between tubular changes and changes in GFR in patients with renal disease (MACKENSEN-HAEN et al. 1981; SCHAINUCK et al. 1970). The relationship between interstitial changes and GFR has also recently been discussed by BOHLE (1982).

In a recent follow-up of workers who had first been examined 13 years previously in 1969, it was found that slight tubular dysfunction was not accompanied by depression of GFR, as indicated by absence of changes in serum creatinine and creatinine clearance. On the other hand, decreases in GFR were observed in a few cases with more severe tubular dysfunction (PISCATOR 1984). This supports the conclusion that GFR may follow tubular and interstitial changes.

E. Diagnosis

It was soon recognized (Friberg 1950) that the proteinuria in chronic cadmium poisoning had some unusual features and that common diagnostic procedures were not suitable for its detection. Friberg (1950) found that the nitric acid test (Heller's test) and the picric acid test (Esbach's test) were not sensitive enough, whereas trichloroacetic acid seemed to give more reliable qualitative estimates.

Piscator (1962 b) studied several quantitative and qualitative methods for determination of protein in urine. It was found that a reagent used by Tsuchiya (1908) and modified by Lehmann (1947) gave complete precipitation of even the small amounts of protein occurring in normal urine. The colorimetric determination was done by a biuret method at a wavelength of 330 µm (Goa 1953).

By comparing quantitative and qualitative results, Friberg's findings were confirmed. Nitric acid gave positive results only at relatively high protein concentrations, whereas trichloroacetic acid gave positive readings near the upper normal level of protein in urine. It was also seen that dipsticks were inferior to trichloroacetic acid. An explanation for these findings was found when concentrated urine proteins were examined by several separation and identification procedures (Piscator 1962 a, 1966 a, b). The majority of the urine proteins were of low molecular weight, albumin constituted a relatively small part, and immunoglobulin chains were present.

For some time, determination of total protein and electrophoretic analysis of concentrated urine proteins were the best methods for establishing the cadmium proteinuria, but soon specific determination of β_2-m became a valuable addition to the diagnostic set (Peterson et al. 1969; Evrin et al. 1971).

In most studies on relationships between Cd exposure and biologic effects, urine β_2-m has been the parameter measured and related to urine excretion of cadmium or concentrations of cadmium in liver or kidney. Simultaneous determination of β_2-m and creatinine in serum and urine has also made it possible to determine the relative clearance of β_2-m, which is a more sensitive measurement than the urine excretion alone. An increase in the excretion of β_2-m is of course not specific for cadmium poisoning; it may occur in many conditions, but in most of them it will be a reversible effect. A persistent increase in the urinary excretion of β_2-m combined with a high renal burden of cadmium is a sure sign of renal tubular dysfunction caused by cadmium. It should be noted that in advanced cases of chronic cadmium poisoning the excretion of β_2-m may be very high and the renal burden of cadmium relatively low, owing to renal losses of cadmium.

There are, however, some disadvantages to using β_2-m. The dependence on urine pH is troublesome. The urine pH should be kept between 6 and 7 and to avoid the need for discarding samples with lower pH it is recommended that oral doses of bicarbonate be given before urine collection. Some of the disadvantages of using β_2-m have been discussed by Bernard and Lauwerys (1981). They suggested that the determination of retinol-binding protein (RBP) is a better way of establishing tubular proteinuria than the use of β_2-m, since the pH dependence is avoided, Bernard et al. (1982 a) showed that RBP is stable in urine down to pH 4.5. They compared the urinary excretion of RBP and β_2-m and found that at pH > 5.6 both proteins were similar with regard to sensitivity and specificity for detecting tubular dysfunction. Both proteins were estimated by a latex immunoassay (BERNARD et al. 1981, 1982b) instead of the earlier commonly used radioimmunoassay (EVRIN et al. 1971). Determination of albumin can also provide useful additional information about type and degree of proteinuria. Excretion of albumin is, however, more easily influenced by physiologic factors than is that of β_2-m or RBP (e.g., posture, time of day, water loading, exercise).

Electrophoresis of concentrated urine proteins still remains a sensitive tool, but the sensitivity falls below that of the quantitative determination of specific proteins. Total protein in urine has been found useful when evaluating long-term trends in cadmium workers (PISCATOR 1983, 1984).

Since an effect on protein reabsorption is an early sign of the nephrotoxic action of cadmium, and as even very small changes can be detected by present methods, determination of amino acids, glucose, phosphorus, concentrating capacity, and acidification capacity gives very little additional information, especially since such studies must be performed under more controlled conditions. Such studies should be used for clinical examination of more severe cases.

Among urine enzymes, N-acetyl-β-glucosaminidase (NAG) has been suggested as a suitable effect parameter, but according to NOGAWA et al. (1983) the increase in NAG activity was not as marked as the increase in urine β_2-m among cadmium-exposed people.

Recently developed methods for the quantitative determination of metallothionein have made it possible to study the urine excretion of this protein. CHANG et al. (1980) determined metallothionein in urine of cadmium-exposed workers. Metallothionein levels were about the same in workers with and without renal dysfunction. The highest level was found in a worker with relatively short exposure and the authors postulated that long-standing renal dysfunction would cause lower levels in urine owing to renal losses of Cd–metallothionein; this explanation agrees with the fact that urine cadmium levels may also decrease.

In studies on Japanese women, TOHYAMA et al. (1982) found that patients with confirmed or suspected itai-itai disease excreted more metallothionein than women with normal renal function. However, the cadmium concentrations in the latter group were not reported and it is thus difficult to compare that report with the one by CHANG et al. (1980). In both studies there was, as expected, a good correlation between urine Cd and metallothionein.

GFR should be monitored by determination of serum creatinine, but as mentioned earlier, small changes in GFR will not be detected until relatively late compared with what can be achieved by determination of proteins. Some aspects of the general problems in studies on renal effects of toxic substances have recently been considered by PISCATOR et al. (1985).

F. Prognosis

Once tubular proteinuria has been established, it seems to be irreversible (PISCATOR 1962a, b, 1966a, 1983, 1984; PISCATOR and PETTERSSON 1977; ROELS et al. 1982). Since cadmium has an extremely long biologic half-life, it is obvious that once an effect has occurred it will take a long time before it disappears. Possibly, minor disturbances in the reabsorptive capacity may eventually return to normal, but there are at present no data available that allow such conclusions. In a recent follow-up of workers originally examined in 1969 (PISCATOR 1984) all workers with slight proteinuria in 1969 showed further slight or moderate increases in protein excretion in 1982, whereas workers with normal renal function in 1969 still excreted proteins at normal rates. A slow progression thus occurs, but long observation times are needed to verify it.

The main problem associated with renal Cd intoxication is not the proteinuria, since even in advanced cases the protein losses are relatively small (<2 g/day). Other disturbances in tubular function may be of greater importance for health, such as the changes in mineral metabolism leading to renal stones (male European workers) or osteomalacia (Japanese women). It is obvious that kidneys with high concentrations of cadmium may have less reserve capacity to handle stress and that they will be more sensitive to such phenomena as changes in bone metabolism, e.g., release of calcium from bone during immobilization.

As mentioned earlier, the fall in GFR may result from tubular interstitial changes. Generally, the decrease in GFR is relatively moderate, even in cases with pronounced tubular dysfunction, and far from the level at which dialysis may be needed.

G. Prevention

Since even slight tubular dysfunction caused by cadmium seems to be irreversible and may progress, it is obvious that this dysfunction should be prevented. This can only be achieved by not letting the cadmium concentrations in the kidney reach toxic levels. The concentration of Cd in the renal cortex (about 200 mg/kg) or the total amount in the kidneys (30–40 mg) or urine excretion (10 µg per gram creatinine) represent potentially critical values. Only the latter estimate can be generally used since the in vivo neutron activation methods cannot be applied everywhere, and should not be used on female workers. Urinary excretion should not be permitted to exceed 5 µg Cd per gram creatinine if low molecular weight proteinuria is to be avoided.

References

Adams RG, Harrison JF, Scott P (1969) The development of cadmium-induced proteinuria, impaired renal function, and osteomalacia in alkaline battery workers. Q J Med 38:425–443

Agus ZS, Goldfarb S, Wassterstein A (1979) Calcium transport in the kidney. Rev Physiol Biochem Pharmacol 90:155–169

Ahlmark A, Axelsson B, Friberg L, Piscator M (1961) Further investigations into kidney function and proteinuria in chronic cadmium poisoning. Proc 13th Int Congr Occup Health 201–203

Axelsson B (1963) Urinary calculus in long-term exposure to cadmium. Proc 14th Int Congr Occup Health 939–942

Axelsson B, Piscator M (1966) Renal damage after prolonged exposure to cadmium. Arch Environ Health 12:360–373

Axelsson B, Dahlgren SE, Piscator M (1968) Renal lesions in the rabbit after long-term exposure to cadmium. Arch Environ Health 17:24–28

Backman U, Danielson BG, Johansson G, Lunghall S, Wikström B (1980) Incidence and clinical importance of renal tubular defects in recurrent renal stone formers. Nephron 25:96–101

Battle DC, Arruda JAL (1981) Renal tubular acidosis syndromes. Miner Electrolyte Metab 5:83–99

Bernard AM, Lauwerys RR (1981) Retinol binding protein in urine: A more practical index than urinary β_2-microglobulin for the routine screening of renal tubular function. Clin Chem 27:1781–1782

Bernard A, Roels H, Hubermont G, Buchet JP, Masson PL, Lauwerys RR (1976) Characterization of the proteinuria in cadmium-exposed workers. Int Arch Occup Environ Health 38:19–30

Bernard AM, Buchet JP, Roels H, Masson P, Lauwerys RR (1979) Renal excretion of proteins and enzymes in workers exposed to cadmium. Eur J Clin Invest 9:11–22

Bernard AM, Vyskocil A, Lauwerys RR (1981) Determination of β_2-microglobulin in human urine and serum by latex immunoassay. Clin Chem 27:832–837

Bernard AM, Moreau D, Lauwerys RR (1982a) Comparison of retinol-binding protein and β_2-microglobulin determination in urine for the early detection of tubular proteinuria. Clin Chim Acta 126:1–7

Bernard AM, Moreau D, Lauwerys RR (1982b) Latex immunoassay of retinol-binding protein. Clin Chem 28:1167–1171

Bohle A (1982) Die Bedeutung des Niereninterstitiums für die Nierenfunktion. Klin Wochenschr 60:1186–1190

Buchet JP, Roels H, Bernard A, Lauwerys RR (1980) Assessment of renal function of workers exposed to inorganic lead, cadmium or mercury vapor. J Occup Med 22:741–750

Butler EA, Flynn FV (1958) The proteinuria of renal tubular disorders. Lancet II:978–980

Butler EA, Flynn FV, Harris H, Robson EB (1962) A study of urine proteins by two-dimensional electrophoresis with special reference to the proteinuria of renal tubular disorders. Clin Chim Acta 7:34–41

Chan JCM (1981) Nutrition and acid-base metabolism. Fed Proc 40:2423–2428

Chan W-Y, Rennert OM (1981) Cadmium nephropathy. Ann Clin Lab Sci 11:229–238

Chang CC, Lauwerys A, Bernard A, Roels H, Buchet JP, Garvey JS (1980) Metallothionein in cadmium-exposed workers. Environ Res 23:422–428

Clarkson TW, Kench JE (1956) Urinary excretion of amino acids by men absorbing heavy metals. Biochem J 62:361–372

Cohen JJ, Barac-Nieto M (1973) Renal metabolism of substances in relation to renal function. In: Orloff J, Berliner RW (eds) Renal physiology, Handbook of physiology, vol 3. American Physiological Society, Washington 8:909–1001

Deen WM, Satvat B (1981) Determinants of the glomerular filtration of proteins. Am J Physiol 241:F162–F170

Ekström B, Peterson PA, Berggård I (1975) A urinary and plasma α_1-glycoprotein of low molecular weight: Isolation and some properties. Biochem Biophys Res Commun 65:1427–1433

Ellis KJ, Morgan WD, Zanzi I, Yasumura S, Vartsky D, Cohn SH (1981) Critical concentrations of cadmium in human renal cortex: Dose-effect studies in cadmium smelter workers. J Toxicol Environ Health 7:691–703

Evrin P-E, Peterson PA, Wide L, Berggård I (1971) Radioimmunoassay of β_2-microglobulin in human biological fluids. Scand J Clin Lab Invest 28:439–443

Falck FY Jr, Fine LJ, Smith RG, Garvey J, Schork A, England B, McClatchey KD, Linton J (1983a) Metallothionein and occupational exposure to cadmium. Br J Ind Med 40:305–313

Falck FY Jr, Fine LJ, Smith RG, McClatchey KD, Annesley T, England B, Schork AM (1983b) Occupational cadmium exposure and renal status. Am J Ind Med 4:541–549

Foulkes EC (1978) Apparent competition between myoglobin and metallothionein for renal reabsorption. Proc Soc Exp Biol Med 159:321–323

Foulkes EC (1982) Tubular reabsorption of low molecular weight proteins. Physiologist 25:56–59

Friberg L (1950) Health hazards in the manufacture of alkaline accumulators with special reference to chronic cadmium poisoning. Acta Med Scand [Suppl 240] 138:1–124

Friberg L, Vahter M (1983) Assessment of exposure to lead and cadmium through biological monitoring: Results of a UNEP/WHO global study. Environ Res 30:95–128

Friberg L, Piscator M, Nordberg GF, Kjellström T (1974) Cadmium in the environment, 2nd edn. CRC, Cleveland

Goa J (1953) A micro biuret method for protein determination. Scand J Clin Lab Invest 5:218–222

Hall PW, Dammin GJ (1978) Balkan nephropathy. Nephron 22:281–300

Iwao S, Tsuchiya K, Sakurai H (1980) Serum and urinary β_2-microglobulin among cadmium-exposed workers. J Occup Med 22:399–402

Joshi BC, Dwivedi C, Powell A, Holscher M (1981) Immune complex nephritis in rats induced by long-term exposure to cadmium. J Comp Pathol 91:11–15

Kazantzis G (1980) Renal tubular dysfunction and osteopathy in cadmium workers. In: Shigematsu I, Nomiyama K (eds) Cadmium-induced osteopathy. Japan Public Health Association, pp 60–65

Kazantzis G, Flynn FV, Spowage JS, Trott DG (1963) Renal tubular malfunction and pulmonary emphysema in cadmium pigment workers. Q J Med 32:165–192

Kjellström T (1979) Exposure and accumulation of cadmium in populations from Japan, the United States, and Sweden. Environ Health Perspect 28:169–197

Kjellström T, Shiroishi K, Evrin P-E (1977) Urinary β_2-microglobulin excretion among people exposed to cadmium in the general environment. Environ Res 13:318–344

Kojima S, Haga Y, Kurihara T, Yamawaki T, Kjellström T (1977) A comparison between fecal cadmium and urinary β_2-microglobulin, total protein and cadmium among Japanese farmers. Environ Res 14:436–451

Lauwerys RR, Buchet JP, Roels HA, Brouwers J, Stanescu D (1974) Epidemiological survey of workers exposed to cadmium. Arch Environ Health 28:145–148

Lauwerys RR, Roels H, Regniers M, Buchet JP, Bernard A, Goret A (1979) Significance of cadmium concentration in blood and in urine in workers exposed to cadmium. Environ Res 20:375–391

Lehmann J (1947) Proteinbestämning i serum respetive plasma och urin. Nord Med 33:338–345

Maack T, Johnson V, Kau ST, Figueiredo J, Sigulem D (1979) Renal filtration, transport, and metabolism of low-molecular weight proteins: a review. Kidney Int 16:251–270

Mackensen-Haen S, Bader R, Grund KE, Bohle A (1981) Correlations between renal cortical interstitial fibrosis, atrophy of the proximal tubules and impairment of the glomerular filtration rate. Clin Nephrol 15:167–171

Mogensen CE, Sölling K (1977) Studies on renal tubular protein reabsorption: partial and near complete inhibition by certain amino acids. Scand J Clin Lab Invest 37:474–477

Murray T, Walker BR, Spratt DM, Chappelka R (1981) Cadmium nephropathy. Monitoring for early evidence of renal dysfunction. Arch Environ Health 36:165–171

Nicaud P, Lafitte A, Gros A (1942) Les troubles de l'intoxication chronique par le cadmium. Arch Mal Prof 4:192–202

Nogawa K, Ishizaki A, Kobayashi E (1979) A comparison between health effects of cadmium and cadmium concentration in urine among inhabitants of the Itai-itai disease endemic district. Environ Res 18:397–409

Nogawa K, Kobayashi E, Honda R, Ishizaki A, Kawano S, Matsuda H (1980) Renal dysfunctions of inhabitants in a cadmium-polluted area. Environ Res 23:13–23

Nogawa K, Yamada Y, Honda R, Tsuritani I, Ishizaki M, Sakamoto M (1983) Urinary N-acetyl-β-D-glucosaminidase and β_2-microglobulin in "Itai-itai" disease. Toxicol Lett 16:317–322

Nordberg M, Elinder C-G, Rahnster B (1979) Cadmium, zinc and copper in horse kidney metallothionein. Environ Res 20:341–350

Pesce AJ, First MR (1979) Proteinuria. Dekker, New York, p 294

Pesce AJ, Clyne DH, Pollak VE, Kant SK, Foulkes EC, Selenke WM (1980) Renal tubular interactions of proteins. Clin Biochem 13:209–215

Peterson PA, Berggård I (1971) Isolation and properties of a human retinol-transporting protein. Biochemistry 10:25–33

Peterson PA, Evrin PH, Berggård I (1969) Differentiation of glomerular, tubular and normal proteinuria: Determinations of urinary excretion of β_2-microglobulin, albumin and total protein. J Clin Invest 48:1189–1198

Piscator M (1962a) Proteinuria in chronic cadmium poisoning. I. An electrophoretic and chemical study of urinary and serum proteins from workers with chronic cadmium poisoning. Arch Environ Health 4:607–621

Piscator M (1962b) Proteinuria in chronic cadmium poisoning. II. The applicability of quantitative and qualitative methods for the demonstration of cadmium proteinuria. Arch Environ Health 5:325–332

Piscator M (1966a) Proteinuria in chronic cadmium poisoning. III. Electrophoretic and immunoelectrophoretic studies on urinary proteins from cadmium workers, with special reference to the excretion of low molecular weight proteins. Arch Environ Health 12:335–344

Piscator M (1966b) Proteinuria in chronic cadmium poisoning. IV. Gelfiltration and ion-exchange chromatography of urinary proteins from cadmium workers. Arch Environ Health 12:345–359

Piscator M (1983) Renale Wirkungen von Cadmium. In: Zumkley H (ed) Spurenelemente. Grundlagen-Ätiologie-Diagnose-Therapie. Thieme, Stuttgart, pp 81–97

Piscator M (1984) Long-term observations on tubular and glomerular function in cadmium exposed persons. Environ Health Perspect 54:175–179

Piscator M, Axelsson B (1970) Serum proteins and kidney function after exposure to cadmium. Arch Environ Health 21:604–608

Piscator M, Lind B (1972) Cadmium, zinc, copper, and lead in human renal cortex. Arch Environ Health 24:426–431

Piscator M, Pettersson B (1977) Chronic cadmium poisoning – diagnosis and prevention. In: Brown SS (ed) Clinical chemistry and chemical toxicology of metals. Elsevier/North-Holland, Amsterdam, pp 143–155

Piscator M, Björck L, Nordberg M (1981) β_2-microglobulin levels in serum and urine of cadmium exposed rabbits. Acta Pharmacol Toxicol (Copenh) 49:1–7

Piscator M, Foulkes EC, Hammond PB (1985) Early detection of renal disease (to be published)

Roels HA, Lauwerys RR, Buchet JP, Bernard A, Chettle DR, Harvey TC, Al-Haddad IK (1981) In vivo measurement of liver and kidney cadmium in workers exposed to this metal. Its significance with respect to cadmium in blood and urine. Enrion Res 26:217–240

Roels HA, Djubgang J, Buchet J-P, Bernard A, Lauwerys RR (1982) Evolution of cadmium-induced renal dysfunction in workers removed from exposure. Scand J Work Environ Health 8:191–200

Roels HA, Lauwerys RR, Dardenne AN (1983) The critical level of cadmium in human renal cortex: A reevaluation. Toxicol Lett 15:357–360

Ryan GB (1981) The glomerular sieve and mechanism of proteinuria. Aust NZ J Med 11:197–206

Saito H, Shioji R, Hurukawa Y, Arikawa T, Saito T, Nagai K, Furuyama T, Yoshinaga K (1977a) Chronic cadmium poisoning induced by environmental cadmium pollution. Renal lesions (multiple proximal tubular dysfunctions) identified in residents of cadmium-polluted Hosogoe, Kosako Town, Akita prefecture, Japan. Jpn J Med 16:2–13

Saito H, Shioji R, Hurukawa Y, Nagai K, Arikawa T, Saito T, Sasaki Y, Furuyama T, Yoshinaga K (1977b) Cadmium-induced proximal tubular dysfunction in a cadmium-polluted area. Contrib Nephrol 6:1–12

Sakurai H (1980) Epidemiological approach to subclinical effects of metals in long-term occupational exposures. In: Holmstedt B, Lauwerys RR, Mercier M, Roberfroid M (eds) Mechanisms of toxicity and hazard evaluation. Elsevier/North-Holland Biomedical, Amsterdam, pp 293–305

Schainuck LI, Striker GE, Cutler RE, Benditt EP (1970) Structural-functional correlations in renal disease. Part 2: The correlations. Hum Pathol 1:631–641

Scott R, Mills EA, Fell GS, Husain FER, Yates AJ, Paterson PJ, McKirdy A, Ottoway JM, Fitzgerald-Finch OP, Lamont A (1976) Clinical and biochemical abnormalities in coppersmiths exposed to cadmium. Lancet II:396–398

Scott R, Paterson PJ, Burns R, Ottoway JM, Hussain FER, Fell GS, Dumbya S, Iqbal J (1978) Hypercalciuria related to cadmium exposure. Urology 11:462–465

Simpson DP (1983) Citrate excretion: A window on renal metabolism. Am J Physiol 244:F223–F234

Smith TJ, Anderson RJ, Reading JC (1980) Chronic cadmium exposures associated with kidney function tests. Am J Ind Med 1:319–337

Sumpio BE, Maack T (1982) Kinetics, competition, and selectivity of tubular absorption of proteins. Am J Physiol 243:F379–F392

Sutton RAL (1983) Disorders of renal calcium excretion. Kidney Int 23:665–673

Tohyama C, Shaikh ZA, Nogawa K, Kobayashi E, Honda R (1982) Urinary metallothionein as a new index of renal dysfunction in "Itai-Itai" disease patients and other Japanese women environmentally exposed to cadmium. Arch Toxicol 50:159–166

Tsuchiya I (1908) Eine neue volumetrische Eiweißbestimmung mittels der Phosphorwolframsäure. Zentralbl Inn Med 29:105–115

Tsuchiya K (1978) Cadmium studies in Japan. A review. Elsevier/North-Holland Biomedical, Amsterdam

CHAPTER 7

Cadmium and the Cardiovascular System

J. KOPP

A. Preface

The dedication of an entire chapter to the subject of the cardiovascular actions
of cadmium implies that cadmium exhibits some degree of selectivity for cardiovascular tissues. Hypothetically, this tissue specificity may be benign or induce
changes in the functional properties of these tissues that are biologically significant. This latter assertion is substantiated by the numerous articles published on
this subject, particularly those which have demonstrated that chronic exposure to
cadmium leads to considerable derangements in cardiovascular system function
in humans and experimental animals (ADAMSKA-DYNIEWSKA et al. 1980a;
BOSCOLO et al. 1980, 1981; DOTTA and FRUSCELLA 1963; IANNACCONE et al. 1979,
1981; KOPP et al. 1978c, 1980a–d, 1982, 1983a, b; PERRY et al. 1977; PERRY and
ERLANGER 1981; PONTEVA et al. 1979; REVIS et al. 1980, 1983; REVIS and ZINS-
MEISTER 1981; SCHROEDER and VINTON 1962; STURKIE 1973; TOMERA and
HARAKAL 1980; VOROBIEVA and EREMEEVA 1980). Before describing the cardiovascular actions of cadmium and the putative cellular sites and mechanisms
believed to be involved in these effects, a brief discourse summarizing the intrinsic
and extrinsic factors that influence and regulate the complex and highly integrated function of the circulatory system is deemed appropriate.

I. Regulatory Aspects of Cardiovascular Function: Intrinsic Considerations

1. Heart

The contractile and excitability characteristics of cardiac muscle and the specialized conduction tissues of the heart are subordinate to the intrinsic structural and
biochemical properties of the cells that comprise these tissues. Excitation–contraction coupling in heart muscle is an ordered activity that coordinates cell-to-
cell communication, the propagation of a depolarizing impulse along fast- and
slow-conducting cell junctions, the stimulation of electrogenically coupled, phos-
phorylation-independent and -dependent ion exchange mechanisms in cell membranes, the activation of fast and slow membrane channels, the release and shift
of ions among various extracellular and intracellular compartments, and the
transduction of chemical energy to mechanical energy (spatial motion–muscle
contraction) through conformational changes in regulatory (troponin) and contractile (actin and myosin) proteins (BERS and LANGER 1979; BRAUNWALD 1982;
LANGER et al. 1974; WALSH et al. 1980). The biophysical events associated with

excitation–contraction coupling in heart muscle are linked to the metabolic processes of the cell in part through changes in intracellular levels of free (ionized) calcium. The release of calcium from membrane-bound sites within the sarcoplasmic reticulum and the sarcolemma serves to trigger the cascade of molecular events which culminate in muscle contraction and force development. Calcium-dependent protein phosphorylation reactions, which require metabolic energy, appear to modulate the extent of the contractile response (BÁRÁNY et al. 1981; KOPP and BÁRÁNY 1979). Conversely, the sequestration of calcium terminates the contractile response and initiates relaxation. The rate of these processes can be modified by changing the kinetics of the calcium release and uptake.

The toxic response to cadmium purportedly is mediated through effects involving various of these cellular sites. Cadmium is a nonessential metal in living systems. The greater affinity generally displayed by cadmium ions for cellular binding sites (BERS and LANGER 1979; LANGER et al. 1974; TROSPER and PHILIPSON 1983) has two primary ramifications: (a) it facilitates the displacement of essential metal cofactors from active sites by cadmium ions; and (b) it renders these sites unresponsive to regulation by the essential metal cofactors that ordinarily interact with these sites in the absence of cadmium ions. In addition, the binding of cadmium ions to critical effector sites may disturb the spatial organization and dynamics of cell structural and biochemical components, causing a disruption of cellular homeostatic mechanisms. An inability to restore the chemical homeostasis of the cell owing to inadequate compensatory responses will affect cellular energy metabolism and repair mechanisms which can lead to cell injury, and ultimately cell death (DHALLA et al. 1978; GIBBS 1978; LANGE and SOBEL 1982; MERIN 1978; OPIE 1976; SINGHAL et al. 1976). The degree of cellular dysfunction that occurs in response to cadmium is proportional to the extent of the injury that was incurred. The actual cellular sites linked to the cardiotoxic behavior of cadmium have not been identified conclusively. Recent evidence indicates that cadmium displaces calcium from cellular binding sites and antagonizes calcium-dependent reactions in the heart by an essentially competitive mechanism (BERS and LANGER 1979; HORIUCHI and HAYASHI 1979; KLEINFELD and STEIN 1968; KOPP and HAWLEY 1976; KOPP and BÁRÁNY 1980; KOPP et al. 1980a, b; LANGER et al. 1974; LEE et al. 1982; LEE and TSIEN 1983; PILATI et al. 1982; PRENTICE 1982; PRENTICE et al. 1984; TODA 1973b; TROSPER and PHILIPSON 1983). Moreover, cadmium exhibits properties analogous to those displayed by organic membrane calcium channel inhibitors (BRAUNWALD 1982; FLECKENSTEIN 1983; LEE et al. 1982; LEE and TSIEN 1983; TSIEN 1983). These latter characteristics suggest that the action of cadmium on myocardial excitation–contraction coupling is linked in part to its antagonism of calcium for membrane transport sites. The antagonism between cadmium and calcium in biologic systems is not limited to the heart, but instead appears to be a characteristic action of cadmium common to many other organ systems as well (ANDO et al. 1977; GRUDEN 1977; HAMILTON and SMITH 1978; SHINO 1976; WASHKO and COUSINS 1976).

The interactions of cadmium with cell membrane constituents in excitable tissues have been documented by direct and indirect measurements (ANTUNES-MADEIRA and CARVALHO 1970; BADER et al. 1970; BERS and LANGER 1979; BLAUSTEIN and GOLDMAN 1968; COOPER and STEINBERG 1977; FORSHAW 1977;

HAFEMANN 1969; HAYASHI and TAKAYAMA 1978; KAMINO et al. 1975; LANGER et al. 1974; LEE et al. 1982; LEE and TSIEN 1983; SATOH et al. 1982; TROSPER and PHILIPSON 1983). In contrast, the reputed intracellular actions of cadmium have been inferred indirectly from biochemical and rate-dependent changes following cadmium exposure (BERS and LANGER 1979; PILATI et al. 1982; PRENTICE 1982; PRENTICE et al. 1984). Direct measures of cadmium flux across the sarcolemma of cardiac cells are nonexistent. Current knowledge regarding the direct actions of cadmium within the interior of the cell has progressed slowly (PASSOW et al. 1961). Cellular uptake of cadmium has been demonstrated, however, in other cellular systems (CORRIGAN and HUANG 1981; FOWLER 1978; POPHAM and WEBSTER 1976; STACEY and KLAASSEN 1980; WONG and KLAASSEN 1980). Indeed, the indirect evidence that has accumulated strongly suggests that intracellular sites are involved in the responses to cadmium (BERS and LANGER 1979; KOPP and BÁRÁNY 1979, 1980; LANGER et al. 1974; PRENTICE et al. 1984; STACEY and KLAASSEN 1980; WAALKES et al. 1983). It would be surprising, for example, if cadmium did not have direct effects on one or more of the following intracellular processes: (a) calcium release and sequestration of calcium by the sarcoplasmic reticulum; (b) mitochondrial function; (c) contractile and regulatory protein function; and (d) high energy phosphate production and utilization in cardiac cells (BERS and LANGER 1979; DIAMOND and KENCH 1974; FUCHS 1971; JACOBS et al. 1956; KOPP et al. 1978 a, b, 1980a; KOPP and BÁRÁNY 1979, 1980; MUSTAFA and CROSS 1971; POOL 1981; RAUCHOVA and DRAHOTA 1979; TROSPER and PHILIPSON 1983; VALLEE and ULMER 1972).

2. Vasculature

Excitation–contraction coupling in vascular smooth muscle is primarily regulated by ionized calcium levels within the cells. Fundamental differences do exist between vascular smooth muscle and cardiac muscle which include the recognition that the contractile state of smooth muscle is regulated principally by the phosphorylation and dephosphorylation of the myosin light chain-2 and that crossbridge formation between actin and myosin is not regulated by troponin (JOHANSSON and SOMLYO 1980). As with the heart, the physiologic properties of vascular tissues are subordinate to the intrinsic structural and biochemical characteristics of the cells that comprise these tissues. A marked biochemical and functional dependence of vascular smooth muscle cells on external calcium fluxes has been demonstrated (FLECKENSTEIN 1983). As a result, vascular smooth muscle exhibits a high degree of sensitivity to agents which inhibit calcium influx (FLECKENSTEIN 1983; VAN BREEMEN et al. 1979). Considering the evidence demonstrating that cadmium is a calcium channel inhibitor in cardiac cells, cadmium would be anticipated to act through a similar mechanism in vascular smooth muscle. The actual experimental findings are conflicting and indicate that the effects of cadmium on vascular tissues are markedly concentration dependent. At low concentrations, cadmium appears to induce vasoconstriction, while at higher doses relaxation (vasodilation) results (FOWLER et al. 1975; GUNN et al. 1966; HATTORI et al. 1983; HAYASHI and TODA 1977; KANISAWA and SCHROEDER 1969; LEVIN and MILLER 1981; NIWA and SUZUKI 1982; PERRY et al. 1967a, b; PRENTICE et al. 1984; THIND et al. 1970b; TODA 1973a; WAITES and SETCHELL 1966). Sodium flux is also a determinant of contraction coupling processes in smooth muscle, purportedly through effects on sarcoplasmic calcium (Ca^{2+}) levels and transmembrane calcium influx (VAN BREEMEN et al. 1979). Cadmium has been shown to inhibit Na, K-ATPase activity in striated muscle and other tissue systems (ANTUNES-MADEIRA and CARVALHO 1970; CHETTY et al. 1980; POOL 1981; VALLEE and ULMER 1972). Inhibition of the Na, K-pump by ouabain has been shown to induce contractions in vascular smooth muscle (VAN BREEMEN et al. 1979). Although direct evidence demonstrating a similar effect of cadmium on vascular smooth muscle has not been demonstrated, a selective inhibition of this enzyme by cadmium at levels below which calcium blockade occurs could conceivably induce a contractile (vasoconstrictor) rather than a relaxation (vasodilator) response. Additional information concerning the effects of cadmium on sodium and calcium homeostasis in smooth muscle cells is required before the apparent contradictory actions of cadmium on vascular smooth muscle can be resolved. Furthermore, except for indications that vascular elasticity may be altered by chronic cadmium exposure (TERPIN and ROACH 1980), the other biochemical and structural effects of cadmium that accompany these physiologic responses have not been delineated.

II. Extrinsic Considerations

Cardiovascular system control is modulated primarily through neural and hormonal effectors which are extrinsic to the myocardium and vascular system. Cellular biophysical properties and biochemical activities are directly influenced by the presence of these effector substances (e.g., neurotransmitters, hormones). Alterations in any or all of the following extrinsic factors would induce significant functional, metabolic, and structural changes in cardiovascular tissues: (a) tonic nerve activity (relative sympathetic–parasympathetic tone); (b) membrane receptor sensitivity and binding affinity (neurotransmitter, hormone); (c) synthesis of effector substances; (d) secretion coupling of processes involved in the release of effector substances; and (e) the rate of effector substance reuptake and degradation.

The information regarding the actions of cadmium on these extrinsic factors and regulators of the cardiovascular system is not abundant, but it appears to be consistent. Cholinergic nerve fibers are affected by direct cadmium exposure in both in situ and in vitro models (FORSHAW 1977; GILES et al. 1983; HAYASHI and TAKAYAMA 1978; SATOH et al. 1982). Cadmium acts primarily on the presynaptic cardiac nerve terminal, blocking the release of acetylcholine. Under the conditions of these experiments, cadmium acts by inhibiting the calcium-activated secretion coupling process involved in the release of acetylcholine (GILES et al. 1983). Postsynaptic effects of cadmium have been detected, as well; however, these responses appear to be relatively nonspecific as evidenced by the relatively high cadmium concentration required to demonstrate this effect (GILES et al. 1983). In addition to its cholinergic effects, prior cadmium exposure has been shown to affect adrenergic neurotransmission as well (COOPER and STEINBERG 1977; WILLIAMS et al. 1978). Studies conducted with isolated nerve–artery preparations from cadmium-exposed animals have demonstrated an increased responsiveness of peripheral arteries to adrenergic nerve fiber stimulation (NECHAY et al. 1978). Subsequent studies by REVIS et al. (1983) concerned with circulating catecholamine levels suggest that the half-life of norepinephrine is increased following chronic cadmium exposure.

Various other endocrine systems have been implicated as sites responsive, either directly or indirectly, to the actions of cadmium, as well. These include the renal kallikrein–bradykinin system (BOSCOLO et al. 1978, 1980, 1981; IANNACCONE et al. 1979, 1981), testicular, adrenal, and thyroid function (DER et al. 1976, 1977; SAKSENA et al. 1977; SHANBAKY et al. 1978), and the endocrine pancreas (GHAFGHAZI and MENNEAR 1973; ITHAKISSIOS et al. 1974a, b). The renal kallikrein–bradykinin system has been proposed as a local hormonal system involved in the regulation of renal blood flow and sodium excretion. Kallikrein, a peptidase, acts on plasma kininogen, an α_2-globulin, to generate a potent peptide vasodilator, bradykinin. Cadmium exposure in humans and experimental animals has been shown to reduce kallikrein activity as evidenced by the decreased urinary kallikrein activity in cadmium-exposed populations (BOSCOLO et al. 1978, 1980, 1981; IANNACCONE et al. 1979, 1981). In addition, following acute exposure to cadmium, decreased plasma thyroid hormone levels (triiodothyronine and thyroxine) have been observed in experimental animals, which are associated with a decrease in the thyroxine secretion rate (DER et al. 1977). Adrenal hypertrophy (zona glomerulosa, zona fasciculata) and testicular degeneration also have been detected following acute cadmium exposure (CHIQUOINE 1964; CLEGG and CARR 1967; DER et al. 1976, 1977; GUNN et al. 1963, 1966, 1968; NIEMI and KORMANO 1965; PAŘÍZEK and ZAHOR 1956; PAŘÍZEK 1957, 1960; SAKSENA et al. 1977; SCHWARTZE and ALSBERG 1923; SETCHELL and WAITES 1970; SUTHERLAND et al. 1974; WAITES and SETCHELL 1966). In conjunction with these effects, circulating blood testosterone and 5α-dihydrotestosterone levels were suppressed, while circulating corticosterone levels were increased (DER et al. 1976, 1977; SAKSENA et al. 1977). Among the other reported endocrinologic responses to cadmium are those which involve effects on pancreatic function. Subacute administration of cadmium has been shown to produce hyperglycemia and glucose intolerance (GHAFGHAZI and MENNEAR 1973). The former response, but not the latter, was prevented by adrenalectomy. Cadmium-induced glucose intolerance was associated with a decreased pancreatic secretory activity and a reduction in circulating serum insulin levels. The cellular biochemical changes that accompany the pathophysiologic alterations in these organs have been reviewed elsewhere (SINGHAL et al. 1976). The extent to which these endocrinologic changes participate in the long-term cardiovascular effects of cadmium are unknown; however, these results suggest that cadmium may influence cardiovascular system function through actions on various extrinsic regulators. A comprehensive understanding of the relationship between these experimental observations and the complex interactions of cadmium in vivo, however, has yet to be achieved.

B. Historical Overview

The ability of cadmium to influence the function of the cardiovascular system was recognized in the nineteenth century (ATHANASIU and LANGLOIS 1895, 1896; MARMÉ 1867; RICHET 1882). Among the early published observations were those by MARMÉ (1867) describing the functional aberrations of the circulatory system following acute cadmium exposure in experimental animals. Generally, these descriptive findings suggested a cardiodepressive action of cadmium, while anatomic evaluation of heart specimens taken from cadmium-treated animals revealed evidence of structural changes characterized by fatty degeneration of the myocardium. Later studies conducted during the next half century reflected an increasing scientific interest in characterizing and quantifying the injurious effects of cadmium on the myocardium (ATHANASIU and LANGLOIS 1895, 1896; RICHET 1882; SALANT and CONNET 1920). Both the contractile function and rhythmicity of the frog heart and isolated turtle heart were shown to be impaired in these studies by cadmium treatment. Although these studies introduced the concept that cadmium was toxic to the heart at rather low doses (approximately 4.4×10^{-6} M Cd, SALANT and CONNET 1920), scientific interest in the cardiotoxicity of cadmium waned, thereafter, except for sporadic reports (PRODAN 1932; WILSON et al. 1941).

Scientific interest in the health effects of cadmium was rekindled following World War II (DECKER et al. 1958; FRIBERG 1948, 1950; FRIBERG et al. 1974; HARRISON et al. 1947; JACOBS et al. 1956; KLEINFELD et al. 1955; PAŘÍZEK 1957; PASSOW et al. 1961; ROTHSTEIN 1959). At this time, an apparent causal relationship was recognized between exposure to high levels of cadmium in the workplace and impaired health of cadmium workers in the metal smelting industry (FRIBERG 1948, 1950). This association was supported by previous experimental and postmortem observations (FRANT and KLEEMAN 1941; PRODAN 1932; STEPHENS 1920–1921; WILSON et al. 1941). The public health concern regarding this relationship stimulated further experimental animal and epidemiologic studies before 1970, interested in defining the toxicologic properties of cadmium in living systems and the potential impact of cadmium exposure on human health (CLEGG and CARR 1967; DECKER et al. 1958; DOTTA and FRUSCELLA 1963; GABBIANI et al. 1967; GUNN et al. 1963; HILL et al. 1963; KENNEDY 1966; KLEINFELD et al. 1966; KLEINFELD and STEIN 1968; PERRY et al. 1961; PERRY and YUNICE 1965; SCHROEDER 1964, 1965; SCHROEDER and BALASSA 1961; SCHROEDER and PERRY 1955; SCHROEDER and VINTON 1962; SKOG and WAHLBERG 1964; TIPTON et al. 1965; WAITES and SETCHELL 1966; WEBER and REID 1969). The propensity for cadmium to accumulate in renal tissue as a function of age and intensity of exposure, combined with demonstrations of impaired renal function in cadmium-exposed workers, focused attention initially on renal actions and related health effects (FRIBERG 1948, 1950; FRIBERG et al. 1974; PERRY et al. 1961). Since cadmium-exposed workers generally were not found to exhibit increased symptoms of cardiovascular damage (FRIBERG 1950), early in vitro and experimental animal findings demonstrating effects on cardiovascular tissues were questioned in terms of their relevance to human health effects (FRIBERG et al. 1974).

Two concepts, one hypothetical and the other experimental, were introduced at this time which fostered a renewed and sustained interest in the cardiovascular actions of cadmium. Initially, a suggestion was made that long-term consumption of infinitesimal amounts of hazardous chemicals (e.g., cadmium) could induce latent, adverse health effects in humans and other living systems (FORBES et al. 1954; SCHROEDER 1956, 1960). This premise was inferred from the then existing literature rather than supported by experimental evidence. Later findings have provided support for this concept (KOPP et al. 1980a–d, 1982, 1983; OHANIAN et al. 1978; OHANIAN and IWAI 1980; PERRY and ERLANGER 1973, 1978, 1980, 1981, 1982; PERRY et al. 1977, 1979, 1980a, b; PERRY and KOPP 1983; REVIS et al. 1981; SCHROEDER and VINTON 1962; SCHROEDER 1964, 1965, 1974). In addition, the unique metal chelation properties of certain antihypertensive drugs (e.g., hydralazine) were recognized at this time (SCHROEDER 1956; SCHROEDER and PERRY 1955), which led to the parallel suggestion that a trace metal might participate in the etiology of essential hypertension in humans. Subsequent studies contributed experimental evidence implicating cadmium as an etiologic factor in hypertension (PERRY et al. 1961; SCHROEDER and PERRY 1955; SCHROEDER and VINTON 1962; SCHROEDER 1964, 1965; SCHROEDER et al. 1970). When considered together, these concepts provided the rationale for suggesting that chronic, subacute cadmium exposure may induce age-dependent and dose-dependent cardiovascular effects. Henceforth, research concerned with the cardiovascular actions of cadmium has focused on two, often divergent issues: overt (acute) and latent (subacute) cadmium toxicity.

Investigations concerned with identifying the toxicologic basis for the deleterious health effects of occupational cadmium exposure have concentrated on the acute actions of cadmium at dosage levels comparable to or greater than those encountered in the industrial workplace (CLEGG and CARR 1967; DUDLEY et al. 1982; FAEDER et al. 1977; FOWLER et al. 1975; GABBIANI et al. 1967; GHAFGHAZI and MENNEAR 1973; GUNN et al. 1963, 1966; HALL and HUNGERFORD 1982; HAYES et al. 1976; HRDINA et al. 1976; ITHAKISSIOS et al. 1974a, b; KOPP and HAWLEY 1978; KOTSONIS and KLAASSEN 1977, 1978; LEVIN and MILLER 1981; NATHANSON and BLOOM 1976; PAŘÍŽEK 1957; PERRY et al. 1970; PERRY and YUNICE 1965; POPHAM and WEBSTER 1976; ROACH and DAMUDE 1980; ROHRER et al. 1978; SAKSENA et al. 1977; SINGHAL 1981; SINGHAL et al. 1976; SUZUKI 1980; WAITES and SETCHELL 1966; WATKINS 1980). Testicular necrosis was recognized early as a toxic manifestation of acute cadmium intoxication in experimental animals (PAŘÍŽEK and ZÁHOŘ 1956; PAŘÍŽEK 1957). Subsequent studies appear to have provided rather convincing evidence which suggests that the pathogenic basis for the action of cadmium on the testes is linked to its augmentation of capillary permeability and depression of testicular blood flow (CLEGG and CARR 1967; GUNN et al. 1963, 1966; WAITES and SETCHELL 1966). These studies are discussed in detail later in the chapter (Sect. D.II.3). Similar effects of cadmium on blood flow to other organs have been demonstrated, as well. Overall, these toxicologic investigations indicate that cadmium alters the functional integrity of vascular tissues in various organs, causing effects which are persistent and which initiate secondary degenerative changes in tissues related to a critical reduction in organ blood flow.

The prospect that latent or subacute functional changes could occur in the cardiovascular system in response to chronic cadmium exposure was neither suspected nor considered seriously until the mid-1950s (FORBES et al. 1954; SCHROEDER 1956). The suggestion that a trace metal might be involved as a causative factor in essential hypertension (SCHROEDER and PERRY 1955; SCHROEDER 1956) led to systematic postmortem studies of human tissues to determine whether the absence or presence of particular trace metals in certain organs could be related to a higher incidence of cardiovascular disease or mortality (PERRY et al. 1961; SCHROEDER 1965; TIPTON et al. 1965). Cadmium became a likely candidate for this role when: (a) remarkably high cadmium concentrations were detected in human kidneys that varied markedly as a function of age and geographic origin (PERRY et al. 1961; TIPTON et al. 1965); (b) retrospective evidence was reported which demonstrated a positive correlation between human hypertension and elevated renal cadmium levels (SCHROEDER 1965); and (c) low levels of dietary cadmium were shown to induce hypertension in rats (SCHROEDER and VINTON 1962; SCHROEDER 1964; SCHROEDER et al. 1966). Subsequent epidemiologic and clinical studies have provided conflicting results concerning the relationship between the incidence of human hypertension and cardiovascular mortality and lifelong cadmium exposure (ADAMSKA-DYNIEWSKA et al. 1980a, b; AVTANDILOV 1967; BEEVERS et al. 1980; BOEHME et al. 1979; BORHANI 1981; CARROLL 1966; CUMMINS et al. 1980; DALLY et al. 1979; FRIBERG 1950; HAMMER et al. 1971; HUEL et al. 1981; KHERA et al. 1980; MOSES 1979; ØSTERGAARD 1978; PERRY and KOPP 1983; PERRY et al. 1980b; PONTEVA et al. 1979; PRIBILLA et al. 1980; PRIBILLA and SCHULTEK 1979; PUNSAR et al. 1975; REVIS and ZINSMEISTER 1981; SCHROEDER 1966, 1967, 1974; SHAPER 1979; SHARRETT 1979; TULLY and LEHMANN 1982; VOORS et al. 1982; VOORS and SHUMAN 1977; VOROBIEVA and EREMEEVA 1980; VUORI et al. 1979; WHANGER 1979). Early epidemiologic evidence led to the assertion that cadmium might be the "water factor" responsible for the high incidence of cardiovascular mortality in soft water areas (BIERENBAUM et al. 1975; LENER and BIBR 1971; SCHROEDER 1960, 1966, 1967). Later studies have failed to provide convincing support for this hypothesis (for reviews see FOLSOM and PRINEAS 1982; NERI and JOHANSEN 1978; ROSENMAN 1979; SHARRETT 1979). Instead, magnesium and calcium have moved to the forefront as potential "water factors" (ANDERSON et al. 1969, 1975; CHIPPERFIELD and CHIPPERFIELD 1978; CRAWFORD et al. 1968; ELWOOD et al. 1974; ISERI et al. 1975; MARIER 1978; SHARRETT and FEINLEIB 1975a, b). Although cadmium is not generally considered to be of major importance in the "water factor controversy," convincing evidence exists which indicates that cadmium does cause deleterious effects on the mammalian cardiovascular system at relatively low exposure levels (BOSCOLO et al. 1980; FADLOUN and LEACH 1981; FOWLER et al. 1975; KANISAWA and SCHROEDER 1969; KOPP et al. 1978c, 1980a–d, 1982, 1983a, b; REVIS 1978; REVIS et al. 1981, 1983). The role of cadmium as a factor in human hypertension and its ability to produce hypertension in experimental animals remains unresolved. Indeed, the hypertension controversy has actually hindered the evaluation of other cadmium-induced cardiovascular effects and obscured the significance of recent findings.

Current scientific information about the cardiovascular effects of cadmium are described and summarized in this chapter, including those areas of knowledge that remain controversial or inadequate. Divergent points of view in this field of research are presented and compared, to the extent considered practical without introducing unsubstantiated speculation. Many of the articles which comprise the literature material referred to in this chapter have not been cited or discussed in previous reviews of this subject. Generally, the organizational hierarchy of each of the subsequent sections of this chapter is based on the chronology of the published literature concerned with the subject matter presented. Although somewhat arbitrary, this approach proved advantageous for two reasons: (a) it provided a means for presenting the historical foundations and the progression of scientific knowlege in this field of research; and (b) it avoided judgment of the subject matter based on subjective assessments of the relative importance of individual topics. It is hoped that through this overall approach a more complete perspective can be obtained concerning the cardiovascular actions of cadmium.

C. Actions of Cadmium on the Myocardium

Generally, in vitro tissue incubation and isolated heart perfusion techniques have been adopted to investigate the direct actions of cadmium on the myocardium under controlled conditions. This approach has facilitated not only a comprehensive evaluation of cadmium's effects on myocardial excitability, contractility, and metabolism, but has also enabled an examination of other dependent variables that contribute to, or antagonize the toxicity of cadmium in the heart. Studies of this nature have demonstrated that at relatively low concentrations, cadmium causes significant, dose-dependent changes in myocardial function and energy metabolism, which rapidly become irreversible, unless control conditions are restored. Cadmium appears to act primarily through a mechanism involving a competitive antagonism with calcium. In this regard, cadmium has been shown to attenuate the slow inward calcium current during diastolic depolarization through an inhibition of sarcolemmal calcium channels (LEE and TSIEN 1982; TROSPER and PHILIPSON 1983). Chronic cadmium exposure in vivo in experimental animals, again at comparatively low exposure levels, has been shown more recently to elicit many of the same types of responses as those observed in isolated heart preparations; however, the overall magnitude of these changes often is less pronounced (KOPP et al. 1983a, b). These cardiotoxic characteristics ascribed to cadmium, which have been based on experimental animal studies, are similar qualitatively to the cardiovascular functional changes which have been described in humans exposed to cadmium oxide in the workplace (VOROBIEVA and EREMEEVA 1980). Thus, evidence exists to indicate that the human myocardium, like that of other animal species, is susceptible to the toxic actions of cadmium. Moreover, the pathophysiologic and metabolic alterations induced experimentally in animal models, as described later, may be more typical than not of the responses which may be anticipated following chronic human exposure to cadmium.

I. Actions of Cadmium Affecting Myocardial Inotropism

1. Introduction

The ability of cadmium to disrupt the rhythmicity and contractile strength of the myocardium was demonstrated (ATHANASIU and LANGLOIS 1895, 1896; PANSERI 1904; RICHET 1882) long before the vascular actions of cadmium were recognized (FOWLER et al. 1975; GUNN et al. 1963; KANISAWA and SCHROEDER 1969; PAŘÍŽEK 1960; PERRY et al. 1967a, b; THIND et al. 1970a; TODA 1973c). These early studies were reported during the same era that RINGER's (1883a, b) classical experiments were published, in which he identified the dependence of cardiac muscle contraction on external calcium. This historical coincidence might be dismissed as anecdotal, if it were not for the fact that a century later cadmium would be recognized as a potent antagonist of calcium-mediated cellular events in the heart. In this context, cadmium has been shown to induce physiologic responses which generally have paralleled those observed by RINGER (1883b) under conditions when calcium was omitted from the supporting medium. The virtually simultaneous publication and the methodological parallelism which exists between these reports suggests that these investigators (Athanasiu, Langlois, Richet, and Ringer) shared a common interest regarding the influence of inorganic cations on myocardial function. Although certain similarities do exist between these studies, the underlying objectives which encouraged these scientists to undertake these experiments appear to have been different. As clearly stated in his articles, Ringer was concerned with identifying the inorganic and organic factors contained in the blood which were required to sustain heart contractile activity. In contrast, Richet and Athanasiu and Langlois were motivated by an interest in the toxicologic, rather than physiologic, properties of various metal salts and their comparative toxicity, as determined by their ability to disrupt myocardial mechanical events.

These early experiments, which were conducted in the hearts of frog (ATHANASIU and LANGLOIS 1896; RICHET 1882; RINGER 1883a, b), tortoise (ATHANASIU and LANGLOIS 1896), and dog (ATHANASIU and LANGLOIS 1896) provided the first definitive experimental evidence demonstrating that myocardial function was directly influenced by external cations, and that these effects varied according to the metal ion involved. Cadmium, as shown by certain of these early investigators, proved to be a remarkably potent inhibitor of the physiologic activity of the heart. Subsequent studies have confirmed and extended these initial observations to include more quantitative appraisals of the action of cadmium on the myocardium and the mechanistic basis for these effects. Indeed, the depressant actions of cadmium on myocardial function have been described in hearts of vertebrate animals representing the avian (MARSH 1976; PADERI 1896; STURKIE 1973), reptilian (ATHANASIU and LANGLOIS 1896), amphibian (ATHANASIU and LANGLOIS 1895, 1896; HORIUCHI and HAYASHI 1979; KLEINFELD et al. 1955; PADERI 1896; PANSERI 1904; RICHET 1882; SALANT and CONNET 1920), osteichthyan (teleost) (PANSERI 1904); and mammalian taxons (ATHANASIU and LANGLOIS 1896; BERS and LANGER 1979; DOTTA and FRUSCELLA 1963; HAWLEY and KOPP 1975; KLEINFELD et al. 1966; KLEINFELD and STEIN 1968; KOPP and HAWLEY 1976, 1978; KOPP et al. 1978a, b; KOPP and BÁRÁNY 1979, 1980; LANGER et al. 1974; PILATI et al. 1982; TODA 1973b, c). The consistency of the reported experimental findings concerning the action of cadmium on the heart suggests that the vertebrate heart responds to appropriate cadmium concentrations in a manner which is similar, irrespective of phylogenetic considerations.

2. Early Studies

RICHET (1882) was among the first toxicologists to observe that the addition of neutral chloride salts of various metals to the external surface of the heart resulted in profound changes in myocardial rhythmicity and contractile vigor. These experiments performed on the frog heart in situ depended on uptake and diffusion of the test metals which were applied dropwise (four drops at 15-min intervals) to the epicardial surface of the heart. The effective dose was shown to vary for each metal tested. The physiologic responses, which were determined by observational criteria, provided an objective basis for comparing the toxicologic properties of these metals based on their ability to induce complete systolic (e.g., calcium, barium, strontium) or diastolic (e.g., magnesium, potassium, cobalt) arrest of the heart within a 2-h experimental period. Using this semiquantitative comparison, cadmium was shown to be the most cardiotoxic metal tested. Reportedly, myocardial arrest was induced by epicardial administration of cadmium at a concentration of 2×10^{-3} M. Contractile activity ceased at a point in the cardiac cycle intermediate between systole and diastole. Clearly, diffusion distances and diffusion rate are major determinants in an experiment such as this. These diffusion considerations affect the rate of the response and the magnitude of the response. As is readily apparent throughout, the dose–effect relationships for cadmium can vary substantially, depending upon the tissue preparation used to study the effect.

Intraperitoneal (or lymph sac) injection of cadmium (3×10^{-3} mol $CdSO_4$ per kilogram body weight) in the frog was shown later (ATHANASIU and LANGLOIS 1896) to cause a marked diminution in the amplitude of the myocardial contractions during peak systole, and a slowing in the periodicity of these weakened contractions. An alternating 3–4–3 contraction rhythm was commonly associated with the cadmium treatment. A diastolic pause equal to the time of one contraction cycle was observed in the repeating periods which had fewer contractions. These effects on the strength and periodicity of myocardial contractions in the frog were consistent with those subsequently observed in the tortoise heart. The arrhythmic pattern suggests a second-degree heart block, which, as will be described in a following section, can be induced by acute cadmium exposure.

A single intravenous bolus injection of cadmium (2×10^{-5} mol $CdSO_4$) into the jugular vein of the tortoise caused a progressive reduction in the vigor of the myocardial contractions during a 3-min period after the cadmium had been administered. The initial negative inotropic interval was followed by a restoration of contractile force and an acceleration in rate which surpassed that observed prior to the cadmium injection. Repeated intravenous cadmium injections abolished this overshoot recovery response. Although this latter phenomenon was first described by ATHANASIU and LANGLOIS (1896), their observations have essentially gone unnoticed by subsequent investigators. The pattern of this secondary recovery phase, as described by these authors, is remarkably similar to the time-dependent hypotensive–hypertensive rebound response in systolic blood pressure that was reported many years later following intravenous cadmium administration (FADLOUN and LEACH 1981; PERRY and YUNICE 1965; PERRY et al. 1970). The mechanistic basis for the secondary rebound phase of the response to intravenous cadmium infusion remains undefined. Presumably, the initial cardiodepression represents the direct action of cadmium on the heart, while the recovery and overshoot phenomena may represent responses mediated by central or peripheral neural and/or hormonal factors.

Cadmium exposure caused a generalized cardiodepressive reaction in the turtle heart, both in situ and when isolated from the body. This observation demonstrated that the in vivo response of the heart to cadmium was direct and not mediated through any secondary toxic factor or neural influence. These treated hearts maintained their chronotropic responsiveness to increases in surface temperature. This finding suggests that the temperature sensitivity of the spontaneous cardiac pacemaker cells was not influenced by the exposure to cadmium.

Isolated heart experiments similar to those performed with the turtle heart were conducted by SALANT and CONNET (1920) using the perfused frog heart. Their observations provided supportive evidence attesting to the marked cardiotoxicity displayed by cadmium as compared with other potentially toxic metal ions. These experiments assessed the actions of various heavy metals on the contractile activity of the perfused frog heart and demonstrated that a significant decline in the strength of contraction was induced by 5×10^{-6} M Cd $(CH_3COO)_2$. A tenfold increase in the perfusate cadmium concentration caused virtual contractile paralysis, intermediate between systole and diastole. This condition was partially reversible by control reperfusion, but was irreversible when the perfusate cadmium concentration was increased above this level (5×10^{-5} M Cd^{2+}). This report by SALANT and CONNET (1920) provided a qualitative account of the depressant effects of cadmium on the amphibian heart. Their findings were entirely compatible with those reported earlier by ATHANASIU and LANGLOIS (1896). Thereafter, between the years 1920 and 1955, research characterizing the actions of cadmium on the heart appears to have ceased. It is possible that the remarkable consistency of these early findings created a certain scientific complacency about the need for further studies concerning the cardiotoxic properties of cadmium.

3. Isolated Perfused Heart Studies

A 35-five year hiatus intervened before KLEINFELD et al. (1955) ushered in the contemporary era of scientific inquiry into the actions of cadmium on the myocardium. As is readily apparent in the sections that follow, the breadth of interest in the cardiotoxic properties of cadmium since Kleinfeld's work has extended beyond the qualitative accounts of the past. The original studies of the late nineteenth and early twentieth centuries provided the original impetus for pursuing this problem by describing the overt effects, but the more recent studies have addressed the subtler effects of cadmium on the heart and provided the experimental facts needed to begin to explain the mechanistic basis for the cardiotoxic actions of cadmium. This refinement in understanding has been made possible by the trend toward incorporating more sophisticated techniques and instrumentation in experimental designs used to investigate the responses of the myocardium to cadmium. This latter aspect reflects the increasingly more complex technologic resources available to modern laboratory scientists. Generally, the result has been that a broader perspective of the problem has been obtained which includes recognition of probable intracellular sites of action and putative cellular mechanisms which define the basis for the actions of cadmium on the myocardium.

The studies conducted in 1955 by KLEINFELD et al. provided actual quantitative interpretations regarding the action of cadmium on the frog heart which confirmed the observations reported in earlier studies (ATHANASIU and LANGLOIS 1896; RICHET 1882; SALANT and CONNET 1920). Perfusion of the isolated frog heart with the cadmium-containing buffer ($5 \times 10^{-5} M$ $CdCl_2$) resulted in a progressive time-dependent decline in mechanical activity, which culminated in complete ventricular arrest in diastole. The sequence of changes generally followed a reproducible pattern. Ventricular dilation was evident after 4 min perfusion with cadmium, and cardiac output was decreased at this time. Cardiac output was decreased further at 6 min (below 50% of the control value). Between 8 and 10 min, the cardiac output was less than 25% of control and continued to decrease to zero after 10 min perfusion, concomitant with diastolic arrest of the ventricles. A noteworthy point regarding the changes in cardiac output induced by cadmium was that heart rate was constant during this interval. Thus, the conclusion was reached that cadmium reduced the cardiac output by decreasing the stroke volume. Qualitatively similar findings were obtained from parallel injection studies (1.4 and 2.8×10^{-5} mol $CdCl_2$ per kilogram) performed in situ in the frog.

KOPP et al. (1978 a, b) were the first investigators to describe the dose-dependent negative inotropic actions of cadmium in the intact mammalian heart (rat). These studies demonstrated that the mammalian heart is as sensitive to the actions of cadmium (based on the rate of onset of the negative inotropic response) as the amphibian and reptilian heart. A dose–effect relationship was defined which indicated that 3×10^{-5} and $3 \times 10^{-6} M$ $CdCl_2$ both produced significant changes in myocardial mechanical activity, but that a cadmium concentration of $3 \times 10^{-8} M$ ($CdCl_2$) was without significant effect. Subsequent investigations (KOPP and BÁRÁNY 1980) were directed toward elucidating the extent to which this cadmium-induced negative inotropism could be prevented by the addition of known positive inotropic agents. The cardiodepressive actions of cadmium ($6 \times 10^{-6} M$ $CdCl_2$) were partially counteracted by the administration of either 6.5 mM $CaCl_2$ or $7 \times 10^{-7} M$ isoproterenol together with the cadmium. Although these agents partially restored myocardial contractile strength in the presence of cadmium, it should be noted that the normal positive inotropic activation of the heart which accompanied administration of these agents to the heart was abolished by cadmium. The addition of cadmium ($6 \times 10^{-6} M$ $CdCl_2$) to the perfusate containing 6.5 mM $CaCl_2$ reduced the amplitude of the contractile tension generated by the heart to 55% of the response induced by the high calcium alone. Similarly, cadmium added to the isoproterenol-containing perfusate attenuated the positive inotropic, but not the chronotropic reaction to isoproterenol, resulting in a mechanical response that was only 47% of that induced by isoproterenol alone.

a) Calcium Dependence

The parallelism between the actions of cadmium on myocardial inotropism and the known effects of low extracellular calcium, combined with the demonstration that increasing the extracellular calcium concentration could attenuate the magnitude of the effect of cadmium, led to the hypothesis that cadmium may act to depress myocardial contractility through a cellular mechanism involving a competition with calcium. Until recently, this hypothesis had not been examined experimentally in the intact heart. PRENTICE (1982) and PRENTICE et al. (1984) have demonstrated that varying the extracellular calcium concentration (0.9–5.0 mM $CaCl_2$) at a fixed perfusate cadmium concentration ($3 \times 10^{-6} M CdCl_2$) produces a negative inotropic response in the isolated perfused rat heart that varies inversely as a function of the perfusate calcium concentration. The curve which defines the rate of myocardial tension development as a function of the extracellular calcium concentration was shifted downward and to the right in response to cadmium ($3 \times 10^{-6} M CdCl_2$). This calcium dose–response curve was essentially parallel to the one obtained under control conditions, indicating that the interaction between cadmium and calcium in the intact perfused heart was primarily one of competitive antagonism.

b) Metabolic Consequences

The recognition of the negative inotropic effects of cadmium in the perfused mammalian heart has led to further studies concerned with identifying biochemical processes which might be involved in this pathophysiologic response to cadmium. Several molecular control mechanisms have been proposed as contributing factors involved in the regulation of chemical–mechanical energy transduction in heart muscle. These mechanisms generally are mediated through various calcium-dependent protein phosphorylation–dephosphorylation reactions which include: phospholamban, sarcolemmal membrane proteins, and the myofibrillar proteins – the inhibitory subunit of troponin (TN-I) and the myosin light chain-2 (LC-2) (BÁRÁNY et al. 1981; KOPP and BÁRÁNY 1979, 1980; WALSH et al. 1980). The effects of cadmium on the phosphorylation–dephosphorylation-dependent activity of these putative regulatory phosphoproteins have been examined only in relation to changes in myofibrillar protein phosphorylation. The phosphorylation of the myosin LC-2 subunit has been shown to be calcium dependent (KOPP and BÁRÁNY 1979). These studies revealed that the negative inotropy induced by $3 \times 10^{-6} M CdCl_2$ was associated with a significantly decreased phosphorylation of the myosin LC-2. The magnitude of this depressed myosin LC-2 phosphorylation was proportional to the amplitude of the negative inotropic response. Moreover, subjecting the heart to positive inotropic agents (6.5 mM $CaCl_2$ or $7 \times 10^{-7} M$ isoproterenol) in conjunction with this cadmium dose resulted in a complete inhibition (calcium) or attenuation (isoproterenol) of the increased TN-I phosphorylation that normally accompanied the positive inotropic response to these agents (KOPP and BÁRÁNY 1979). The relative phosphorylation of the myosin LC-2 under these conditions was comparable to the untreated controls, but was markedly diminished as compared with the levels detected in hearts treated with only the positive inotropic agents. Overall, the observed relationship between the contractile activity of the hearts treated with cadmium and the action of cadmium on the phosphorylation of purported regulatory myofibrillar phosphoproteins suggests that cadmium interferes with the regulation of cardiac muscle contraction through a mechanism involving these phosphorylation reactions. The fact that these biochemical regulatory processes respond to extracellular calcium and are either activated by calcium (TN-I) or dependent on calcium (myosin LC-2) provides further support for the hypothesis that cadmium acts in heart muscle primarily through a mechanism linked to its antagonism with cellular calcium.

Clearly, these findings suggest an enzymatic site of action (e.g., myosin light chain kinase) for cadmium; however, this interpretation must be tempered somewhat owing to the demonstration that cadmium also disturbs cellular high energy phosphate metabolism (adenosine triphosphate ATP; phosphocreatine PCr) (PRENTICE 1982; PRENTICE et al. 1984). Hearts perfused with $3 \times 10^{-6} M$ CdCl$_2$ were characterized by reduced high energy phosphate (ATP and PCr) levels and a corresponding accumulation of low energy phosphates (adenosine diphosphate ADP; inorganic phosphate Pi, and inosine monophosphate IMP), that varied in intensity as an inverse function of the perfusate calcium concentration. In conjunction with the effects of cadmium on myocardial energy stores, a secondary accumulation of glycolytic intermediates (e.g., glucose 1-phosphate, glucose 6-phosphate) was observed, as well. These metabolic findings suggest that cadmium interferes with substrate utilization by glycolytic and oxidative pathways of the cell, thereby creating a lower energy state within the myocardial cell. This condition may influence the ability of the cells to maintain phosphorylation-dependent reactions, such as that involved in the myofibrillar protein phosphorylation reactions.

Although cadmium has been shown to influence myocardial energy metabolism in the isolated perfused heart, an additional effect involving myocardial phosphoglyceride metabolism has been deduced as well from the metabolite analyses. This finding may have comparable significance to the effects noted on energy metabolism. These hearts characteristically had elevated glycercol 3-phosphate (G3-P) levels and a decreased glycerol 3-phosphorylcholine (GPC) content, as compared with identically treated controls (Fig. 1). As shown, this effect was calcium dependent. Since the phosphocholine content of these cadmium-treated hearts was not affected significantly by cadmium, the effects on the phosphoglyceride derivatives, GPC and G3-P, cannot be attributed to an increased catabolism of GPC. Instead, these findings are in accordance with the hypothesis that these changes represent a partial inhibition of phosphatidylcholine biosynthesis induced by cadmium. Since increasing the perfusate calcium concentration partially reversed this action of cadmium in the perfused heart, a likely enzymatic site of action for cadmium would be the calcium-regulated enzyme, choline phosphotransferase (Fig. 2; ROSSITER and STRICKLAND 1970).

Disturbances in myocardial phosphoglyceride metabolism induced by cadmium may provide a mechanistic basis for understanding the effect of cadmium on the heart and the changes induced by cadmium in the sensitivity and responsiveness of the myocardium to external calcium. Phosphatidylcholine is a major constituent of the sarcolemmal membrane. Presumably, an inhibition in the for-

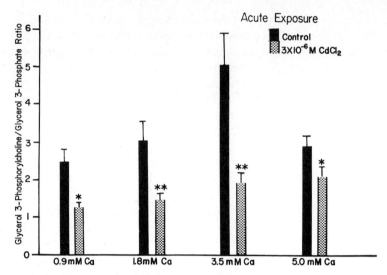

Fig. 1. Dose–response relationship between perfusate calcium concentration and the ratio of glycerol 3-phosphorylcholine (phosphatidylcholine degradation product) to glycerol 3-phosphate (phosphatidylcholine precursor) in the isolated perfused rat heart following 60 min perfusion with or without cadmium (3×10^{-6} M CdCl$_2$). *Asterisks* denote changes significantly different relative to the corresponding control (* $P < 0.05$; ** $P < 0.01$)

mation of this phosphoglyceride would alter the structural and functional characteristics of the cardiac cell membrane (CORR et al. 1981; ROSSITER and STRICKLAND 1970), conceivably leading to: (a) unbalanced calcium influx and extrusion rates; (b) altered bioelectrical and biophysical properties of the membrane which would influence cardiac cell excitability and contractility; and (c) modified receptor site sensitivity which may modify the inotropic responsiveness of the myocardium to adrenergic stimulation. This hypothetical concept is elaborated upon and the proposed sites of action of cadmium are illustrated schematically in Sect. C.I.7.

4. In Vitro Heart Tissue Studies

Generally, papillary muscle, atrial muscle strip, and cardiac cell culture preparations have been utilized, in addition to the perfused heart, to evaluate and characterize the actions of cadmium under a variety of externally controlled conditions. Although these methodological approaches have certain advantages, diffusion distances, which are defined by the cross-sectional diameter of the tissue, and surface diffusion rates are limiting factors that may affect the apparent sensitivity or response rate of these preparations to cadmium. Generally, these considerations are more pertinent to the papillary muscle preparation than for instance, a monolayer of cultured heart cells. Although the concentrations of cadmium required to yield an effect are often greater when diffusion distances are increased, the qualitative interpretations derived from such studies have proven to be consistent with those obtained by other methods. This consistency attests to the va-

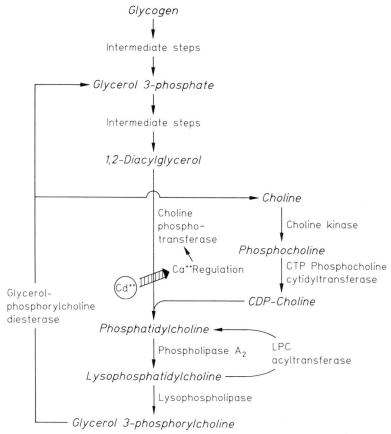

Fig. 2. Simplified schema depicting the biosynthetic and degradation pathway for conversion of glycerol 3-phosphate→phosphatidylcholine→glycerol 3-phosphorylcholine (GPC). The postulated inhibitory site of cadmium (Cd^{2+}) is indicated with the large *hatched arrow*. The proposed site of action has been inferred from indirect evidence (accumulation of glycerol 3-phosphate and decreased GPC content). Apparent activation of this pathway by calcium is shown in Fig. 1. The regulation of choline phosphotransferase by calcium has been reported elsewhere (ROSSITER and STRICKLAND 1970). The known antagonism of cadmium for calcium binding sites suggests that cadmium either directly (actual binding to the enzyme active site), or indirectly (hindrance of calcium activation, i.e., effects on intracellular Ca^{2+} levels) affects the activity of this enzyme. Since the effects of cadmium on this enzyme have not been measured directly, this proposed site of action should be considered tentative

lidity of the interpretations derived from the experimental findings obtained by these approaches. Thus, the reported findings of these studies are presented with emphasis placed on the conceptual aspects and similarities, rather than on absolute quantitative comparisons.

a) Contractile Responses and Calcium Dependence

The initial studies performed by KLEINFELD et al. (1955), which further characterized and confirmed the negative inotropic actions of cadmium using the isolated perfused frog heart, were not pursued using a mammalian heart model until more than a decade later (KLEINFELD and STEIN 1968). Treatment of isolated superfused rat atria at 23 °C with a Tyrode buffer containing 4.5×10^{-5} M $CdCl_2$ caused a significant decrease in the isometric tension generated in response to electrical stimulation. This decline in contractility was apparent within 2 min after the cadmium was administered to the tissue. Within 4–28 min thereafter, the negative inotropic response reached a maximal level, plateauing at a value approaching 10% of the original control tension. Intervention with Tyrode buffer containing twice the calcium concentration (3.6 mM $CaCl_2$) at the point when contractile tension had diminished to 50%–30% of control, resulted in a restoration of contractile tension that approached the control state.

Similar observations were made by TODA (1973 b) in studies conducted on isolated rabbit atrial muscle. The experimental conditions to which these atrial preparations were subjected differed somewhat from those employed by KLEINFELD and STEIN (1968). These isolated atrial preparations were superfused at 30 °C with a physiologic salt solution containing 2.2 mM $CaCl_2$. Moreover, the actions of cadmium were evaluated only after a 30-min equilibration period with the cadmium-containing medium (5×10^{-6}–10^{-4} M $CdCl_2$). Cadmium caused a dose-dependent decrease in the peak isometric tension response to electrical stimulation. Within the effective range of cadmium concentrations (2×10^{-5}–10^{-4} M $CdCl_2$), a negative inotropic effect was manifested within 3 min and progressively increased thereafter, reaching a maximal negative inotropic response within 30 min.

Further characterization of this effect revealed that the force–frequency relationship between peak contractile tension and stimulation frequency of these cadmium-treated cardiac muscle preparations was altered significantly. Varying the stimulation frequency over the range of 30–240 beats/min in atria exposed to 2×10^{-5} M $CdCl_2$ amplified the negative inotropy induced by cadmium. The more pronounced attenuation in peak isometric tension at high stimulation frequencies as compared with lower stimulation rates (below 12 beats/min) suggests that cadmium alters the intrinsic contractile properties of cardiac muscle (e.g., effective refractory period may be prolonged). At the highest cadmium concentration studied (10^{-4} M $CdCl_2$), the force–frequency relationship was abolished completely, with the contractile force remaining essentially constant, though markedly diminished, at all stimulation frequencies. Cysteine (1 mM), glutathione (1 mM), and calcium (4.4 mM) were shown to partially antagonize the negative inotropic actions of cadmium and its effects on the force–frequency curve. At a cadmium concentration of $2 \times 10^{-5} M$, calcium was more effective than cysteine in restoring the contractile responsiveness of the treated atrial preparations to electrical stimulation; however, this situation was reversed at the higher cadmium concentration.

Parallel studies performed on feline papillary muscles have demonstrated that cadmium not only depresses isometric tension development, but also decreases the maximal rate of tension development and slows the maximal rate of relaxation (PILATI et al. 1982). These effects of cadmium were concentration dependent throughout the range of 10^{-6}–10^{-4} M $CdCl_2$. Restoration of control conditions resulted in a complete reversal of the cadmium effect in muscles exposed to

10^{-6} M Cd^{2+}; however, at higher cadmium concentrations this reversal was incomplete. Increasing the extracellular calcium concentration from 2 mM to 5–6 mM (CaCl$_2$) resulted in a restoration in peak tension development to pre-cadmium control levels. Despite this reversal of the cadmium-induced negative inotropy by calcium, the contraction pattern of these muscles remained abnormal. The authors suggest that this latter characteristic may represent a noncompetitive action of cadmium.

In addition to the demonstrations that the actions of cadmium are calcium sensitive, Horiuchi and Hayashi (1979) have shown that the negative inotropic actions of cadmium are also pH sensitive. Using isolated frog atrial muscle, the pH of the supporting buffer was varied from 7.2 to 10 and contractility was evaluated in the presence or absence of cadmium (1.3×10^{-5} M Cd). The negative inotropism induced by a fixed cadmium concentration was found to be inversely related to the extracellular pH. Although the contractile effects of cadmium were diminished at more alkaline pH, these effects remained dose and calcium dependent. At the higher pH values, the ionization of cadmium may be significantly decreased. This chemical property was not considered by the authors, and therefore cannot be ignored as a factor contributing to the reduced biologic responsiveness of these preparations to cadmium under alkaline conditions.

b) Role of Calcium

Although intracellular sites of action cannot be discounted, the characteristics of the observations described suggest that superficial calcium binding sites are involved in the cardiodepressive action of cadmium. Indeed, Langer et al. (1974) have demonstrated that the ability of cadmium to diminish contractile tension of cardiac cells in tissue culture correlates well with its ability to displace calcium from superficial membrane binding sites, and thereby to inhibit further transmembrane calcium influx. These rapidly exchangeable stores of calcium associated with the basement membrane are of crucial importance in the maintenance of excitation–contraction coupling in heart cells. These results indicate that the degree of negative inotropy induced by cadmium depends to a considerable degree on the extent to which it competes with and displaces calcium from these rapidly exchangeable cellular binding sites. Moreover, when jointly considered with the evidence which demonstrates that the effect of cadmium on cardiac contractile function is antagonized by increasing the extracellular calcium concentration (Horiuchi and Hayashi 1979; Kleinfeld and Stein 1968; Kopp and Bárány 1980; Kopp et al. 1980c; Pilati et al. 1982; Prentice 1982; Prentice et al. 1984; Toda 1973b), these findings suggest a unifying mechanistic concept for the action of cadmium on cardiac muscle contraction. This postulated mechanism of action asserts that cadmium competes antagonistically with calcium for membrane calcium binding sites. By displacing calcium from these sites, the slow inward flux (rate and magnitude) of calcium that occurs during the initial phases of excitation–contraction coupling is attenuated, which leads to a diminished contractile response. This latter effect is analogous to the functional response of the myocardium to decremental changes in the extracellular concentration of ionized calcium.

The studies by LANGER and co-workers (BERS and LANGER 1979; LANGER et al. 1974) have demonstrated that membrane-bound calcium levels are significantly decreased following cadmium treatment. As stated, this action of cadmium on membrane-bound calcium presumably would alter the rate and magnitude of inward calcium current during excitation. Recently, TROSPER and PHILIPSON (1983) have contributed experimental evidence that supports and extends this hypothetical concept. Using purified canine cardiac sarcolemmal vesicles, these investigators demonstrated that cadmium inhibits membrane sodium–calcium exchange processes. This inhibition of the calcium influx across the sarcolemmal membrane was concentration dependent within the range examined (10^{-6}–10^{-3} M Cd^{2+}). Reciprocally, cadmium was also shown to stimulate calcium efflux from calcium-loaded vesicles, possibly through a cadmium–calcium exchange mechanism. The relative effectiveness of cadmium in this regard, as compared with other divalent metal ions, was shown to be related to the similarity between the crystal ionic radii of cadmium (0.97 Å) and calcium (0.99 Å). Unfortunately, cadmium uptake by these vesicles was not measured.

Although cadmium uptake was undetermined, certain inferences can be made from the reported findings. Unlike other studies in which the relative concentration of calcium to cadmium in the experimental supporting medium may differ by a factor of 10^3 or 10^4, the action of cadmium on calcium uptake and efflux by these vesicles was examined under conditions in which the ratio of calcium to cadmium outside the membrane was 10 or less. Under these circumstances, cadmium–calcium exchange becomes a meaningful entity which can be readily demonstrated. Thus, the suggestion becomes tenable that a cadmium–calcium exchange mechanism may be operant, thereby contributing to the increased calcium efflux observed in response to cadmium. Moreover, this mechanism implies that cadmium permeates the sarcolemmal membrane, suggesting that cadmium may act through mechanisms which are distinct from its effects on the cell membrane (e.g., intracellular sites of action). Although these findings add credence to the argument that intracellular sites are involved in the action of cadmium on the heart, this and other indirect evidence is not considered conclusive. The ability of cadmium to permeate the cardiac cell membrane has not been convincingly demonstrated by direct measurements. Thus, until additional experimental information is provided, caution should be exercised in attempting to explain the biochemical, biophysical, and functional effects of cadmium on cardiac cells in terms of intracellular sites of action. Furthermore, consideration should be given to the possibility that cadmium ions may not actually enter the cell, but act primarily by mechanisms which interfere with sarcolemmal ion and substrate transport processes.

The rapid onset of the inotropic response to cadmium and the overwhelming disparity in the effective concentrations of cadmium used in most studies relative to the buffer concentration of calcium (Ca/Cd = 10^3–10^4) are inconsistent with the suggestion that cadmium competes on a one-to-one basis for membrane and intracellular calcium binding sites. A more practical interpretation of the available information would be to suggest that the initial effects of cadmium involve cellular structures that have a limited number of accessible binding sites. The calcium channels of the cardiac sarcolemmal membrane are an obvious choice for the primary site of action. The latent effects of cadmium, which are dependent upon the duration of exposure (e.g., reversibility, intracellular biochemical changes), however, may be argued to involve direct or indirect effects on intracellular processes. A recent report by LEE and TSIEN (1983) has provided direct evidence demonstrating that cadmium (10^{-4} M CdCl$_2$) competes with calcium for transport through the membrane calcium channels, causing an attenuation of the slow inward calcium current in single dialyzed heart cells. This effect was demonstrated through a cadmium-induced inactivation of the calcium channel current. Increasing the extracellular calcium concentration from 3 to 30 mM CaCl$_2$ in the presence of 10^{-4} M CdCl$_2$ partially restored the peak calcium current in these heart cells by increasing the number of unblocked channels. In the context of these experiments, cadmium was shown to mimic the actions of organic calcium channel inhibitors (e.g., diltiazem, nitrendipine) in these heart cell preparations completely, except in one respect. Evidence was provided indicating that cadmium was bound to the metal ion coordination site of the calcium channel. In contrast, these organic inhibitors were bound to a site on the membrane associated with calcium channel activity, but which was distinctly different from the coordination site. The functional significance of this difference is not known.

5. Effects Following Chronic Cadmium Exposure In Vivo

Disturbances in myocardial contractile function have not been investigated extensively in the living animal following chronic subacute exposure to cadmium. Indeed, quantitative studies of this nature have only been conducted by one investigative group (KOPP et al. 1980a–d, 1982, 1983a, b). In these studies cadmium was administered by routes and in doses simulating human exposure. The responses were measured by simultaneous analysis of myocardial contractility and excitability in vivo (KOPP 1983).

a) Myocardial Contractile and Metabolic Effects Derived from Ex Vivo Analysis

Oral ingestion of cadmium via the drinking water (4.4×10^{-5} or 8.9×10^{-6} M CdCl$_2$) for variable periods of time (12–20 months) has been shown to induce significant physiologic changes within cardiovascular tissues of rats (KOPP et al. 1978c, 1980a–d, 1982, 1983a, b). These animals were characterized by normal growth and hematologic patterns and lacked any overt signs conventionally ascribed to cadmium intoxication (FRIBERG et al. 1974). Analysis of intact hearts from these animals under ex vivo perfusion conditions has revealed that chronic cadmium exposure was associated with a significant decrease in the magnitude and rate of myocardial tension development. Since these hearts were examined under conditions of constant preload and afterload, the possibility exists that the length–tension characteristics of cardiac muscle may have been altered by cadmium exposure.

The duration of the cadmium exposure appeared to influence the magnitude of the inotropic effects (KOPP et al. 1980b–d). Hearts from rats exposed to 4.4×10^{-5} M CdCl$_2$ for 15 months developed a maximal systolic tension under control conditions that corresponded to only 85% of that generated by control hearts; after 20 months exposure, maximal systolic tension fell to 75% of control values. The reduction in myocardial contractile activity following chronic cadmium exposure was shown to be associated with various biochemical disturbances in the heart. These disturbances parallel those described earlier in the perfused heart. The ATP content and the phosphorylation potential of the myocardium were significantly reduced following chronic cadmium exposure for both 15 and 18 months. The magnitude of these changes correlated directly with the duration of exposure. Myocardial ADP, Pi and PCr stores were not affected significantly after 15 months; however, following 20 months exposure, the level of ADP in hearts from cadmium-treated rats was elevated significantly. In addition to these changes in energy metabolites, GPC levels were decreased and G3-P levels were elevated significantly. With this same approach, similar changes in myocardial contractile activity and metabolite levels were detected in hearts from rats which had received $8.9 \times 10^{-6}\ M$ $CdCl_2$ in their drinking water for 18 months (KOPP et al. 1983a). The overall magnitude of these cardiac functional and metabolic perturbations was comparable to that observed in animals which received the higher dose of cadmium for a 20-month period. This lack of an apparent dose-dependent relationship between the dietary cadmium levels and the resultant physiologic and biochemical disturbances suggests that critical organ concentrations of cadmium may accumulate within the myocardium following relatively low exposures (KOPP et al. 1982). Alternatively, these findings may also indicate that concentration-dependent responses to cadmium were obscured by the prolonged periods of exposure.

Although the precise relationship between these metabolic changes and the depressed contractile activity of the hearts from the cadmium-treated animals cannot be deduced from existing experimental data, the potential functional significance of these changes can be put into perspective. A decline in myocardial ATP stores and a reduction in the phosphorylation potential of cardiac cells would be expected to have an adverse effect on the ability of these hearts to sustain phosphorylation-dependent processes (DHALLA et al. 1978). ATP is the essential driving force in these reactions. The differential phosphorylation of critical regulatory proteins in the cells and membrane structures of the mammalian myocardium purportedly functions as a common regulatory pathway which mediates or modulates myocardial responses to extrinsic (e.g., hormonal) and intrinsic (e.g., myogenic) physiologic effectors (WALSH et al. 1980). Various cellular rate processes (e.g., calcium sequestration by sarcoplasmic reticulum), exchange mechanisms (e.g., sarcolemmal cation transport), membrane receptor activities (e.g., hormone receptor binding), and protein interactions (e.g., actin and myosin) are regulated to a greater or lesser extent by phosphorylation-dependent reactions (BÁRÁNY et al. 1981; WALSH et al. 1980). It should be noted that many of these phosphorylation–dephosphorylation processes of the cell are either activated by an increase, or inhibited by a decrease in ionized calcium levels. Moreover, sarcolemmal calcium transport processes apparently require the phosphorylation of sites within the calcium channel. This observation is especially relevant in terms of the previously described antagonism between calcium and cadmium for membrane calcium-binding sites. Protein phosphorylation thus serves in part as a transduction process for converting chemical energy to mechanical work in the

heart muscle. The mediation of physiologic responses by protein phosphorylation-dependent reactions suggests that factors, such as cadmium, which alter either the reaction rate, or the number of potential phosphorylation sites operant
in the cells, will alter the physiologic responsiveness of the heart.

This hypothetical argument is supported by recent experimental findings from
rats chronically exposed to cadmium (KOPP et al. 1980a). Intact hearts from cadmium-treated rats (4.4×10^{-5} M CdCl$_2$, 15 months duration) were excised and
perfused under externally controlled conditions. The basal contractile activity of
the hearts from the cadmium-treated rats was significantly less than that observed
in the controls. Inotropic stimulation of these hearts with a β-adrenergic agonist
(isoproterenol 7×10^{-7} M) yielded positive inotropic and chronotropic responses
of comparable relative, but not absolute, magnitude in hearts from both groups
of animals; however, the maximal peak tension developed by the cadmium hearts
remained significantly below control levels. In conjunction with these physiologic
analyses, the relative cardiac myofibrillar protein phosphorylation activities were
determined and compared. As can be seen in Table 1, the altered contractile
events in the hearts from cadmium-treated rats were associated with a depressed
phosphorylation of the myosin LC-2. This effect was similar quantitatively to the
response observed in hearts perfused with cadmium (6×10^{-6} M CdCl$_2$). In contrast, unlike the attenuated TN-I phosphorylation detected in cadmium-perfused
hearts, the phosphorylation of TN-I in response to isoproterenol was not significantly affected in hearts from cadmium-fed rats, as compared with the corresponding controls. This disparity suggest that the phosphorylation of the myosin
LC-2 is particularly sensitive to the actions of cadmium and that the inhibition

Table 1. Specific phosphate ^{32}P incorporation into certain cardiac myofibrillar proteins of
heart (mole phosphate ^{32}P/mol specific myofibril protein), mean ± standard error

Groups	TN-I[a]	LC-1[b]	LC-2[c]	References
Control	0.053 ± 0.006	0.029 ± 0.007	0.116 ± 0.006	KOPP and BÁRÁNY (1980)
Control-fed + isoproterenol ($7 \times 10^{-7}M$)	0.184 ± 0.013[h]	0.024 ± 0.003	0.170 ± 0.009[g]	KOPP et al. (1980a)
Cd-fed (4.4×10^{-5} M CdCl$_2$) isoprote- renol (7×10^{-7} M)	0.166 ± 0.019[h]	0.018 ± 0.002	0.131 ± 0.008[d,g]	KOPP et al. (1980a)
Cd-perefused (6×10^{-6} M CdCl$_2$)	0.084 ± 0.004[d,e,f]	0.023 ± 0.001	0.095 ± 0.008[d]	KOPP and BÁRÁNY (1980)

[a] TN-I, troponin inhibitory subunit (29500 daltons)
[b] LC-1, myosin light chain-1 (27000 daltons)
[c] LC-2, myosin light chain-2 (19000 daltons)
[d] Significantly different from isoproterenol control, $P < 0.01$
[e] Significantly different from Cd-fed + isoproterenol, $P < 0.01$
[f] Significantly different from control, $P < 0.02$
[g] Significantly different from control, $P < 0.01$
[h] Significantly different from control, $P < 0.001$

of TN-I phosphorylation may represent a nonspecific response that is manifested at the higher cadmium concentrations used in the perfused heart studies.

b) In Vivo Assessment of Myocardial Contractility and Metabolic Correlates

Myocardial contractility assessments have been performed in vivo in anesthetized rats that had received 8.9×10^{-6} M CdCl$_2$ in their drinking water for 12 months (KOPP et al. 1983 b). As part of these cardiologic evaluations, peak left intraventricular pressure development and the maximal rate of left ventricular pressure development were measured directly and were used to calculate the contractile element shortening velocity V_{ce} and the maximal intrinsic shortening velocity of the heart muscle contractile elements V_{max} (KOPP 1983; MASON 1969; PARMLEY and SONNENBLICK 1967; SONNENBLICK et al. 1969). These latter indices of myocardial contractility minimize any inherent bias attributable to differences in preload (end-diastolic pressure) and afterload (arterial pressure) that may exist between control and cadmium-treated animals. Moreover, these calculated contractile element velocities V_{ce} and V_{max} parallel directly the coupling rates of chemical energy (ATP) to mechanical work by the heart, and the activity of the myosin ATPase (directly proportional to V_{max}, BÁRÁNY 1961).

Cadmium exposure was associated with subtle, but significant negative inotropic effects on the myocardium which involved the velocity components of contraction (KOPP et al. 1983 b). The altered myocardial contractility and dystrophic changes in cardiac muscle of workers chronically exposed to cadmium oxide (0.04–0.5 mg/m^3) (VOROBIEVA and EREMEEVA 1980) corroborates the potential significance of these experimental findings to humans. The contractile element shortening velocity of hearts from cadmium-treated rats (8.9×10^{-6} M CdCl$_2$) was 72% of the control value. Similarly, the maximal intrinsic shortening velocity of the contractile elements was decreased (86% of control) as well. As such, the decreased V_{ce} and V_{max} levels detected in hearts of cadmium-exposed rats appears to represent impaired ATP coupling to mechanical work, which may be related to a partial inhibition, either direct or indirect, of the myosin ATPase activity. Since the contractility characteristics of these hearts were measured in vivo, potential artifactual findings resulting from differential or selective responses to the tissue isolation procedures used in ex vivo and in vitro studies were eliminated. As previously mentioned, procedures that require ex vivo heart perfusion or in vitro tissue superfusion conditions in order to analyze the contractility of hearts from cadmium-treated animals subject the heart cells to brief episodes of ischemia. Intrinsic differences in the relative tolerance of hearts from control and cadmium-exposed animals to this period of ischemia cannot be measured and cannot be discounted in terms of possible selective influences on the subsequent physiologic and metabolic findings and interpretations obtained from such studies. Indeed, differences of this nature have been discovered by comparing the metabolic results obtained by ex vivo and in vivo analytic procedures (Fig. 3).

As described previously, chronic cadmium exposure was associated with significant changes in high energy phosphate levels of hearts which were not artificially perfused (in vivo). The ratios of ATP:ADP, and PCr:Pi, as well as the

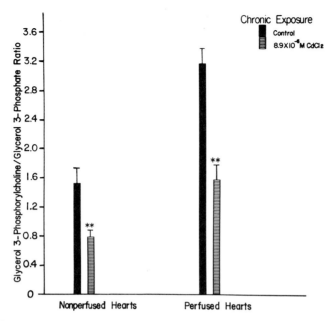

Fig. 3. In vivo versus ex vivo analysis. Molar ratios of glycerol 3-phosphorylcholine : glycerol 3-phosphate in hearts from rats chronically exposed to cadmium for a minimum of 12 months. Cadmium, as the acetate salt, was administered to the rats in the drinking water. The term "nonperfused" signifies that the hearts were not artificially perfused under ex vivo conditions. Instead, these hearts were biopsied while in the animal (see KOPP 1983 for details). Note the increased ratio of these heart metabolites resulting from ex vivo perfusion (1.8 mM CaCl$_2$, glucose as exogenous substrate) of control hearts and the attenuated response exhibited by the hearts from the cadmium-treated rats. *Asterisks* denote significantly different changes relative to the respective controls (** $P < 0.01$)

tissue phosphorylation potential, were significantly reduced relative to control. The magnitude of this effect was not as pronounced as that observed in ex vivo heart perfusion studies. The most prominent feature that distinguished the in vivo findings from those obtained by ex vivo analysis was the effects of cadmium exposure on phosphoglyceride derivatives. Under both conditions, cardiac G3-P levels were elevated and GPC levels were diminished in response to cadmium. The disparity between the results obtained by these two analytic procedures was apparent when the magnitude of the effects on the GPC:G3-P ratios were compared (Fig. 3). Ex vivo perfusion of control hearts resulted in a marked increase in GPC relative to G3-P. The ratio GPC:G3-P increased under these conditions in hearts from control animals. Hearts perfused under external conditions were subjected to an increased extracellular concentration of ionized calcium, as compared with levels normally found in blood. As shown previously in Fig. 1, the ratio GPC:G3-P was responsive to changes in calcium in the control perfused hearts. Myocardial lipolytic activity has been shown to be calcium activated and directly proportional to the external calcium concentration (HRON et al. 1977). Presumably, the lower ratio of these metabolites detected in the control hearts not artifically perfused reflects the difference between the ionized calcium levels of the perfusate and blood. Hearts from cadmium-treated animals had a significantly lower ratio of these metabolites and were less responsive to the calcium activation of these metabolites during external perfusion. This response was similar qualitatively to that shown to occur in isolated heart perfused with 3×10^{-6} M CdCl$_2$ at variable perfusate calcium concentrations (see Fig. 1). As described earlier, these phosphoglyceride derivatives are involved in the metabolism of phosphatidylcholine, a phospholipid constituent of the sarcolemma (see Fig. 2). Since the phosphocholine content of these hearts was not altered in conjunction with the changes involving GPC and G3-P, the changes in the ratio GPC:G3-P cannot be attributed to an increased catabolism of GPC. Instead, the relative accumulation of G3-P and decreased GPC content in hearts from cadmium-treated rats and the decreased responsiveness to calcium stimulation (both perfused and nonperfused) appears to represent a partial inhibition of phosphatidylcholine biosynthesis by cadmium through an effect on the calcium-regulated enzyme, choline phosphotransferase. Alterations in phosphatidylcholine metabolism in the heart have been shown to be associated with significant myocardial functional disturbances (CLARKSON and TEN EICK 1983; CORR et al. 1981). The effect of cadmium on phosphoglyceride metabolism was exacerbated under ex vivo perfusion conditions. In addition, the ability of cadmium to induce significant changes in membrane phospholipids and lipid metabolism is certainly not unprecedented and has been shown in other systems (DATSON 1982; HAYES et al. 1976; HENDERSON et al. 1979; NAKAGAWA et al. 1977; REVIS et al. 1980; SCHROEDER and BALASSA 1965). Overall, these observations indicate that, in addition to competing with calcium for membrane binding sites, cadmium may also affect the phospholipid structure of the sarcolemma, and physiologic responses to cadmium in part reflect these actions of cadmium on the cell membrane (GILES et al. 1983; LANGER et al. 1974; LEE and TSIEN 1983; PASSOW et al. 1961; PRITCHARD 1979; ROTHSTEIN 1959).

6. Consequences of Human Exposure

Based on roentgenologic, electrocardiographic, and blood pressure examinations of workers exposed to cadmium oxide (mean exposure 2 years), the conclusion was reached that the prevalence of cardiac disease was not increased by occupational exposure (FRIBERG 1950). Similarly, a postmortem case study of a worker exposed for 9 years to airborne cadmium in a copper–cadmium foundry did not reveal any remarkable histologic abnormalities of the myocardium (SMITH et al. 1957). In contrast, subsequent experimental and epidemiologic analyses have indicated that, indeed, chronic cadmium exposure may be associated with significant myocardial dysfunction and an increased incidence of cardiovascular disease in occupationally and nonoccupationally exposed humans (ADAMSKA-DYNIEWSKA et al. 1980a, b; BOEHME et al. 1979; KHERA et al. 1980; PONTEVA et al. 1979; REVIS and ZINSMEISTER 1981; TULLY and LEHMANN 1982; VOORS and SHUMAN 1977; VOORS et al. 1982; VOROBIEVA and EREMEEVA 1980). Workers exposed to cadmium oxide in concentrations of 0.04–0.5 mg per m^3 air were characterized by changes in cardiac function consisting of tachycardia, arterial hypertension, altered conductivity and contractility, and dystrophic changes in the myocardium (VOROBIEVA and EREMEEVA 1980). In this study, the incidence of both essential hypertension and renal disorders was higher among workers exposed to cadmium as compared with nonexposed workers. In a similar study, urinary kallikrein activity was reduced by 80% relative to control in young workers (mean age 29 years) exposed occupationally to cadmium (0.02–1.4 mg per m^3 air) (BOSCOLO et al. 1978). Parallel observations have been made in patients suffering from essential hypertension (IANNACCONE et al. 1979), suggesting that changes in the kallikrein–bradykinin system during chronic cadmium exposure may have a role in the etiology of hypertension in the affected cadmium-exposed workers (BOSCOLO et al. 1978). Studies concerned with the incidence of heart disease and blood cadmium levels have shown a significant direct correlation between blood cadmium levels and each of the following conditions: cardiovascular disease (KHERA et al. 1980), coronary artery disease (ADAMSKA-DYNIEWSKA et al. 1980a), and myocardial infarction (PONTEVA et al. 1979). As noted by LEWIS et al. (1972), and others (BEEVERS et al. 1980; CUMMINS et al. 1980; ELLIS et al. 1979; ØSTERGAARD 1978; TULLY and LEHMANN 1982; WARD et al. 1978), blood cadmium levels are increased in cigarette smokers. It should be noted that blood cadmium levels alone are of limited value in predicting soft tissue damage associated with exposure to cadmium (FRIBERG et al. 1974). Hence, the epidemiologic correlations, both positive and negative, involving blood levels of cadmium are informative, but may be of limited predictive value. Postmortem studies have demonstrated a positive correlation between hepatic cadmium concentrations and an increased mortality related to heart disease (VOORS and SHUMAN 1977; VOORS et al. 1982). Similarly, cadmium levels of heart and aortic tissues from hypertensive subjects (postmortem) have been shown to be elevated significantly relative to normotensive controls (BOEHME et al. 1979). Despite these findings, the results to date appear inconclusive with respect to the ability of cadmium to cause significant cardiovascular system pathology. The reported results do indicate, however, that under certain circumstances chronic cadmium exposure is associated with significant functional changes in the heart and vascular system.

7. Conclusions

Overall, the cardiodepressant effects of cadmium have been demonstrated in vivo following chronic exposure in humans and experimental animals, ex vivo in isolated perfused hearts, and in vitro in superfused cardiac tissue preparations, and incubated heart cells. Throughout this broad spectrum of tissue preparations that vary in their complexity, the mechanical responses elicited by cadmium were qualitatively consistent. Moreover, the antagonism with calcium is well documented at all levels examined. Studies of the effects of cadmium on isolated cardiac cells have demonstrated that cadmium exhibits many of the fundamental properties common to organic calcium channel inhibitors. Although the temptation exists to define the actions of cadmium exclusively in terms of its competitive antagonism with calcium, other mechanisms warrant consideration as well. PILATI et al. (1982) demonstrated in isolated papillary muscle studies that although cadmium and calcium are competitive antagonists, noncompetitive mechanisms also contribute to the effect of cadmium. The existence of these, as yet undefined, noncompetitive components was invoked to explain the inability exactly to reverse the contraction pattern of the cadmium-treated muscle preparation by increasing the extracellular calcium concentration. These noncompetitive mechanisms may include intracellular sites of action, which equilibrate more slowly, but whose actions persist thereafter. Cadmium-induced changes of this nature may involve protein-binding sites linked to muscle contraction, as demonstrated by FUCHS (1971), or biochemical processes as indicated by KOPP and BÁRÁNY (1979, 1980) and PRENTICE (1982; PRENTICE et al. 1984).

Considering the diverse metabolic changes that have been reported to occur in conjunction with cadmium exposure (depressed high energy phosphate stores, altered phosphoglyceride metabolism; decreased myofibrillar phosphorylation activity), the absence of direct intracellular actions by cadmium would indeed be surprising. Two schematic illustrations are presented which provide a composite summary of the reported effects and putative cellular sites of action of cadmium (Figs. 4, 5). The specific membrane sites purportedly involved in the activity of cadmium are indicated in Fig. 4. The hypothesis that the primary site of action for cadmium may be the cell membrane is not new. ROTHSTEIN (1959) postulated that the primary site of action of cadmium, and other heavy metals, was the cell membrane. This proposal was based on interpretations and inferences derived from the then existing body of experimental information. The experimental evidence that has accumulated since Rothstein's hypothesis was presented has been consistent with his original proposal. Presumably, the rapid phase of the response to cadmium represents effects on the cell membrane. Subsequent latent effects have been postulated to represent intracellular actions of cadmium.

The intracellular processes reportedly affected either directly or indirectly by cadmium are illustrated in Fig. 5. As stated earlier, the ability of cadmium to permeate the sarcolemma has not been demonstrated directly. As a result, the proposed intracellular actions of cadmium have been inferred from indirect evidence. Presumably, the action of cadmium affecting intracellular sites occurs with a defined latency and may represent the slow, noncompetitive phase of the cadmium effect (BERS and LANGER 1979; PILATI et al. 1982; PRENTICE 1982; PRENTICE et al. 1984). In other cellular systems, cellular uptake of cadmium has been demonstrated (POPHAM and WEBSTER 1976; SKOG and WAHLBERG 1964; WAALKES et al. 1983; WONG and KLAASSEN 1980) and was found to be independent of metallothionein synthesis (STACEY and KLAASSEN 1980). This latter characteristic suggests that the cadmium which enters the cell may be mobile, rather than necessarily sequestered by metallothionein, thus facilitating interactions with other intracellular structural and enzymatically active binding sites.

Although progress has been made in recent years toward defining the biochemical mechanisms and cellular structures that participate in the pathophysiologic responses of the heart to cadmium, various other avenues of research need to be explored as well. Included among these future areas of research are intracellular localization studies designed to identify the subcellular organelles which are sites of cadmium action in the living cell. The results obtained from such studies will help resolve the issue of whether the actions of cadmium in the heart involve subcellular sites, or whether the biologically significant interactions of the cardiac cell with cadmium are limited to superficial sites within the cell membrane. Furthermore, initial indications are that cadmium exposure, both acute and chronic,

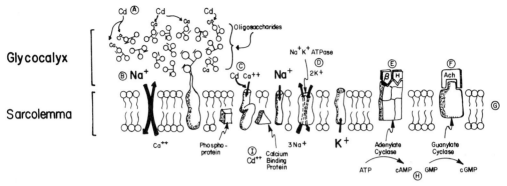

Fig. 4. Schematic model illustrating the generally recognized structural components that comprise the cardiac muscle cell sarcolemma (modified from SOLARO 1982). The phospholipid–lipid matrix that forms the hydrophobic backbone of the membrane is depicted interspersed between the membrane proteins, cation transport channels, and receptor binding sites. The glycocalyx forms the outer surface of the sarcolemma (only shown over a portion of the membrane surface) and is negatively charged. The membrane sites which have been shown to be affected by Cd^{2+} or potential sites of action are indicated by the *circled letters* Ⓐ–Ⓘ. Ⓐ LANGER et al. (1974) and BERS and LANGER (1979) have demonstrated that cadmium displaces calcium from rapidly exchangeable Ca^{2+} binding sites of the cardiac sarcolemma (glycocalyx). Ⓑ TROSPER and PHILIPSON (1983) have shown that Cd^{2+} inhibits $Na^+–Ca^{2+}$ exchange processes in canine sarcolemmal vesicles. In addition, Cd^{2+} stimulated Ca^{2+} efflux from these vesicle preparations. Ⓒ Evidence indicating a Cd^{2+}-induced Ca^{2+} channel inhibition has been presented by LEE and TSIEN (1983). The results suggest that Cd^{2+} binds to the metal cation coordination site (LEE et al. 1982; LEE and TSIEN 1983). Ⓓ Cd^{2+} has been shown in various muscle and nonmuscle preparations to inhibit the activity of the Na^+, K^+-ATPase (ANTUNES-MADEIRA and CARVALHO 1970; BADER et al. 1970; CHETTY et al. 1980; POOL 1981). This effect has not been demonstrated per se in cardiac cells and, therefore, should be considered as a potential site of action. Ⓔ Physiologic evidence (KOPP and BÁRÁNY 1980; KOPP et al. 1980a) suggests that the inotropic responsiveness of cardiac muscle to β-adrenergic stimulation is reduced. The mechanism for this effect (e.g., receptor binding, loss of receptor sensitivity, changes in adenylate kinase activity) has not been defined. Ⓕ The actions of cadmium on postsynaptic cholinergic receptors have been demonstrated; however, the concentrations required to produce an effect are considerably higher than those needed to produce presynaptic inhibition (GILES et al. 1983). Ⓖ Initial evidence demonstrating changes in phosphoglyceride metabolism in cardiac muscle suggests a decrease in phosphatidylcholine production. These findings are consistent with reported effects from other organ systems (DATSON 1982; HAYES et al. 1976; REVIS et al. 1980; SCHROEDER and BALASSA 1965). This response to cadmium suggests an altered pattern of phospholipid turnover in these cells which may affect the phospholipid composition of the sarcolemma. Ⓗ Biochemical studies (NATHANSON and BLOOM 1976; POOL 1981; SINGHAL et al. 1976; SINGHAL 1981; SUTHERLAND et al. 1974) have suggested that the effects of cadmium on adenylate cyclase activity vary according to the tissue model examined. Effects of cadmium on cardiac cyclic nucleotide and receptor activity have not been definitively described; hence, these sites of action should be considered tentative. Ⓘ Cd^{2+} may compete with Ca^{2+} for inner membrane surface calcium-binding sites. No experimental evidence has been presented to support this site of action; therefore, this site represents a possible cadmium interactive site

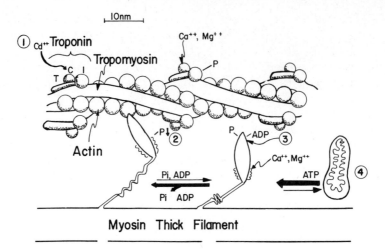

Fig. 5. Schema depicting the thin and thick filament structural components of striated muscle fibrils that are involved in the contractile process (modified from SOLARO 1982). The *circled numbers* indicate myofibril and organelle sites potentially affected by cadmium, based on published reports. Although direct interactions of cadmium with these sites cannot be excluded, the absence of definitive evidence demonstrating that cadmium actually enters cardiac cells suggests that the actions of cadmium may be indirect, as well. The indirect effects would be linked to a cadmium-induced inhibition of calcium influx through the membrane calcium channel. This effect would attenuate the Ca^{2+}-induced Ca^{2+} release within the cell, thereby reducing the Ca^{2+} available for activation of the contractile elements. Alternately, cadmium (Cd^{2+}) may act intracellularly, blocking calcium-binding sites coupled to the contractile process. ① Cd^{2+} has been shown to displace $^{45}Ca^{2+}$ from purified troponin of striated muscle (FUCHS 1971). The biologic activity of this complex is unknown; however, Fuchs does indicate that unpublished results obtained at that time suggested that Cd^{2+} can activate ATPase activity of natural actomyosin. The binding of Cd^{2+} to troponin has not been demonstrated in intact cardiac tissue preparations. ② The phosphorylation of the myosin light chain-2 (mol ^{32}P phosphate/mol light chain-2 protein) has been shown to be decreased in hearts (isoproterenol-activated) from cadmium-fed animals (KOPP et al. 1980a) and hearts perfused with cadmium (KOPP and BÁRÁNY 1980). The myosin light chain kinase that catalyzes this reaction is a calcium-activated enzyme. The reduced phosphorylation of this enzyme is linked to decreased cardiac muscle inotropy and may result from indirect effects of Cd^{2+} on intracellular Ca^{2+} levels or direct actions on the enzyme active site. ③ Based on in vivo myocardial contractility determinations, chronic cadmium exposure was shown to be associated with a decreased maximal intrinsic shortening velocity V_{max} of the cardiac muscle contractile elements (KOPP et al. 1983b). Since V_{max} is directly proportional to the myosin ATPase activity (BÁRÁNY 1961), these results suggest that cadmium exposure may directly or indirectly cause a decreased myosin ATPase activity. ④ The ATP content of cardiac muscle from cadmium-exposed animals or cadmium-perfused hearts has been shown to be reduced significantly (KOPP et al. 1978c, 1980b–d, 1983a, b; PRENTICE 1982; PRENTICE et al. 1984). Cadmium appears to affect mitochondrial oxidative phosphorylation; however, the site of action is not known

causes significant disturbances in myocardial metabolism. These studies need to be expanded to facilitate a broader understanding of the metabolic pathways and rate-limiting enzymatic steps which are influenced by cadmium exposure in the living cell. As demonstrated by ex vivo and in vitro studies, the responsiveness of cadmium-treated hearts to physiologic stressors is compromised. The extent to which these and other observations reflect the actions of cadmium in vivo need to be identified before the potential significance of chronic cadmium exposure can be approximated in living systems. Recent assessments of myocardial function following chronic exposure to cadmium in humans and experimental animals have detected significant pathophysiologic changes which are qualitatively similar to one another and to the findings obtained by ex vivo and in vitro methods. Overall, these results obtained by diverse methodological approaches indicate that cadmium is cardiotoxic at very low levels and that further studies are needed to assess the impact of chronic cadmium exposure from environmental and industrial sources on human health.

II. Actions of Cadmium Affecting Cardiac Excitability

1. Overview of Cadmium Effects on Heart Excitability

Although researchers in the nineteenth century demonstrated that cadmium exposure slowed the spontaneous contraction rate of the heart (ATHANASIU and LANGLOIS 1895, 1896; MARMÉ 1867; PANSERI 1904; RICHET 1882), the electrophysiologic foundations of these cadmium-induced disturbances in myocardial rhythmicity were not identified until the mid-twentieth century (DOTTA and FRUSCELLA 1963; HAWLEY and KOPP 1975; KLEINFELD et al. 1955, 1966; KOPP and HAWLEY 1976, 1978; KOPP et al. 1978 a–c, 1980 b–d, 1983 a, b; PRENTICE 1982; PRENTICE et al. 1984; STURKIE 1973; TODA 1973 b, c; VOROBIEVA and EREMEEVA 1980). KLEINFELD et al. (1955), using the isolated perfused frog heart, were among the first research groups to investigate the effects of cadmium on myocardial excitability. Subsequent studies concerned with the effects of cadmium on the surface electrocardiogram and intracardiac electrical recordings have demonstrated significant cadmium-induced cardiac conduction disturbances in mammals, birds, and amphibians. Generally, the results obtained from isolated perfused heart preparations have agreed qualitatively with the findings obtained in vivo following chronic exposure to cadmium. In conjunction with these studies, cadmium has been shown to alter the excitability of specific anatomic sites preferentially within the cardiac conduction system (KOPP et al. 1978 a, b, 1980 a–d, 1983 a). The specificity of these responses has been shown to decrease with increasing cadmium concentrations. Moreover, increasing the extracellular calcium concentrations has been shown to antagonize these effects of cadmium (PRENTICE 1982; PRENTICE et al. 1984). Recently, the effects of cadmium on ventricular muscle excitability have been investigated in vivo and ex vivo. The results indicate that the conduction velocity of the ventricular muscle mass is depressed following exposure to cadmium (KOPP et al. 1983 b; PRENTICE 1982; PRENTICE et al. 1984).

Attempts to elucidate the cellular basis for the cardiac conduction disturbances associated with acute cadmium exposure have focused on identifying the characteristics of transmembrane action potentials recorded from various heart preparations during cadmium exposure (KLEINFELD et al. 1955, 1966; TODA 1973b). Collectively, the results have demonstrated that cadmium is a potent depressor of myocardial excitability. The mechanistic basis for the cadmium-induced decline in myocardial excitability appears to be related to changes in membrane sodium and calcium conductance. Conceptually, changes of this nature are associated with an increased arrhythmogenicity (HAUSWIRTH and SINGH 1979). A decrease in the rate of depolarization of pacemaker cells within the sinoatrial node and a slowing of atrioventricular conduction can often trigger latent pacemaker activity. If too frequent, the resultant ectopic arrhythmias may compromise cardiac hemodynamics.

In human studies, the reported electrocardiographic findings from workers exposed to cadmium in the workplace have been inconclusive. FRIBERG (1950) reported that of the 57 workers examined, 7 had electrocardiographic disturbances: 5 cases were attributed to coronary insufficiency, 1 case to intraventricular impairment of conduction, and in 1 case the PQ interval was prolonged. However, the study concluded that workers exposed to cadmium oxide fumes in the workplace for an average of 2 years did not exhibit an increased incidence of electrocardiographic abnormalities as compared with sawmill workers. In contrast, VOROBIEVA and EREMEEVA (1980) have reported that myocardial conductivity was significantly altered in workers exposed to cadmium oxide fumes (0.04–0.5 mg per m^3 air). These reported findings are consistent in that cardiac conduction disturbances were detected in cadmium-exposed workers. The disparity between these studies is one of interpretation and concerns the incidence of electrocardiographic abnormalities in the respective control groups compared with cadmium-exposed workers.

2. Cadmium-Induced Effects on Electrical Events

a) Perfused Hearts

KLEINFELD et al. (1955), using in situ and isolated perfused frog heart preparations, reported that cadmium induced electrocardiographic changes consisting of a prolongation in the PR interval, T wave inversion, increased QRS duration, and decreased voltage of the QRS complex. The dose of cadmium administered in situ by injection into the aorta, ventricle, or ventral abdominal vein was either 1.4×10^{-5} or 2.8×10^{-5} mol CdCl$_2$ per kilogram body weight. Hearts perfused with cadmium were exposed to 5×10^{-5} M CdCl$_2$. Analysis of single fiber action potentials recorded simultaneously with the bipolar electrocardiograms were characterized by: (a) a shortening of the action potential (AP) duration; (b) a decrease in the AP voltage; (c) impaired rate of depolarization; and (d) a decrease in the plateau phase of the AP which hastened the rate of repolarization. The consistent effects of cadmium in situ and in the isolated perfused heart provided evidence suggesting that the response of the heart was directly related to the cellular actions of cadmium in the heart, rather than mediated through central nervous system effects. Pretreatment of the hearts with cysteine delayed, but did not prevent the cadmium-induced changes. Treatment of hearts with cysteine after cadmium had induced significant electrical effects was ineffective in reversing the effects of cadmium.

Studies concerned with the actions of cadmium on the electrical events of the intact mammalian heart were not performed until two decades later (HAWLEY and KOPP 1975; KOPP and HAWLEY 1976; KOPP et al. 1978 a, b). Electrocardiographic analysis of intact, isolated perfused rat hearts revealed a dose-dependent prolongation of the PR interval (first-degree heart block) that was progressive with time at each cadmium concentration examined (3×10^{-8}–3×10^{-5} M $CdSO_4$). The progressive increase in the PR interval was accompanied by an increase in the QRS duration (by as much as 33%) followed by partial block of ventricular activation (second-degree heart block) and culminated in complete atrioventricular heart block (third-degree heart block) at cadmium concentrations greater than 3×10^{-6} M. Although a cadmium-induced bradycardia was noted, particularly at the higher dosage levels, atrial electrical events, characterized by the persistence of rhythmical P wave activity, continued for an extended period after ventricular electrical activity had ceased. The specificity exhibited by cadmium for prolonging the PR interval of the ECG was interpreted to represent a strong affinity of cadmium for binding sites within the atrioventricular node and His–Purkinje system, which resulted in a depression of this portion of the heart conduction system.

Additional studies (KOPP and HAWLEY 1976), were undertaken to characterize further the external factors that contributed to the responsiveness of the mammalian myocardium to cadmium. The effect of cadmium (3×10^{-5} M $CdSO_4$) on the PR interval of the ECG was shown to vary as an inverse function of the perfusate pH within the range 6.8–7.6. These pH studies suggested that within a very narrow range slightly acidic conditions favored the interaction of cadmium with membrane and cellular binding sites of cells within the atrioventricular node His–Purkinje system, resulting in a decreased excitability. Comparison of the responses induced by cadmium with those produced by changing the perfusate calcium concentration (from 2.4 to 0.005 mM $CaCl_2$) revealed conduction system disturbances that paralleled each other. Decreasing the perfusate calcium concentration caused a progressive increase in the PR interval. This pattern was most pronounced at 37- and 370-fold dilutions of the original perfusate calcium concentration. The parallelism between these findings suggested that cadmium acted on the atrioventricular node His–Purkinje cells of the cardiac conduction system by displacing calcium from cellular binding sites. When combined with the information obtained from the pH studies, these findings suggested that a possible antagonism existed between cadmium and calcium for cellular binding sites which was pH dependent, favoring cadmium binding at pH < 7.0.

The effect of cadmium on the cardiac conduction system was subsequently localized to the atrioventricular node through the use of His bundle electrogram (HBE) recording techniques (KOPP et al. 1978 a, b). Intact isolated rat hearts were perfused in a modified apparatus that facilitated access to the intra-atrial septum for His bundle electrode placement. Exposure to cadmium (3×10^{-5}, 3×10^{-6}, 3×10^{-8} M $CdCl_2$) caused an increase in the atrio–His interval of the HBE at all cadmium concentrations studied and complete heart block at the higher cadmium concentrations. This response was selective at low levels of cadmium, was not related to heart rate effects, and was progressive with time. The conduction disturbances caused by cadmium proximal to the His bundle could denote depressed conduction at the atrial junction of the atrioventricular node (upper nodal cells), within the atrioventricular node (nodal cells), or within the upper portion of the His bundle (nodal His cells). At the higher cadmium concentrations, the His–ventricular interval (essentially representing conductivity of the His–Purkinje system) was also significantly increased in response to cadmium. This effect was dose dependent and appeared to be a nonspecific response. Attempts to reverse the suppression of atrioventricular node excitability with norepinephrine were unsuccessful. In contrast, the responsiveness of the sinoatrial node to norepinephrine was not affected by prior cadmium treatment.

b) In Vitro Actions On Cardiac Cell Action Potentials

Some 11 years after describing the actions of cadmium on the action potentials of the frog heart, Kleinfeld and co-workers (KLEINFELD et al. 1966; KLEINFELD and STEIN 1968) presented their findings from work performed with the canine false tendon–papillary muscle preparation and the isolated, superfused rat atrium. Analysis of Purkinje and ventricular fiber action potentials recorded from electrically paced (60 beats/min) false tendon–papillary muscle preparations (KLEINFELD et al. 1966) revealed that cadmium (1.8×10^{-4} M CdCl$_2$) induced effects common to both cell types. These effects consisted of an attenuation of the phase 2 (plateau phase) component of the action potential, a reduction in the height of the plateau phase (increase in the phase 1 component), a decrease in the overall duration of the action potential, and a decrease in the velocity of the phase 3 (repolarization) component. The voltage characteristics of the membrane potential (amplitude of the action potential, membrane resting potential, overshoot) were not affected appreciably by cadmium treatment. In addition, a slight reduction in the velocity of the action potential phase 0 component was observed in the recordings from the ventricular cells.

Parallel studies performed with the isolated rat atrium (KLEINFELD and STEIN 1968) yielded findings that were quantitatively similar to those observed in the ventricular cells. Since the atrial muscle action potential has a plateau phase (phase 2) with a relatively short duration, the actions of cadmium on this aspect of the atrial action potential were inferred from the duration at constant phase 3 voltage (50 mV below zero potential). Atrial preparations exposed to cadmium (4.5×10^{-5} M CdCl$_2$) and electrically stimulated at a rate of 120 beats/min were characterized by a decrease in the duration of the action potential (-32% relative to control), the membrane action potential, resting membrane potential, and overshoot voltages were not significantly affected by cadmium exposure. Collectively, the results obtained from atrial, ventricular, and Purkinje cells were consistent and indicated that the primary effect of cadmium on the cardiac cell action potential is on the action potential duration (phase 2). This phase component of the action potential corresponds to the opening of the slow calcium channels of the sarcolemma and the slow inward current of calcium and sodium.

The experimental findings reported by KLEINFELD et al. (1955, 1966) and by KLEINFELD and STEIN (1968) provided initial insights into the underlying disturbances in the electrical properties of the cardiac cells responsible for the negative dromotropic responses to cadmium. These studies involved only single doses of cadmium which were known to induce relatively rapid and reproducible effects. As such, the specificity of these responses was undetermined. In subsequent studies, TODA (1973 b, c) examined the specificity of these responses by determining the dose-dependent effects of cadmium on the electrophysiologic properties of atrial muscle and sinoatrial node pacemaker cells. The efficacy of potential cadmium antagonists was evaluated as a basis for determining the reversibility of the cadmium-induced effects on the transmembrane potentials of atrial muscle cells. In addition, the functional integrity of adrenergic and histaminergic membrane receptor sites was evaluated in pacemaker cells of the sinoatrial node. These latter experiments were undertaken to clarify the extent to which cadmium interferes with amine receptor binding at the membrane surface. In isolated rabbit left atria paced at a frequency of 60 beats/min, the addition of cadmium (2×10^{-5}–5×10^{-4} M $CdCl_2$) caused a dose-dependent decrease in the action potential amplitude (overshoot) relative to control. At cadmium concentrations of 10^{-4} and 5×10^{-4} M, the resting potential was decreased significantly as well. Cadmium exposure also shortened the action potential duration (2×10^{-5} and 10^{-4} M $CdCl_2$), while the rate of depolarization (phase 0) of the action potential was slowed in addition at the highest concentration (5×10^{-4} M $CdCl_2$). The effects of cadmium on the voltage characteristics of the action potential differed from those reported by KLEINFELD and STEIN (1968). The disparity between the results from these two studies may represent concentration differences; however, certain differences in the experimental conditions may have been contributing factors as well; e.g., the experiments conducted by TODA (1973 b) were performed at 30 °C, while those performed by KLEINFELD and STEIN (1968) were done at 23 °C.

Approximately 50% of the atrial preparations superfused with 5×10^{-4} M $CdCl_2$ for 40 min were refractory to electrical stimulation. Increasing the intensity of the electrical stimulation was ineffective in regenerating action potentials from atrial tissues so affected. The addition of cysteine (1 mM), 1,4-dithiothreitol (1 mM), calcium (4.4 mM), or EGTA (2 mM, ethyleneglycol-bis(β-aminoethyl ether)-N,N,N',N'-tetraacetic acid) to the bathing medium caused a partial restoration of atrial excitability in these and other preparations affected to a lesser extent by cadmium. Parallel studies (TODA 1973 c) concerned with the effects of cadmium on the transmembrane potential of sinoatrial nodal pacemaker cells revealed that cadmium (10^{-4} and 5×10^{-4} M $CdCl_2$) induced significant, dose-dependent decreases in the maximal diastolic potential, the threshold potential, and overshoot components of the pacemaker action potential. Moreover, the action potential duration was prolonged and the slope of the diastolic depolarization was decreased in a dose-dependent manner. In 90% of the preparations treated with 5×10^{-4} M $CdCl_2$, the pacemaker potential was completely abolished. The inhibitory effects of cadmium were partially reversed by the addition of cysteine (1 mM) to the bathing medium. Calcium (4.4 mM) was ineffective in reversing the depressant effects of cadmium on sinoatrial node pacemaker potentials; however, calcium pretreatment of atrial preparations was effective in preventing the cadmium-induced changes. The dose–response relationship between norepinephrine and rate of sinoatrial node pacemaker discharge was suppressed markedly in the presence of 2×10^{-5} and 10^{-4} M $CdCl_2$. Norepinephrine sensitivity was partially restored in these cadmium-treated preparations by the addition of calcium

(4.4 mM) and/or cysteine (1 mM). The sensitivity of atrial preparations to histamine stimulation was attenuated in the presence of cadmium, and partially reversed in the presence of calcium and/or cysteine.

Overall, these findings indicate that cadmium alters the electrophysiologic properties of cardiac muscle cells (atrial and ventricular) and specialized cells within the cardiac conduction system (sinoatrial node pacemaker cells, Purkinje fiber cells) in a concentration-dependent manner. Based on the known ionic and biophysical properties of cardiac cells (HAUSWIRTH and SINGH 1979) and the reported electrophysiologic evidence, cadmium appears to act by altering the slow inward current of calcium and sodium through interactions at the membrane surface. The inability of elevated extracellular calcium concentrations to reverse completely the depressive effects of cadmium on the transmembrane potentials suggests that the affinity of cadmium ions for these surface binding sites exceeds that of calcium. It should be noted that under the described experimental conditions the relative ratio of calcium to cadmium was between 10:1 and 100:1. The ability of thiol reagents (e.g., cysteine) to restore the excitability of these cadmium-exposed cells indicates that the affinity of cadmium ions for SH groups exceeds the affinity of cadmium ions for these membrane binding sites. Moreover, these findings also lend credence to the interpretation that cadmium binding to sites on the surface of the membrane is relatively rapid and constitutes a primary mechanism through which cadmium depresses the excitability of cardiac cells. The postulated action of cadmium on membrane binding sites is consistent with evidence presented previously indicating that cadmium acts as a membrane calcium channel inhibitor in cardiac cells.

c) In Vivo Effects On Myocardial Excitation

DOTTA and FRUSCELLA (1963) published the first definitive report describing the electrocardiographic manifestations of chronic cadmium toxicity (intraperitoneal injections, CdCl$_2$ 1.6×10^{-5} mol kg^{-1} day^{-1}) and acute (1.1×10^{-4} mol/kg administered intraperitoneally). Daily cadmium injections induced an increase in P wave and R wave voltages and a 50% increase in the PR interval. The modifications in ventricular activity occurred in 80% of the cadmium-treated rats and were interpreted to represent a verticalization of the electrical axis. These alterations were maximal at 10 days and persisted without significant modification thereafter during the remaining 22 days of the exposure period. Sinus rhythm was maintained and heart rate was not significantly affected by cadmium exposure. When electrocardiographic evaluations were performed immediately after injecting cadmium, several transient changes were observed. A second-degree heart block (2:1 atrioventricular heart block) with intermittent arrhythmic complexes characterized by P waves of irregular frequency (atrial flutter) was typically observed. Histologic evaluation of hearts from these cadmium-treated rats revealed myofibrillar distortion in both atrial and vetricular muscle fibers and a moderate sarcoplasmic vacuolation of specialized conduction cells.

Acute administration of cadmium resulted in pronounced electrocardiographic changes within the first few minutes after injection (CdCl$_2$ 1.1×10^{-4} mol/kg i.p.). Heart rate decreased with a concurrent increase in atrioventricular conduction time (prolongation of the PR interval), which was progressive with time. Complete atrioventricular dissociation was manifested after 20 min, which was accompanied by a progressive sinus bradycardia. These changes occurred prior to the onset of respiratory paralysis.

Electrocardiographic disturbances associated with cadmium injections in chickens ($CdCl_2$ 1.1×10^{-5} mol kg^{-1} day^{-1} i.p.) (STURKIE 1973) were essentially in accord with those described in rats by DOTTA and FRUSCELLA (1963). Within 33 days after initiating the daily cadmium injections 20% of the chickens (1 of 5) exhibited atrioventricular heart block. The most prevalent electrocardiographic anomaly detected in these animals was a persistent inversion of the T wave. At autopsy, gross examination of hearts from cadmium-treated birds revealed varying degrees of myocardial infarction. Heart enlargement was also commonly observed.

Oral administration of cadmium to rats at doses which were overtly toxic (1.17×10^{-3} M $CdCl_2$ in the drinking water) and doses which were not (8.9×10^{-5} M $CdCl_2$ in the drinking water), based on growth and hematologic effects, produced electrocardiographic changes that were progressive with the duration of exposure (KOPP and HAWLEY 1978). The PR interval steadily increased during the 75-day period of exposure. The magnitude of the increased atrioventricular conduction time was correlated neither with the concentration of cadmium in the drinking water nor with the blood cadmium concentration.

Subsequent chronic, low level feeding studies have been conducted under rigorously controlled conditions for considerably longer exposure periods (12–24 months) using lower dietary cadmium concentrations (4.4×10^{-5}–8.9×10^{-6} M $Cd(CH_3COO)_2$) in drinking water (KOPP et al. 1978c, 1980a–d, 1983a, b). These studies attempted in part to elucidate the cardiac conduction disturbances associated with chronic exposure to cadmium at levels that frequently are encountered by the human population. Chronic cadmium exposure was shown consistently to cause PR interval prolongation at these doses. Through the application of His bundle electrocardiographic recording techniques, this effect was localized to the atrioventricular nodal region of the cardiac conduction system. A trend toward a greater increase in atrioventricular conduction time as a direct function of the exposure duration was noted (KOPP et al. 1978c, 1980a–d, 1983a, b). Microscopic analysis of the atrioventricular nodal region in hearts from cadmium-fed rats (4.4×10^{-5} M $Cd(CH_3COO)_2$ for 24 months) revealed evidence of structural damage within the atrioventricular node, consisting of an accumulation of dense bodies adjacent to foci of vacuolation in cells of this region (KOPP et al. 1978c).

Prolongation of the PR interval and anatomic localization of the depressed conductivity to the atrioventricular nodal region has been a finding common to all of the in vivo, in situ, and ex vivo heart studies that have been reported (DOTTA and FRUSCELLA 1963; HAWLEY and KOPP 1975; KLEINFELD et al. 1955; KOPP and HAWLEY 1976, 1978; KOPP et al. 1978a–c, 1980a–d, 1983a, b; STURKIE 1973), except one (KOTSONIS and KLAASSEN 1978). In this latter study, exposure to cadmium (8.9×10^{-5}, 2.7×10^{-4}, 8.9×10^{-4} M $CdCl_2$ in the drinking water) for 24 weeks was ineffective in inducing significant changes in the PR interval of the electrocardiogram.

3. Conclusions

The selective actions of cadmium on the various cells of the myocardium included effects involving virtually every electrophysiologic property of the cells which have a significant dependence on inward calcium currents. These effects were demonstrated in tissues from multiple animal models (dog, rabbit, rat, frog) and were consistent in the various types of tissues examined (ventricular muscle, atrial muscle, Purkinje fibers, and sinoatrial node pacemaker cells). Generally, these depressive actions of cadmium on membrane depolarization rate and membrane conductance were manifested as prolonged conduction intervals in the surface electrocardiogram and the intracardiac electrogram. Indeed, a consistent finding common to virtually all intact heart studies was the cadmium-induced prolongation of electrocardiographic conduction intervals, particular within the region corresponding to conduction through the atrioventricular node (PR interval). As with many chemical agents, the specificity of cadmium for certain cells diminished and more cells responded to the effect of cadmium as the tissue preparation was exposed to higher cadmium concentrations. The nonspecific effects of cadmium in certain cells (e.g., decreased diastolic depolarization rate in pacemaker cells) were evident at both the cell and intact tissue level as bradycardia and atrial arrhythmias. These responses to cadmium appear to represent acute toxicity effects. Conversely, the specific negative dromotropic effects of cadmium, which were evident at low cadmium exposure levels, indicate that cadmium acts preferentially on the cells of the atrioventricular node and ventricular muscle cells. Both of these cell types have a significant calcium dependence that is essential to sustaining membrane excitability. Overall, the reported electrophysiologic and electrocardiographic findings describing the actions of cadmium on myocardial excitability were consistent and compatible with the interpretation that the action of cadmium involves an antagonism with calcium for surface binding sites of the membrane. These responses to cadmium were demonstrable following low exposures to cadmium and appeared to represent subacute phases of cadmium toxicity. It should be noted, as well, that the dose of cadmium required to induce significant changes in the electrocardiogram were at least 10–100 times below that required for contractile effects (in perfused hearts). These findings, and those which have demonstrated that the response to cadmium was inversely proportional to the extracellular pH within a very narrow range (pH 6.8–7.6), suggest that the heart is remarkably sensitive to the actions of cadmium at levels that are not acutely toxic. The possibility exists that chronic human exposure to cadmium may affect adversely the excitability and conductivity of the myocardium, particularly in response to circumstances that increase tissue acidosis. The toxicologic manifestations of acute cadmium exposure appear to represent nonspecific tissue responses which are likely to occur only after acute exposures, and not after chronic subacute exposures to cadmium (e.g., depressed sinoatrial node automaticity and bradycardia).

D. Vascular Actions of Cadmium

I. Introduction

Before addressing the reported actions of cadmium on vascular tissue, it is necessary to discuss briefly the current concepts regarding vascular smooth muscle contraction–relaxation mechanisms (for reviews see FLECKENSTEIN 1983; JOHANSSON and SOMLYO 1980; VAN BREEMEN et al. 1979). Fundamental differences exist between the physiologic and biochemical properties of cardiac and smooth muscle. These intrinsic differences must be kept in mind when attempting to define the cellular mechanisms of cadmium common to both types of muscle. As already discussed, the concentration of intracellular ionized calcium (Ca^{2+}) regulates the contraction–relaxation cycle in cardiac muscle; a property shared by vascular smooth muscle. Despite this similarity, the mechanisms which participate in the regulation of smooth muscle contraction are quite different from those which predominate in cardiac muscle. In addition, two basic types of plasma membrane calcium channels have been proposed which are responsible for calcium influx in vascular smooth muscle cells. These reputed membrane sites are the potential-dependent channels, activated by membrane depolarization, and the receptor-operated channels associated with, and activated by membrane receptors that respond to vasoactive substances independently of membrane voltage changes. Activation of one or the other type of channel likely corresponds to the processes known as electromechanical and pharmacomechanical coupling, respectively. Pharmacomechanical coupling has been defined as a process or processes through which drugs can cause contraction or relaxation of smooth muscle without a requisite voltage-dependent change in the membrane potential. The mechanism of pharmacomechanical coupling is not well understood; however, this process may be mediated by: (a) extracellular calcium influx; (b) release of calcium from intracellular binding sites within the sarcoplasmic reticulum and mitochondria in response to changes in surface membrane calcium coupling (calcium influx); and (c) a direct action of the drug in intracellular calcium sequestration sites. These postulated mechanisms are not considered to be mutually exclusive. To some extent the degree to which any of these mechanisms are involved in the response to a vasoactive substance depends on the source of the vascular tissue under study and the properties of the chemical agent. Considerable heterogeneity exists between various smooth muscle preparations (e.g., aorta, coronary artery, mesenteric artery) in that there are intrinsic differences (e.g., calcium kinetics) in the properties of vascular smooth muscle from different vascular beds within the same animal and between different animal species. These differences in part represent anatomic variations in the structure of the vessels. Moreover, vascular beds from hypertensive donors differ considerably in their responsiveness to vasoactive substances and dependence on external calcium as compared with the same vessels obtained from normotensive donors. These differences suggest that caution must be exercised when defining generalized mechanisms of action of various vasoactive substances on vascular smooth muscle. Seemingly conflicting results, therefore, probably are more a reflection of deficiencies in current knowledge about fundamental smooth muscle processes and an inability to interpret the significance of subtle differences in the experimental methods, than an index of the validity of the experimental findings.

As stated, the triggering event which activates the sequence leading to smooth muscle contraction is an increase in sarcoplasmic free calcium (Ca^{2+}) levels. The rise in sarcoplasmic Ca^{2+} levels may be caused by an increased influx of extracellular calcium owing to activation of voltage-dependent and/or receptor-operated calcium channels in the cell membrane. It should be noted that inhibition of the electrogenic Na, K-pump may result in activation of the voltage-dependent calcium channels leading to a net Ca^{2+} uptake (van Breemen et al. 1979). Release of Ca^{2+} from intracellular storage sites (sarcoplasmic reticulum, mitochondria) may participate and can initiate the activation process, as well. The increased levels of sarcoplasmic Ca^{2+} activate the myosin light chain kinase through the formation of an active ternary complex with calmodulin (Ca^{2+}–calmodulin–myosin light chain kinase) which results in the phosphorylation of the myosin P-light chain (LC-2). The phosphorylation of the myosin head (P-light chain) promotes actin myosin interaction, facilitating cross-bridge formation and thereby producing contraction of the smooth muscle cell. In addition, the increased sarcoplasmic Ca^{2+} levels may also influence contraction through thin filament (actin)-linked regulation. At present this latter mechanism is not well defined. Thus, agents which affect the potential-dependent and/or receptor-operated calcium channels of the cell membrane, or which influence intracellular calcium release and sequestration processes will have a profound impact on the contractile dynamics of vascular smooth muscle.

II. Vascular Responses to Cadmium

1. Overview

Although the effects of cadmium on vascular tone and reactivity have been intensively investigated, no overall unifying concepts have yet emerged which define the mechanistic basis for the vascular actions of cadmium. The ability of cadmium to accumulate and persist in vascular tissues, and to alter the function of vascular smooth muscle seems unquestionable; however, the confusing aspect of this effect is that cadmium has been shown to elicit both apparent vasodilator and vasoconstrictor responses in different studies (Amacher and Ewing 1975; Fowler et al. 1975; Hayashi and Toda 1977; Kanisawa and Schroeder 1969; Levin and Miller 1981; Nechay et al. 1978; Niwa and Suzuki 1982; Perry et al. 1967a, b; Prentice et al. 1984; Thind and Fischer 1975; Thind et al. 1970b; Toda 1973a). In part, the confusion concerning the actions of cadmium on vascular smooth muscle is linked to the incompletely defined mechanisms which purportedly regulate the excitation–contraction and vasodilation processes in vascular smooth muscle. The inconsistent and often contradictory experimental results obtained in studies concerned with the vascular actions of cadmium may represent: (a) the specificity (low concentrations) and nonspecificity (high concentrations) of the cadmium effect as determined by the response of the tissue to the applied concentration of cadmium; (b) the differential responsiveness of different vascular tissue models; and (c) variations attributable to differences in the external conditions applied to the tissue. As indicated, evidence exists that suggests that cadmium may act directly on the vascular bed to induce vasoconstriction. Although this effect has been observed in vitro in isolated tissue preparations (NIWA and SUZUKI 1982; PERRY et al. 1967 a), generally, evidence of this response is observed only indirectly in vivo and in intact organ preparations (FOWLER et al. 1975; KANISAWA and SCHROEDER 1969; LEVIN and MILLER 1981; NECHAY et al. 1978; PRENTICE 1982; PRENTICE et al. 1984). In contrast, vasodilator responses are reported frequently in isolated smooth muscle preparations following cadmium treatment (HAYASHI and TODA 1977; THIND et al. 1970 b; TODA 1973 a).

The intent of this and subsequent sections of this chapter is to classify and summarize the reported vascular responses to cadmium. An understanding of the mechanisms through which cadmium acts to alter vascular smooth muscle tone and its reactivity to vasoactive substances is critically important if the effects of cadmium on systemic circulation are to be understood. However, it is clear that our current knowledge about the biochemical events that regulate smooth muscle functions are not sufficiently well defined to interpret all of the reported effects of cadmium. Resolution of the controversy which surrounds the vascular actions of cadmium must await further progress in our understanding of the biochemical and biophysical principles that define smooth muscle function.

2. Direct Actions of Cadmium on Isolated Tissue Preparations

Table 2 summarizes the contractile responses of various isolated artery preparations to externally applied cadmium in the range $10^{-4}-10^{-8}$ M Cd. Helically cut arterial strips were evaluated under conditions of externally imposed isometric tension applied by stretching the arterial strips. A decrease in the recorded isometric tension from that applied externally was interpreted to represent vascular smooth muscle relaxation. Conversely, an increase in isometric tension was interpreted to represent smooth muscle contraction. As is readily apparent from Table 2, the ability of cadmium to act by direct or indirect mechanisms to induce vascular smooth muscle contraction or relaxation has not been extensively studied. The responses observed by PERRY et al. (1967 a) and THIND et al. (1970 b) were inconclusive, although a relaxation response predominated in the study by Thind. In 56% of the aortic strips studied, cadmium exposure resulted in a decrease in initial isometric tension. The response to cadmium was not correlated with the buffer cadmium concentration. The observations reported by TODA (1973 a) were consistent with the interpretation that cadmium induces smooth muscle relaxation at concentrations greater than 2×10^{-5} M.

In studies using calcium-depleted arterial preparations (HAYASHI and TODA 1977), the response to cadmium was similar to that reported by TODA (1973 a). The relaxation response reportedly was not dependent upon the cadmium concentration applied to the preparation. An important methodological consideration concerning the results of this study is that the response to cadmium was measured in arterial strips that were depolarized by potassium (25 mM) and calcium depleted. Conceptually, depolarizing the arterial smooth muscle would activate the voltage-dependent calcium channel, thus enabling an assessment of smooth muscle responsiveness to externally applied calcium. Thus, the results ob-

Table 2. Direct action of cadmium on vascular smooth muscle

Blood vessel bioassay model	Cadmium concentration (M)	Measured response	Inferred contractile response	References
Helical strips of thoracic aorta (rabbit)	10^{-4}	Inconsistent: slow contractions noted	Some vasconstrictor effect	PERRY et al. (1967a)
Helical strips of thoracic aorta (rabbit)	5.5×10^{-7}– 5.5×10^{-3}	Unchanged 39%; contraction 5%, relaxation 56%, (no apparent dose-response relationship)	Inconsistent	THIND et al. (1970b)
Helical strips of thoracic aorta (rabbit)	2×10^{-5}, 10^{-4}	Decreased tension (dose-dependent)	Muscle relaxation vasodilator response	TODA (1973a)
Calcium-depleted helical strips of various arteries (dog)	5×10^{-6}, 2×10^{-5}, 10^{-4}	Cerebral artery Decreased tension	Slight persistent relaxation, vasodilator response	HAYASHI and TODA (1977)
	5×10^{-6} 2×10^{-5}, 10^{-4}	Coronary artery Unchanged Decreased tension		
	5×10^{-6} 2×10^{-5}, 10^{-4}	Mesenteric artery Unchanged Decreased tension		
Helical strips of thoracic aorta (rat)	9×10^{-8}– 9×10^{-5} 9×10^{-4}	Increased tension Decreased tension	Vascoconstriction at low doses which dissipates upon repeated administration (maximum response at $10^{-7} M$ $CdCl_2$) Vasodilation at higher doses ($> 9 \times 10^{-5} M$	NIWA and SUZUKI (1982)
	9×10^{-7}	Decreased tension with lower calcium concentrations (1.0, 0.4, 0.2 mM $CaCl_2$) relative to response at 2.2 mM $CaCl_2$	Cadmium contractions dependent on external calcium	
Calcium-depleted helical strips of thoracic aorta (rat)	9×10^{-4}	Cadmium-induced contractions	Direct activation of smooth muscle contraction by cadmium	
Helical strips of thoracic aorta (rabbit)	10^{-4}	Decreased ^{45}Ca uptake under basal and stimulated (30 m M KCl) conditions	Calcium influx, but not efflux, altered in the presence of cadmium	HATTORI et al. (1983)

Table 2 (continued)

Blood vessel bioassay model	Cadmium concentration (M)	Measured response	Inferred contractile response	References
Coronary arteries of intact perfused heart (rat)	3×10^{-6}	Coronary flow rate decreased in conjunction with reductions in perfusate calcium (5.0, 3.5, 1.8, 0.9 m M CaCl$_2$)	Cadmium-induced coronary vasoconstriction inversely related to external calcium	PRENTICE et al. (1984)

tained when cadmium was added to the medium in the absence of calcium relate to the ability of cadmium to substitute for calcium, rather than the ability of cadmium to induce calcium-mediated smooth muscle excitation–contraction coupling. These results indicated that cadmium cannot substitute directly for calcium to initiate contraction. Furthermore, this experimental approach demonstrated that cadmium (5×10^{-6}–10^{-5} M) specifically inhibited calcium-activated smooth muscle contraction via the voltage-dependent calcium channel (HAYASHI and TODA 1977). This effect of cadmium was concentration dependent, as demonstrated by the graded attenuation of isometric tension development with increasing cadmium concentration. The sensitivity of various artery preparations to this action by cadmium was greater in cerebral than carotid and mesenteric arteries. Cysteine (1 mM cysteine hydrochloride) partially reversed the response to cadmium, suggesting a superficial site of action with a binding affinity for cadmium lower than the affinity of cadmium for SH groups. Subsequent studies have demonstrated that cadmium (10^{-4} M) acts to suppress calcium-activated vascular smooth muscle contraction by attenuating calcium (^{45}Ca) influx through the voltage-dependent calcium channels (HATTORI et al. 1983). Rapid and slow calcium efflux were not affected by cadmium administration.

In contrast to the reported relaxant effects of cadmium on vascular smooth muscle (THIND et al. 1970 b; TODA 1973 a), NIWA and SUZUKI (1982) have demonstrated that low concentrations of cadmium (9×10^{-8}–9×10^{-5} M) induced isometric contractions in normal helically cut strips from the thoracic aorta of the rat. This effect of cadmium was dependent directly on the calcium concentration of the supporting medium (Locke's solution) and was abolished at a buffer calcium concentration of 0.1 mM CaCl$_2$. As indicated in Table 2, the maximal effective concentration for inducing peak contractile responses was 9×10^{-7} M CdCl$_2$. Increasing the cadmium concentration beyond this level diminished the force of the isometric contraction until at 9×10^{-4} M CdCl$_2$ relaxation was manifested. Repeated administration (30-min intervals) of cadmium (9×10^{-7} M CdCl$_2$) to the same arterial muscle preparation caused a decrement in the magnitude of the contractile response induced by cadmium, ending in complete abolition of this effect. However, the responsiveness of these preparations to norepinephrine persisted at a level comparable to control. Voltage-dependent activation of these arterial smooth muscle preparations by varying concentrations of potassium was enhanced by cadmium at low levels (9×10^{-7} and 9×10^{-8} M) and suppressed at higher concentrations (9×10^{-6} and 9×10^{-5} M). Similar responses were observed following receptor-dependent activation of these arterial preparations by variable doses of norepinephrine. The sensitivity to barium-induced activation of smooth muscle contraction was also increased at these low cadmium concentrations and attenuated by higher doses (9×10^{-6} and 9×10^{-5} M). This augmented sensitivity to barium at low cadmium concentrations suggests that at low doses cadmium facilitates barium influx. Overall, the effects of low cadmium concentrations on the sensitivity of voltage-dependent and receptor-dependent processes that activate smooth muscle contractions suggest that cadmium may act to accelerate calcium entry through these membrane calcium channels. Conversely, at higher cadmium concentrations, cadmium appears to inhibit calcium entry through both voltage-dependent and receptor-operated calcium channels.

Recently, PRENTICE (1982) and PRENTICE et al. (1984) have demonstrated that cadmium (3×10^{-6} M $CdCl_2$) caused a pronounced coronary vasoconstriction in the isolated perfused rat heart. In contrast to the findings of NIWA and SUZUKI (1982), the vasoconstrictor effect of cadmium was most pronounced at low perfusate calcium concentrations (0.9 and 1.8 mM $CaCl_2$) and was partially reversed at elevated perfusate calcium levels (3.5 and 5.0 mM). This cadmium-induced coronary vasoconstriction was manifested in hearts which were characterized by depressed contractility and prolonged diastolic intervals. Thus, increased ventricular wall compression of the coronary vessels was not a factor in this effect. The site of action of cadmium in this tissue preparation (e.g., arteries, arterioles) is uncertain. Moreover, since coronary vascular resistance is under significant local metabolic control, the possibility exists that the vasoconstrictor response to cadmium may be mediated indirectly or partially by local metabolic factors. This assertion is especially pertinent in view of the pronounced changes in myocardial energy metabolism induced by cadmium, which were inversely related to the perfusate calcium concentration.

Overall, these experimental findings suggest that cadmium has significant, direct effects on smooth muscle contractile processes. These actions appear to be concentration dependent, with low doses eliciting a constrictor response, while higher doses induce a vasodilator response. The fact that the evidence indicating a cadmium-induced vasoconstrictor response arises from only one species (rat) is somewhat disconcerting and indicates the need for additional studies in different species. The rather small number of studies concerned with the direct actions of cadmium on vascular smooth muscle contractile processes precludes any conclusive remarks.

3. In Vivo Studies

Circulatory disorders associated with chronic or acute cadmium administration have been observed in renal, testicular, adrenal, uteroplacental, and neural tissues (CHIQUOINE 1964; CLEGG and CARR 1967; FOWLER et al. 1975; GABBIANI et al. 1967; GUNN et al. 1963, 1966, 1968; JOHNSON 1969; KANISAWA and SCHROEDER 1969; LEVIN and MILLER 1981; MASON et al. 1964; NIEMI and KORMANO 1965; SCHLAEPFER 1971; SETCHELL and WAITES 1970; WAITES and SETCHELL 1966;

WONG and KLAASSEN 1982). As shown in many of these studies, the degenerative changes in the capillary endothelium do not occur uniformly. This apparent differential sensitivity to cadmium may be caused by a number of factors, including capillary diffusion gradients determined by local metabolic factors, which would affect the relative membrane surface area of the endothelial cells exposed to cadmium, and quantitative and qualitative differences in the chemical composition and properties of the membrane, which would affect intrinsic diffusion characteristics and reactivity. The structural changes in the vascular beds of these tissues that occur following cadmium-treatment generally lead to a decreased organ perfusion due to a restriction in blood flow. Early functional evidence derived from studies concerned with the effects of cadmium on the testes (CHIQUOINE 1964; CLEGG and CARR 1967; GUNN et al. 1963, 1966, 1968; JOHNSON 1969; NIEMI and KORMANO 1965; WAITES and SETCHELL 1966) indicated that acute cadmium exposure produced a pronounced vascular constriction that primarily affected the artery of the ductus deferens, the internal spermatic artery, and the pampiniform plexus. This observation led to the hypothesis of two distinct mechanisms for the action of cadmium. The endothelial mechanism proposed that the primary site of action was the capillary endothelium and that the associated vascular damage was a secondary effect. Functional disturbances is endothelial permeability characteristics caused by an increase in the intercellular gaps of the endothelium would lead to interstitial fluid retention and edema, ultimately leading to increased interstitial pressure and compression of capillary and possibly arteriolar beds. The resultant effect, it was argued, would be a decrease in effective organ perfusion, a decline in nutritive blood flow, cellular ischemia, and necrosis (PAŘÍZEK and ŽAHOŘ 1956; PAŘÍZEK 1957). Alternatively, the vascular mechanism asserts that cadmium acts primarily on the vasculature, causing vasoconstriction and vascular injury, which leads to secondary endothelial damage, interstitial fluid accumulation, and ultimately, necrotic changes in the tissue (GUNN et al. 1963).

The chronology of the functional and structural changes that occur following cadmium treatment has been investigated to assess the validity of these mechanistic hypotheses. It should be noted that both vascular and endothelial damage were manifested in response to cadmium in these studies; the chronological sequence of changes was evaluated to define which occurred first. Functional (CLEGG and CARR 1967; JOHNSON 1969; SETCHELL and WAITES 1970; WAITES and SETCHELL 1966), angiographic (NIEMI and KORMANO 1965), and microscopic (CHIQUOINE 1964; CLEGG and CARR 1967; JOHNSON 1969) evidence is consistent with the interpretation that the vascular bed and the blood flow of the testes are altered very soon after injection. No direct evidence has been presented demonstrating a direct vasoconstrictor action of cadmium on testicular circulation. Instead, the experimental findings support the concept that cadmium acts primarily to increase capillary permeability by affecting the intercellular gap junction distances and thereby promoting fluid leakage from the vascular compartment (endothelial mechanism). Concomitant with these changes, tissue blood flow is restricted. This interpretation is consonant with the reported actions of cadmium in other vascular beds (e.g., adrenal artery, uteroplacental circulation, neuronal vasculature (LEVIN and MILLER 1981; SCHLAEPFER 1971). For example, uteroplacental and adrenal blood flow have been shown to be diminished in pregnant rats following acute cadmium administration (LEVIN and MILLER 1981). During the early phase of the cadmium-induced depression in fetoplacental and adrenal blood flow, maternal cardiac output was unaffected. These observations suggest a vascular action of cadmium on the uteroplacental and adrenal arteries, rather than an effect secondary to a cardiodepressive action on the maternal circulatory system. Since organ blood flow is proportional to its arteriovenous pressure gradient and inversely related to the vessel resistance, the diminished organ blood flow reported in this study would be predicted to represent the direct or indirect effect of cadmium on arterial resistance, assuming a constant or even a moderately increased systemic blood pressure. As before, in the studies concerned with the action of cadmium on testicular circulation, the possibility exists that cadmium may cause an increased interstitial fluid pressure through effects on capillary permeability, thereby contributing to the reduced organ perfusion. Alternatively, cadmium may act directly to increase smooth muscle tone, thereby increasing arterial resistance. The actual mechanistic basis for the actions of cadmium on these vascular beds cannot be determined with certainty from existing information. Overall, the vascular effects caused by acute injections of cadmium at toxic doses demonstrate that cadmium can directly influence the functional properties of vascular tissue, thereby altering organ blood flow which leads to cellular and tissue degeneration.

The vascular effects of cadmium following chronic, subacute exposures have not been extensively investigated; however, those studies which have been published suggest that cadmium induces significant morphological changes that have functional significance (FOWLER et al. 1975; KANISAWA and SCHROEDER 1969). Significant, age-dependent structural changes were detected in the renal vasculature of rats administered cadmium in the drinking water ($4.4 \times 10^{-5} M$ $Cd(CH_3COO)_2$) from 15 to 42 months (KANISAWA and SCHROEDER 1969). These lesions were most pronounced in kidneys from cadmium hypertensive rats and consisted primarily of a "... generalized thickening of the renal arterioles, and small-and-medium-sized arteries, with proliferation of endothelial cells, subintimal fibroblasts, and especially the smooth muscle cells of the media. The lumina were narrowed. These changes were confined to subinternal and medial areas of the vessels, and were similar in small arteries and arterioles ..." (KANISAWA and SCHROEDER 1969) of the kidney, spleen, testes, and interstitial tissue of the pancreas.

In a parallel study by FOWLER et al. (1975), rats treated with cadmium ($1.8 \times 10^{-6}, 1.8 \times 10^{-5}, 1.8 \times 10^{-4}, 1.8 \times 10^{-3} M$ $CdCl_2$) for 5 weeks were characterized by significant changes in the morphology of renal blood vessels. This chronic cadmium exposure produced renal arteriolar constriction, mild dilation of the larger arteries, and a diffuse capillary fibrosis at all dose levels. These changes were interpreted to suggest that effective renal circulation would decrease with time in conjunction with the pathologic changes. The actions of cadmium on the renal vasculature were independent of the cadmium dose administered to the rats. The consistent findings reported in these studies suggest that chronic cadmium exposure, even at very low doses ($1.8 \times 10^{-6} M$), may induce significant morphological changes in the arterial vasculature of the kidney, especially smooth muscle hypertrophy. Changes of this nature, which influence renal blood flow, will have profound effects on blood flow autoregulation in the kidney, and possibly systemic circulation as well. KANISAWA and SCHROEDER (1969) found that these vascular morphological changes were not confined to renal blood vessels. In addition, these chronic exposure studies demonstrated, rather convincingly, that cadmium acts on vascular tissue through distinctly different mechanisms when administered chronically, as opposed to acutely. This marked disparity between the vascular effects of acute and chronic doses of cadmium may provide some insights concerning the general systemic circulatory responses (hypotension versus hypertension) to similar doses of cadmium.

III. Reactivity of Vascular Tissue Following Chronic or Acute Cadmium-Treatment

1. Responses to Vasoactive Agents Activating Receptor-Operated Calcium Channels

Appendix A provides a compendium of the literature pertaining to experimental conditions and the reported effects of chronic and acute exposures to cadmium on vascular reactivity to norepinephrine, epinephrine, tyramine, histamine, angiotensin, and bradykinin. In the studies concerned with the systemic responses to intravenously or intra-arterially administered doses of vasoactive substances, the effects were inferred from the pressor (blood pressure) changes relative to the control groups (untreated with cadmium). The majority of both the in vivo and in vitro studies have indicated that the sensitivity of cadmium-exposed vascular tissue to catecholamine (and vasoactive peptide agent) stimulation is either decreased or unchanged (IANNACCONE et al. 1981; NIWA and SUZUKI 1982; PORTER et al. 1975; SCHROEDER et al. 1970; THIND et al. 1970 a, b; TODA 1973 a; WILLIAMS et al. 1978). Several notable exceptions have been reported that involve methodological modifications in the conditions under which the responses were measured (FADLOUN and LEACH 1981; NECHAY et al. 1978; PERRY et al. 1967).

FADLOUN and LEACH (1981) are the only investigators to have reported an increased vascular response (blood pressure) to norepinephrine in cadmium-treated animals. The responses to norepinephrine were made in pithed rats pretreated for 12 days with intraperitoneal cadmium injections (10^{-6} M $CdCl_2$). Correlative studies performed in these same animals demonstrated that in response to stimulation of the lower sympathetic spinal efferents (T-10 to L-1) the systemic pressor effect was significantly less in cadmium-treated rats than controls. A second methodological variant of interest is that reported by WILLIAMS et al. (1978). Unlike the other studies in which arterial smooth muscle preparations were preincubated with cadmium for varying periods of time, these investigators observed an increased contractile response to norepinephrine when it was administered concurrently with very low cadmium concentrations (10^{-7}–10^{-6} M). At higher cadmium concentrations, the reactivity of these preparations was diminished. Although these latter observations are instructive in terms of future areas of research, the consensus of the results from the literature is that vascular smooth muscle from animals either pretreated with cadmium or exposed to cadmium in vitro is somewhat less responsive to stimulants which activate smooth muscle contraction by promoting increased calcium influx through receptor-operated calcium channels. TOMERA and HARAKAL (1980) have demonstrated in cadmium-hypertensive rabbits that the cyclic adenosine monophosphate content of vascular tissue (aorta) was diminished markedly (decreased by 95%) in response to cadmium exposure. The ability of cadmium to influence cellular cyclic nucleotide levels has been observed in other tissues, as well (NATHANSON and BLOOM 1976; SINGHAL et al. 1976; SINGHAL 1981). This effect of cadmium on cyclic nucleotide metabolism may contribute to the diminished reactivity of cadmium-treated smooth muscle to norepinephrine and other vasoactive hormones. These observations would tend to suggest that higher circulating catecholamine levels and increased adrenergic neurosecretion might be required to maintain sympathetic vascular tone. Indeed, increased circulating levels of norepinephrine have been reported in response to cadmium exposure (REVIS and ZINSMEISTER 1981; REVIS et al. 1981).

2. Responses to Calcium Agonists or Agents Activating Voltage-Dependent Calcium Channels

The vascular reactivity of cadmium-treated vascular smooth muscle preparations to potassium and barium is summarized in Appendix A. NIWA and SUZUKI (1982) have reported that the isometric force developed by isolated aortic strips in response to both high potassium and barium was increased in the presence of low cadmium levels (9×10^{-8} and 9×10^{-7} M) and was decreased by the addition of high amounts of cadmium (9×10^{-6} and 9×10^{-5} M). This latter response was in accordance with the effects of cadmium reported by THIND et al. (1970b) and Toda and his coinvestigators (HATTORI et al. 1983; HAYASHI and TODA 1977; TODA 1973a). Generally, these latter studies have utilized 20–6,000 times the dose of cadmium described by NIWA and SUZUKI (1982) as having vasoconstrictor effects. These findings are consistent with earlier observations that suggest that the contradictory vascular responses to cadmium may in part be related to specific and nonspecific actions manifested at low and high concentrations, respectively. These actions of cadmium would appear to involve smooth muscle activation mechanisms which are linked to voltage-activated calcium channels, rather than receptor-activated calcium channels. Recall that within a similar concentration range (10^{-6}–10^{-4} M), cadmium produced a dose-dependent decrease in vascular reactivity to norepinephrine, an activator of the receptor-operated calcium channels (WILLIAMS et al. 1978).

Overall, cadmium at relatively high doses acts to depress the responsiveness of vascular smooth muscle preparations to vasoactive substances that stimulate calcium influx through an activation of voltage-dependent or receptor-operated calcium channels. In this regard, these effects of cadmium are consistent with the earlier described interpretation that cadmium acts as a calcium channel inhibitor. However, the low dose effects of cadmium on vascular tissue are not consistent with this interpretation and suggest that the actions of cadmium at these levels are mediated through an as yet undescribed mechanism. It should be noted that in the study by NIWA and SUZUKI (1982) the supporting medium was Locke's solution. The classical Locke's solution does not contain magnesium (LOCKWOOD 1961), and as such, represents a methodological variant from other studies using similar vascular tissue preparations. Another significant feature of this study was that the calcium : cadmium ratio in the supporting medium (at vasoconstricting cadmium doses) was between $2.4 \times 10^3 : 1$ and $2.4 \times 10^4 : 1$. This ratio is considerably higher than that employed in studies which demonstrated an inhibitory effect (240–0.4). This observation suggests that a competitive interaction between calcium and cadmium may favor calcium when the Ca : Cd ratio is high, thereby permitting calcium influx through these channels. This ratio is also higher than that generally required for organic calcium channel blocker activity (11,000–500) (HAYASHI and TODA 1977). Further studies are required before the low-level effects of cadmium and the sites of action in vascular smooth muscle can be clarified.

E. The Cadmium Hypertension Controversy

The ability of cadmium to induce hypertension in experimental animals and its possible role in human essential hypertension have long been enigmas to scientists and nonscientists alike. The magnitude of the blood pressure increases reported by SCHROEDER and VINTON (1962) and by SCHROEDER (1964) were most extraordinary; however, when other investigators were unable to reproduce effects of similar magnitude, skepticism about this relationship became somewhat pervasive within the scientific and clinical communities. As a result, a common perception of the effects of cadmium on blood pressure is that cadmium-induced hypertension is an esoteric finding that manifests itself in only a few laboratories and only in highly selected animal populations. In defense of this posture the early observations of Schroeder were indeed misleading and have contributed to the subsequent confusion about the magnitude of the potential effect of cadmium on systemic blood pressure. The studies reported in 1962 and 1964 grouped the blood pressures from the cadmium-treated populations and divided them into two categories: hypertensive (responders); and normotensive (nonresponders). Thus, the average pressures for the cadmium-exposed population represented only the subpopulation that responded to cadmium by developing hypertension. The inherent bias of this approach was recognized by Schroeder, and in his subsequent work only average pressures for the entire groups of cadmium-exposed rats were reported. These average pressures were consistently 25–50 mm Hg above the average control values, but far below the 80–120 mm Hg differences reported in his early studies (SCHROEDER and VINTON 1962; SCHROEDER 1964; SCHROEDER et al. 1966, 1970; SCHROEDER and BUCKMAN 1967). Obviously, changing the method of reporting the blood pressure responses rationalizes some, but not all, of the differences in the magnitude of the pressure responses to cadmium observed by Schroeder and other investigators (BOSCOLO et al. 1980, 1981; DOYLE et al. 1974; EAKIN et al. 1980; FINGERLE et al. 1982; FRICKENHAUS et al. 1976; HADLEY et al. 1979; KOPP and HAWLEY 1978; KOPP et al. 1978c, 1980a–d, 1983a, b; KOTSONIS and KLAASSEN 1977; LOESER and LORKE 1977a, b; OHANIAN et al. 1978; PERRY and ERLANGER 1974; PERRY et al. 1976, 1977, 1979, 1982; PETERING et al. 1979; REVIS

1978; Revis et al. 1981, 1983; Tomera and Harakal 1980). A summary of the existing literature on cadmium and its relationship to hypertension is presented in the pages that follow in an attempt to resolve some of the misconceptions that surround this controversial issue.

I. Experimental Animal Studies

1. Chronic Oral Exposure

Appendix B summarizes the conditions and experimental findings of studies concerned with the effects of oral cadmium exposure on the systemic blood pressure of experimental animals. Cadmium-induced hypertension has been reported from nine laboratories (Boscolo et al. 1980, 1981; Hadley et al. 1979; Kopp et al. 1980a–d, 1983a, b; Ohanian et al. 1978; Perry and Erlanger 1974, 1982; Perry et al. 1976, 1977, 1979, 1980; Revis 1978; Revis et al. 1981, 1983; Schroeder and Vinton 1962; Schroeder 1964; Schroeder and Buckman 1967; Walker and Moses 1979), while a similar number of laboratories have reported that cadmium exposure was not associated with a significant pressor response (Doyle et al. 1974; Eakin et al. 1980; Fingerle et al. 1982; Frickenhaus et al. 1976; Kotsonis and Klaassen 1978; Loeser and Lorke 1977a, b; Petering et al. 1979). The report by Walker and Moses (1979) was excluded from Appendix B owing to a lack of reported statistical evaluation of the data. The authors reported that female Sprague-Dawley rats maintained on laboratory chow diets and cadmium-supplemented distilled water (4.2×10^{-5} M Cd(NO$_3$)$_2$) for 9 months had systolic blood pressures of 155 mm Hg compared with 96 mm Hg for the control group. Generally, in studies where cadmium exposure was not associated with a significant pressor effect, the duration of the exposure period was relatively short, often less than 6 months (Table 3). Closer inspection of the blood pressures in the male populations that comprised the control groups in these studies has yielded an interesting observation (Table 3). Where cadmium had no significant effect on the blood pressures of treated rats, the corresponding control populations averaged 15–20 mm Hg above those in studies in which a hypertensive response to cadmium was described. A similar comparison of the female control populations did not reveal any major difference. The differences between the male control populations are somewhat disconcerting, considering that the magnitude generally represents that of the pressor response induced by cadmium in recent studies (Boscolo et al. 1980, 1981; Hadley et al. 1979; Kopp et al. 1980a–d, 1982, 1983a, b; Ohanian et al. 1978; Perry and Erlanger 1974, 1982; Perry et al. 1976, 1977, 1979, 1980; Revis 1978; Revis et al. 1981, 1983; Tomera and Harakal 1980). This disparity in the male control populations points to a fundamental problem that relates to the hypertension controversy, namely that the significance of high control blood pressures should be taken into consideration when interpreting the effects of cadmium on systemic blood pressures. Often, this consideration is overlooked when concluding that an insignificant effect was produced. Under these circumstances such an interpretation may be misleading. The absence of a standardized control population common to these studies precludes interlaboratory comparisons of control blood pressures to assess the effects contributed by exter-

Table 3. Comparison of systolic blood pressures in control rat populations in which hypertension was or was not induced by cadmium

Exposure period (months)	Systolic blood pressure (mmHg)				References
	Cadmium hypertension		Nonsignificant cadmium effect		
	Male	Female	Male	Female	
6–8	112[a]	112[a]			Schroeder and Vinton (1962)[f]
30	109[a]	116[a]			Schroeder (1964)[f]
13–14		84[a]			Schroeder and Buckman (1967)[f]
12		110[a]			Perry and Erlanger (1974)[f]
5–6			118[a]	107[a]	Doyle et al. (1974)[g]
3				112[d]	Frickenhaus et al. (1976)[h]
6–12	118[a]	103[a]/91[b]			Perry et al. (1976)[f]
3			121[d]	106[d]	Loeser and Lorke (1977a)[g]
18		114[a]			Perry et al. (1977)[f]
2		NR[o]			Revis (1978)[j]
2–3			157[b]		Kopp and Hawley (1978)[k]
24				116[a]	Kopp et al. (1978c)[f]
5–6			127[b]		Kotsonis and Klaassen (1978)[k]
6–18	118[a]	91[a]			Perry et al. (1979)[f]
12	114[d]				Hadley et al. (1979)[j]
9			121[b]	100[b]	Petering et al. (1979)[k]
15		96[a]			Kopp et al. (1980a)[f]
15		101[a]			Kopp et al. (1980b)[f]
15/18		103[a]/102[a]			Kopp et al. (1980c)[f]
18		110[a]			Kopp et al. (1980d)[f]
12/18		101[a]/113[a]			Perry et al. (1980a)[f]
20–21			145[e]		Eakin et al. (1980)[l]
5–6		132[b]			Boscolo et al. (1980)[k]
5–6		134[b]			Boscolo et al. (1981)[k]
14	101[a,f]		113[a,m]/108[a,n]		Perry and Erlanger (1982)
3–4			150[b]	136[b]	Fingerle et al. (1982)[k]
6		137[b]/133[c]	149[d]		Revis et al. (1983)[j]
18		100[a]			Kopp et al. (1983a)[f]
12		116[a]			Kopp et al. (1983b)[f]

Rat strains:
[a] Long-Evans
[b] Sprague-Dawley
[c] Fischer
[d] Wistar
[e] Oregon State University brown

Diets:
[f] Rye-based diet
[g] Purified basal diet: glucose, vegetable oil, egg white base
[h] Powdered food obtained commercially
[j] Dietary conditions not specified
[k] Commercial pelletized chow diet
[l] Purified basal diet: casein, glucose, vegetable oil base
[m] Commercial chow diet, mineral-fortified water
[n] Commercial chow diet, deionized water
[o] Actual pressure not reported; results reported as increase above control

nal and internal factors (e.g., diet, housing conditions, extraneous environmental cadmium exposures).

The findings summarized in Appendix B and Table 3 indicate that cadmium-induced hypertension has been demonstrated in various animal species: rats, rabbits (THIND 1970a; TOMERA and HARAKA 1980), dogs (THIND and FISCHER 1975), a variety of rat strains (Long-Evans, Sprague-Dawley, and Fischer 344, but not Wistar and Oregon State University brown), in rats of both sexes, and in studies which have utilized rye-based and commercial chow diets, mineral-fortified water (SCHROEDER and VINTON 1962), and deionized water. The differences in composition and mineral contents of the various diets used in these studies are detailed in the footnotes of Appendix B. The cross-species findings add credence to the possibility that similar effects may occur in humans. Hypertension has not been reported in response to cadmium either in studies which have used purified diets (DOYLE et al. 1974; EAKIN et al. 1980) or in studies in which cadmium was administered in the food as $CdCl_2$ (LOESE and LORKE 1977a, b) or as CdS (FRICKENHAUS et al. 1976). It should be noted that in the studies involving dogs (LOESER and LORKE 1977b), the blood pressure values correspond to results obtained from only two animals. These findings indicate that the ability of cadmium to induce hypertension is not necessarily strain, sex, or diet specific. Although considerable information about the experimental conditions of these studies is provided, the rationale for the ability or inability of cadmium to induce hypertension is not readily apparent.

The conditions under which these studies were conducted are considered important determinants of the pressor response to cadmium. Recent reviews summarize the known relationships (PERRY and ERLANGER 1982; PERRY and KOPP 1983; PERRY et al. 1976). A noteworthy consideration regarding the ability of cadmium to induce hypertension is the concentration of cadmium administered to the experimental animals. As shown in Fig. 6, the pressor response to cadmium has a defined dietary maximum, which if exceeded, leads to a diminution of the effect (KOPP et al. 1982). This observation is contrary to intuitive expectations that a large dose of cadmium should yield a greater effect than a lower dose. Thus, the administered dose of cadmium is an important consideration in the pressor response produced.

The mechanistic basis for the hypertension associated with chronic cadmium exposure has not been elucidated. To some extent, the complex pluricausal etiology of hypertension contributes to the difficult task of defining the contributing mechanisms (BEYER and PEULER 1983). Without a well-defined understanding of the functional relationships involved in this response, the potential role of cadmium in human hypertension remains obscure. Various mechanisms have been proposed to explain the cadmium-induced hypertension following chronic exposure in various animal models (BOSCOLO et al. 1980, 1981; CAPRINO and TOGNA 1979; FADLOUN and LEACH 1981; FOWLER et al. 1975; IANNACCONE et al. 1981; NIWA and SUZUKI 1982; PERRY et al. 1967b; PERRY and ERLANGER 1981; REVIS 1978; REVIS et al. 1983; SCHROEDER and BALASSA 1965). These postulated mechanisms are based on experimental findings which indicate that cadmium induces changes that are common to known risk factors in human hypertension. These include: (a) sodium retention (DOYLE et al. 1974; PERRY and ERLANGER 1980,

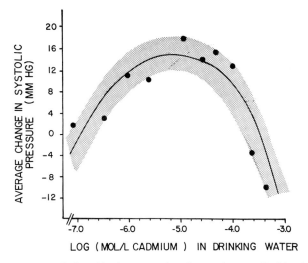

Fig. 6. Dose–response relationship between the change in systolic blood pressure (compared with control) after 18 months exposure to cadmium, plotted against the logarithm of the cadmium concentration (M) added to the drinking water (8.9×10^{-8}–4.4×10^{-4} M $Cd(CH_3COO)_2$). Each *point* corresponds to an average of 16 or more rats per exposure group with a total population of 520 rats represented. The least squares regression curve which approximates this relationship is indicated by the *solid line*. The *shaded area* corresponds to the standard deviation about the regression curve. The apex of the curve depicting the maximal pressor response to cadmium occurred at a cadmium concentration of 4.4×10^{-6} M Cd added to the drinking water. The increased blood pressure at this cadmium concentration corresponds to a 20% increase above control (KOPP et al. 1982)

1981); (b) increased plasma renin activity which leads presumably to increased conversion of angiotensinogen to angiotensin I and subsequently to angiotensin II, a potent vasoconstrictor (PERRY and ERLANGER 1973); (c) increased total peripheral resistance due to cadmium-induced arterial vasoconstriction (NIWA and SUZUKI 1982; PRENTICE 1982; PRENTICE et al. 1984); (d) reduced endogenous kinin activity reflecting an attenuation of the kallikrein–bradykinin system (BOSCOLO et al. 1980, 1981; IANNACCONE et al. 1981); (e) diminished vascular tissue prostaglandin (prostacyclin, PGI_2) production (CAPRINO and TOGNA 1979); (f) altered norepinephrine metabolism leading to an increased plasma half-life (REVIS 1978; REVIS et al. 1983); and (g) promotion of atherosclerotic plaque formation (REVIS et al. 1981; SCHROEDER and BALASSA 1965). Although these individual observations suggest various structure–function relationships, as yet, no mechanism has been proposed that incorporates these pathophysiologic consequences of chronic cadmium exposure into a unified conceptual framework. These observations are interrelated and interdependent in many instances; however, their relative importance (e.g., primary, secondary, tertiary) as contributing factors to the systemic hypertension response cannot be assessed at present. As shown in several human studies, various observations associated with cadmium exposure in experimental animals have been demonstrated in humans exposed to cadmium (BOSCOLO et al. 1978; IANNACCONE et al. 1979; REVIS et al. 1981; VOROBIEVA and EREMEEVA 1980).

This clinical evidence lends credence to the proposed mechanisms derived from the experimental animal studies and suggests that further work with these animal models may provide new insights in this area.

2. Chronic and Acute Injection

Intraperitoneal injections of cadmium were shown to induce hypertension following both chronic and acute administration (Fig. 7; see Appendix B for details). The threshold dose for this response was approximately 10^{-6} mol Cd per kilogram body weight. As shown by HALL and HUNGERFORD (1982), the cadmium-induced increase in systemic blood pressure was more pronounced in the animals while anesthetized as opposed to the conscious state. In isolated instances, hypertension was not induced (PORTER et al. 1974) or was transient (ROACH and DAMUDE 1980). In the chronic injection studies, evidence was presented suggesting a dose–response relationship within a very narrow range of administered cadmium concentrations (1.3×10^{-7}–4.4×10^{-6} mol/kg) (FADLOUN and LEACH 1981; HALL and HUNGERFORD 1982). The ability of cadmium to induce a significant pressor response has been demonstrated in many rat strains (Long-Evans, Sprague-Dawley, Fischer 344, Wistar–Kyoto normotensive, Wistar–Kyoto spontaneously hypertensive, Dahl sensitive – but not resistant) and in New Zealand white rabbits (FADLOUN and LEACH 1981; HALL and HUNGERFORD 1982; HALL and NASSETH 1980; OHANIAN et al. 1978; PERRY and ERLANGER 1973; REVIS 1978; ROACH and DAMUDE 1980; SCHROEDER et al. 1966, 1970; THIND et al. 1970a; WATKINS 1980). Overall, intraperitoneal cadmium injections at low doses were associated with a significant increase in arterial pressure (measured directly or indirectly) through an, as yet, unspecified mechanism. This effect was evident in both short-term and chronic studies and was apparently unaffected by experimental conditions, except for possible anesthetic contributions (HALL and HUNGERFORD 1982).

Intra-arterial and intravenous infusion of cadmium produced responses which were concentration dependent and variable with time. Generally, hypotension was induced during the initial period after injection, but the result was a persistent pressor response at low cadmium doses (9×10^{-7}–4.4×10^{-6} mol/kg intravenously), or a sustained hypotension at higher doses (2.7×10^{-6}–2.8×10^{-5} mol/kg, see Appendix B for details). As first described by ATHANASIU and LANGLOIS (1896), in dogs, intravenous injection of cadmium (1.4×10^{-4} mol/kg) caused transient hypotensive responses followed by latent restorative or hypertensive responses which persisted thereafter. Repeated administration of cadmium abolished this effect. This phasic response to single intravenous cadmium doses has been observed since then by other investigators (FADLOUN and LEACH 1981; PERRY and YUNICE 1965; PERRY et al. 1970). In contrast to the hypotensive effect induced by intravenous cadmium doses, intra-arterial cadmium injection has been reported to produce hypertension without the early hypotensive phase (8.9×10^{-7}–7.1×10^{-6} mol/kg) (PERRY and YUNICE 1965; PERRY et al. 1970). Since cadmium administered intravenously would not be filtered through the hepatic and renal beds before perfusing the heart, the heart may be exposed to a higher concentration of cadmium under these circumstances. As indicated pre-

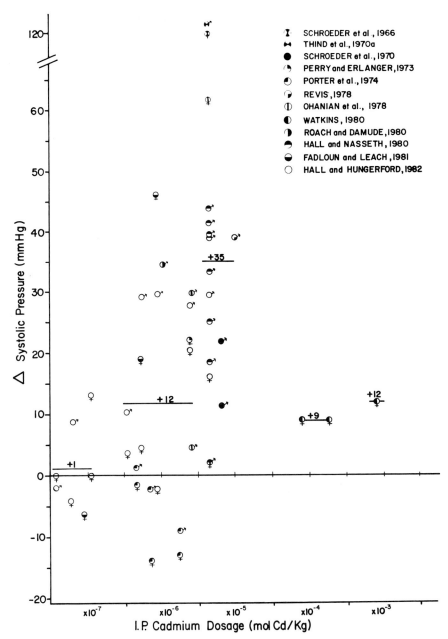

Fig. 7. Graph depicting the changes in the systolic blood pressure induced by chronic intra-peritoneal injection of cadmium at the doses indicated. Detailed information concerning the experimental protocol used in each study is summarized in Appendix B. The numerical value listed above each *horizonal bar* corresponds to the average systolic pressure change reported for the specific doses of cadmium bracketed within the width of each *horizonal bar*. These averaged values are presented only to illustrate the qualitative aspects of the apparent relationship observed between the dose of cadmium administered by intraperitoneal injection and the resultant blood pressure response. Note the qualitative similarity between the apparent hyperbolic nature of this response and the one illustrated in Fig. 6, which depicts the effects of oral cadmium doses on systolic blood pressure

viously, cadmium is a proven negative inotropic agent on the myocardium which suggests that the intravenous dose of cadmium may be sufficient to cause a transient depression of myocardial excitability and contractility. This cardiodepression would be expected to elicit compensatory responses mediated through the sympathetic nervous system, resulting in an elevation in systemic blood pressure. The increased heart rate that has been shown to follow the transient hypotension phase supports the contention that cardiac sympathetic tone is increased during, and contributes to, the period of elevated blood pressure.

Acknowledgments. This work was supported by US Public Health Service grant ES-02397 from the National Institute of Environmental Health Sciences, the Chicago Community Trust Fund, and an award from the Max Goldenberg Foundation. Special thanks go to Ms. Rose Sage, Mrs. Yvette E. Baker, and Mrs. Kay Keenan for typing the manuscript, Ms. Janice M. Feliksik for her technical assistance, Ms. June P. Tow for her technical assistance and for preparing the figures, and Ms. Ruth Zelkha for the fine illustrations. This chapter is dedicated to the memory of Professor Louis S. D'Agrosa, scientist, teacher, and beloved friend.

Appendix A. Summary of reported responsiveness of cadmium-treated (chronic or acute) vascular tissue to vasoactive agents*

Animal, strain, and sex	Vasoactive agent dose	Pressor or contractile response	Method of cadmium administration	References
A. Catecholamines and precursors				
I. Norepinephrine				
1. Systemic responses				
Long-Evans, Blu: (LE) rat, ♂	4.0–5.0×10^{-8} mol/kg i.v.[1]	Decreased	Oral pretreatment[2]	SCHROEDER et al. (1970)
	4.0–5.0×10^{-8} mol/kg i.v.	Unchanged	Acute i.p. injection[3]	
Sprague-Dawley rat, ♀	1.6×10^{-9} mol/kg i.v.	Decreased	Injection pretreatment[4]	PORTER et al. (1975)
Holtzman rat, ♀	3×10^{-9}–3×10^{-8} mol/kg i.v.	Decreased (1.5–3×10^{-8} mol/kg) Unchanged (3×10^{-9} mol/kg)	High-dose injection pretreatment[5]	NECHAY et al. (1978)
	3×10^{-10}–3×10^{-8} mol/kg i.v.	Increased; prolonged duration (3×10^{-10}–1.5×10^{-8} mol/kg) Unchanged (3×10^{-8} mol/kg)	Low-dose injection pretreatment 1–4 weeks after last dose[5,6] Low-dose injection pretreatment 20 weeks after last dose	
Sprague-Dawley, CFE rat, ♀	7×10^{-9}–3×10^{-8} mol/kg i.v.	Increased (7×10^{-9} –1.5×10^{-8} mol/kg in 10^{-6} M CdCl$_2$-pretreated rats) Unchanged (all other treatment groups)	Injection (i.p.) pretreatment[7]	FADLOUN and LEACH (1981)
Sprague-Dawley rat, ♂	2.4×10^{-9} mol/kg i.v.	Decreased	Oral pretreatment[8]	IANNACCONE et al. (1981)
2. Isolated vascular tissue: isolated artery responses				
Holtzman rat, ♀	10^{-10}–10^{-6} M	Increased; sensitivity increased (thoracic aorta)	Cadmium pretreatment (low-dose regimen) 1–4 weeks[9]	NECHAY et al. (1978)
New Zealand white rabbit, ♂	5×10^{-7} M	Dose-dependent decrease with increasing cadmium concentration	Cadmium ($[\text{CdCl}_2] = 7.5 \times 10^{-8}$ –2.5×10^{-4} M) added to muscle bath for 3 s preincubation	WILLIAMS et al. (1978)

Appendix A (continued)

Animal, strain, and sex	Vasoactive agent dose	Pressor or contractile response	Method of cadmium administration	References
Rat, strain and sex unspecified	$7 \times 10^{-7} M$	Unchanged (thoracic aorta)	Cadmium added to muscle chamber[10] 9×10^{-7}, $9 \times 10^{-8} M$ CdCl$_2$ 9×10^{-5}, $9 \times 10^{-6} M$ CdCl$_2$	NIWA and SUZUKI (1982)
New Zealand white rabbit, ♂	$4.9 \times 10^{-8} M$ $4.9 \times 10^{-8} M$	Decreased (thoracic aorta) Unchanged Decreased (no difference between responses of aortic strips from normotensives and cadmium hypertensives to exogenous cadmium) (thoracic aorta)	Injection pretreatment[11] Cadmium ([CdCl$_2$] = 1.1×10^{-4}, 1.4×10^{-4}, $2.2 \times 10^{-4} M$) added to muscle bath 30, 120, 30 min preincubation, respectively)[12]	THIND et al. (1970a)
New Zealand white rabbit, ♂	$4.9 \times 10^{-8} M$	Unchanged Decreased Irreversible effect	Cadmium added to muscle bath 30 min preincubation [CdCl$_2$] = $5.5 \times 10^{-5} M$ [CdCl$_2$] > $5.5 \times 10^{-5} \leqq 5.4 \times 10^{-4} M$ [CdCl$_2$] = $5.5 \times 10^{-4} M$	THIND et al. (1970b)
Albino rabbit, random sex	$2.5 \times 10^{-6} M$	Unchanged Decreased	Cadmium added to muscle bath preincubated 20 min[14] [CdCl$_2$] = $10^{-4} M$ [CdCl$_2$] = $5 \times 10^{-4} M$	TODA (1973a)
New Zealand white rabbit, ♂	$5 \times 10^{-7} M$	Unchanged Decreased Increased	Cadmium added to muscle bath preincubation $2.5 \times 10^{-6} M$ Concurrent addition of cadmium with norepinephrine	WILLIAMS et al. (1978)
II. Epinephrine *1. Systemic responses*				
Sprague-Dawley rat, ♀	2.7×10^{-9} mol/kg i.v.	Unchanged	Injection pretreatment[4]	PORTER et al. (1975)
Sprague-Dawley rat, ♂	6.8×10^{-10} mol/kg i.v. 2.7×10^{-9} mol/kg i.v.	Decreased[15] Decreased[16]	Oral pretreatment[8]	IANNACCONE et al. (1981)

2. Isolated vascular tissue: thoracic aorta responses

Sprague-Dawley rat, ♀	$10^{-9} \times 10^{-5}$ M	Decreased	Injection pretreatment[17]	Porter et al. (1975)
New Zealand white rabbit, ♀	10^{-7} M	Decreased	Cadmium added to muscle bath[18] (no preincubation period specified)	Perry et al. (1967a)
New Zealand white rabbit, ♂	5.4×10^{-8} M	Unchanged after 30 and 75 min preincubation	Cadmium added to muscle bath[13] 6.5×10^{-5} M CdCl$_2$ (30 min preincubation)	Thind et al. (1970b)

III. Tyramine

1. Systemic response

Sprague-Dawley CFE rat, ♀	$3.5, 7.0, 14 \times 10^{-8}$ mol/kg i.v.	Decreased (0.5 and 1 μM Cd-treated groups)	Injection pretreatment[7]	Fadloun and Leach (1981)

2. Isolated vascular tissue: thoracic aorta response

Sprague-Dawley rat, ♀	10^{-6}–10^{-3} M	Decreased	Injection pretreatment[17]	Porter et al. (1975)

B. Vasoactive peptides

I. Angiotensin

1. Systemic responses

Long-Evans, Blu (LE) rat, ♂	$6.3-8 \times 10^{-12}$ mol/kg i.v.[19] (angiotensin I*) $6.3-8 \times 10^{-12}$ mol/kg i.v.[19]	Decreased Unchanged	Oral pretreatment[2] Acute i.p. injection[3]	Schroeder et al. (1970)
Sprague-Dawley rat, ♂	8×10^{-10} mol/kg i.v. (angiotensin I*) $5-10 \times 10^{-10}$ mol/kg i.v. (angiotensin II)	Decreased Unchanged	Oral pretreatment[8]	Iannaccone et al. (1981)

2. Isolated vascular tissue: thoracic aorta responses

Sprague-Dawley rat, ♀	10^{-9}–10^{-6} M (angiotensin amide)	Decreased	Injection pretreatment[17]	Porter et al. (1975)

Appendix A (continued)

Animal, strain, and sex	Vasoactive agent dose	Pressor or contractile response	Method of cadmium administration	References
New Zealand white rabbit, ♀	$2\times10^{-8}\,M$	Increased	Cadmium added to muscle bath[18] (no preincubation period specified)	Perry et al. (1967a)
New Zealand white rabbit, ♂	$9.7\times10^{-9}\,M$	Decreased	Injection pretreatment[11]	Thind et al. (1970a)
	$9.7\times10^{-9}\,M$	Decreased (no difference between responses of aortic strips from normotensives and cadmium hypertensives to exogenous cadmium)	Cadmium ($[CdCl_2]=5.5\times10^{-6}$ and $5.5\times10^{-4}\,M$) added to muscle bath for 240 and 30 min preincubation, respectively[12]	
		Unchanged	Cadmium ($[CdCl_2]=5.5\times10^{-5}\,M$) added to muscle bath for 120 min preincubation[12]	
New Zealand white rabbit, ♂	$9.7\times10^{-9}\,M$	Unchanged	Cadmium added to muscle bath[13] $\leqq 1.1\times10^{-4}\,M$ Cd 30 and 60 min preincubation)	Thind et al. (1970b)
		Decreased (irreversible)	$5.5\times10^{-6}\,M$ Cd (240 min preincubation)	
		Decreased (irreversible only at $5.5\times10^{-3}\,M$ $CdCl_2$)	$\geqq 2.7\times10^{-4}\,M$ Cd (30 min preincubation)	
		Decreased (irreversible)	$5.5\times10^{-4}\,M$ Cd (120 min preincubation)	
Albino rabbit, random sex	$2\times10^{-8}\,M$	Unchanged	Cadmium added to muscle bath[14] preincubated 20 min $[CdCl_2]=10^{-4}\,M$	Toda (1973a)
		Decreased	$[CdCl_2]=5\times10^{-4}\,M$	

II. *Bradykinin*

1. Systemic responses

Animal, strain, and sex	Vasoactive agent dose	Pressor or contractile response	Method of cadmium administration	References
Sprague-Dawley rat, ♂	1.4×10^{-9} mol/kg i.v.	Decreased	Oral pretreatment[8]	Iannaccone et al. (1981)

C. Other vascoactive agents

I. Potassium

1. Isolated vascular tissue responses

Preparation	Concentration	Response	Conditions	Reference
Rat, strain, and sex unspecified	0.13 M	Increased	Cadmium added to muscle chamber[10] [CdCl$_2$]=9×10⁻⁸–9×10⁻⁷ M	Niwa and Suzuki (1982)
New Zealand white rabbit, ♂	0.1 M	Decreased	[CdCl$_2$]=9×10⁻⁶–9×10⁻⁵ M Cadmium added to muscle bath[13] 30 min preincubation	Thind et al. (1970b)
		Decreased (essentially irreversible)	5.5×10⁻⁴ and 5.5×10⁻³ M CdCl$_2$	
		Caused relaxation of K⁺-induced contracture	2.7×10⁻⁴ M CdCl$_2$	
Albino rabbit, random sex	0.025 M	Decreased (dose-dependent with increasing cadmium concentration)	Cadmium added to muscle bath preincubation for 20 min[14] 2×10⁻⁵–5×10⁻⁴ M CdCl$_2$	Toda (1973a)
Albino rabbit, radom sex	0.025 M KCl plus 2.2 M CaCl$_2$	Dose-dependent inhibition of calcium-induced contracture in K⁺-depolarized muscles	5×10⁻⁴ M CdCl$_2$ added to calcium-depleted aortic strips preincubated for 20 min[14,22]	Toda (1973a)
Albino rabbit, random sex	0.030 M	Caused relaxation of K⁺-induced contracture	Cadmium (5×10⁻⁴ M CdCl$_2$) added to muscle bath[20]	Hattori et al. (1983)
Mongrel dogs, random sex	0.025 M KCl plus 2.2 mM CaCl$_2$ stimulation	Decreased calcium-activated contraction in calcium-depleted aortic strips. Susceptibility of arteries to cadmium effect: cerebral > coronary > mesenteric	Cadmium 5×10⁻⁶–5×10⁻⁴ M CdCl$_2$[21]	Hayashi and Toda (1977)

II. Barium

1. Isolated vascular tissue responses

Preparation	Concentration	Response	Conditions	Reference
Sprague-Dawley rat, ♀	10⁻⁶–10⁻³ M Ba(OH)$_2$	Decreased	Injection pretreatment[4]	Porter et al. (1975)
Rat, strain and sex unspecified	0.016 M (BaCl$_2$)	Increased / Decreased	Cadmium added to muscle bath[10] 9×10⁻⁸, 9×10⁻⁷ M CdCl$_2$ 9×10⁻⁶, 9×10⁻⁵ M CdCl$_2$	Niwa and Suzuki (1982)

Appendix A (continued)

Animal, strain, and sex	Vasoactive agent dose	Pressor or contractile response	Method of cadmium administration	References
Albino rabbit, random sex	0.002 M (BaCl₂)	Decreased	Cadmium added to muscle bath[14] preincubation for 20 min 10^{-4}, 5×10^{-4} M CdCl₂	TODA (1973a)
	0.002 M (BaCl₂)	Decreased		
III. Histamine				
1. Isolated vascular tissue response				
Albino rabbit, random sex	5.4×10^{-5} M	Unchanged	Cadmium added to muscle bath[14] preincubation for 20 min 10^{-4} M CdCl₂	TODA (1973a)
		Decreased	5×10^{-4} M CdCl₂	

* Whenever necessary, the administered doses of cadmium and the reported vasoactive agents were converted to concentrations (M/l or mol/kg body weight) using the molecular weights shown:

Angiotensin I	1296	Cadmium acetate	266.53	Norepinephrine	169.18
Angiotensin II (angiotensin II amide 5-valine)	1031.2	Cadmium chloride	183.32	Norepinephrine bitartrate	319.27
Bradykinin	1060.25	Epinephrine	183.2	Norepinephrine HCl	205.64

[1] Dose administered was not expressed per kg; chemical form of norepinephrine was not specified. Calculations based on a body weight of 0.34 kg (stated range 300–380 g) and a norepinephrine formula weight = 205.64 (norepinephrine HCl)

[2] Responses derived from direct arterial blood pressure measurements (femoral artery) performed under sodium pentobarbital anesthesia (40 mg/kg) on rats that had received 10 ppm Cd in their drinking water for 3–6 months

[3] 3×10^{-5} mol Cd(CH₃COO)₂/kg injected i.p. prior to analysis of vasular reactivity. Direct arterial blood pressure responses were monitored from the femoral artery under sodium pentobarbital anesthesia (40 mg/kg) 20 min after blood pressure stabilized

[4] Cadmium pretreatment consisted of one 1.8×10^{-5} mol Cd(CH₃COO)₂/kg and one 8.9×10^{-6} mol Cd(CH₃COO)₂/kg dose injected i.p. 21 days apart. In vivo studies were conducted 14–27 days after last dose. Responses were based on direct arterial blood pressure measurements (carotid artery) performed under Dial-urethane anesthesia (0.6–0.8 ml/kg, i.p.). Responsiveness to acetylcholine (4×10^{-10} mol/kg i.v.), isoproterenol (4×10^{-11} mol/kg), atropine (7×10^{-7} mol/kg), and propranolol (3.4×10^{-6} mol/kg) were also analyzed in this study. The depressor response to acetylcholine was diminished significantly in cadmium-pretreated rats. The reactivity to the other vasoactive agents was unchanged relative to control

[5] High-dose regimen consisted of a series of evenly spaced injections of 6×10^{-6} mol CdCl₂/kg (total dose 7×10^{-5} mol CdCl₂/kg) administered during a 2-week period. Low-dose regimen consisted of a series of evenly spaced injections of 2×10^{-6}–4×10^{-6} mol CdCl₂/kg (total dose 9×10^{-6}–2×10^{-5} mol CdCl₂/kg) administered, respectively, during a 1- to 2-week period. In each instance, route of cadmium administration

was i.p. with 3 mequi. cysteine. Responses were based on direct arterial (carotid artery) blood pressure recording obtained under Dial-urethane anesthesia 1–4 weeks after last administered dose of cadmium

6 20 weeks after administering the last dose of cadmium in the low-dose groups, the pressor responses and the duration of the responses were comparable among control and cadmium-treated rats. A temporal change that was not discussed in this reference relates to the reported results for the control groups. The duration of the pressor response to 1.5 and 3×10^{-8} mol norepinephrine per kilogram in the control groups was increased substantially at this time relative to the corresponding control values at 1–4 weeks. The duration of the pressor response to these norepinephrine doses also increased in the cadmium-treated rats (approximately 25 and 55 s for 1.5 and 3×10^{-8} mol norepinephrine per kilogram, respectively; however, the magnitude of this temporal effect was far less than the corresponding increases observed in the control population (approximately, 80 and 70 s, respectively). Thus, the duration of the blood pressure response to norepinephrine was not diminished with time, but actually was increased 20 weeks after the last cadmium dose was administered. The absence of a significant difference between control and cadmium populations at this time appears to be related more to a change in the responsiveness of the control group to these norepinephrine doses, such that the control population could not be distinguised from the cadmium-treated rats

7 Cadmium as $CdCl_2$ was injected i.p. in doses of 4.4×10^{-7}, 2.2×10^{-6}, or 4.4×10^{-6} mol/kg daily for 12 consecutive days. Responses were determined from direct arterial (carotid artery) blood pressure measurements performed in rats under sodium pentobarbitone anesthesia, artifically respirated and pithed

8 Cadmium (10 or 20 ppm) was administered via the drinking water for a period of 160 days. Responses to vasoactive agents were determined from direct systemic arterial pressure (carotid artery) recordings obtained under sodium pentothal anesthesia (50 mg/kg i.p.)

9 Contractile responses of 5-mm aortic ring segments from rats pretreated with cadmium (see footnote 5) determined relative to control

10 Developed isometric contractile force of spirally cut aortic strips determined in presence or absence of cadmium (9×10^{-8}–9×10^{-5} M $CdCl_2$) in the muscle bath. Following the addition of cadmium to the bath and the stabilization of the subsequent contractile response to cadmium alone, the vasoactive agent was added to the medium. The relative contractile responses of in vitro cadmium-treated aortic strips to vasoactive agents were based on a comparison with control strips not treated with cadmium

11 Rabbits received a series of weekly i.p. injections of 7.5×10^{-6} mol $Cd(CH_3COO)_2$/kg for an average of 8–9 weeks until animals exhibited a sustained hypertension for 1–2 consecutive weeks. The isometric contractile force developed by helical aortic strips from cadmium hypertensives and normotensive controls in response to various vasoactive agents was compared

12 Helical aortic strips were obtained, as before,[11] from cadmium hypertensives and normotensive controls. The norepinephrine- and angiotensin-induced isometric contractile force developed by these aortic strips when pretreated exogenously with cadmium (5.5×10^{-6}–5.5×10^{-4} M $CdCl_2$) for various incubation times (30–240 min) was determined and compared

13 Helical aortic strips from normotensive controls were incubated with various concentrations of exogenously administered cadmium (5.4×10^{-9}–5.4×10^{-3} M $CdCl_2$) for a 30-min preincubation period prior to analysis of reactivity to vasoactive agents. Reversibility of the cadmium-induced changes in vascular responsiveness was determined 40–60 and 120–200 min after removal of cadmium from the muscle bath. Irreversible effect denotes an incomplete restoration of contractile responsiveness after 200 min postincubation in control medium

14 The isometric contractile force developed by helically cut aortic strips obtained from untreated animals in response to vasoactive agents was assessed 20 min after administering the cadmium dose to the muscle bath

15 This dose of epinephrine induced a significant decrease relative to control in both systolic and diastolic blood pressure in the rats treated with 10 µg/ml (10 ppm) cadmium. The pressure response of the rats given 20 µg/ml (20 ppm) in the drinking water did not differ substantially from control

16 The diminished pressor response was more pronounced in the rats treated with 10 ppm in the drinking water

17 Cadmium pretreatment consisted of one 1.8×10^{-5} mol $Cd(CH_3COO)_2$/kg and one 8.9×10^{-6} mol $Cd(CH_3COO)_2$/kg dose injected i.p. 21 days apart. In vitro studies were conducted 9–37 days after last dose. Analyses were based on differential isometric contractile responsiveness of spirally cut aortic strips from cadmium- and control-treated rats to vasoactive agents

18 Developed isometric contractile force of spirally cut aortic strips in response to vasoactive agents determined in the presence or absence of cadmium (10^{-4} M cadmium salt unspecified)

19 Specified as "angiotensin amide (Hypertensin)". The inferred molecular weight of this substance (1031.2) was used to approximate the molarity of the injected solution

20 Isometric contractions induced by K^+ were monitored in the presence or absence of cadmium. Primary focus of this study was to examine effects of cadmium on ^{45}Ca uptake by isolated helical aortic strips during K^+-induced contracture (5 and 120 min after ^{45}Ca added to supporting medium). Determined that ^{45}Ca uptake was attenuated by cadmium. The efflux of ^{45}Ca from these cadmium-treated aortic strips was unchanged

21 Isometric contractile force generated by various isolated calcium-depleted arterial muscle preparations were compared in response with KCl and $CaCl_2$ stimulation in the presence and absence of cadmium. Helical arterial strips from cerebral (basilar and middle cerebral branch) coronary (left ventral intraventricular branch), and mesenteric (distal portion of superior mesenteric) arteries were equilibrated in control buffer for 90–120 min. Arterial strips were then stimulated with 0.025 M KCl to provide a control reference for contractile response (100%). After 35–45 min reequilibration, a 40-min incubation period in calcium-free medium followed, during which time the buffer was replaced every 20 min. Subsequently, cadmium (5–100 μM $CdCl_2$) was added to the arterial muscle preparations for a 20-min preincubation period. The cadmium-treated strips were depolarized with 0.025 M KCl (except cerebral arteries) and, upon stabilization, stimulated with 2.2 mM $CaCl_2$. Comparative responsiveness to calcium stimulation was determined. Findings demonstrated a dose-dependent attenuation of the calcium-induced contractions by cadmium. The susceptibility of the various arteries to the action of cadmium differed

22 Calcium-depleted aortic strips were prepared by incubating tissues in calcium-free media containing 1 mM EGTA for 40 min followed by incubation for an additional 20 min in calcium-free buffer without EGTA. These tissue preparations do not contract in response to 25 mM KCl; however, the addition of 2.2 mM $CaCl_2$ in combination with the KCl induces a 50%–70% maximal response (Toda 1973a)

Appendix B. Summary of experimental animal studies of effects of cadmium on arterial blood pressure following chronic or acute exposure

Animal, sex, strain	Cadmium dosage[1]	Method of blood pressure measurement	Systolic/diastolic pressure difference from control (mmHg)[2]	Cadmium effect	References
A. Chronic oral exposure					
Rats, ♀ and ♂, Long-Evans (weanlings)	4.4×10^{-5} mol/Cd/l "basic water"[3] $(CdCl_2)$ ad lib. 180–240 days[4]	Indirect[5] sodium pentobarbital anesthesia (45 mg/kg, i.p.)	♂ (+NaCl) +27[6] ♀ (+NaCl) +88, (−NaCl) +112	Hypertensive Hypertensive	SCHROEDER and VINTON (1962)
Rats, ♀ and ♂, Long-Evans (weanlings)	4.4×10^{-5} mol/l "basic water"[3] $(Cd(CH_3COO)_2)$ ad lib. 30 months[4]	Indirect[5] sodium pentobarbital anesthesia (45 mg/kg i.p.)	♂ +76[7] ♀ +81[7]	Hypertensive Hypertensive	SCHROEDER (1964)
Rats, ♀, Long-Evans (weanlings)	4.4×10^{-5} mol Cd/l "basic water"[3] $(Cd(CH_3COO)_2)$ ad lib. 400 days[4]	Indirect[5] sodium pentobarbital anesthesia (45 mg/kg i.p.)	+43[8]	Hypertensive	SCHROEDER and BUCKMAN (1967)
Rats, ♀ Long-Evans (weanlings)	8.9×10^{-6}, 2.2×10^{-5}, 4.4×10^{-5}, 8.9×10^{-5}, 2.2×10^{-4}, 4.4×10^{-4} mol Cd/l "basic water"[3] $(Cd(CH_3COO)_2)$ ad lib. 12 months[4]	Indirect sodium pentobarbital anesthesia (35 mg/kg i.p.)	+19 (lowest dose) +14 +27 +5 +9 −12 (highest dose)	Hypertensive Normotensive Hypotensive	PERRY and ERLANGER (1974)
RATS, ♂ and ♀ Long-Evans (weanlings)	4.4×10^{-5} mol Cd/l ad lib. 171 days[9]	Indirect[5] sodium pentobarbital anesthesia (35 mg/kg i.p.)	♂ +7[10] ♀ +9	Normotensive	DOYLE et al. (1974)
Rats, ♀ Stamm FW49 Wistar (150 g)	2.3, 3.6×10^{-4} mol Cd/kg food (CdS) 12 weeks	Indirect[5] conscious animals	0 (lowest dose) +6 (highest dose)	Normotensive	FRICKENHAUS et al. (1976)
Rats, ♂, Long-Evans (LE) ♀ Long-Evans and Sprague-Dawley (SD) (weanlings)	4.4×10^{-5} mol Cd/l "fortified water" $(Cd(CH_3COO)_2)$ Long-Evans 12 months Sprague-Dawley 6 months	Indirect sodium pentobarbital anesthesia (35 mg/kg i.p.)	♂ +17 ♀ LE +11 SD +10	Hypertensive	PERRY et al. (1976)

Appendix B (continued)

Animal, sex, strain	Cadmium dosage[1]	Method of blood pressure measurement	Systolic/diastolic pressure difference from control (mmHg)[2]		Cadmium effect	References
Rats, ♂ and ♀, SPF–Wistar (weanlings)	8.9×10^{-6}, 2.7×10^{-5}, 8.9×10^{-5}, 2.7×10^{-4} mol Cd/g food (CdCl$_2$) ad lib. 3 months[11]	Indirect[5] conscious animals	♂	+ 3 (lowest dose) 0 + 5 0 (highest dose)	Normotensive	Loeser and Lorke (1977a)
			♀	− 3 (lowest dose) − 2 − 5 − 2 (highest dose)	Normotensive	
Dogs, ♂ and ♀, beagle (4–6 months old)	8.9×10^{-6}, 2.7×10^{-5}, 8.9×10^{-5}, 2.7×10^{-4} mol Cd/g food (CdCl$_2$) 3 months[12]	Intra-arterial, catheterization (carotid artery) ether anesthesia	♂	+18/+2[13] −7/−5 +23/+12 +10/+12	Normotensive	Loeser and Lorke (1977b)
			♀	+7/+8[13] +20/+20 0/+8 +10/+10	Normotensive	
Rats, ♀, Long-Evans (weanlings)	8.9×10^{-6}, 2.2×10^{-5}, 4.4×10^{-5}, 8.9×10^{-5}, 2.2×10^{-4}, 4.4×10^{-4} mol Cd/l "basic water"[3] (Cd(CH$_3$COO)$_2$) 18 months[3,4,14]	Indirect[5] sodium pentobarbital anesthesia (35 mg/kg i.p.)		+14 (lowest dose) +16 +17 − 4 −17 −12 (highest dose)	Hypertensive at low doses; normotensive to hypotensive trend at higher doses	Perry et al. (1977)
Rats, ♂, Sprague-Dawley (50–70 days old)	3×10^{-5} mol Cd/l drinking water (CdCl$_2$) ad lib. 60 days	Intra-arterial catheterization (femoral artery) sodium pentobarbital anesthesia (40 mg/kg s.c.)		+25	Hypertensive	Revis (1978)
Rats, ♂, Sprague-Dawley (40–60 days old)	1.1×10^{-3} and 8.9×10^{-5} mol Cd/l drinking water (CdCl$_2$) (0.5% NaCl) ad lib. 71 days[15]	Intra-arterial catheterization (carotid artery) sodium pentobarbital anesthesia (25 mg/kg i.p.)		− 8/−11 (lowest dose) −25/−30 (highest dose)	Normotensive, hypotensive trend	Kopp and Hawley (1978)

Animal	Dose/treatment	Method	Blood pressure change	Result	Reference
Rats, ♀, Long-Evans (weanlings)	4.4×10^{-5} mol Cd/l "basic water"[3] ($Cd(CH_3COO)_2$) ad lib. 24 months	Indirect[5] sodium pentobarbital anesthesia (25 mg/kg i.p.)	+13	Normotensive	Kopp et al., (1978c)
Rats, ♂ and ♀, Sprague-Dawley Dahl, HR, Dahl, HS (weanlings)	8.9×10^{-6}, 2.2×10^{-5}, 4.4×10^{-5}, 8.9×10^{-5} mol Cd/l drinking water ($Cd(CH_3COO)_2$) orally ad lib. 28 weeks[16]	Indirect,[5] ether anesthesia	HS[17] +24 (lowest dose), +20, +14, +8 (highest dose)	Hypertensive / Normotensive	Ohanian et al. (1978)
			HR[17] +5 (lowest dose), +5, +5, +3 (highest dose)	Normotensive	
Rats, ♂, Sprague-Dawley (50–70 days old)	8.9×10^{-5}, 2.7×10^{-4}, 8.9×10^{-4} mol Cd/l deionized water ($CdCl_2$) ad lib. 24 weeks[18]	Intra-arterial catheterization (femoral artery) urethane anesthesia (900 mg/kg i.p.)	+5/+3 (low dose), +7/+6, +14/+14 (highest dose)	Normotensive	Kotsonis and Klaassen (1978)
Rats, ♀, Long-Evans	8.9×10^{-8}, 2.7×10^{-7}, 8.9×10^{-7}, 2.2×10^{-6}, 4.4×10^{-6}, 8.9×10^{-6}, 4.4×10^{-5}, 2.2×10^{-4}, 8.9×10^{-5}, 4.4×10^{-4} mol Cd/l "basic water" ($Cd(CH_3COO)_2$) 18 months[3,4]	Indirect[5] sodium pentobarbital anesthesia (25 mg/kg i.p.)	0 (lowest dose), +1, +18, +19	Normotensive	Perry et al. (1979)
			+14, +14, +16, +22	Hypertensive	
			+7	Normotensive	
			−17	Hypotensive	
			−12 (highest dose), +14	Hypertensive	
Rats, ♂, Wistar, SPF (70 days old)	5.3×10^{-7} mol Cd/l air (CdO) for 30 min examined 1 year postexposure to cadmium aerosol[19]	Indirect[5] no anesthesia specified	+14	Hypertensive	Hadley et al. (1979)
Rats, ♂ and ♀, Sprague-Dawley (weanlings)	3.8×10^{-5}, 7.6×10^{-5}, 1.5×10^{-4} mol Cd/l drinking water ($CdCl_2$) ad lib. 39 weeks[20]	Indirect[4] sodium pentobarbital anesthesia (35 mg/kg i.p.)	♂ −9 (lowest dose), +11, +15 (highest dose)	Normotensive / Hypertensive	Petering et al. (1979)
			♀ −3 (lowest dose), +6, −9 (highest dose)	Hypertensive / Normotensive	

Appendix B (continued)

Animal, sex, strain	Cadmium dosage[1]	Method of blood pressure measurement	Systolic/diastolic pressure difference from control (mmHg)[2]	Cadmium effect	References
Rats, ♀, Long-Evans (weanlings)	4.4×10^{-5} mol Cd/l "basic water",[3,4] ($Cd(CH_3COO)_2$) ad lib. 15 months	Indirect[5] sodium pentobarbital anesthesia (25 mg/kg i.p.)	+19	Hypertensive	Kopp et al. (1980a, b)
Rats, ♀, Long-Evans (weanlings)	4.4×10^{-5} mol Cd/l "basic water",[3,4] ($Cd(CH_3COO)_2$) ad lib. 18–20 months	Indirect[5] sodium pentobarbital anesthesia (25 mg/kg i.p.)	+27	Hypertensive	Kopp et al. (1980c, d)
Rabbits, ♀, New Zealand white	8.9×10^{-6} mol Cd/l ($Cd(CH_3COO)_2$) drinking water ad lib. 34 days	Not stated	+54 (mean arterial pressure difference)	Hypertensive	Tomera and Harakal (1980)
Rats, ♀, Long-Evans (weanlings)	2.2×10^{-5}, 8.9×10^{-5} mol Cd/l "basic water",[3,4] ($Cd(CH_3COO)_2$) ad lib. 12 or 18 months	Indirect[5] sodium pentobarbital anesthesia (25 mg/kg i.p.)	15 (lower dose) +13 (higher dose)	Hypertensive	Perry et al. (1980a)
Rats, ♂, OSU brown (weanlings)	8.9×10^{-4} mol Cd/l distilled water, ad lib. 16 weeks[21]	Indirect[5] conscious animals	−29	Hypotensive	Eakin et al. (1980)
	8.9×10^{-5}, 1.8×10^{-4} mol/l distilled water; given ad lib. 88 weeks[22]	As above	−2 (lower dose) −3 (higher dose)	Normotensive	
Rats, ♂, Sprague-Dawley	1.8×10^{-4} mol Cd/l commercial diet deionized water ($Cd(CH_3COO)_2$) ad lib. 160–180 days[23]	Intra-arterial catheterization (carotid artery) sodium pentobarbital anesthesia (40 mg/kg i.p.)	+34	Hypertensive	Boscolo et al. (1980)
Pigeon, ♂, white Carneau (3 months old)	5.3×10^{-6} mol Cd/l double-deionized water ($CdCl_2$) ad lib. 6 months[24]	Intra-arterial catheterization (pectoral artery to aorta) unanesthetized	+33 +18	Hypertensive	Revis et al. (1981)
Rats, ♂, Sprague-Dawley (adults)	8.9×10^{-5}, 1.8×10^{-4} mol Cd/l deionized water ($Cd(CH_3COO)_2$) ad lib. 160 days[24,25]	Intra-arterial catheterization (carotid artery) sodium pentobarbital anesthesia (40 mg/kg i.p.)	+19/+20 +30/+29	Hypertensive	Boscolo et al. (1981)

Animal	Dose / Administration	Method	Change	Result	Reference
Rats, ♀, Longs-Evans (weanlings)	8.9×10^{-7}, 8.9×10^{-6} mol/l "basic water"[3,4] (Cd(CH$_3$COO)$_2$) ad lib. 14 months[26]	Indirect[5] sodium pentobarbital anesthesia (25 mg/kg i.p.)	Rye diet +10 (low dose) +13 (High dose); Commercial diet −5 (low dose) −1 (low dose)	Hypertensive; Normotensive	PERRY and ERLANGER (1982)
Rats, ♂ and ♀, Sprague-Dawley (weanlings)	4.4×10^{-5}, 1.1×10^{-4}, 2.8×10^{-4} mol Cd/l demineralized water (CdCl$_2$) 4.4×10^{-5} mol Cd/l "basic water"[3] (CdCl$_2$) ad lib. 14 weeks[27]	Indirect[5] conscious animals	♂ −7 (lowest dose)[28] −3 −6 (highest dose) −8 (+basic water) ♀ 0[29] +4 +7 −5	All Normotensive	FINGERLE et al. (1982)
Rats, ♂, (4 months old) multiple strains: Wistar (normotensive)	4.4×10^{-5} mol Cd/l distilled drinking water (CdCl$_2$) ad lib. 6 months	Intra-arterial catheterization sodium pentobarbital anesthesia (45 mg/kg s.c.)	−50/−8	See below; Hypotensive	REVIS et al. (1983)
Wistar (hypertensive) Sprague-Dawley Fischer			−38/+3 +20/+23 +21/+20	Hypotensive Hypertensive Hypertensive	
Rats, ♀, Long-Evans (weanlings)	8.9×10^{-6} mol Cd/l "basic water" (CdCH$_3$COO)$_2$) ad lib. 18 months[3,4,14]	Indirect[5] sodium pentobarbital anesthesia (25 mg/kg i.p.)	+31	Hypertensive	KOPP et al. (1983a)
Rats, ♀, Long-Evans (weanlings)	8.9×10^{-6} mol Cd/l "basic water" (Cd(CH$_3$COO)$_2$) ad lib. 12 months[3,4,14]	Indirect[5] conscious animals	+13	Hypertensive	KOPP et al. (1983b)

B. Injection studies

1. Intraperitoneal administration

Animal	Dose / Administration	Method	Change	Result	Reference
Rats, ♀, Long-Evans 120 days old	1.8×10^{-5} mol Cd/kg body weight Cd$_3$(C$_6$H$_5$O$_7$)$_2$. Single injection, after 3 weeks second injection; 1 week later blood pressure measured	Indirect[5] sodium pentobarbital anesthesia (45 mg/kg i.p.)	+120	Hypertensive	SCHROEDER et al. (1966)

Appendix B (continued)

Animal, sex, strain	Cadmium dosage[1]	Method of blood pressure measurement	Systolic/diastolic pressure difference from control (mmHg)[2]	Cadmium effect	References
Rabbits, ♂, New Zealand white	1.8×10^{-5} mol Cd/kg body weight (Cd(CH₃COO)₂). Single injection for 9 weeks	Indirect[30] conscious	+122	Hypertensive	THIND et al. (1970a)
Rats, ♂, Long-Evans 26 months or 110–180 days	3×10^{-5} mol/kg body weight (Cd(CH₃COO)₂). Single, acute injection; responses measured during 20-min stabilization period	Indirect[5] sodium pentobarbital anesthesia 40 mg/kg i.p.)	+21 (26 months) / +11 (110–180 days)	Hypertensive / Normotensive	SCHROEDER et al. (1970)
Rats, ♀, Wistar 180–200 g	9×10^{-6} mol Cd/kg body weight (Cd(CH₃COO)₂). Single, acute injection; responses measured after 10 min	Intra-arterial catheterization (femoral artery) under sodium pentobarbital anesthesia (45 mg/kg i.p.)	+23	Hypertensive	PERRY and ERLANGER (1973)
Rats, ♀ and ♂, Sprague-Dawley 78 days	1.9×10^{-6}, 3.7×10^{-6}, 7.5×10^{-6} mol Cd/kg body weight (Cd(CH₃COO)₂). Single injections at 10-days intervals for 8 doses or 6 doses (highest exposure group)	Indirect ether anesthesia	♀: − 1 (lowest dose) / − 14 / − 13 (highest dose) / ♂ + 1 / − 2 / − 9	Normotensive / Normotensive	PORTER et al. (1974)
Rats, ♂, Sprague-Dawley 200–300 g	$3{-}5 \times 10^{-5}$ mol Cd/kg body weight (CdCl₂). Single, acute injection; responses measured after 5–10 min	Intra-arterial catheterization under sodium pentobarbital anesthesia (40 mg/kg s.c.)	+38	Hypertensive	REVIS (1978)
Rats, ♀ and ♂, Dahl R, S, Sprague-Dawley ancestors,[31] 16 weeks	1.8×10^{-5} mol Cd/kg body weight (Cd(CH₃COO)₂). Single injection; at 3 weeks and 23 weeks 9×10^{-6} mol Cd/kg body weight injected, responses measured weekly during 27 weeks period after first injection	Indirect[5] ether anesthesia	♀ R + 2 / S +62 / ♂ R + 4 / S +29	Normotensive[32] / Hypertensive / Normotensive / Hypertensive	OHANIAN et al. (1978)

Animal	Dose	Method	Response (change)	Effect	Reference
Rats, ♀, Sprague-Dawley 250 g	$4 \times 10^{-4}, 8 \times 10^{-4}, 4 \times 10^{-3}$ mol Cd/kg body weight (Cd(CH₃COO)₂); responses measured every 2–3 days for 15 days	Indirect[5] conscious	+9 (lowest dose), +9, +12	Hypertensive[33] (transient)	WATKINS (1980)
Rats, ♂, Sprague-Dawley 170–200 g	5.3×10^{-6} mol Cd/kg body weight (CdCl₂) daily for 5-day periods during 6-week period; responses measured daily	Indirect[5] conscious	NR[34]	Hypertensive[35] (transient); Normotensive (sustained)	ROACH and DAMUDE (1980)
Rats, ♂, various strains 5 weeks	1.8×10^{-5} mol/kg body weight (CdCl₂) injected weekly; responses measured 15 and 30 min postinjection	Indirect both conscious and anesthetized (30 mg/kg i.p. sodium pentobarbital)	Anesthetized at 3 weeks[36] — SD: +41, F344: +33, WKY: +44, SHR: +38. Conscious at 6 weeks — SD: +39, F344: +25, WKY: +2, SHR: +18	Hypertensive, Hypertensive, Hypertensive, Hypertensive, Hypertensive, Hypertensive, Normotensive, Hypertensive	HALL and NASSETH (1980)
Rats, ♀, Sprague-Dawley CFE 200–250 g	$4.4 \times 10^{-7}, 2.2 \times 10^{-6}$, 4.4×10^{-6} mol Cd/kg body weight (CdCl₂) injected daily for 12 consecutive days	Intra-arterial catheterization (common carotid artery) anesthetized (60 mg/kg sodium pentobarbitone); rats artificially respirated and pithed	−7 (lowest dose), +18, +46 (+40) (highest dose)	Normotensive, Hypertensive, Hypertensive	FADLOUN and LEACH (1981)
Rats, ♀, Sprague-Dawley 200–250 g	$1.3 \times 10^{-7}, 2.8 \times 10^{-7}, 5.6 \times 10^{-7}, 1.1 \times 10^{-6}, 2.2 \times 10^{-6}, 4.4 \times 10^{-6}, 8.9 \times 10^{-6}, 1.8 \times 10^{-5}$ mol Cd/kg body weight (CdCl₂); responses measured 15 min after injection	Indirect both conscious and anesthetized (30 mg/kg i.p. sodium pentobarbital)	Conscious — 0 (lowest dose), −4, 0, +3, +4, −2, +20, +16 (highest dose)	Normotensive, Normotensive, Normotensive, Normotensive, Normotensive, Normotensive, Hypertensive, Hypertensive	HALL and HUNGERFORD (1982)

Appendix B (continued)

2. Intra-arterial and intravenous administration

Animal, sex, strain	Cadmium dosage[1]	Method of blood pressure measurement	Systolic/diastolic pressure difference from control (mmHg)[2]	Cadmium effect	References
Cats, sex, strain, and age not identified	2.7×10^{-6}–4.4×10^{-6} mol/kg body weight ($CdSO_4$) intravenous injection, effects noted 0–3 min after dose given	Intra-arterial catheterization (carotid artery) anesthesia induced by ether sustained by α-chloralose (60 mg/kg i.v.)	Anesthetized[37] − 2 + 8 + 13 + 10 + 28 + 29 + 27 + 29 − 15 to − 45	Normotensive Hypertensive Hypertensive Hypertensive Hypertensive Hypertensive Hypertensive Hypertensive Hypotensive	DALHAMN and FRIBERG (1954)
Rats, ♀, Sprague-Dawley 200–250 g	8.9×10^{-7}, 3.6×10^{-6}, 7.1×10^{-6}, 2.8×10^{-5} mol/kg body weight ($CdCl_2$ and $CdSO_4$) intra-arterial injection; effects on diastolic pressure noted during 8-min interval postinjection	Intra-arterial catheterization (femoral artery) under anesthesia (30 mg/kg sodium pentobarbital i.p.)	1 min postinjection[38] + 30 (lowest dose) + 25 − 4 − 10 (highest dise) 8 min postinjection + 13 + 11 + 8 + 6	Hypertensive Hypertensive Normotensive Hypotensive Hypertensive Hypertensive Normotensive Normotensive	PERRY and YUNICE (1965)
Rats, ♀, Wistar 180–220 g	1.8×10^{-6} mol/kg body weight ($CdCl_2$) injected either intra-arterially (femoral artery) (i.a.), or intravenously (femoral vein) (i.v.); responses (diastolic pressure change) ... continuously for	Intra-arterial catheterization (femoral artery) under sodium pentobarbital anesthesia (35 mg/kg i.p.)	1 min postinjection + 26 (i.a.) − 11 (i.v.) 8 min postinjection + 13 (i.a.) + 15 (i.v.)	Hypertensive Hypotensive Hypertensive Hypertensive	PERRY et al. (1970)

Animal	Dosage[1]	Method[5]	Response[2]	Classification[2]	Reference
Rats, ♀, Sprague-Dawley 103 g	1.8×10^{-5} mol/kg body weight injected intravenously; responses (systolic pressure) determined 15 and 30 min postinjection	Indirect under sodium pentobarbital anesthesia (30 mg/kg i.p.)	+33 (15 min) +30 (30 min)	Hypertensive Hypertensive	HALL and NASSETH (1980)
Rats, ♀, Sprague-Dawley CFE 200–250 g	4.4×10^{-7}, 2.2×10^{-6}, 4.4×10^{-6} mol/kg body weight (CdCl$_2$) injected intravenously; responses – systolic (diastolic) pressures – determined at successive times for 32 min postinjection	Intra-arterial catheterization (common carotid artery) anesthetized (60 mg/kg sodium pentobarbitone); rats artifically respirated and pithed	1 min postinjection [39] + 1 (+2) + 4 (+4) − 1 (−9) 8 min postinjection + 2 (+ 4) + 5 (+ 7) +16 (+13)	Normotensive Normotensive Systolic normotensive Diastolic hypotensive Normotensive Normotensive Hypertensive	FADLOUN and LEACH 1981

[1] The standard expression of dosage in these studies is generally ppm (μg Cd/g(ml) H_2O; however, since concentrations are expressed uniformly as molarities throughout this chapter, the reported ppm values were converted to M to maintain consistency. A value of $8.9 \times 10^{-6} M$ Cd is equivalent to 1 ppm Cd. The cadmium salt used in each study is shown in parentheses

[2] These values correspond to those reported at the conclusion of the experiment. Unless otherwise specified, multiple consecutive measurements were performed on each animal and the average of these was computed to determine the blood pressure for each animal. The increase or decrease in blood pressure was based on the group means. The term "hypertensive" is used to denote a significant increase; "normotensive" is used to denote a nonsignificant change; and "hypotensive" refers to a significant decrease in blood pressure

[3] The term "basic or fortified water" refers to deionized water (resistance $> 1 M\Omega$) with added trace elements: $1.7 \times 10^{-5} M$ Co (1 ppm); $1.0 \times 10^{-5} M$ Mo (1 ppm), $1.8 \times 10^{-4} M$ Mn (10 ppm), $7.6 \times 10^{-4} M$ Zn (50 ppm), $7.9 \times 10^{-5} M$ Cu (5 ppm). These levels of trace metals approximate the amounts normally ingested from standard commercial rat foods, if 30 ml water was consumed per rat per day (SCHROEDER and VINTON 1962)

[4] The rats were maintained on a prepared diet consisting of coarsely ground flour 60%; dried skim milk 30%; corn oil 9%; and sodium chloride 1%; enriched with ferrous sulfate and vitamins (50 mg niacin; 10 mg pantothenic acid; 1.0 g choline chloride; 100 mg pyridoxine; 5,000 IU vitamin A; 1,000 IU vitamin D per kilogram food). The level of cadmium contained in the food was below the detection limit ($< 1.8 \times 10^{-10}$ mol Cd (0.02 μg)/g food

[5] Indirect refers to various plethysmographic methods involving the noninvasive measurement of arterial pressure from the caudal tail artery

[6] Various amounts of NaCl were added to the fortified drinking water: 0, 0.5%, 1.0%, and 1.5%. The results do not specify blood pressures according to the different NaCl regimens, but instead are expressed according to diets with, and without NaCl, and without NaCl. No blood pressures for the male rats without NaCl were presented

7 When the author presented the original results, the systolic pressure values for "normotensives" and "hypertensives" from both the control and cadmium-treated groups were reported separately. Since this practice of reporting subpopulation findings has not been generally adopted and is considered, therefore, to be a nonstandard method of expression, the differences in the mean systolic blood pressure values for the control and cadmium-treated rats are based on the average of all control and all cadmium-treated rats at 30 months, irrespective of whether or not they were defined as hypertensive or normotensive

8 Systolic blood pressures reported in this study for "cadmium-fed normal" and "cadmium-fed elevated" were averaged and the differences presented here are based on group averages

9 Chromium was added to the drinking water (8.6 × 10^{-5} M Cr, 4.5 ppm Cr). The quality of the drinking water (e.g., deionized, distilled, tap) was not specified. The water was not otherwise fortified with essential minerals. The basal diet contained as mol/kg diet (ppm): Se 6.3 × 10^{-7} (0.05 ppm); Cu 8.8 × 10^{-5} (5.6 ppm); Zn 2.0 × 10^{-4} (13 ppm); Fe 6.3 × 10^{-4} (35 ppm); Mn 8.2 × 10^{-4} (45 ppm); Mg 1.6 × 10^{-2} (400 ppm); K 5.1 × 10^{-2} (2,000 ppm); Na 1.7 × 10^{-1} (3,935 ppm); Ca 1.3 × 10^{-1} (5,200 ppm); P 1.3 × 10^{-1} (4,000 ppm)

10 "The systolic blood pressure was taken as the lowest of 3 consecutive measurements within 6 mmHg" (Doyle et al. 1974)

11 Rats were maintained on tap water and given a diet of powdered Altromin (Altrogge, Lage/Lippe) ad lib. The cadmium was mixed with the powdered feed

12 Dogs were maintained on tap water and given a diet of powdered Altromin H ad lib. The cadmium was mixed with the powdered feed and given to the animals in weighed aliquots

13 Reported blood pressures represent the average values for two animals at each exposure level

14 Pressures are presented at 18 months, rather than 30 months, owing to the increased mortality that occurred among all groups, particularly the treated populations during the last 12 months of the study period. The mineral composition of the rye-based diet was analyzed and presented in this study. The average amounts detected were as follows, mol per kilogram food: Zn 5.4 × 10^{-4} (35 ppm); Hg <2.5 × 10^{-8} (<0.005 ppm); Se 4.7 × 10^{-6} (0.37 ppm); Fe 7.5 × 10^{-4} (42 ppm); Mn 4.2 × 10^{-4} (23 ppm); Cu 5.2 × 10^{-5} (3.3 ppm); Ni 4.9 × 10^{-6} (0.29 ppm); Cr <9.6 × 10^{-7} (<0.05 ppm); Na 2.6 × 10^{-1} (5,900 ppm); Ca 9.5 × 10^{-2} (3,800 ppm); K 1.9 × 10^{-1} (7,600 ppm); Mg 5.8 × 10^{-2} (1,400 ppm); Cd 1.2 × 10^{-7} (0.0137 ppm). These values are relevant for later studies conducted by Perry et al. and collaborative studies with Kopp et al. The added vitamins include calciferol 1.25 mg; calcium pantothenate 2.5 mg; retinol palmitate 5 mg; niacin 12.5 mg; pyridoxine monohydrate 25 mg; and choline chloride 250 mg (Perry and Erlanger 1982)

15 Rats were maintained on a commercial diet (Purina chow) ad lib.

16 Rats were maintained on a special diet (Agway Inc., Country Foods Division, Syracuse, New York) found to contain 7 × 10^{-4} mol Cd per gram food. The control water contained 5.3 × 10^{-6} M Cd/l

17 Values were not reported according to the sex of the animals

18 Rats were maintained on a commercial diet (Purina rat chow) ad lib. The cadmium content of the diet was not reported

19 Dietary conditions were not specified

20 Rats were maintained on a commercial diet (source unspecified) which contained per kilogram food less than 3 ppm Cd (2.7 × 10^{-5} mol), 53–60 ppm Zn (8.1–9.2 × 10^{-4} mol); 11–17 ppm Cu (1.7–2.7 × 10^{-4} mol), 200 ppm Fe (13.6 × 10^{-3} mol) in addition to "optimal amounts of other mineral, vitamins, and protein" (Petering et al. 1979)

21 Rats in this study were maintained on a purified basal diet consisting of casein, glucose monohydrate, vegetable oil, and vitamins. Analysis of the diet indicated the presence (per kilogram food) of 20 ppm Zn (3.1 × 10^{-4} mol), 10 ppm Cu (1.6 × 10^{-4} mol), 60 ppm Fe (1.1 × 10^{-3} mol), 0.1 ppm Cd (8.9 × 10^{-7} mol); 0.6 ppm Ni (1.0 × 10^{-5} mol), 0.2 ppm Se (2.5 × 10^{-6} mol)

22 The blood pressure of the control group was 145 mmHg after 88 weeks on the specified dietary regimen [20]

24 ...rats were maintained on a standard laboratory chow containing (per kilogram food), 50 ppm Zn (7.6×10^{-4} mol); 60 ppm Cu (9.4×10^{-4} mol), 290 ppm Fe (5.2×10^{-3} mol). These elements were the only ones specifically identified

25 The reported cadmium content of the diet was <0.27 ppb (2.4×10^{-9} mol per kilogram food)
The rats were maintained on a standard laboratory chow diet

26 The constituents which comprise the individual rye-based and Purina chow diets were reported in this study. The mineral composition of the chow feed is as follows in mol per kilogram food (ppm): Cd 1.1×10^{-6} (0.12 ppm); Pb 1.7×10^{-6} (0.357 ppm); Zn 8.9×10^{-4} (58 ppm); Fe 3.6×10^{-3} (198 ppm); Mn 9.3×10^{-4} (51 ppm); Cu 2.8×10^{-4} (18 ppm); Se 2.8×10^{-4} (0.22 ppm); Co 6.8×10^{-6} (0.4 ppm); Na 2.1×10^{-1} (4,900 ppm); Ca 3×10^{-1} (12,000 ppm); K 2.1×10^{-1} (8,200 ppm); Mg 1.1×10^{-1} (2,600 ppm); P 3×10^{-1} (9,400 ppm). For comparison with the rye-based diet see footnote 14. In addition, the water (37% rye-based, 0% chow), protein (14% rye-based, 24% chow), fat (4.8% rye-based, 4.3% chow), carbohydrate (39% rye-based, 60% chow), ash (3.2% rye-based, 7.3% chow), and fiber (2.3% rye-based, 5.2% chow) content of the respective diets were presented

27 The animals were given a pelletized commercial diet (Eggersmann, Rinteln). According to the manufacturer, this diet contained 20% raw protein, 6% raw fat, 4% raw fiber. The food contained vitamin A 10,000 IU; vitamin D 1,000 IU; vitamin E 150 mg; vitamin K_3 10 mg; vitamin C 100 mg; vitamin B 20 mg; vitamin B_2 30 mg; vitamin B_6 100 mg; vitamin B_{12} 30 μg; calcium pantothenate 40 mg; choline chloride 1000 mg; folic acid 5 mg; inositol 5 mg; biotin 80 μg. The reported mineral composition of the food was as follows as mol per kilogram food (ppm): Ca 3.3×10^{-1} (13,200 ppm); K 2.8×10^{-1} (11,000 ppm); P 3×10^{-1} (9,200 ppm); Na 1.7×10^{-1} (3,900 ppm); Mg 7.4×10^{-2} (1,800 ppm); Mn 1.5×10^{-3} (80 ppm); Zn 7.6×10^{-4} (50 ppm); Fe 7.0×10^{-4} (39 ppm); Cu 3.2×10^{-4} (20 ppm); Cd 1.8×10^{-6} (0.2 ppm). For comparison with other diets see footnotes 14 and 25

28 The control systolic blood pressure of the male rats averaged 150 mmHg at the conclusion of the experiment

29 The control systolic blood pressure of the female rats averaged 136 mmHg at the conclusion of the experiment

30 Indirect blood pressure measured from the central artery of the ear

31 Dahl R and S lines refer to hypertension-resistant (R) and -sensitive (S) responsiveness to putative hypertension-inducing stimuli

32 Blood pressure values correspond to those recorded at the conclusion of the experiment (+27 weeks)

33 Maximal blood pressure response during 3–6 days after the first injected dose. The pressor response was not sustained at a significant level; however, blood pressures generally remained elevated above control during the succeeding 15-day postinjection period

34 The values were not reported as group means, but instead were reported for individual rats (total of six rats)

35 When blood pressures were recorded within several hours after injection, they were elevated significantly. In contrast, within 24 h, pressures were within the normal range. Authors attribute pressor response to "mesenteric irritation rather than to some metabolic effect of the cadmium

36 Rat strain abbreviations: SD Sprague-Dawley; F344 Fischer 344; WKY Wistar-Kyoto normotensive; SHR Wistar-Kyoto spontaneously hypertensive

37 Responses to cadmium were compared by the authors with blood pressures of these animals recorded under anesthesia to correct for the effects of the anesthetic on the systemic blood pressure

38 Cadmium doses less than 8.9×10^{-7} mol/kg were usually inert. Similar doses of organic cadmium compounds did not exert a pressor effect

39 Peak hypotensive responses to intravenous cadmium (2.2×10^{-6}, 4.4×10^{-6} mol/kg) occurred within the first minute, recovering to control levels at 1 min. Thereafter the blood pressures of rats treated with these cadmium doses increased, reaching a maximum at 4 min followed by an equilibration to a steady state which remained elevated in each instance, but which was significant only for the highest exposure group. A slight, but significant hypotensive response was induced by the lowest cadmium dose (4.4×10^{-7} mol/kg) which was evident 0.5 min after administering the Cd

References

Adamska-Dyniewska H, Bala T, Florczak H, Trojanowska B, Trzcinka M (1980a) Blood cadmium level changes in patients with coronary artery disease in relation to risk factors (in Polish). Kardiol Pol 23:467–473

Adamska-Dyniewska H, Bala T, Trojanowska B, Trzcinka M (1980b) Studies on blood cadmium changes in chronic circulatory failure (in Polish). Pol Tyg Lek 35:1173–1175

Amacher DE, Ewing KL (1975) Cadmium deposition in canine heart and major arteries following intravascular administration of cadmium chloride. Bull Environ Contam Toxicol 14:457–464

Anderson TW, LeRiche WH, Mackaw JS (1969) Sudden death and ischemic heart disease. Correlation with hardness of local water supply. N Engl J Med 280:805–807

Anderson TW, Neri LC, Schreiber CB, Talbot FDF, Zdrojewski A (1975) Ischemic heart disease, water hardness and myocardial magnesium. Can Med Assoc J 113:199–203

Ando M, Sayato Y, Tonomura M, Osawa T (1977) Studies on excretion and uptake of calcium by rats after continuous oral administration of cadmium. Toxicol Appl Pharmacol 39:321–327

Antunes-Madeira MC, Carvalho AP (1970) Effects of zinc and cadmium on the surface adenosine triphosphatase of frog skeletal muscle. Mem Estud Museu Zool Univ Coimbra 312:1–17

Athanasiu J, Langlois P (1895) De l'action comparée des sels de cadmium et de zinc. C R Soc Biol (Paris) 47:496–497

Athanasiu J, Langlois P (1896) Recherches sur l'action comparée des sels de cadmium et de zinc. Arch Physiol Norm Pathol 8:251–263

Avtandilov GC (1967) Trace element content in normal and atherosclerosis-affected portions of human aorta connected with age. Arkh Patol 29:40–42

Bader H, Wilkes AB, Jean DH (1970) The effect of hydroxylamine, mercaptans, divalent metals and chelators on $(Na^+ + K^+)$-ATPase. Biochim Biophys Acta 198:583

Bárány M (1961) ATPase activity of myosin correlated with speed of muscle shortening. J Gen Physiol 50:197–218

Bárány M, Bárány K, Barron JT, Kopp SJ, Doyle DD, Hager SR, Schlesinger DH, Homa F, Sayers ST (1981) Protein phosphorylation in live muscle. Cold Spring Harbor Conferences on cell proliferation 8:869–886

Beevers DG, Cruickshank JK, Yeoman WB, Carter GF, Goldberg A, Moore MR (1980) Blood-lead and cadmium in human hypertension. J Environ Pathol Toxicol 4:251–260

Bers DM, Langer GA (1979) Uncoupling cation effects on cardiac contractility and sarcolemmal Ca^{2+} binding. Am J Physiol 237:H332–H341

Beyer KH, Peuler JD (1983) Hypertension: perspectives. Pharmacol Rev 34:287–313

Bierenbaum ML, Fleischman AI, Dunn J, Arnold J (1975) Possible toxic water factor in coronary heart-disease. Lancet I:1008–1010

Blaustein MP, Goldman DE (1968) The action of certain polyvalent cations on the voltage-clamped lobster axon. J Gen Physiol 51:279–291

Boehme DH, Sampson LT, Marks N (1979) Cadmium and hypertension: tissue levels in human heart, aorta, and brain. Fed Proc 38:120

Borhani NO (1981) Exposure to trace elements and cardiovascular disease. Circulation 63:260A–263A

Boscolo P, Cecchetti G, Iannaccone A, Porcelli G, Salimei E (1978) La callicreina urinaria nell'esposizione professionale al cadmio. Ann Ist Super Sanita 14:597–600

Boscolo P, Carmignani M, Porcelli G, L'Abbate N, Ripanti G (1980) Cardiovascular function and urinary kallikrein excretion in rats chronically exposed to mercury, arsenic, lead, cadmium or cadmium and lead. Acta Med Rom 18:211–217

Boscolo P, Porcelli G, Carmignani M, Finelli VN (1981) Urinary kallikrein and hypertension in cadmium-exposed rats. Toxicol Lett 7:189–194

Braunwald E (1982) Mechanism of action of calcium-channel-blocking agents. N Engl J Med 307:1618–1627

Caprino L, Togna G (1979) Inhibition of prostacyclin-like material formation by cadmium. Toxicol Appl Pharmacol 48:529–531

Carroll RE (1966) The relationship of cadmium in the air to cardiovascular disease death rates. JAMA 198:267–269

Chetty KN, Drummond L, Desaiah D (1980) Effect of cadmium on ATPase activities in rats fed on iron-deficient and sufficient diets. J Environ Sci Health 15:379–393

Chipperfield B, Chipperfield JR (1978) Differences in metal content of the heart muscle in death from ischemic heart disease. Am Heart J 95:732–737

Chiquoine AD (1964) Observations on the early events of cadmium necrosis of the testis. Anat Rec 149:23–36

Clarkson CW, Ten Eick RE (1983) On the mechanism of lysophosphatidylcholine-induced depolarization of cat ventricular myocardium. Circ Res 52:543–556

Clegg EJ, Carr I (1967) Changes in the blood vessels of the rat testis and epididymus produced by cadmium chloride. J Pathol Bacteriol 94:317–322

Cooper GP, Steinberg D (1977) Effects of cadmium and lead on adrenergic neuromuscular transmission in the rabbit. Am J Physiol 232:C128–C131

Corr PB, Lee BI, Sobel BE (1981) Electrophysiological and biochemical derangements in ischemic myocardium: interactions involving the cell membrane. Acta Med Scand 210:59–68

Corrigan AJ, Huang PC (1981) Cellular uptake of cadmium and zinc. Biol Trace Element Res 3:197–216

Crawford MD, Gardner MJ, Morris JN (1968) Mortality and hardness of local water supplies. Lancet I:827–831

Cummins PE, Dutton J, Evans CJ, Morgan WD, Sivyer A, Elwood PC (1980) An in-vivo study of renal cadmium and hypertension. Eur J Clin Invest 10:459–461

Dalhamn T, Friberg L (1954) The effect of cadmium on blood pressure and respiration and the use of dimercaprol (BAL) as antidote. Acta Pharmacol Toxicol (Copenh) 10:199–203

Dally S, Maury P, Boidard D, Bacle S, Gaultier M (1979) Blood cadmium level and hypertension in humans. Clin Toxicol 13:403–408

Datson GP (1982) Toxic effects of cadmium on the developing rat lung. II. Glycogen and phospholipid metabolism. J Toxicol Environ Health 9:51–61

Decker LE, Byerrum RU, Decker CF, Hoppert CA, Langham RF (1958) Chronic toxicity studies. I. Cadmium administered in drinking water to rats. Arch Ind Health 18:228–231

Der R, Fahim Z, Yousef M, Fahim M (1976) Environmental interaction of lead and cadmium on reproduction and metabolism of male rats. Res Commun Chem Pathol Pharmacol 14:689–713

Der R, Yousef M, Fahim Z, Fahim M (1977) Effects of lead and cadmium on adrenal and thyroid functions in rats. Res Commun Chem Pathol Pharmacol 17:237–253

Dhalla NS, Das PK, Sharma GP (1978) Subcellular basis of cardiac contractile failure. J Mol Cell Cardiol 10:363–385

Diamond EM, Kench JE (1974) Effects of cadmium on the respiration of rat liver mitochondria. Environ Physiol Biochem 4:280–283

Dotta F, Fruscella R (1963) Le alterazioni miocardiche da intossicazione sperimentale da cadmio: reperti istologici cardiopolmonari, reperti elettrocardiografici. Rass Med Ind Ig Lav 32:559–567

Doyle JJ, Bernhoft RA, Sandstead HH (1974) The effects of a low level of dietary cadmium on some biochemical and physiological parameters in rats. In: Hemphill DD (ed) Trace substances in environmental health, vol VIII. University of Missouri Press, Columbia, pp 403–409

Dudley RE, Svoboda DJ, Klaassen CD (1982) Acute exposure to cadmium causes severe liver injury in rats. Toxicol Appl Pharmacol 65:302–313

Eakin DJ, Schroeder LA, Whanger PD, Weswig PH (1980) Cadmium and nickel influence on blood pressure, plasma renin, and tissue mineral concentrations. Am J Physiol 238:E53–E61

Ellis KJ, Vartsky D, Zanzi I, Cohn SH (1979) Cadmium: in vivo measurement in smokers and nonsmokers. Science 205:323–325

Elwood PC, Abernathy M, Morton M (1974) Mortality in adults and trace elements in water. Lancet II:1470–1472

Fadloun Z, Leach GDH (1981) The effects of cadmium ions on blood pressure, dopamine-β-hydroxylase activity and on the responsiveness of in vivo preparations to sympathetic nerve stimulation, noradrenaline and tyramine. J Pharm Pharmacol 33:660–664

Faeder EJ, Chaney SQ, King LC, Hinners TA, Bruce R, Fowler BA (1977) Biochemical and ultrastructural changes in livers of cadmium-treated rats. Toxicol Appl Pharmacol 39:473–487

Fingerle H, Fischer G, Classen HG (1982) Failure to produce hypertension in rats by chronic exposure to cadmium. Food Chem Toxicol 20:301–306

Fleckenstein A (1983) History of calcium antagonists. Circ Res [Suppl 1] 52:3–16

Folsom AR, Prineas RJ (1982) Drinking water composition and blood pressure: a review of the epidemiology. Am J Epidemiol 115:818–832

Forbes RM, Cooper AR, Mitchell HH (1954) On the occurrence of beryllium, boron, cobalt and mercury in human tissues. J Biol Chem 209:857–865

Forshaw PJ (1977) The inhibitory effect of cadmium on neuromuscular transmission in the rat. Eur J Pharmacol 42:371–377

Fowler BA (1978) General subcellular effects of lead, mercury, cadmium, and arsenic. Environ Health Perspect 22:37–41

Fowler BA, Jones HS, Brown HW, Haseman JK (1975) The morphologic effects of chronic cadmium administration on the renal vasculature of rats given low and normal calcium diets. Toxicol Appl Pharmacol 34:233–252

Frant S, Kleeman I (1941) Cadmium "food poisoning". JAMA 117:86–89

Friberg L (1948) Proteinuria and kidney injury among workmen exposed to cadmium and nickel dust. J Ind Hyg Toxicol 30:32–36

Friberg L (1950) Health hazards in the manufacture of alkaline accumulators with special reference to chronic cadmium poisoning. Acta Med Scand [Suppl 240] 138:1–124

Friberg L, Piscator M, Nordberg GF, Kjellström T (1974) Systemic effects and dose-response relationships. In: Friberg L, Piscator M, Nordberg GF, Kjellström T (eds) Cadmium in the environment, 2nd edn. CRC, Boca Raton, pp 23–135

Frickenhaus B, Lippal J, Gordon T, Einbrodt HJ (1976) Blutdruck und Pulsfrequenz bei oraler Belastung mit Cadmiumsulfid im Tierversuch. Zentralbl Bakteriol Mikrobiol [B] 161:371–376

Fuchs F (1971) Ion exchange properties of the calcium receptor sites of troponin. Biochim Biophys Acta 245:221–229

Gabbiani G, Baic D, Déziel C (1967) Toxicity of cadmium for the central nervous system. Exp Neurol 18:154–160

Ghafghazi T, Mennear JH (1973) Effects of acute and subacute cadmium administration on carbohydrate metabolism in mice. Toxicol Appl Pharmacol 26:231–240

Gibbs CL (1978) Cardiac energetics. Physiol Rev 58:174–254

Giles W, Hume JR, Shibata EF (1983) Presynaptic and postsynaptic actions of cadmium in cardiac muscle. Fed Proc 42:2994–2997

Gruden N (1977) Influence of cadmium on calcium transfer through the duodenal wall in rats. Arch Toxicol 37:149–154

Gunn SA, Gould TC, Anderson WAD (1963) The selective injurious response of testicular and epididymal blood vessels to cadmium and its prevention by zinc. Am J Pathol 42:685–702

Gunn SA, Gould TC, Anderson WAD (1966) Protective effect of thiol compounds against cadmium-induced vascular damage to testis. Proc Soc Exp Biol Med 122:1036–1039

Gunn SA, Gould TC, Anderson WAD (1968) Mechanisms of zinc, cysteine and selenium protection against cadmium-induced vascular injury to mouse testis. J Reprod Fertil 15:65–70

Hadley JG, Conklin AW, Sanders CL (1979) Systemic toxicity of inhaled cadmium oxide. Toxicol Lett 4:107–111

Hafemann DR (1969) Effects of metal ions on action potentials of lobster giant axons. Comp Biochem Physiol 29:1149–1161

Hall CE, Hungerford S (1982) Influence of dosage, consciousness, and nifedipine on the acute pressor response to intraperitoneally administered cadmium. J Toxicol Environ Health 9:953–962

Hall CE, Nasseth D (1980) Factors affecting the acute pressor response to bolus cadmium injections. Physiol Behav 24:373–380

Hamilton DL, Smith MW (1978) Inhibition of intestinal calcium uptake by cadmium and the effect of a low calcium diet on cadmium retention. Environ Res 15:175–184

Hammer DI, Finklea JF, Creason JP, Sandifer SH, Keil JE, Priester LE, Stara JF (1971) Cadmium exposure and human health effects. In: Hemphill DD (ed) Trace substances in environmental health, vol 5. University of Missouri Press, Columbia, pp 269–276

Harrison HE, Bunting H, Ordway NK, Albrink WS (1947) The effects and treatment of inhalation of cadmium chloride aerosols in the dog. J Ind Hyg Toxicol 29:302–314

Hattori K, Shimoura K, Toda N (1983) Modification by cadmium ions of ^{45}calcium uptake by isolated rat aortae. Jpn J Pharmacol 33:655–658

Hauswirth O, Singh BN (1979) Ionic mechanisms in heart muscle in relation to the genesis and the pharmacological control of cardiac arrhythmias. Pharmacol Rev 30:5–63

Hawley PL, Kopp SJ (1975) Extension of PR interval in isolated rat heart by cadmium. Proc Soc Exp Biol Med 150:669–671

Hayashi H, Takayma K (1978) Inhibitory effects of cadmium on the release of acetylcholine from cardiac nerve terminals. Jpn J Physiol 28:333–345

Hayashi S, Toda N (1977) Inhibition by Cd^{2+}, verapamil and papaverine of Ca^{2+} induced contractions in isolated cerebral and peripheral arteries of the dog. Br J Pharmacol 60:35–43

Hayes JA, Snider GL, Palmer KC (1976) The evolution of biochemical damage in the rat lung after acute cadmium exposure. Am Rev Respir Dis 113:121–130

Henderson RF, Rebar AH, Pickrell JN, Newton GJ (1979) Early damage indicators in the lung. III. Biochemical and cytological response of the lung to inhaled metal salts. Toxicol Appl Pharmacol 50:123–136

Hill CH, Matrone G, Payne WL, Barber CW (1963) In vivo interactions of cadmium with copper, zinc and iron. J Nutr 80:227–235

Horiuchi E, Hayashi H (1979) Effects of cadmium on the contractility of a frog cardiac muscle in relation to pH of external solution. Jpn J Physiol 29:569–583

Hrdina PD, Peters DAV, Singhal RL (1976) Effects of chronic exposure to cadmium, lead and mercury on brain biogenic amines in the rat. Res Commun Chem Pathol Pharmacol 15:483–493

Hron WT, Jermok GJ, Lombardo YB, Menahan LA, Lech JJ (1977) Calcium dependency of hormone stimulated lipolysis in the perfused rat heart. J Mol Cell Cardiol 9:733–748

Huel G, Boudene C, Ibrahim MA (1981) Cadmium and lead content of maternal and newborn hair: relationship to parity, birth weight, and hypertension. Arch Environ Health 36:221–227

Iannaccone A, Porcelli G, Boscolo P (1979) The urinary kallikrein activity in cadmium exposure. Adv Exp Med Biol 120B:683–684

Iannaccone A, Carmignani M, Boscolo P (1981) Reattività cardiovascolare nel ratto dopo cronica esposizione a cadmio o piombo. Ann Ist Super Sanita 17:655–660

Iseri LT, Freed J, Bures AR (1975) Magnesium deficiency and cardiac disorders. Am J Med 58:837–846

Ithakissios DS, Kessler WV, Arvesen JN, Born GS (1974a) Differences in uptake of cadmium in selected organs of normal and alloxan-diabetic rats. Toxicol Appl Pharmacol 28:235–239

Ithakissios DS, Kessler WV, Arvesen JN, Born GS (1974b) Effect of multiple doses of cadmium on glucose metabolism in the rat. J Pharm Sci 63:146–149

Jacobs EE, Jacob M, Sanadi DR, Bradley LB (1956) Uncoupling of oxidative phosphorylation by cadmium ion. J Biol Chem 223:147–156

Johansson B, Somlyo AP (1980) Electrophysiologic and excitation-contraction coupling. In: Bohr DF, Somlyo AP, Sparks HV Jr (eds) The cardiovascular system, vol II. American Physiological Society, Bethesda, pp 301–323

Johnson MH (1969) The effect of cadmium chloride on the blood-testis barrier of the guinea pig. J Reprod Fertil 19:551–553

Kamino K, Inouye K, Ogawa M, Uyesaka N, Inouye A (1975) Calcium-binding of synaptosomes isolated from rat brain cortex. III. Binding with some divalent heavy metal ions and calcium-binding sites. J Membr Biol 23:21–31

Kanisawa M, Schroeder HA (1969) Renal arteriolar changes in hypertensive rats given cadmium in drinking water. Exp Mol Pathol 10:81–98

Kennedy A (1966) Hypocalcaemia in experimental cadmium poisoning. Br J Ind Med 23:313–317

Khera AK, Wibberley DG, Edwards KW, Waldron HA (1980) Cadmium and lead levels in blood and urine in a series of cardiovascular and normotensive patients. Int J Environ Stud 14:309–312

Kleinfeld M, Stein E (1968) Action of divalent cations on membrane potentials and contractility in rat atrium. Am J Physiol 215:593–599

Kleinfeld M, Greene H, Stein E, Magin J (1955) Effect of the cadmium ion on the electrical and mechanical activity of the frog heart. Am J Physiol 181:35–38

Kleinfeld M, Stein E, Aguillardo D (1966) Divalent cations on action potentials of dog heart. Am J Physiol 211:1438–1442

Kopp SJ (1983) Vascular intracardiac catheterization technique for multiphasic evaluation of rat heart in vivo. Toxicol Appl Pharmacol 70:273–282

Kopp SJ, Bárány M (1979) Phosphorylation of the 19,000-dalton light chain of myosin in perfused rat heart under the influence of negative and positive inotropic agents. J Biol Chem 254:12007–12012

Kopp SJ, Bárány M (1980) Influence of isoproterenol and calcium on cadmium- or lead-induced negative inotropy related to cardiac myofibrillar protein phosphorylations in perfused rat heart. Toxicol Appl Pharmacol 55:8–17

Kopp SJ, Hawley PL (1976) Factors influencing cadmium toxicity in A-V conduction system of isolated perfused rat heart. Toxicol Appl Pharmacol 37:531–544

Kopp SJ, Hawley PL (1978) Cadmium feeding: apparent depression of atrioventricular-His Purkinje conduction system. Acta Pharmacol Toxicol (Copenh) 42:110–116

Kopp SJ, Baker JC, D'Agrosa LS (1978a) Simultaneous recording of His bundle electrogram, electrocardiogram, and systolic tension from intact modified Langendorff rat heart preparations. II. Dose-response relationship of cadmium. Toxicol Appl Pharmacol 46:489–497

Kopp SJ, Baker JC, D'Agrosa LS, Hawley PL (1978b) Simultaneous recording of His bundle electrogram, electrocardiogram, and systolic tension from intact modified Langendorff rat heart preparations. I. Effects of perfusion time, cadmium, and lead. Toxicol Appl Pharmacol 46:475–487

Kopp SJ, Fischer VW, Erlanger M, Perry EF, Perry HM Jr (1978c) Electrocardiographical, biochemical and morphological effects of chronic low level cadmium feeding on the rat heart. Proc Soc Exp Biol Med 159:339–345

Kopp SJ, Bárány M, Erlanger M, Perry EF, Perry HM Jr (1980a) The influence of chronic low-level cadmium and/or lead feeding on myocardial contractility related to phosphorylation of cardiac myofibrillar proteins. Toxicol Appl Pharmacol 54:48–56

Kopp SJ, Glonek T, Erlanger M, Perry EF, Bárány M, Perry HM Jr (1980b) Altered metabolism and function of rat heart following chronic low level cadmium/lead feeding. J Mol Cell Cardiol 12:1407–1425

Kopp SJ, Glonek T, Erlanger M, Perry EF, Perry HM Jr, Bárány M (1980c) Cadmium and lead effects on myocardial function and metabolism. J Environ Pathol Toxicol 4:205–227

Kopp SJ, Perry HM Jr, Glonek T, Erlanger M, Perry EF, Bárány M, D'Agrosa LS (1980d) Cardiac physiologic-metabolic changes after chronic low-level heavy metal feeding. Am J Physiol 239:H22–H30

Kopp SJ, Glonek T, Perry HM Jr, Erlanger M, Perry EF (1982) Cardiovascular actions of cadmium at environmental exposure levels. Science 217:837–839

Kopp SJ, Perry HM Jr, Perry EF, Erlanger M (1983a) Cardiac physiologic and tissue metabolic changes following chronic low-level cadmium and cadmium plus lead ingestion in the rat. Toxicol Appl Pharmacol 69:149–160

Kopp SJ, Perry HM Jr, Feliksik JM, Erlanger M, Perry EF (1983b) In vivo assessment of cardiac contractility following chronic dietary cadmium or cadmium plus lead ingestion in the rat. In: Hemphill DD (ed) Trace substances in environmental health, vol 17. University of Missouri Press, Columbia, pp 165–173

Kotsonis FN, Klaassen CD (1977) Toxicity and distribution of cadmium administered to rats at sublethal doses. Toxicol Appl Pharmacol 41:667–680

Kotsonis FN, Klaassen CD (1978) The relationship of metallothionein to the toxicity of cadmium after prolonged oral administration to rats. Toxicol Appl Pharmacol 46:39–54

Lange LG, Sobel BE (1982) Pharmacological salvage of myocardium. Annu Rev Pharmacol Toxicol 22:115–143

Langer GA, Serena SD, Nudd LM (1974) Cation exchange in heart cell culture: correlation with effects on contractile force. J Mol Cell Cardiol 6:149–161

Lee KS, Tsien RW (1983) Mechanism of calcium channel blockade by verapamil, D600, diltiazem and nitrendipine in single dialyzed heart cells. Nature 302:790–794

Lee KS, Lee EW, Tsien RW (1982) Comparison between Ca^{2+} channel block by Cd^{2+} and D600 in single mammalian heart cells. Biophys J 37:342a

Lener J, Bibr B (1971) Cadmium and hypertension. Lancet I:1970

Levin AA, Miller RK (1981) Fetal toxicity of cadmium in the rat: decreased uteroplacental blood flow. Toxicol Appl Pharmacol 58:297–306

Lewis GP, Jusko WJ, Coughlin LL, Hartz S (1972) Contribution of cigarette smoking to cadmium accumulation in man. Lancet I:291–292

Lockwood APM (1961) "Ringer" solutions and some notes on the physiologic basis of their ionic composition. Comp Biochem Physiol 2:241–289

Loeser E, Lorke D (1977a) Semichronic oral toxicity of cadmium. 1. Studies on rats. Toxicology 7:215–224

Loeser E, Lorke D (1977b) Semichronic oral toxicity of cadmium. 2. Studies on dogs. Toxicology 7:225–232

Marier JR (1978) Cardioprotective contribution of hard waters to magnesium intake. Rev Can Biol 37:115–125

Marmé W (1867) Über die giftige Wirkung und den Nachweis einiger Cadmiumverbindungen. Z Rat Med 29:125–128

Marsh NA (1976) The effect of divalent cations on the isolated chicken heart. J Physiol (Lond) 256:17P–18P

Mason DT (1969) Usefulness and limitations of the rate of rise of intraventricular pressure (dP/dt) in the evaluation of myocardial contractility in man. Am J Cardiol 23:516–527

Mason KE, Brown JA, Young JO, Nesbit RR (1964) Cadmium-induced injury of the rat testis. Anat Rec 149:135–148

Merin RG (1978) Myocardial metabolism for the toxicologist. Environ Health Perspect 26:169–174

Moses HA (1979) Trace elements: an association with cardiovascular diseases and hypertension. J Natl Med Assoc 71:227–228

Mustafa M, Cross CE (1971) Pulmonary alveolar macrophage. Oxidative metabolism of isolated cells and mitochondria and effect of cadmium ion on electron- and energy transfer reactions. Biochemistry 10:4176–4184

Nakagawa M, Takamura M, Kojima S (1977) Some heavy metals affecting the lecithin-cholesterol acyltransferase reaction in human plasma. J Biochem 81:1011–1016

Nathanson JA, Bloom FE (1976) Heavy metals and adenosine cyclic 3′,5′-monophosphate metabolism: possible relevance to heavy metal toxicity. Mol Pharmacol 12:390–398

Nechay BR, Williams BJ, Steinsland OS, Hall CE (1978) Increased vascular response to adrenergic stimulation in rats exposed to cadmium. J Toxicol Environ Health 4:559–567

Neri LC, Johansen HL (1978) Water hardness and cardiovascular mortality. Ann NY Acad Sci 304:203–219

Niemi M, Kormano M (1965) An angiographic study of cadmium-induced vascular lesions in the testis and epididymus on the rat. Acta Pathol Microbiol Scand 63:513–521

Niwa A, Suzuki A (1982) Effects of cadmium on the tension of isolated rat aorta (a possible mechanism for cadmium induced hypertension). J Toxicol Sci 7:51–60

Ohanian EV, Iwai J (1980) Etiological role of cadmium in hypertension in an animal model. J Environ Pathol Toxicol 4:229–241

Ohanian EV, Iwai J, Leitl G, Tuthill R (1978) Genetic influence on cadmium-induced hypertension. Am J Physiol 235:H385–H391

Opie LH (1976) Metabolic regulation in ischemia and hypoxia. Effects of regional ischemia on metabolism of glucose and fatty acids. Circ Res [Suppl 1] 38:52–74

Østergaard K (1978) Renal cadmium concentration in relation to smoking habits and blood pressure. Acta Med Scand 203:379–383

Paderi C (1896) Sur l'action physiologique du cadmium. Arch Ital Biol Napoli 25:283

Panseri A (1904) L'action du rubidium et du cadmium sur le coeur. Arch Ital Biol Napoli 41:306

Pařížek J (1957) The destructive effect of cadmium ion on testicular tissue and its prevention by zinc. J Endocrinol 15:56–63

Pařížek J (1960) Sterilization of the male by cadmium salts. J Reprod Fertil 1:294–309

Pařížek J, Záhoř Z (1956) Effect of cadmium salts on testicular tissue. Nature 177:1036–1037

Parmley WW, Sonnenblick EH (1967) Series elasticity in heart muscle. Its relation to contractile element velocity and proposed muscle models. Circ Res 20:112–123

Passow H, Rothstein A, Clarkson TW (1961) The general pharmacology of the heavy metals. Pharmacol Rev 13:185–224

Perry HM Jr, Erlanger MW (1973) Elevated circulating renin activity in rats following doses of cadmium known to induce hypertension. J Lab Clin Med 82:399–405

Perry HM Jr, Erlanger M (1974) Metal induced hypertension following chronic feeding of low doses of cadmium and mercury. J Lab Clin Med 83:541–547

Perry HW Jr, Erlanger MW (1978) Pressor effects of chronically feeding cadmium and lead together. In: Hemphill DD (ed) Trace substances in environmental health, vol 12. University of Missouri Press, Columbia, pp 268–275

Perry HM Jr, Erlanger MW (1980) Cadmium as both an antinariuretic and a pressor agent. In: Hemphill DD (ed) Trace substances in environmental health, vol 14. University of Missouri Press, Columbia, pp 280–286

Perry HM Jr, Erlanger MW (1981) Sodium retention in rats with cadmium-induced hypertension. Sci Total Environ 22:31–38

Perry HM Jr, Erlanger M (1982) Effect of diet on increases in systolic pressure induced in rats by chronic cadmium feeding. J Nutr 112:1983–1989

Perry HM Jr, Kopp SJ (1983) Does cadmium contribute to human hypertension. Sci Total Environ 26:223–232

Perry HM Jr, Yunice A (1965) Acute pressor effects of intra-arterial cadmium and mercuric ions in anesthetized rats. Proc Soc Exp Biol Med 120:805–808

Perry HM Jr, Tipton IH, Schroeder HA, Steiner RL, Cook MJ (1961) Variation in the concentration of cadmium in human kidney as a function of age and geographic origin. J Chron Dis 14:259–271

Perry HM Jr, Schoepfle E, Bourgoignie J (1967a) In vitro production and inhibition of aortic vasoconstriction by mercury cadmium, and other metal ions. Proc Soc Exp Biol Med 124:485–490

Perry HM Jr, Erlanger M, Yunice A, Perry EF (1967b) Mechanism of the acute hypertensive effect of intra-arterial cadmium and mercury in anesthetized rats. J Lab Clin Med 70:963–972

Perry HM Jr, Erlanger M, Yunice A, Schoepfle E, Perry EF (1970) Hypertension and tissue metal levels following intravenous cadmium, mercury, and zinc. Am J Physiol 219:755–761

Perry HM Jr, Erlanger MW, Perry EF (1976) Limiting conditions for the induction of hypertension in rats by cadmium. In: Hemphill DD (ed) Trace substances in environmental health, vol X. University of Missouri Press, Columbia, pp 459–467

Perry HW Jr, Erlanger M, Perry EF (1977) Elevated systolic blood pressure following chronic low-level cadmium feeding. Am J Physiol 232:H114–H121

Perry HM Jr, Erlanger M, Perry EF (1979) Increase in the systolic pressure of rats chronically fed cadmium. Environ Health Perspect 28:251–260

Perry HM Jr, Erlanger MW, Perry EF (1980a) Inhibition of cadmium-induced hypertension in rats. Sci Tot Environ 14:153–166

Perry HM Jr, Perry EF, Erlanger MW (1980b) Possible influence of heavy metals in cardiovascular disease: introduction and overview. J Environ Path Toxicol 4:195–203

Petering HG, Murthy L, Sorenson JRJ, Levin L, Stemmer KL (1979) Effect of sex on oral cadmium dose responses in rats: blood pressure and pharmacodynamics. Environ Res 20:289–299

Pilati CF, Ewing KL, Paradise NF (1982) Effects of cadmium on contractility and calcium concentration in isolated heart muscle. Proc Soc Exp Biol Med 169:480–486

Ponteva M, Elomaa I, Bäckman H, Hansson L, Kilpiö J (1979) Blood cadmium and plasma zinc measurements in acute myocardial infarction. Eur J Cardiol 9:379–391

Pool ML (1981) Exposure and health effects of cadmium. Part 3. Effects of cadmium on enzyme activities. Toxicol Environ Chem Rev 4:179–203

Popham JD, Webster WS (1976) The ultrastructural localization of cadmium. Histochemistry 46:249–259

Porter MC, Miya TS, Bousquet WF (1974) Cadmium: inability to induce hypertension in the rat. Toxicol Appl Pharmacol 27:692–695

Porter MC, Miya TS, Bousquet WF (1975) Cadmium and vascular reactivity in the rat. Toxicol Appl Pharmacol 34:143–150

Prentice RC (1982) Calcium dependent cadmium and lead effects in the isolated perfused rat heart. Doctoral thesis, Department of Physiology and Biophysics, University of Illinois Graduate College, Chicago

Prentice RC, Hawley PL, Glonek T, Kopp SJ (1984) Calcium-dependent effects of cadmium on energy metabolism and function of perfused rat heart. Toxicol Appl Pharmacol 75:198–210

Pribilla O, Schultek T (1979) Blei-, Cadmium-, Chrom-, Mangan- und Zinkgehalt arteriosklerosefreier menschlicher Aorten. Z Rechtsmed 83:273–281

Pribilla O, Darmstadter H, Schultek T (1980) Blei-, Cadmium-, Chrom-, Mangan- und Zinkgehalt atherosklerotisch veränderter menschlicher Aorten. Z Rechtsmed 85:127–137

Pritchard JB (1979) Toxic substances and cell membrane function. Fed Proc 38:2220–2225

Prodan L (1982) Cadmium poisoning. II. Experimental cadmium poisoning. J Ind Hyg 14:174–196

Punsar S, Erametsa O, Karvonen MJ, Rhyanen A, Hilska P, Vornamo H (1975) Coronary heart disease and drinking water. J Chron Dis 28:259–287

Rauchova H, Drahota Z (1979) Activation of the beef heart mitochondrial ATPase by cadmium ions. Int J Biochem 10:735–738

Revis N (1978) A possible mechanism for cadmium-induced hypertension in rats. Life Sci 22:479–488

Revis NW, Zinsmeister AR (1981) The relationship of blood cadmium level to hypertension and plasma norepinephrine level: a Romanian study. Proc Soc Exp Biol Med 167:254–260

Revis NW, Major TC, Horton CY (1980) The effects of calcium, magnesium, lead or cadmium on lipoprotein metabolism and atherosclerosis in the pigeon. J Environ Pathol Toxicol 4:293–304

Revis NW, Zinsmeister AR, Bull R (1981) Atherosclerosis and hypertension induction by lead and cadmium ions: an effect prevented by calcium ion. Proc Natl Acad Sci USA 78:6494–6498

Revis NW, Major TC, Horton CY (1983) The response of the adrenergic system in the cadmium-induced hypertensive rat. J Am Coll Toxicol 2:165–174

Richet C (1882) De l'action chimique des différents métaux sur le coeur de la grenouille. C R Acad Sci 94:742–743

Ringer S (1883 a) A further contribution regarding the influence of the different constituents of the blood on the contraction of the heart. J Physiol 4:29–42

Ringer S (1883 b) A third contribution regarding the influence of the inorganic constituents of the blood on the ventricular contraction. J Physiol 4:222–225

Roach MR, Damude LR (1980) The effect of daily injections on cadmium on the systolic pressure of conscious rats. J Environ Pathol Toxicol 4:443–449

Rohrer SR, Shaw SM, Lamar CH (1978) Cadmium induced endothelial cell alterations in the fetal brain from prenatal exposure. Acta Neuropathol (Berl) 44:147–149

Rosenman KD (1979) Cardiovascular disease and environmental exposure. Br J Ind Med 36:85–97

Rossiter RJ, Strickland KP (1970) Metabolism of phosphoglycerides. In: Lijtha A (ed) Metabolic reactions in the nervous system. Plenum, New York, pp 467–489 (Handbook of neurochemistry, vol 3)

Rothstein A (1959) Cell membrane as site of action of heavy metals. Fed Proc 18:1026–1035

Saksena SK, Dahlgren L, Lau IF, Chang MC (1977) Reproductive and endocrinological features of male rats after treatment with cadmium chloride. Biol Reprod 16:609–613

Salant W, Connet H (1920) The influence of heavy metals of the isolated frog heart. J Pharmacol Exp Ther 15:217–232

Satoh E, Asai F, Itoh K, Nishimura M, Urakawa N (1982) Mechanism of cadmium-induced blockage of neuromuscular transmission. Eur J Pharmacol 77:251–257

Schlaepfer WW (1971) Sequential study of endothelial changes in acute cadmium intoxication. Lab Invest 25:556–564

Schroeder HA (1956) Trace metals and chronic diseases. Adv Intern Med 8:259–303

Schroeder HA (1960) Relation between mortality from cardiovascular disease and treated water supplies. 172:1902–1908

Schroeder HA (1964) Cadmium hypertension in rats. Am J Physiol 207:62–66

Schroeder HA (1965) Cadmium as a factor in hypertension. J Chron Dis 18:647–656

Schroeder HA (1966) Municipal drinking water and cardiovascular death rates. JAMA 195:81–85

Schroeder HA (1967) Cadmium, chromium, and cardiovascular disease. Circulation 35:570–582

Schroeder HA (1974) The role of trace elements in cardiovascular diseases. Med Clin North Am 58:381–396

Schroeder HA, Balassa JJ (1961) Abnormal trace metals in man: cadmium. J Chron Dis 14:236–258

Schroeder HA, Balassa JJ (1965) Influence of chromium, cadmium, and lead on rat aortic lipids and circulating cholesterol. Am J Physiol 209:433–437

Schroeder HA, Buckman J (1967) Cadmium hypertension. Its reversal in rats by a zinc chelate. Arch Environ Health 14:693–697

Schroeder HA, Perry HM Jr (1955) Antihypertensive effects of metal binding agents. J Lab Clin Med 46:416–422

Schroeder HA, Vinton WH Jr (1962) Hypertension induced in rats by small doses of cadmium. Am J Physiol 202:515–518

Schroeder HA, Kroll SS, Little JW, Livingston PO, Myers MAG (1966) Hypertension in rats from injection of cadmium. Arch Environ Health 13:788–789

Schroeder HA, Baker JT, Hansen NM Jr, Size JG, Wise RA (1970) Vascular reactivity of rats altered by cadmium and a zinc chelate. Arch Environ Health 21:609–614

Schwartze EW, Alsberg CL (1923) Studies on the pharmacology of cadmium and zinc with particular reference to emesis. J Pharmacol Exp Ther 21:1–22

Setchell BP, Waites GMH (1970) Changes in the permeability of the testicular capillaries and of the 'blood-testis barrier' after injection of cadmium chloride in the rat. J Endocrinol 47:81–86

Shanbaky IO, Borowitz JL, Kessler WV (1978) Mechanisms of cadmium- and barium-induced adrenal catecholamine release. Toxicol Appl Pharmacol 44:99–105

Shaper AG (1979) Cardiovascular disease and trace metals. Proc R Soc Lond [Biol] 205:135–143

Sharrett AR (1979) The role of chemical constituents of drinking water in cardiovascular diseases. Am J Epidemiol 110:401–419

Sharrett AR, Feinleib M (1975a) Possible toxic water factor in coronary heart-disease. Lancet II:76

Sharrett AR, Feinleib M (1975b) Water constituents and trace elements in relation to cardiovascular diseases. Prev Med 4:20–36

Shino H (1976) Mechanisms of the contracting action of K, acetylcholine and Ba and of the antispasmodic action of Cd and Mn on the pyloric antrum strip of rat's stomach, particularly in relation to Ca (in Japanese). Folia Pharmacol Jpn 72:95–104

Singhal RL (1981) Testicular cyclic nucleotide and adrenal catecholamine metabolism following chronic exposure to cadmium. Environ Health Perspect 38:111–117

Singhal RL, Merali Z, Hrdina PD (1976) Aspects of the biochemical toxicology of cadmium. Fed Proc 35:75–80

Skog E, Wahlberg JE (1964) A comparative investigation of the percutaneous absorption of metal compounds in the guinea pig by means of the radioactive isotopes: ^{51}Cr, ^{58}Co, ^{65}Zn, ^{110}Ag, ^{115m}Cd, ^{203}Hg. J Invest Dermatol 43:187–192

Smith JC, Kench JE, Smith JP (1957) Chemical and histological post-mortem studies on a workman exposed for many years to cadmium oxide fume. Br J Ind Med 14:246–249

Solaro RJ (1982) The role of calcium in the contraction of the heart. In: Flaim SF, Zelis R (eds) Calcium blockers. Mechanisms of action and clinical applications. Urban and Schwarzenberg, Munich, pp 21–36

Sonnenblick EH, Parmley WW, Urschel CW (1969) The contractile state of the heart as expressed by force-velocity relations. Am J Cardiol 23:488–503

Stacey NH, Klaassen CD (1980) Cadmium uptake by isolated rat hepatocytes. Toxicol Appl Pharmacol 55:448–455

Stephens GA (1920/1921) Cadmium poisoning. J Ind Hyg 2:129–132

Sturkie PD (1973) Effects of cadmium on electrocardiogram, blood pressure, and hematocrit of chickens. Avian Dis 17:106–110

Sutherland DJB, Tsang BK, Merali Z, Singhal RL (1974) Testicular and prostatic cyclic AMP metabolism following chronic cadmium treatment and subsequent withdrawal. Environ Physiol Biochem 4:205–213

Suzuki Y (1980) Cadmium metabolism and toxicity in rats after long-term subcutaneous administration. J Toxicol Environ Health 6:469–482

Terpin T, Roach MR (1980) The effects of cadmium on the structure and elastic properties of carotid arteries from rats. J Environ Pathol Toxicol 3:449–464

Thind GS, Fischer GM (1975) Cadmium and zinc distribution in cardiovascular and other tissues of normal and cadmium-treated dogs. Exp Mol Pathol 22:326–334

Thind GS, Karreman G, Stephan KF, Blakemore WS (1970a) Vascular reactivity and mechanical properties of normal and cadmium-hypertensive rabbits. J Lab Clin Med 76:560–568

Thind GS, Stephan KF, Blakemore WS (1970b) Inhibition of vasopressor responses by cadmium. Am J Physiol 219:577–583

Tipton IH, Schroeder HA, Perry HM Jr, Cook MJ (1965) Trace elements in human tissue Part III Subjects from Africa, the Near and Far East and Europe. Health Phys 11:403–451

Toda N (1973a) Influence of cadmium ions on contractile response of isolated aortas to stimulatory agents. Am J Physiol 225:350–355

Toda N (1973b) Influence of cadmium ions on the transmembrane potential and contractility of isolated rabbit left atria. J Pharmacol Exp Ther 186:60–66

Toda N (1973c) Inhibition by cadmium ions of the electrical activity of sinoatrial nodal pacemakers fibers and their response to norepinephrine. J Pharmacol Exp Ther 184:357–365

Tomera JF, Harakal C (1980) Cyclic nucleotide changes in aortic segments derived from hypertensive rabbits. Eur J Pharmacol 68:505–508

Trosper TL, Philipson KD (1983) Effects of divalent and trivalent cations on Na^+-Ca^{2+} exchange in cardiac sarcolemmal vesicles. Biochim Biophys Acta 731:63–68

Tsien RW (1983) Calcium channels in excitable cell membranes. Annu Rev Physiol 45:341–358

Tully RT, Lehmann HP (1982) Method for the simultaneous determination of cadmium and zinc in whole blood by atomic absorption spectrophotometry and measurement in normotensive and hypertensive humans. Clin Chim Acta 122:189–202

Vallee BL, Ulmer DD (1972) Biochemical effects of mercury, cadmium and lead. Annu Rev Biochem 41:91–128

Van Breemen C, Aaronson P, Loutzenhiser R (1979) Sodium-calcium interactions in mammalian smooth muscle. Pharmacol Rev 30:167–208

Voors AW, Shuman MS (1977) Liver cadmium levels on North Carolina residents who died of heart disease. Bull Environ Contam Toxicol 17:692–696

Voors AW, Johnson WD, Shuman MS (1982) Additive statistical effects of cadmium and lead on heart-related disease in a North Carolina autopsy series. Arch Environ Health 37:98–102

Vorobieva RS, Eremeeva EP (1980) Cardiovascular function in workers exposed to cadmium (in Russian). Gig Sanit 10:22–25

Vuori E, Huunan-Seppälä A, Kilpiö JO, Salmela SS (1979) Biologically active metals in human tissues. II. The effect of age on the concentration of cadmium in aorta, heart, kidney, liver, lung, pancreas and skeletal muscle. Scand J Work Environ Health 5:16–22

Waalkes MP, Watkins JB, Klaassen CD (1983) Minimal role of metallothionein in decreased chelator efficacy for cadmium. Toxicol Appl Pharmacol 68:392–398

Waites GMH, Setchell BP (1966) Changes in blood flow and vascular permeability of the testes, epididymis and accessory reproductive organs of the rat after the administration of cadmium chloride. J Endocrinol 34:329–342

Walker HL, Moses HA (1979) Cadmium: hypertension induction and lead mobilization. J Natl Med Assoc 71:1187–1189

Walsh MP, LePeuch CJ, Vallet B, Cavadore J-C, Demaille JG (1980) Cardiac calmodulin and its role in the regulation of metabolism and contraction. J Mol Cell Cardiol 12:1091–1101

Ward RJ, Fisher M, Tellez-Yudilevich M (1978) Significance of blood cadmium concentrations in patients with renal disorders or essential hypertension and the normal population. Ann Clin Biochem 15:197–200

Washko PW, Cousins RJ (1976) Metabolism of ^{109}Cd in rats fed normal and low-calcium diets. J Toxicol Environ Health 1:1055–1066

Watkins BE (1980) Effects of cadmium injections on arterial pressure regulation in the rat. Clin Exp Hypertens 2:153–162

Weber CW, Reid BL (1969) Effect of dietary cadmium on mice. Toxicol Appl Pharmacol 14:420–425

Whanger PD (1979) Cadmium effects in rats on tissue iron, selenium, and blood pressure; blood and hair cadmium in some Oregon residents. Environ Health Perspect 28:115–121

Williams BJ, Laubach DJ, Nechay DJ, Steinsland OS (1978) The effects of cadmium on adrenergic neurotransmission in vitro. Life Sci 23:1929–1934

Wilson RH, DeEds F, Cox AJ Jr (1941) Effects of continued cadmium feeding. J Pharmacol Exp Ther 71:222–235

Wong K-L, Klaassen CD (1980) Tissue distribution and retention of cadmium in rats during postnatal development: minimal role of hepatic metallothionein. Toxicol Appl Pharmacol 53:343–353

Wong K-L, Klaassen CD (1982) Neurotoxic effects of cadmium in young rats. Toxicol Appl Pharmacol 63:330–337

CHAPTER 8

Role of Metallothionein in Cadmium Metabolism

M. Webb

A. Introduction

Induction of the synthesis of the metal-binding protein, thionein, is not only a particularly interesting feature of the biochemistry of the cadmium (Cd) ion, but also of considerable importance in relation to its metabolism and chronic toxicity. As Cd is neither an abundant element, nor readily absorbed through the mammalian gastrointestinal tract, normally only small amounts of it are transmitted through the food chain to animals and humans. Nevertheless, much of the absorbed Cd is retained, principally in the liver and kidneys and, even in uncontaminated environments, long-lived animal species may accumulate appreciable body burdens during their lifetimes. Earlier studies, reviewed by VALLEE (1979) had shown the presence of Cd in a wide variety of biological tissues, relatively high concentrations usually being present in human and equine renal cortex. A search for a possible biochemical function of this seemingly biologically ubiquitous element led to the isolation from horse kidney of a low molecular weight protein, deficient in aromatic amino acids, which not only had a high content of Cd (20–25 mg per gram protein), but also contained most of the Cd in the tissue (MARGOSHES and VALLEE 1957). Subsequent preparations of the metalloprotein by improved methods (KÄGI and VALLEE 1960, 1961) were found to contain 5% Cd, 2.2% Zn, 0.4% Fe, 0.18% Cu, 14.9% N, and 8.5% S. Because of the presence of several metals, in addition to Cd and the high sulphur content KÄGI and VALLEE (1960) named the metalloprotein "metallothionein", i.e. a metallo-derivative of the sulphur-rich protein, thionein. This terminology has both disadvantages and limitations; thionines are phenthiozine dyes (see, e.g. SCHMIDT 1936), thionins are plant peptides of high sulphur content (see, e.g. CARRASCO et al. 1981). Whilst, as recommended by the plenum of the First International Metallothionein Meeting (KÄGI and NORDBERG 1979), the retention of the prefix "metallo" reduces the possible ambiguity, it is known now that metallothioneins can be induced by various metals, both essential and nonessential, do not necessarily contain Cd and exist in isomeric forms. Thus, ideally, the metal composition and form needs to be defined, e.g. (Cd, Zn, Cu)isometallothionein-1 or, when the atomic ratio of metals is known, by additional subscripts (e.g. $(Cd_{4.7}, Zn_{2.0}, Cu_{0.5})$isometallothionein-1), the metallic ions being listed in order of relative abundance. Whilst, in this chapter, efforts are made to conform to convention, metallothionein is abbreviated to MT and the term CdMT is used either when the contents of secondary cations are not defined in the original publications, or the bound Cd is the only relevant ion.

B. Historical Background and Chemistry of the Metallothioneins

Much of the earlier work on these metalloproteins, which followed the discovery by Piscator (1964) of the progressive accumulation, without toxic manifestations, of high concentrations of MT-bound Cd in the livers and kidneys of rats and rabbits, repeatedly injected with low doses of Cd, was concerned with their synthesis and function in response to the administration of this and certain other toxic metals, principally with the rat as the experimental animal (see, e.g. Webb 1979 a). The dramatic, rapid, dose-dependent accumulation and retention of MT-bound Cd, particularly in the liver after parenteral dosing, which could be followed by an extremely simple technique (see Sect. C) thus became a popular topic for study, specifically in relation to the detoxification of the metallic ion (see, e.g. Kägi and Nordberg 1979; Webb 1979 a; Kotsonis and Klaassen 1981). These investigations established that thionein is an inducible protein, the synthesis of which is controlled at the transcriptional level (but cf. Sect. K) and, at chronic exposure, increases in both the liver and kidney with the organ content of Cd. At all times, the protein occurs in combination with Cd and other metals (Zn and/or Cu) as the heat-stable metallothionein, apparently unassociated with other cellular components (Bakka et al. 1982) and free thionein is not detectable (see Webb 1979 a).

The observation that hepatic MT synthesis occurred in the rat in response to the parenteral administration of high doses of Zn, the isolation and characterization of ZnMT from human and equine liver, of (Zn,Cu)MT from the livers of pigs, sheep and calves, the livers and kidneys of rats, the variations in the contents of these metalloproteins with the dietary intakes of Zn and Cu and the demonstration of excessively high concentrations of ZnMT or (Zn,Cu)MT in the livers of foetal and newborn animals (see, e.g. Webb 1979 a; Bremner 1982; and also Sect. K), established that thionein functions in the metabolic regulation of certain essential, but potentially toxic ions. Induction of metallothioneins by Cd, Hg and Au thus seems to be an extension of the normal homeostatic function (Webb and Cain 1982) to foreign metals, which also bind with high affinity to thiol groups. The widespread occurrence of metallothioneins not only in terrestrial animals, but also in normal, or metal-exposed aquatic mammals, crustaceans, fish, birds, blue-green algae, moulds, yeasts and, possibly, plants indicates that this normal function is of considerable antiquity and fundamental biological importance in terms of evolutionary development (Kägi and Nordberg 1979; Bremner 1982). Moreover, many recent studies, particularly with cell culture systems, have shown that ZnMT synthesis can be stimulated by dexamethasone and other glucocorticoids, even in the absence of Zn uptake. Such hormonal effects, perhaps erroneously, have been regarded as of little relevance to the role of MT in the metabolism of Cd and have been omitted from the present discussion. Although a detailed review of the subject is not available, a number of recent publications (e.g. Etzal et al. 1979; Karin and Herschman 1981; Karin et al. 1981; Brady 1981) give extensive summaries of the literature.

In most of the species that have been studied in detail the endogenous or Cd-induced metallothioneins consist of at least two isometallothioneins. These differ slightly in their primary structures and can be separated by procedures that exploit the charge differences of the isoforms (i.e. ion exchange chromatography, electrophoresis and isoelectric focusing; see e.g. WEBB 1979a). Isoform-2 of (Cd,Zn)MT from the livers of Cd-dosed rats has a greater Stokes radius (17 Å) than isoform-1 (16.2 Å), differs from the latter in its ability to reconstitute apo-carbonic anhydrase (see Sect. J) and, after cleavage of the NH_2 terminal acetylmethionine residue (a characteristic feature of these metalloproteins), in the sequence of certain amino acids in the first 25 residues (WINGE and MIKLOSSY 1982a). Although two genes that code for isoMT-1 and isoMT-2 have been detected in mouse liver and the nucleotide sequence of one of them (the isoMT-1 gene) has been determined (GLANVILLE et al. 1981; see also DURNAM et al. 1980; DURNAM and PALMITER 1981; KARIN and RICHARDS 1982, for the recent developments in this field), even these isometallothioneins are heterogeneous and can be resolved by reverse-phase high pressure liquid chromatography (HPLC) into several isoproteins, which may differ only by the substitution of one amino acid (e.g. Ser) for another (e.g. Leu) in the peptide chain (KLAUSER et al. 1983). Although PRINS and VAN DEN HAMER (1981, 1982) consider, from somewhat inadequate evidence, that isoMT-1 and isoMT-2 in the kidneys of normal brindled mice are involved in metal (specifically Cu) transport and storage, respectively, the reasons for the existence of MT isomers remain to be established.

In the early investigations on the (Cd,Zn)MT of equine renal cortex all of the thiol groups of the cysteine residues (30% of the total residues) were found to be involved in metal coordination, the atomic sulphur : metal ($\Sigma Cd + Zn$) ratio being approximately 3:1 (KÄGI and VALLEE 1961). The same ratio has been found in the (Cd,Zn)metallothioneins from other mammalian species and in the isometallothioneins, separated therefrom by ion exchange chromatography or electrophoretic techniques (see, e.g. WEBB 1979a). In CuMT (e.g. from the liver of the Cu-loaded rat), in which the bound cation is monovalent, the ratio of thiol groups : bound metal is less, usually 1.5–2.0:1 (see, e.g. GELLER and WINGE 1982) and thus is indicative of a different conformation (see also WINGE and MIKLOSSY 1982a). Replacement of Cd and Zn in a (Cd,Zn)MT by Hg, which differs in complex geometry and ionic radius from either of the endogenous metals, also causes structural changes in the MT molecule (SOKOLOWSKI et al. 1974).

Once the amino acid sequences of several of the mammalian (Cd,Zn)MT or ZnMT had been determined (see KÄGI and NORDBERG 1979), it was clear that irrespective of the source, isomeric form and of minor differences in amino acid composition, the positions of the 20 cysteine residues in the polypeptide chain were conserved. (Metallothioneins from nonmammalian sources, e.g. the crab *Scylla serrata* and the mould *Neurospora crassa,* may differ from those of mammalian tissues in chain length and number of cysteine residues per molecule (see KÄGI and NORDBERG 1979). The invariant distribution of the cysteine residues and thus of the functional thiol groups in the mammalian metallothioneins, coupled with model studies with synthetic peptides that contained three cysteinyl residues, but no aromatic amino acids (YOSHIDA et al. 1979), the early physico-chemical investigations of KÄGI and VALLEE (1961) and the confirmation by ^{1}H-NMR (GALDES et al. 1978a, b; VAŠÁK et al. 1980) that other amino acid residues did not participate in the binding of Zn and Cd ions, established that the metal–thiolate complexes were essential for the maintenance of the structure and probably function of these metalloproteins. Further studies by ^{113}Cd-NMR spectrometry on (^{113}Cd,Zn)MT (Sadler et al. 1978; Otvos and Armitage 1979, 1980; Nicholson et al. 1983) and by spectrophotometry, measurements of magnetic circular dichroism and X-ray photoelectron specta of (Cd,Zn)MT, CuMT (Weser and Rupp 1979; Vašák et al. 1981) and CoMT (obtained by cation replacement from (Cd,Zn)MT, Vašák et al. 1981), determination of extended X-ray absorption fine spectra on yeast CuMT (Bordas et al. 1982) and sheep liver ZnMT (Garner et al. 1982), showed each metal atom to be coordinated to four sulphur atoms in a tetrahedral arrangement. Since, at least in a (Cd,Zn)MT, the ratio of sulphur : metal atoms is 3 : 1, it follows that some of the 20 sulphur atoms in such a fully metal-saturated mammalian MT must bridge across two or more metal atoms.

An important development from this work has been the discovery that the complex ^{113}Cd-NMR spectra of the isometallothioneins from the livers of ^{113}Cd-doses rabbits, which are considered to indicate heterogeneity (i.e. mixtures of molecules with different relative amounts of Zn and Cd), become simpler when the protein-bound Zn is replaced by ^{113}Cd in vitro. Analysis of the spectroscopic data for these preparations showed the presence of two separate metal clusters (A and B) in each isoMT, one of which (A) contained four and the other (B) three Cd ions. These two cluster arrangements were observed also in human liver isoZnMT after in vitro substitution of ^{113}Cd for Zn and, because of the sequence homologies and, in particular, the conservation of the positions of the cysteinyl residues in the peptide chains, are considered likely to be common to all mammalian metallothioneins (Otvos and Armitage 1979, 1980; Boulanger and Armitage 1982). In contrast, the MT from crab hepatopancreas (18 cysteine residues in a 58-amino acid peptide chain) contains two three-metal clusters (Otvos et al. 1982).

Studies (Briggs and Armitage 1981) with native calf liver (Zn,Cu)MT (atomic Cu : Zn ratio = 0.75 : 1), after selective replacement of Zn with ^{113}Cd, showed each isoprotein to have a simple ^{113}Cd-NMR spectrum, the four Cd atoms being located in cluster A. Thus from the stoichiometry of the bound metals in the native MT, it appeared that Cu(I) ions were bound selectively to the three-metal cluster, or B sites. Winge and Miklossy (1982 b) also have produced evidence of site-selective binding of Cd and Zn in a preparation of (Cd$_{4.7}$,Zn$_{2.0}$)MT from the livers of Cd-dosed rats. Thus treatment of this MT with 1 mM EDTA at pH 7.8 removed the Zn ions and destabilized the three-metal cluster (B). The product of this reaction, in contrast with the native MT, was cleaved by proteolysis into a 32-residue polypeptide (residues 30–61 of the parent molecule) that contained four Cd ions. Thus the three-metal cluster (B) seems to be located in the NH$_2$ terminal half and the four-metal cluster in the COOH terminal portion of the MT molecule.

C. Determination of Metallothionein Concentrations in Mammalian Tissues

There is no simple, sensitive chemical method for the analysis of tissue homogenates for MT. Usually the concentration of the metalloprotein is estimated by measurement of the total metal content of the MT fraction after its separation by gel filtration from a known weight of tissue (see, e.g. WEBB 1979a). When Cd and/or Zn are the only bound metals, the content of the apoprotein can be calculated on the basis of 7 mol metal per mol protein of molecular weight 6,500, the limit of detection being about 5–10 µg thionein (BRADY and KAFKA 1979). Although MT-bound Zn is more labile than MT-bound Cd, (Cd,Zn)MT usually can be isolated by gel filtration without significant loss of Zn, provided that fresh tissue extracts are processed immediately. Storage of soluble fractions for some days at 4 °C, or dialysis after heat treatment (60 °C for 1 min) to remove labile proteins before gel filtration, results in partial loss of Zn, followed by oxidation and the formation of either MT polymers, or disulphide conjugates with other thiol-proteins. Such oxidized cytosolic fractions yield Zn-deficient monomers on treatment with mercaptoethanol (MINKEL et al. 1980). Also SUZUKI and YAMAMURA (1980a) have found small amounts of three dimers, which yield only isoMT-1, a mixture of isoMT-1 and isoMT-2, and only isoMT-2 on reduction with mercaptoethanol, in addition to the much larger amounts of the monomers, in the livers of rabbits after multiple doses of Cd. On occasions, therefore, the low molecular weight MT fraction from a gel filtration column may not contain all the cytosolic metalloprotein. Also reports that: (a) ZnMT, when isolated by this method from certain tissues, is undersaturated with metal ions (see Sect. F.II); and (b) the isoZnMT-2 from the residual liver of the partially hepatectomized rat contains 8.2 mol Zn per mol and has a thiol : Zn ratio of 2.5 : 1 (OHTAKI and KOGA 1979) illustrate other possible errors of this method. To overcome the former PROBST et al. (1977) treat the soluble fraction of the tissue with Cd before gel filtration. Separation and analysis (by Cd determination) of isoCdMT-1 and isoCdMT-2 in tissue-soluble fractions, that contain less than 1 µg MT-bound Cd per millilitre, can be achieved rapidly by an HPLC method, in which the gel permeation column is connected to the nebulizer tube of an atomic absorption spectrophotometer (SUZUKI 1980).

Metallothioneins that contain Cu, Hg, Au and Bi are even more difficult to determine accurately by metal analysis; first, because the limits of detection of these metals by atomic absorption spectrophotometry are much higher than those of Zn and Cu, and, second, because the metal-binding stoichiometry either is not known accurately, or may be altered during fractionation (see WEBB 1979a). Purified, anaerobically prepared CuMT from the livers of Cu-doses rats, for example, contains 10.1 ± 1.2 mol Cu per mol in the diamagnetic state and 18 titratable thiol groups. Under aerobic conditions, however, the Cu(I) ions are oxidized to Cu(II) and the number of reactive thiol groups falls to 10–12/mol (GELLER and WINGE 1982).

Other chemical procedures have included the use of ^{203}Hg- and ^{109}Cd-binding assays in which high molecular weight metal-binding proteins are eliminated by trichloroacetic acid precipitation (PIOTROWSKI et al. 1973) or heat treatment without or with the addition of a haemolysate of rat red blood cells (the Cd-haem method) to remove other ^{109}Cd-binding proteins and excess ^{109}Cd (CHEN and GANTHER 1975; ONOSAKA and CHERIAN 1982a) respectively. Although these methods are not specific for either MT, or thiol groups (OLAFSON and SIM 1979), KOTSONIS and KLAASSEN (1977a) first reported the ^{203}Hg procedure of PIOTROW-SKI et al. (1973) to be reliable and to give similar results to those obtained by saturation of the MT with ^{109}Cd before gel filtration; in later studies (KOTSONIS and KLAASSEN 1979) however, some ^{203}Hg, bound to components of molecular weight $<$ MT, was found to be a source of error.

Amongst various physical methods of analysis, pulse polarography was used for the determination of MT by LEBER and MIYA (1976) and ONOSAKA and CHERIAN (1982a) and was shown by OLAFSON and SIM (1979) to provide a very sensitive and rapid method of assay, when applied to either crude or, if necessary, partially fractionated tissue homogenates. In comparative studies with different strains of mice, HATA et a. (1978) isolate the isometallothioneins by ion exchange chromatography and, after removal of salts, estimate the protein concentration spectrophotometrically, on the assumption that the absorption coefficient, determined for a known concentration of one preparation, is the same for all preparations from the same species.

Probably the most significant recent advance in MT analysis has been the development of quantitative radioimmunoassays of high sensitivity and specificity. As (a) synthesis of metallothioneins, which show only minor differences in amino acid composition, is common to all mammalian species (see Sect. B) and (b) isolated MT, when injected into animals of the same or different species, is cleared rapidly from the blood by filtration in the kidneys (see Sect. G), these metalloproteins usually are not good antigens (WEBB 1982). Although BRADY and KAFKA (1979) and MADAPALLIMATAM and RIORDAN (1977) successfully raised antibodies to rat ZnMT and CdMT in rabbits, others have found the immune response to the native metalloproteins to be poor and, in consequence, have used isometallothioneins, either self-polymerized with glutaraldehyde (VANDER MALLIE and GARVEY 1978, 1979), or coupled to methylated bovine serum albumin (ABEL and OHNESORGE 1980) and, after separation by disc electrophoresis, an emulsion of the appropriate polyacrylamide gel slices (TOHYAMA and SHAIKH 1978) as antigens in rabbits, and isoMT-1 rabbit IgG conjugates as antigens in sheep (MEHRA and BREMNER 1983). Antisera raised to one isoMT usually cross-react with others from different memmalian species, but not with crab hepatopancreas MT (TOHYAMA and SHAIKH 1981) which, as mentioned previously, differs from mammalian metallothioneins in chain length and amino acid composition. Although antisera usually are reported to show no specificity for either the organ source of, or bound metal in the MT, the high titre antibodies obtained by MEHRA and BREMNER (1983) were specific for isoMT-1.

Essentially, the radioimmunoassay, described in detail in the original publications, involves an initial incubation of the diluted antiserum with an unlabelled MT, followed by the addition of the same MT that was used as antigen, but labelled with ^{125}I (e.g. VANDER MALLIE and GARVEY 1978, 1979), or with ^{109}Cd to high specific activity by replacement of the endogenous Zn (BRADY and KAFKA 1979). The immune complex then is precipitated, either together with other proteins by ammonium sulphate at pH 8.6 (TOHYAMA and SHAIKH 1978), or with an antibody to the host serum (VANDER MALLIE and GARVEY 1978, 1979; BRADY and KAFKA 1979) or immunoglobulins (i.e. anti-sheep IgG from donkey serum; MEHRA and BREMNER 1983), the precipitates being analysed for ^{125}I or [109]Cd. The assay, which has a detection range of 1–300 ng protein, i.e. thionein (VANDER MALLIE and GARVEY 1979), or 1–36 ng MT per millilitre in plasma and urine (TO-HYAMA and SHAIKH 1981) has been used to determine the urinary excretion of MT in itai-itai disease patients and other Japanese women environmentally exposed to Cd (TOHYAMA et al. 1982), MT levels in plasma and urine of Cd workers (CHANG et al. 1980) and of experimental animals (TOHYAMA and SHAIKH 1978; MEHRA and BREMNER 1983), to analyse the translation products from the livers of Cd-dosed rats (CHERIAN et al. 1981) and in the cellular localization of MT by immunofluorescence (KOJIMA and HAMASHIMA 1978) and other immunohisto-chemical methods (BANERJEE et al. 1982; DANIELSON et al. 1982). If, as much of the evidence summarized in the preceding paragraph suggests, the antigenic deter-minants in the isometallothioneins usually are sequential, rather than conforma-tional, the use of radioimmunoassay methods alone in the screening of (human) Cd exposure may have limitations.

D. Metallothionein and the Metabolism of Cadmium

Irrespective of the route of exposure, Cd enters the blood and associates loosely and reversibly with plasma proteins, particularly albumin. A single parenteral dose of Cd, therefore, is cleared rapidly from the blood and distributes amongst most organs of the body (Table 1). Most of the body burden, 45%–75% accord-ing to the dose, species (and strain), sex and nutritional status, accumulates in the liver, mainly in the parenchymal cells (CAIN and SKILLETER 1980, 1983; SCIORTINO et al. 1982) and only a small amount (1%–4% of the dose) is taken up directly by the kidneys (TANAKA et al. 1975; FRAZIER and PUGLESE 1978; WEBB 1979a; FRAZIER 1980, 1982). Uptake by these and other organs is influenced considerably by Zn deficiency; consumption of a Zn-deficient diet from the 5th to the 13th day of gestation in Holtzman rats increases the retention of Cd in all maternal organs at 24 h after the intraperitoneal administration of Cd (Table 1) on the 13th day (ROHRER et al. 1978). Also in Zn-sufficient Ehrlich ascites cells in vivo, Cd accu-mulation is much less than in Zn-deficient cells (KOCH et al. 1980).

FRAZIER and PUGLESE (1978), in agreement with the earlier work of WEBB (1972a) and CEMPEL and WEBB (1976), identify two separate processes, i.e. accu-mulation and redistribution, in the short-term kinetics of Cd in the liver after the intravenous injection of a supposedly nontoxic dose. Redistribution, which re-sults in the transfer of Cd from the particulate components (membranes, nuclei, mitochondria, microsomes) and the high molecular weight (hmw) proteins of the cytosol to MT (Fig. 1), begins after a lag phase of about 3 h (TANAKA et al. 1974; CEMPEL and WEBB 1976; YOSHIKAWA and SUZUKI 1976; SUZUKI and YAMAMURA 1980b). The Cd-induced synthesis of MT, as measured by the rate of cysteine ^{3}H incorporation, is maximal at 4 h after a single injection of Cd and returns to the control level within 16 h (ANDERSEN et al. 1978). The high binding affinity of MT

Table 1. Distribution of Cd in the rat

Organ	Intravenous			Intraperitoneal		Subcutaneous		Oral	Pregnant female[g]
	Virgin female[a]	Virgin female[b]	Pregnant female[b]	Pregnant female Zn-deficient[c]	Pregnant female Zn-sufficient[c]	Male[d]	Male[e]	Male[f]	
	Cd (μg per gram wet tissue weight)						% of dose	Cd (ng per organ)	Cd (μg per gram wet tissue weight)
Liver	4.05±0.05	27.04±0.44	24.80±0.32	22.75 ±4.76	9.46 ±1.18	17.61	69.3	63.5 + 6.7	27.94 ±5.61
Kidney	1.13±0.03	8.26±0.34	4.63+0.52	4.00 ±0.33	1.83 ±0.23	13.86	8.5	217.0 ±22.2	
Pancreas	0.96±0.01					4.76	1.3	3.19± 0.6	
Spleen	0.38±0.02					2.61	0.2	0.79± 0.1	
Heart	0.23±0.01	1.88±0.20	2.36±0.30			0.333	0.2	0.43± 0.11	
Brain	0.03±0.00					0.066		0.16± 0.04	
Testis						0.115	0.07	1.07± 0.25	
Lung		1.75±0.20	2.41±0.32			0.400	0.3	0.91± 0.19	
Intestine							2.3	66.9 ± 0.60	
Thymus		1.38±0.20	1.39±0.18						
Adrenal		4.92±0.46	4.97±0.24			0.242			
Skelet muscle							3.8		
Placenta			5.54±0.3	1.08 ±0.15	0.66 ±0.18				0.483±0.281
Blood	0.69±0.04		0.91±0.08	0.057±0.003	0.029±0.007		0.4		9.91 ±3.44

[a] At 18 h after injection of 1.0 mg Cd per kilogram body weight (WEBB and VERSCHOYLE 1976)
[b] At 8 h after injection of 1.58 mg Cd per kilogram body weight (SAMARAWICKRAMA and WEBB 1981)
[c] At 24 h after injection of 0.75 mg Cd per kilogram body weight on the 13th day of gestation (ROHRER et al. 1978)
[d] At 26 days after injection of 2.24 mg Cd per kilogram body weight (LUCIS et al. 1972)
[e] At 14 days after administration of a tracer dose of ¹⁰⁹Cd (SAMARAWICKRAMA 1979)
[f] After 2 years at a dietary Cd intake of 2.1 μg/day in food and water (SABBIONI et al. 1978)
[g] On the 21st day of gestation after the administration of 20 mg Cd per kilogram body weight per day on days 7–16 of gestation (BARAŃSKI et al. 1982)

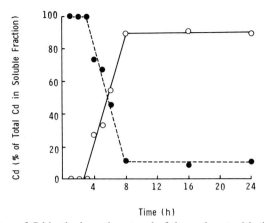

Fig. 1. Redistribution of Cd in the hepatic cytosol of the male rat with time after the injection of Cd (1.6 mg/kg i.v.). The figure is drawn from the results of CEMPEL and WEBB (1976). Cd bound to hmw protein (—●—) and to MT (—○—) is shown

for Cd, implied by the redistribution of the metal in the liver, is also shown by the change in biliary Cd excretion with time after the parenteral administration of a single dose. Excretion by this route decreases with the onset of MT synthesis and terminates when most of the intracellular Cd is in this protein-bound form (see FRAZIER 1982). Also in animals in which hepatic MT is preinduced by pretreatment with Cd or Zn, even the initial phase of biliary excretion of [109]Cd (and of Hg, Cu, and Ag, but not of As, Mn or MeHg) is reduced, or eliminated (CHERIAN 1977; KLAASSEN 1978).

In male rats, given total doses of 20, 200 and 1,000 µg Cd by intravenous injection (FRAZIER and PUGLESE 1978), or 27–3,350 µg Cd intraperitoneally (SABBIONI and MARAFANTE 1975), the fraction of the dose accumulated by the liver decreases with increase in dose, whilst that accumulated by the kidney increases. According to FRAZIER and PUGLESE (1978) this change in distribution indicates partial saturation of the ability of the liver to accumulate Cd at higher dose levels. It seems more likely, however, that hepatic uptake and/or retention are decreased because the liver is damaged. At the highest dose level (1,000 µg Cd) used by FRAZIER and PUGLESE (1978), for example, the hepatic Cd concentration was maximal at 1 h and then decreased, whereas, after doses of 20 and 200 µg Cd the concentration reached a maximum and then remained constant. Also their observation that the rate of Cd incorporation into hepatic MT shows saturation kinetics with respect to dose could have been due to altered liver function (e.g. protein synthesis) since, in rats given daily intraperitoneal injections of Cd (277 µg per animal) for 8 days, the hepatic concentrations of total and MT-bound Cd increase in proportion with the total dose (Table 2). In mice of different strains (closed colonies), given the same cumulative dose of $CdCl_2$ (550 µg) over a period of 9 days, the total MT concentration and the ratio of isoMT-1 to isoMT-2 in the liver appear to vary with the strain (Table 3, HATA et al. 1978). The use of the spectrophotometric method of analysis (see Sect. C) in this work seems to have been justified since: (a) the amino acid compositions of the MT isomers did not

Table 2. Concentrations of total and MT-bound Cd in the livers of rats at different times during the administration of 277 µg Cd per animal every day for 8 days (Sabbioni and Marafante 1975)

Number of Cd injections	Time interval between first injection and death (days)	Total cumulative dose of Cd (µg)	Total liver Cd (µg)	Total liver Cd (% of total dose)	MT-bound Cd (µg)	MT-bound Cd (% of total Cd in liver)
1	0.5	277	141	51	125	88.7
1	1.0	277	150	54	114	76.0
2	2.0	554	266	48	222	83.5
4	4.0	1,108	543	49	443	81.6
8	8.0	2,216	1,219	55	931	76.4

Table 3. Concentrations of isoMT-1 and isoMT-2 in the livers of five strains of mice after treatment with 550 µd $CdCl_2$ over a period of 9 days (Hata et al. 1978)

Strain	IsoMT-1 (mg per gram liver)	IsoMt-2 (mg per gram liver)	IsoMT-1 / IsoMT-2
DDY	0.66	0.21	3.1
DDN	0.43	0.33	1.3
DDY (N)	0.24	0.06	3.8
STD-DDY	0.32	0.21	1.5
SWR	0.36	0.26	1.4

differ between strains; and (b) both isoforms from all strains contained 4 atoms Cd per molecule and differed only slightly in their Zn contents.

The reason why Cd, in contrast with, for example, Hg, accumulates initially in the liver, not in the kidney, probably is determined by the strength of binding to metal carrier proteins in the blood. It is apparent that MT synthesis is a response to, not the cause of the hepatic uptake. Thus the organ distribution of Hg, which has a much greater affinity than Cd for the metal-binding sites of thionein in vitro (Kägi and Vallee 1960), is not altered appreciably by the presence of preinduced MT in the liver (Webb and Magos 1976). From studies with rat hepatocyte primary cultures, Gerson and Shaikh (1982) conclude that: (a) these liver cells differentiate between Cd and Hg and preferentially accumulate the former; and (b) when incorporated intracellularly, Hg, in contrast to Cd, is only a weak inducer of MT, since it binds predominantly to membranous (particulate) fractions of the hepatocyte. As only three concentrations of each metallic ion (3, 10, and 30 μM) were used in this work, some of the results are insufficiently detailed for quantitative assessment. Scatchard plots, derived from the limited data for the concentrations of total and non-protein-bound metals, however, show clearly that Cd and Hg differ considerably in their binding affinities to components of the serum-supplemented culture medium (Fig. 2). It is likely, therefore,

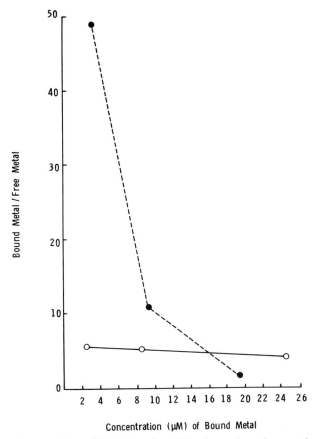

Fig. 2. Binding characteristics of Cd (—o—) and Hg (—●—) to the protein components of Dulbecco modified Eagle's (DME) culture medium, supplemented with 10% calf serum. The Scatchard plots are derived from the data of Gerson and Shaikh (1982)

that the significantly greater uptake of Cd, relative to that of Hg, which was observed at each of the three concentrations (molar Cd:Hg uptake ratios of 8:1, 7.9:1, and 1.4:1, respectively), was not due to cellular discrimination between the two metals, but to the decreased availability of Hg, in consequence of its stronger binding to protein components of the culture medium. This would explain why the uptake of Hg increased disproportionately with the increase in concentration of total Hg from 10 to 30 μM, but was linear with respect to "free" Hg (Fig. 3). Differences in the availability of Cd and Hg from the culture medium also would explain the observation that, at the highest concentration (30 μM) Cd, but not Hg, was cytotoxic. It is apparent from the results of Gerson and Shaikh (1982), however, that the responses to intracellularly incorporated Cd and Hg are very different. Thus exposure to the lowest Cd concentration (3 μM) caused a time-dependent induction of MT, which led to a significant redistribution of intracellular Cd between 6 and 24 h. At a medium concentration of 30 μM Hg, uptake

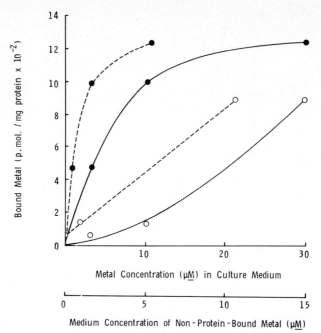

Fig. 3. Cellular uptake (pmol per milligram cell protein $\times 10^{-2}$) of Cd ($\bullet$) and Hg ($\circ$) in relation to the concentrations of total (—) and non-protein-bound (----) metal in the hepatocyte culture medium. The figure is drawn from the results of GERSON and SHAIKH (1982)

of Hg was 1.9 times greater than that of Cd at 3 μM concentration, but did not cause the induction of MT.

Cadmium is known to be transferred slowly from the liver to the kidney, probably through the liberation of hepatic MT and at either prolonged low-level exposure, or several months after a single dose (in rats and rabbits) the renal concentration is likely to exceed the hepatic concentration (see Sect. H). In rats 2–14 days after a single oral dose of Cd in the range 25–150 μg/kg, however, the concentration of Cd remains constant in the liver, increases in the kidney and decreases by approximately 50% in spleen, heart, testes, muscle and brain and by 90% in the intestine (KOTSONIS and KLAASSEN 1977b). It seems, therefore, that soon after exposure the kidney accumulates Cd that is eliminated from extrahepatic organs. It is not known, however, if the transfer from these organs is a direct process, or occurs indirectly via the liver. Possibly the latter is less likely, since the constancy of the hepatic concentration during the 12-day period (see also Table 5), implies that, at any dose level, loss of Cd from the liver would be equal to its uptake from other sources. Also, when multiple doses of Zn (4 mg/kg) are administered parenterally to rats that have been maintained for 30 weeks on a diet supplemented with 100 ppm Cd, the concentration of MT-bound Cd remains essentially constant in the liver (i.e. 19.1 and 18.2 μg Cd MT per gram wet weight in the Zn-treated and control animals, respectively), but increases appreciably (from 17.7 to 31.1 μg/g) in the kidney (Fig. 4). These results show that it is not

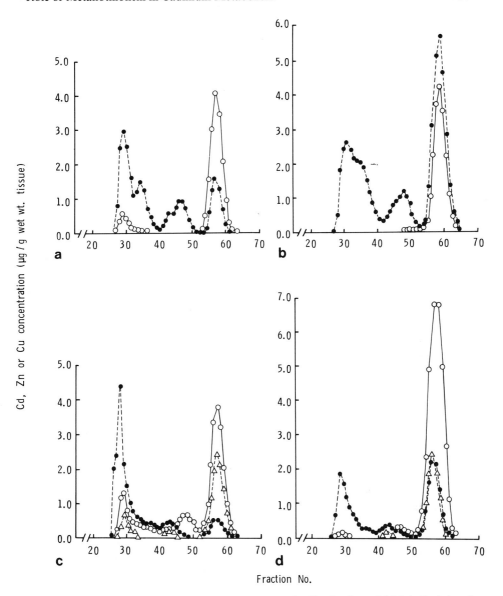

Fig. 4a–d. Effect of parenterally administered Zn on the distribution of Cd (○), Zn (●) and Cu (△) in the soluble fractions from the livers (**a, b**) and kidneys (**c, d**) of female rats, maintained on a diet supplemented with 100 ppm Cd for 30 weeks from weaning. During the last week five animals were given Zn (4 mg/kg s.c.) every 24 h for 5 days and were killed after a further 48 h. Soluble fractions were prepared from the pooled livers and kidneys of the control (**a, c**) and Zn-treated groups (**b, d**) and fractionated by gel filtration. Metal concentrations were determined by atomic absorption spectrophotometry (M. WEBB 1975, previously unpublished work)

Table 4. Concentrations of MT in various organs and tissues of the rat, given total doses of 6.4, 12.0 and 24.0 mg Cd per kilogram body weight over a 16-day period and the relationships between MT concentration and total Cd dose and tissue or organ Cd concentration (Onosaka and Cherian 1981)

Organ or tissue	MT concentration (µg per gram wet weight)[a]				Relationship between MT concentration (µg per gram wet weight) and	
	Total Cd dose (mg per kilogram body weight)					
	0 (control)	6.4	12.0	24.0	Dose (mg/kg)	Cd concentration (µg/g)
Brain	32 ± 12	41 ± 2	37 ± 2	45 ± 10		
Lung	19 ± 8	32 ± 4	33 ± 5	44 ± 8		$5.86\,\text{Cd} + 19.7$
Heart	5 ± 2	64 ± 4^{b}	79 ± 8^{b}	149 ± 36^{b}	$5.7\,\text{Cd} + 13^{c}$	$16.0\ \text{Cd} + 6.6$
Liver	20 ± 8	$1,600 \pm 40^{b}$	$2,190 \pm 12^{b}$	$4,700 \pm 624^{b}$	$190\ \ \text{Cd} + 116^{b}$	$16.6\ \text{Cd} + 40.7$
Kidney	61 ± 14	534 ± 29^{b}	857 ± 35^{b}	$1,430 \pm 102^{b}$	$56\ \ \text{Cd} + 125^{b}$	$10.4\ \text{Cd} + 112$
Stomach	23 ± 6	48 ± 8^{b}	75 ± 12^{b}	102 ± 6^{b}	$3.3\,\text{Cd} + 27^{c}$	$16.3\ \text{Cd} + 20.7$
Small intestine	40 ± 4	59 ± 16	65 ± 16	112 ± 14^{b}	$3.0\,\text{Cd} + 27^{c}$	$20.0\ \text{Cd} + 35.1$
Pancreas	39 ± 6	323 ± 65^{b}	529 ± 70^{b}	674 ± 50^{b}	$26\ \ \text{Cd} + 118^{c}$	$16.7\ \text{Cd} + 73.6$
Spleen	8 ± 4	55 ± 2^{b}	73 ± 6^{b}	125 ± 6^{b}	$4.7\,\text{Cd} + 116^{c}$	$9.84\,\text{Cd} + 8.0$
Testis[d]	179 ± 8	171 ± 5	137 ± 22	60 ± 32		
Muscle	4 ± 0	5 ± 2	5 ± 2	12 ± 0		

[a] Analyses were made on the tissues and organs from three animals by the Cd-haem method (see Sect. C)
[b] $P < 0.01$
[c] $P < 0.05$
[d] The dose-dependent decrease in MT concentration was due to testicular necrosis

possible to eliminate MT-bound Cd from either the liver or kidney by administration of a large dose of Zn, since Zn incorporated into these organs causes further MT synthesis, and thus suggest that Cd in (certain) other organs, which is transferred to the kidney as a result of Zn treatment, must be stored in a different form. Nevertheless, by the Cd-haem and radioimmunoassay methods (Sect. C), the presence of MT has been demonstrated in various organs, in addition to the liver, kidney and intestine, of the Cd-dosed experimental animal (Table 4). It is not known, however, if these organs liberate CdMT to the blood. Whilst synthesis of CdMT has been reported in the lungs of animals exposed to Cd aerosols (see Sect. E) and Prigge (1978) has found higher kidney : liver concentration ratios in rats after exposure to Cd by inhalation than by gastric gavage, other evidence suggests that CdMT liberation from the lungs either is not significant, or MT-bound Cd is replaced by Cu in the blood (see Sect. G) and becomes bound to albumin. Thus, in studies with rabbits exposed to aerosols of $CdCl_2$, Post et al. (1982) found a subsequent slow transfer of Cd from the lung to both the liver and kidney; the Cd concentration, however, was higher in the former than in the latter organ for at least 17 days after termination of the exposure.

Normally the liver and, subsequently, the kidney are the major internal organs that accumulate high concentrations of Cd (Table 1) and, even at prolonged low level exposure the amounts in other body organs, with the exception of the intestine, are small. Only a few attempts have been made, therefore, to investigate whether Cd causes MT synthesis at other sites in the body. The results of Table 4, coupled with the further characterization of the Cd- (and Zn)-induced pancreatic metallothioneins by their resolution into isoMT-1 and isoMT-2 (ONOSAKA and CHERIAN 1981, 1982 b), thus provide additional evidence not only to confirm the tentative identification of the Cd-binding proteins in the spleen (AMACHER and EWING 1975) and pancreas (BREMNER and DAVIES 1974; SABBIONI et al. 1979) as metallothioneins, but also to suggest that dose-dependent MT synthesis occurs also in response to Cd in the heart and stomach. Synthesis (or accumulation) of MT in the testes, not observed by ONOSAKA and CHERIAN (1981) because of the Cd-induced atrophy of this organ (see Sect. J) has been reported by NORDBERG (1971), CHEN et al. (1972), SINGH and NATH (1972), and SINGH et al. (1974) and in the placenta by LUCIS et al. (1972) and SAMARAWICKRAMA and WEBB (1981). Synthesis also has been established in primary and clonal cultures of many different cell types (see, e.g. WEBB 1979 a; KOCH et al. 1980; GICK et al. 1981, for later literature summaries). By immunohistochemical methods (see Sect. C) DANIELSON et al. (1982) and BANERJEE et al. (1982) have demonstrated endogenous MT (or thionein) in rat hepatocytes, renal collecting duct epithelium and distal convoluted tubular epithelia. Repeated administration of Cd leads to either increased amounts, or the appearance of MT in the liver, kidneys, respiratory epithelial cells of the lung, the surface columnar epithelial cells of the intestinal villi, the Paneth cells of the small intestine and in the Sertoli and interstitial cells of the testis, but not in the vascular endothelial cells, fibroblasts, leucocytes and spermatogonia. In the liver both the nuclei and cytoplasm of hepatocytes show high intensity staining and the bile duct epithelium also gives a positive reaction. In the kidney, the proximal convoluted tubules and the lumina of these tubules, collecting duct epithelium and, according to BANERJEE et al. (1982), in contrast to DANIELSON et al. (1982), the glomerular, mesangial and visceral epithelial cells also contain MT.

From the regression equations (Table 4) ONOSAKA and CHERIAN (1981) conclude that the uptake of 1 μg Cd per gram wet tissue will induce almost the same amount of MT (16–17 μg/g) in the liver, pancreas, stomach and heart and 20 μg/g in the small intestine. In kidney, spleen and lung, induction is considered to be less effective, i.e. 10.4, 9.8, and 5.9 μg/g, respectively, in response to a Cd concentration of 1 μg/g. These results imply that, in contrast to the observations of others (see, e.g. WEBB 1979 a): (a) there is no threshold Cd concentration below which MT synthesis does not occur in any of the responsive tissues and organs; and (b) the concentration of MT is proportional to the tissue concentration of Cd, irrespective of the concentrations of Zn and Cu in the metalloprotein. Nevertheless the same authors (ONOSAKA and CHERIAN 1982 b) have shown that a threshold concentration of Zn, which may differ from tissue to tissue, has to be exceeded before MT synthesis occurs in response to this metal.

In animals exposed to low dietary levels of Cd, the concentrations of MT-bound Cd in the livers and kidneys increase in parallel with the organ concentrations of the metal throughout most of their lifetimes (see, e.g. SABBIONI et al. 1979; WEBB 1979 a). After multiple parenteral doses, the MT concentration in the liver also increases with the total dose; e.g. from 69 to 530 μg per gram wet weight in stepwise increments in response to the subcutaneous injection of 0.25 μg Cd per kilogram body weight in the rat every 48 h for 1 week (Klaassen 1978; see also Table 2). The Cd-induced MT in the mammalian liver, however, always seems to contain appreciable amounts of Zn, whereas that from the kidney contains either Zn or Cu as the major "secondary" metal. Whilst the accumulation of MT-bound Cu in the kidneys of the brindled mutant mouse (an animal model of Menkes' disease) is well documented (see, e.g. Prins and van den Hamer 1982), Suzuki (1979) has shown that multiple doses of Cd in rats and guinea-pigs, but not in mice, hamsters and rabbits, lead to the accumulation of Cu, in addition to Cd, in the renal MT. Thus, although the content of MT-bound Zn increases in the kidneys of the five species, the increase is much greater in the last three.

According to Elinder et al. (1981) the concentration of MT-bound Cd in equine liver (about 80% of the total hepatic burden accumulated from environmental sources) is related to that of MT-bound Zn by the equation

$$\text{ZnMT (}\mu\text{mol)} = 2.5 \, [\text{CdMT (}\mu\text{mol)}] + 0.26$$

a relationship which implies that, in this species, incorporation of every Cd atom into the hepatic MT is accompanied by the incorporation of 2.5 atoms Zn and, at all times the Cd-induced MT contains 5 atoms Zn and 2 atoms Cd per molecule. After a single acute dose of Cd in experimental animals, however, hepatic uptake and MT binding of Cd precede the uptake and binding of Zn by several hours or days, according to the route of administration. Thus in mice after a single subcutaneous dose of Cd (2.5 mg per kilogram body weight) the hepatic concentration of Cd is maximal at about 10 h (Table 5; Sugawara 1977). The hepatic Zn concentration at this time, however, is the same as that in the untreated control animal and does not increase significantly until 6 days after dosing. The increase in kidney Cd concentration, which continues slowly over a 20-day period, is not associated with any change in either hepatic Cd, or renal Zn concentration. These results, in agreement with the earlier observations of Webb (1972 a) and Cempel and Webb (1976) and the later studies of Frazier and Puglese (1978) and Winge et al. (1978) with intravenously dosed rats, show that Cd administration has little or no immediate effect upon the total hepatic Zn concentration. It does, however, alter the distribution of Zn between cytoplasmic macromolecules and, in particular, causes an initial displacement of this metal from

Table 5. Hepatic and renal concentrations of Cd and Zn in mice at different times after the subcutaneous injection of 2.5 mg Cd per kilogram body weight (Sugawara 1977)

Organ	Metal	Time after Cd injection						
		0 (control)	0.5 h	4 h	10 h	24 h	6 days	20 days
		Metal concentration (µg per gram wet tissue weight)						
Liver	Cd		5.3 ± 2.6	15.9 ± 6.0	23.3 ± 2.8	22.1 ± 3.7	25.8 ± 7.5	22.9 ± 5.3
	Zn	21.7 ± 2.2	22.1 ± 1.9	20.4 ± 5.2	22.0 ± 4.1	29.1 ± 5.1	41.3 ± 8.5	43.4 ± 4.9
Kidney	Cd		1.8 ± 0.1	3.0 ± 0.6	3.1 ± 0.9	5.0 ± 0.8	11.4 ± 3.2	12.9 ± 1.6
	Zn	15.0 ± 2.0	16.0 ± 0.3	14.0 ± 1.3	17.0 ± 1.2	13.1 ± 2.1	17.0 ± 3.0	20.7 ± 2.3

the hmw protein fraction. Accumulation of MT-bound Zn, however, seems to begin only after most, if not all of the cytoplasmic Cd has been transferred from its initial binding sites to the induced thionein. In consequence, the atomic ratio of MT-bound Cd:Zn alters with time, e.g. from more than 8:1 within a few hours of the intravenous injection of rats with 2 mg Cd per kilogram body weight to 2–3:1 at 12 h (WINGE et al. 1978) and from 5.5:1 at 4 h to 0.8:1 at 6 days after the subcutaneous injection of 2.5 mg/kg in mice (SUGAWARA 1977). WINGE et al. (1978) consider that although increased intestinal uptake may contribute to the increase in total and MT-bound Zn in the liver of the Cd-dosed animal, decreased excretion, possibly owing to the Cd-induced reduction in biliary elimination of metals, mentioned earlier in this section, is the main reason for the hepatic accumulation of Zn.

Although the results of SUGAWARA (1977) and of WINGE et al. (1978) show that, in contrast to Zn-induced MT (SUZUKI and YAMAMURA 1980c), the elevated content of Zn in the Cd-induced MT is maintained for up to 6 months after dosing, WHANGER et al. (1980) have observed the Zn:Cd ratio in both hepatic and renal MT to decrease at 80 days after Cd injection. Also CHEN et al. (1975) found the amount of Zn in association with the MT of rat liver to be maximal at 4 days after the subcutaneous injection of 3 mg Cd per kilogram body weight. Thus, the loss of Zn from the Cd-induced hepatic MT, which is accompanied by changes in the ratios of isoMT-1:isoMT-2 and of Zn:Cd in these isomers (SUZUKI and

Table 6. Amino acid compositions of intestinal and hepatic isometallothioneins from Cd-exposed rats

Amino acid residue	Content (% of total residues)					
	Intestinal (Cd, Zn) MT		Hepatic (Cd, Zn) MT			
	TAGUCHI and NAKAMURA (1982)		WINGE et al. (1975)		ANDERSEN et al. (1978)	
	Isoform 1	Isoform 2	Isoform 1	Isoform 2	Isoform 1	Isoform 2
Asp	6.9	6.8	8.5	8.4	6.7	6.6
Thr	5.3	3.2	6.2	4.0	6.0	3.2
Ser	14.3	13.7	17.5	15.7	17.2	16.4
Glu	4.4	5.8	3.9	7.3	2.0	4.9
Pro	0	0	3.4	3.7	3.7	3.4
Gly	12.3	8.5	10.3	7.2	10.0	6.6
Ala	6.7	10.3	6.1	8.8	5.0	8.0
Cys	27.6	26.3	28.8	25.4	31.1	33.3
Val	6.6	5.9	1.7	1.4	3.3	1.9
Met	0	0	1.3	1.2	1.5	1.5
Ile	0.9	1.9		0.7		1.3
Leu	1.1	1.0	0.6	0.7		
Phe	1.0	0.5				
Lys	13.0	16.1	11.6	14.1	13.4	12.9

Yamamura 1980 b; Suzuki et al. 1981), probably is dependent upon nutritional status, as well as time and Cd dose.

Both parenteral and oral administration of Cd result in the retention of Cd in the intestine (see Table 1). The Cd-binding protein, isolated from the intestinal mucosae of rats at 24 h after an oral dose of 100 mg Cd per kilogram body weight, has been resolved into two major electrophoretically homogeneous isoprotein fractions (Taguchi and Nakamura 1982). The high cysteine, serine, glycine and lysine contents of these proteins (Table 6) identify them as isometallothioneins. Nevertheless, their amino acid compositions not only differ from those of rat hepatic iso(Cd,Zn)MT-1 and iso(Cd,Zn)MT-2, particularly with regard to proline and methionine (Table 6), but indicate minimum molecular weights, which are much greater than those (i.e. 6,500–7,000) usually accepted as typical of liver isometallothioneins (see Kägi and Nordberg 1979). It seems unfortunate that as Taguchi and Nakamura (1982) did not determine the amino acid compositions of the isometallothioneins from the livers of their animals, comparison between the compositions of the intestinal and hepatic proteins is dependent upon the results of others, which show considerable interlaboratory variation (Webb 1979 a). Nevertheless, all previously reported analyses show proline and methionine (the normal NH_2 terminal amino acid) contents of 2.8%–6.9% (mean 4.0%) and 0.4%–1.7% (mean 1.3%) respectively. The absence of these amino acids from the intestinal isometallothioneins obtained by Taguchi and Nakamura (1982), therefore, could be significant, particularly in relation to the immunohistochemical localization of MT in the intestine with antibodies which, as discussed in Sect. C, are raised against the hepatic metalloprotein.

E. Metallothionein Synthesis in Relation to the Chronic Toxicity of Cadmium

The defence, or detoxification function of MT synthesis, originally proposed by Piscator (1964) to explain the progressive accumulation of high, but apparently nontoxic renal and hepatic burdens of Cd in rats and rabbits in response to the repeated administration of low doses of Cd, has been established unequivocally by a multiplicity of subsequent studies (see, e.g. Webb 1979 a, b). The ability of MT to prevent significant interactions of Cd with sensitive cellular targets is illustrated by the observations of Suda et al. (1974) that accumulation of appreciable amounts of Cd in the kidneys of rats, as in chickens, has no effect on the mitochondrial 1-hydroxylation of 25-hydroxyvitamin D_3, a reaction which in vitro is inhibited completely by 25 μM $CdCl_2$, but is unaffected by the same concentration of Cd, when added as (Cd,Zn)MT. Also Cd, but not (Cd,Zn)MT at the same molar Cd concentration, strongly and irreversibly inhibits the acyl-CoA-acyltransferases of rat liver microsomes in vitro (Waku et al. 1980). The claim by Minkel et al. (1980) that the effects of chronic Cd exposure on liver function in the rat must be attributed to CdMT, not to non-MT-bound Cd, thus is not supported by these enzyme studies.

In animals that continually ingest Cd from their diets, the critical concentration of Cd in the kidney, the critical organ at chronic exposure, is high (200–

600 μg per gram wet weight according to species; NOMIYAMA and NOMIYAMA 1982) since, although Cd accumulates progressively, most of the renal burden is bound to MT. At least until an appreciable kidney Cd concentration has been accumulated, the concentration of MT-bound Cd increases in proportion to the organ concentration of Cd and the amount of non-MT-bound metal, the presumptive toxic species, in the particulate components and other cystosolic proteins of the tubular cell, probably remains below 20% of the total (CAIN and WEBB 1983). It has yet to be established if this proportionality is maintained and the onset of renal damage is coincident with a critical concentration of non-MT-bound Cd, or whether the capacity for MT synthesis is limited. A complicating factor is the loss of MT from the kidney to the urine with the onset of renal damage (SHAIKH and HIRAYAMA 1979; VANDER MALLIE and GARVEY 1979; TOHYAMA and SHAIKH 1981). Although RAGHAVEN and GONICK (1980) conclude that the ability of MT to bind Cd must be exhausted before there is sufficient "free" Cd to inhibit renal cortical Na, K-ATPase, which they consider to be the cause of renal tubular dysfunction, their results are equally explicable by a progressive increase in non-MT-bound Cd, in parallel with that of CdMT, to a critical level.

Sex differences, as shown by approximately twofold greater concentrations of total and MT-bound Cd in the livers, but not in the kidneys, of female as compared with male rats, fed a diet supplemented with 100 ppm Cd, were reported by STONARD and WEBB (1976). In later work, PETERING et al. (1979) found that, in rats exposed to Cd in the drinking water, the accumulation of Cd in the livers and kidneys, of Cu in the kidneys, and possibly of Zn in the livers, was greater in females than in males (Table 7). The dose-related increases in Cd concentrations in the heart, lung, pancreas and gonads also were higher in females than in males. An important contributory factor to these differences was the consumption of about twice as much water and thus twice as much Cd by the female as by the male rats. Observations that, at 6 days after the second of two subcutaneous injections of Cd (2.5 mg per kilogram body weight), the renal concentration of CdMT is higher in male than in female rats (WEBB and MAGOS 1976), re-

Table 7. Mean concentrations of Zn, Cu and Cd in the livers and kidney of rats exposed to Cd (4.3, 8.6, and 17.2 μg/ml) in the drinking water for 39 weeks (PETERING et al. 1979)

Organ	Metal	Metal concentration (μg per gram dry tissue weight)							
		Males				Females			
		Cd concentration (μg/ml) in drinking water							
		0.0	4.3	8.6	17.2	0.0	4.3	8.6	17.2
Liver	Zn	100	96	106	114	105	114	118	144
	Cu	13.5	13.6	12.8	13.3	17.8	18.0	17.3	19.5
	Cd	0.2	2.1	7.2	20.4	0.3	6.8	17.9	39.4
Kidney	Zn	88	117	114	121	102	127	126	148
	Cu	23.4	28.8	33.8	35.5	46.7	75.8	52.6	114.8
	Cd	0.6	16.2	41.8	83.3	1.1	27.5	63.3	163.9

tention of dietary Cd is less in intact males than in normal females, or in gonad-ectomized rats of either sex (KELLO et al. 1979 a), the half-lives of Cd in the kidney and salivary glands, although influenced by age, invariably are longer in females than in males (TAGUCHI and SUZUKI 1981) and Cd pretreatment prolongs the hexobarbital-induced sleep time in male, but not in female rats (HICKS et al. 1976; PENCE et al. 1977) provided evidence that Cd metabolism in this species is influenced by sex hormones. Such effects are not unexpected; Cu metabolism in the rat, for example is known to be influenced by hormonal factors, the sex-linked variations in plasma Cu concentration being reflected in greater renal concentrations of total and MT-bound Cu in female than in male animals (BREMNER et al. 1981). Ovariectomized and orchiectomized rats lose the ability to regulate effectively the plasma levels of Zn and Cu (CHOUDHURY et al. 1974), and, in 13-week-old female rats, ovariectomized at 7 weeks of age, the kidney Cu concentration is reduced from 27.8 ± 1.7 µg per gram wet weight in normal animals (21.3 ± 1.6 in the sham-operated controls) to 13.9 ± 1.3 µg/g (BREMNER et al. 1981). The latter authors also point out that the sex-linked difference in kidney Cd accumulation in the rat cannot be explained entirely by the greater Cd intake in the female and suggest that, as the accumulation of Cd probably occurs by the processes normally used for Cu metabolism, susceptibility to Cd intoxication possibly could be related to sex, as well as to age. BREMNER et al. (1981) emphasize, however, that the changes in Cu metabolism and renal CuMT concentration are secondary, not direct responses to sex hormones and, furthermore, may be restricted to certain species (see, e.g. Sect. D). In human beings, for example, the results of ANKE and SCHNEIDER (1974) show that major changes in kidney Cu content are not associated with either age or sex. Also in comparable age groups, urinary excretion of Cd is greater (SUZUKI and TAGUCHI 1970) whilst kidney concentrations are less (ANKE et al. 1979) in women than in men. Other evidence, summarized by ANKE et al. (1979) shows faecal excretion of Cd in quail cocks to be lower than in hens, but to become similar to that in the latter after treatment with oestrogens, whilst in goats, fed 500 ppm Cd in the diet, Cd concentrations in the kidney, liver, aorta and skeletal muscle are higher in males than in females. Thus the sex differences in Cd retention and, in particular, renal Cd concentration are not consistent between species and probably are influenced by genetic factors, as well as by hormonal status (ANKE et al. 1979).

As discusses in Sect. D, the MT induced by Cd usually, if not invariably contains Zn and/or Cu as secondary metals. In the kidneys of horses (NORDBERG et al. 1979), as in human beings (PISCATOR and LUND 1972), the concentration of Zn, but not of Cu, increases in almost equimolar proportion with the increase in Cd concentration until the latter exceeds 0.6 mmol per kilogram wet weight. This additional Zn is located in the renal MT, which also contains most (65%) of the kidney Cd (ELINDER et al. 1981). The molar ratio of MT-bound Zn : MT-bound Cd is constant at renal Cd concentrations below 0.1 mmol/kg, but then falls as the latter increases (NORDBERG et al. 1979). If, however, this change in ratio is due to the limited capacity of the kidney to synthesize MT, it might be expected that, as Cu binds to thionein with greater affinity than Cd, species in which Cu is the major secondary metal in the renal MT would be more susceptible to Cd-induced nephrotoxicity. Such species differences in response, however, are not apparent.

In the kidney of the Cd-exposed rat, for example, the increase in renal Cd concentration ultimately leads to a decrease in the concentration of Cu (and of Zn), relative to that of Cd in the MT fraction (KOTSONIS and KLAASSEN 1978; SATO and NAGAI 1982). Changes in the metal ratio of the renal MT thus may not be of any great significance, but a consequence of the normal turnover of the protein, coupled with the increase in Cd concentration in the kidney.

SATO and NAGAI (1980, 1982) have reported that at the time of onset of renal damage in rats in response to the repeated subcutaneous injection of Cd, the rates of increase in the Cd concentrations in mitochondria, lysosomes and hmw protein fraction of the cytosol are greater than that in MT. These authors also claim that when the kidney concentration of Cd is elevated appreciably, Cd is associated with four additional fractions of the cytosol. It is apparent from their results, however, that the amount of Cd associated with any of these fractions never exceeds 4.3% of the total soluble Cd and, even at kidney concentrations near 200 µg per gram wet weight, there is no significant clear-cut increase in their Cd contents. Earlier COLUCCI et al. (1975) observed the appearance of two additional Cd-binding protein fractions in the liver cytosol of rats with high hepatic burdens of Cd and proposed that these fractions could be important in the development of physiological changes in this organ. It was shown by FAEDER et al. (1977), however, that Cd binding to these (or similar) fractions in the liver was not dose related and did not correlate with any observable change, either biochemical, or morphological. SUZUKI et al. (1981) also have detected small increases in the Cd contents of certain cytoplasmic components other than MT in the livers of rats, repeatedly exposed to Cd (4×3.0 mg/kg^{-1} week^{-1} s.c. for up to 4 weeks), but give little or no sound evidence to support their conclusions that: (a) some of these are metallothioneins of shorter than normal chain length; and (b) alterations in hepatic function are related to the amount of Cd associated with the heat-labile hmw protein fraction of the cytosol.

The experiments summarized in the preceding paragraph are not ideal models of chronic Cd exposure, since the dose levels are excessive and invariably lead to high liver burdens of Cd. The same criticism applies to the studies of NOMIYAMA and NOMIYAMA (1982), in which male rabbits were given subcutaneous injections of 0.5 mg Cd per kilogram body weight for 6 days per week over a period of 21 weeks. After 8 weeks the concentrations of total and MT-bound Cd in the livers of these animals were 580 and 510 µg per gram wet weight, respectively. The latter value suggests, first, that the capacity of the liver for MT synthesis is not saturated at a hepatic Cd concentration of almost 600 µg/g and, second, that transfer of CdMT from the liver to the kidney which, presumably, is dependent upon the hepatic MT content, could be excessively high. Thus NOMIYAMA and NOMIYAMA's (1982) estimates of the critical concentrations of total and non-MT-bound Cd in the kidneys of rabbits as 280 and 65 µg/g, respectively, may not be relevant to continual low-level dietary ingestion of Cd, the normal route of exposure in humans.

Continual exposure to Cd has been reported to cause not only renal tubular damage, but also glomerular dysfunction in both industrially exposed human beings (LOUWERYS et al. 1979) and experimental animals (BERNARD et al. 1980). TOHYAMA and SHAIKH (1981) suggest that this glomerulonephritis may be an immune complex nephritis that results from autoantibody production in response to the release to the blood of hepatic MT during Cd exposure.

In relation to human Cd exposure by inhalation, which is (or was) an industrial problem, synthesis of a metalloprotein, tentatively identified as CdMT, in the lungs of Syrian hamsters exposed to $CdCl_2$ aerosols was considered by BENSON and HENDERSON (1980) to provide a possible early defence mechanism. Two and 40-fold increases in MT concentration (determined immunochemically with antibodies to rat liver or kidney MT) in the lungs of rats have been detected after continuous inhalation of CdO fumes (25 mg/m^3 for 50 days) and ZnO (625 mg/m^3 for 23 days) by OBERDÖRSTER and KÖRDEL (1981). Metallothioneins or, at least, Cd-binding proteins, which resemble MT in their behaviour on gel filtration, also have been isolated after in vitro culture of cells derived from pulmonary tissue, e.g. alveolar macrophages (COX and WATERS 1978), lymphocytes (HILDEBRAND and CRAM 1979) and fibroblasts (HART and KEATING 1980). Inhalation of $CdCl_2$ aerosols (800 and 1,600 µg/m^3 for 2 h on alternate days during a 5-day period), however, was found by POST et al. (1982) to lead to the appearance of at least three low molecular weight Cd-binding proteins in the lungs of rabbits. Although two of these proteins were chromatographically, electrophoretically and spectrophotometrically similar to the isoforms of rabbit liver (Cd,Zn)MT, they accounted for only 25% of the total Cd in the lung cytosol at 24 h after the last exposure. Most (75%) of the soluble, protein-bound Cd in the lung did not bind to DEAE–Sephadex, even after treatment with mercaptoethanol, and thus appeared to be neither a polymer of MT, nor related to MT. The apparent induction of this protein by inhalation exposure, however, was considered to indicate a protective function, similar to that of MT in other organs.

At dietary exposure, Cd uptake through the intestine is limited and, according to species, probably only about 0.3%–5% of the amount ingested enters the systemic circulation (see, e.g. BREMNER 1979). Intestinal retention, however, is high. As it is probable that Cd has no specific transport mechanism, uptake is likely to occur by carrier systems that operate for certain essential metals. Studies by STARCHER (1969), and EVANS et al. (1970) led to the concept that synthesis of MT in the intestinal mucosa functions to regulate the absorption and/or transport of Zn and Cu and that the antagonistic interactions of these metals, either between themselves, or with Cd, could be explained by competition for the thiol binding sites of MT. The interaction between various metals at the level of intestinal absorption is further considered in Chap. 3.

Whilst the more recent results of DAVIES and CAMPBELL (1977), however, indicate that MT has a minimal role in the regulation of Cu absorption in rats, increased concentrations of ZnMT in the intestinal mucosa, as well as in the liver, follow the administration of Zn (RICHARDS and COUSINS 1976). A direct relationship between Zn binding to MT and the reduction of Zn flux from the intestinal lumen to the plasma (SMITH and COUSINS 1979), coupled with earlier observations, reviewed by COUSINS (1979), led to the suggestion (COUSINS 1979) that the inducible synthesis of MT controls the efflux of Zn and, possibly, Cd from the mucosal cells. Whilst there is no doubt that MT synthesis in these cells is influenced by Zn status, at normal dietary levels of Zn, the mucosal MT concentration is very small (HALL et al. 1979). Also STARCHER et al. (1980) point out that the experiments of RICHARDS and COUSINS (1976), which led to the concept of an inverse relationship between dietary [65]Zn absorption and the intestinal concentration of ZnMT, did not allow for isotope dilution by endogenous Zn and, when corrections are made for this, Zn absorption is directly proportional to the intestinal concentration of ZnMT. These results, coupled with the observed inhibition by actinomycin D of both the induction of MT and the increase in [65]Zn absorption, which follows the subjection of the animals to mild stress, suggests either a direct role of MT in Zn absorption, or that the dose-dependent synthesis of intestinal ZnMT drives Zn absorption by a gradient effect (STARCHER et al. 1980). The second of these alternatives suggests that MT synthesis would result in the retention of Zn and provide some restraint on absorption at high dietary intakes.

In normal rats after a single intragastric dose of Cd the percentage absorbed is independent of the dose (KOTSONIS and KLAASSEN 1977a); MT becomes a major binding component of the intestine only at 5 h after dosing with 100 mg Cd per kilogram body weight, although it is a primary acceptor of Cd in animals that have been pretreated orally with 20 mg/kg 24 h previously (SQUIBB et al. 1976). The suggestion by these authors, reiterated by CHERIAN et al. (1978), KOTSONIS and KLAASSEN (1978), McGIVERN and MASON (1979) and TAGUCHI and NAKAMURA (1982), that intestinal MT may function to regulate (or prevent) the absorption of Cd, however, is difficult to reconcile with the observation that, relative to the normal control, such pretreatment increases the uptake of Cd from a subsequent higher dose into the liver, kidney and testis, but decreases intestinal retention by 66% (SQUIBB et al. 1976). The possibility that, by analogy with the hypothesis of STARCHER et al. (1980) for Zn transport, intestinal CdMT drives Cd absorption by a gradient effect, is unlikely, since pretreatment with Cd increases the absorption of [109]Cd (ENGSTRÖM and NORDBERG 1979), an observation which implies little or no equilibration of the labelled metallic ion with MT-bound Cd.

Clear evidence that MT in the jejunal mucosa is not a determinant in Cd absorption has been obtained from perfusion experiments in situ with low concentrations of Cd (10–20 μM CdCl$_2$) in glucose saline (KELLO et al. 1979b). Elevation of the MT in the mucosal tissue from the normal level (40 µg per gram wet weight) to 144 µg/g (as determined by the [109]Cd saturation method, Sect. C), by preexposure of rats to 50 ppm Cd in the drinking water for 9 days, had no effect on [109]Cd transport to the body and caused only a marginal increase in the accumulation of [109]Cd in the mucosal tissue. Also, although the Cd-binding capacity of the intestinal MT of both preexposed and control animals greatly exceeded the actual binding of newly absorbed Cd (i.e. each MT presumably contained excess Zn), binding was not restricted to this fraction of the mucosal cytosol. Thus after perfusion of control rats, most of the [109]Cd retained in the mucosal segments was bound to the hmw proteins, even though MT was present in excess. In pretreated rats the Cd distribution was different; most of the metal in the soluble fraction was associated with MT.

F. Metallothionein Synthesis in Relation to the Acute Toxicity of Cadmium

Reference may here be made to the involvement of MT in cellular resistance to Cd, as discussed in Chap. 11.

I. Normal Animals

After a single parenteral dose of Cd, at or above the LD_{50}, a number of animals die from respiratory failure during the acute phase which, in rats, lasts for 20–30 min. Those that survive exhibit a progressive decrease in activity, impaired coordination and food intake and may die within the next 48 h (see, e.g. SAMARAWICKRAMA 1979). At post-mortem examination, pathological changes are apparent in many organs and thus it is obvious that Cd interacts with a multiplicity of target sites. Since parenterally administered Cd is cleared rapidly from the blood (see SAMARAWICKRAMA 1979), it is probable that, after either lethal or sublethal acute doses of Cd, these interactions occur rapidly and hence the subsequent onset of MT synthesis, principally in the liver and intestine under these conditions, is of little or no consequence in relation to the toxic response. Simultaneous administration of excess cysteine with Cd (1.12 mg/kg) in rats, for example, increases appreciably the kidney uptake of Cd and leads to death from renal failure. The onset of tubular damage occurs rapidly; pathological changes are obvious by light microscopy at 4 h and the synthesis of MT, which occurs between 2 and 7 h after dosing, does not prevent their progressive increase with time (MURAKAMI and WEBB 1981).

It has been claimed, however, that strain differences in susceptibility to Cd in mice are correlated with differences in the rates of MT synthesis. Thus TSUNOO et al. (1979) and HATA et al. (1980) reported that, after the subcutaneous injection of 30 μmol $CdCl_2$ per kilogram body weight, the rate of hepatic MT synthesis in male C_3H mice was significantly less than that in either BALB/c or DBA/2 mice, although liver uptake of Cd was essentially the same in the three strains (Table 8). At 6 h after dosing, severe haemorrhage, zonal hepatocyte necrosis and congestion were seen consistently in the livers of C_3H mice, but seldom in the livers of the other strains. Most (80%) of the C_3H mice died within 15 h, whereas all of the DBA/2 and 70% of the BALB/c mice survived for at least 48 h. As, at 6 h after dosing, the amount of Cd bound as MT was less, whilst the amounts associated with the particulate cellular components and cytosolic hmw proteins were greater in the C_3H mouse than in either the BALB/c, or DBA/2 mouse, mortality was considered to be related inversely to the rate of hepatic MT synthesis, the induction of which was determined by genetic predisposition. The validity of this conclusion, however, is questionable. Thus, as extensive liver damage was apparent histologically in the C_3H strain at 6 h, it seems reasonable to suppose that the biochemical interactions, responsible for these pathological changes, occurred earlier, probably during, or immediately following the uptake of Cd, which was essentially complete within 2 h (Table 8). At 4 h after treatment, however, the concentrations of MT-bound Cd were similar in the three strains and were small in relation to the total Cd contents of the livers (Table 8). It seems more likely,

Table 8. Contents of total and MT-bound Cd in the liveres of male C_3H, BALB/c and DBA/2 mice at different times after the subcutaneous administration of 30 μmol $CdCl_2$ per kilogram body weight (HATA et al. 1980)

Time after Cd injection (h)	Total liver Cd (% of dose)			Content of MT-bound Cd (% of dose)		
	C_3H[a]	BALB/c	DBA/2	C_3H[a]	BALB/c	DBA/2
2	35.9 ± 5.0	42.7 ± 3.2	37.3 ± 3.0	0.1 ± 0.1	1.9 ± 1.7	0.9 ± 0.9
3	36.6 ± 4.9	41.2 ± 5.5	34.1 ± 3.2	1.2 ± 0.4	4.1 ± 3.3	1.1 ± 0.6
4	37.4 ± 2.8	41.9 ± 5.7	34.9 ± 1.4	4.1 ± 1.7	5.7 ± 2.6	5.1 ± 1.6
6	37.2 ± 3.3	40.4 ± 2.3	36.1 ± 4.6	7.6 ± 4.2	15.3 ± 3.2	20.4 ± 5.3
24		40.3 ± 6.5	39.6 ± 4.2		29.8 ± 5.3	30.9 ± 2.6
48		34.4 ± 8.8	39.8 ± 5.0		26.7 ± 7.4	32.0 ± 4.5

[a] The mice of this strain died within 15 h

therefore, that the reduced synthesis of MT in the liver of the C_3H mouse which, because of the high mortality in this strain, was apparent only at 6 h, was a consequence, not the cause of the tissue damage. Support for this conclusion is provided by the observation that the C_3H, BALB/c, and DBA/2 mouse strains, which are available in the United Kingdom, do not differ significantly in response to Cd doses that are insufficient to cause histologically detectable damage to the liver. At 15 h after the injection of Cd (2.1 mg/kg i.p.) into C_3H and DBA/2 mice, for example, the concentrations of hepatic MT-bound Cd are similar and account for about 90% (88.2% in the C_3H strain; 94.1% in the DBA/2 strain) of the total cytosolic Cd (D. HOLT and M. WEBB 1980, unpublished work).

In the experimental animal, Cd, when administered alone as a single acute dose, accumulates initially in the liver, and kidney uptake is small (Table 1). Neither renal failure nor appreciable renal damage occurs, therefore, under these conditions of exposure. The pregnant female in late gestation, however, is an exception to this generalization. In such animals, the placentae provide additional sites of Cd binding and, soon after intravenous injection, accumulate higher concentrations than all other organs except the liver (Table 1). About 40%–60% of the placental Cd is bound to MT (see Sect. K). In the pregnant rat between the 17th and 21st day of gestation, an acute dose of Cd leads to placental degeneration and haemorrhage and also to extensive damage to the kidneys (PAŘÍZEK 1964, 1965; CHIQUOINE 1965). Severely affected animals die from uraemia, which follows bilateral renal necrosis (PAŘÍZEK 1965). There is good evidence, however, that this toxic response is a consequence of the haemorrhagic shock (MAGOS and WEBB 1983) and is not due to the transfer of Cd, either as CdMT, or in any other form, from the damaged placentae to the kidney (SAMARAWICKRAMA and WEBB 1981).

At acute Cd exposure, the mammalian scrotal testis is a target organ of toxicity. A single parenteral dose of Cd (2–4 mg/kg) in rats, hamsters and gerbils (GUNN and GOULD 1970; BERLINER and JONES-WITTERS 1975; WADA et al. 1982), causes haemorrhagic necrosis followed by testicular atrophy and permanent sterility. Inbred strains of mice differ in susceptibility (CHIQUOINE and SUNTZEFF

1965; Gunn et al. 1965; Lucis and Lucis 1969), the differences being determined by a single autosomal recessive gene (Taylor et al. 1973). In the gerbil (Berliner and Jones-Witters 1975), as in the rat (see Gunn and Gould 1970), oedema and haemorrhage, which occur in the caput epididymidis as well as in the testis, result from greatly increased vascular permeability, probably by direct insult to the vasculature, rather than by the release of histamine or hyaluronidase (see Samarawickrama 1979). Damage is likely to be initiated during the testicular uptake of Cd, not by the chemical form of the relatively small amount of Cd that is accumulated (see Table 1 and, e.g. Kotsonis and Klaassen 1977a). Thus contrary to the conclusions of Chen et al. (1972), endogenous ZnMT probably is neither a target of, nor a protective agent against Cd toxicity in the testis. Indeed, Waalkes et al. (1984) have shown that, at least in the rat, the low molecular weight metal-binding testicular protein is not a MT, although it behaves as such on ion exchange chromatography.

Recent studies have examined the relationship of strain differences in susceptibility to Cd-induced testicular necrosis and differences in organ distribution of Cd, particularly in hepatic MT synthesis. In apparent agreement with the observations of Lucis and Lucis (1969) on susceptible (DBA/IJ) and resistant (C57BL/6J) strains of mice, Hata et al. (1980) reported that testicular uptake of Cd was maximal at 2 h after injection and, in the sensitive DBA/2 mouse, was approximately double that in the resistant (BALB/c) animal. Thereafter, the testicular Cd concentration decreased with time and, at 48 h, was similar in both strains. These differences in initial concentrations and in the rates of loss of Cd, however, were not correlated with either the liver uptake, or MT synthesis in the sensitive and resistant strains (see Table 8). Also, in previous work, Hata et al. (1978) claimed that certain mouse strains, which did not differ in susceptibility to testicular damage when exposed to the same dose of Cd, differed as much as threefold in inducibility of hepatic MT. Meisler et al. (1979), however, could find no quantitative differences in Cd uptake into the liver, kidneys and testes of resistant (C57BL/6J) and sensitive (DBA/2J) strains of mice after the intraperitoneal injection of a nontoxic dose of Cd. In the immature rat it is clear that preinduced hepatic MT does not reduce the amount of Cd transported to the testis. Thus, although the hepatic ZnMT concentration is 20 times greater in the newborn rat than in the adult, the testicular concentration of Cd at 2 h after the intravenous injection of 1 mg Cd per kilogram body weight is 5 times greater in the former than in the latter (Wong and Klaassen 1980a). Despite this difference in uptake, the testes of the 2-week-old, or younger rat, in contrast to those of rats aged 6 weeks or more, are undamaged at this dose level. This resistance is not correlated with differences in concentration of endogenous, testicular MT. It seems, therefore that the species, strain and age variations in sensitivity to Cd-induced testicular damage are not related to either the endogenous concentration, or the rate of synthesis of MT in the liver and/or testis.

II. Cd-Pretreated Animals

Pretreatment with a low dose of Cd protects the experimental animal against a subsequent, normally lethal dose (see, e.g. Terhaar et al. 1965; Leber and Miya

1976; WEBB and VERSCHOYLE 1976; PROBST et al. 1977). Pretreatment also induces tolerance to Cd-induced testicular necrosis, placental haemorrhage, teratogenic malformations, inhibition of insulin secretion and inhibition of xenobiotic metabolism (see, e.g. SAMARAWICKRAMA 1979; WEBB 1979 b; ROBERTS and SCHNELL 1981). Pretreatment with a higher dose of Zn also protects against most, if not all of these acute toxic effects of Cd (see, e.g. WEBB 1979 b). Understandably, therefore, it has been proposed repeatedly that protection results from the preinduction of (Cd,Zn)MT, or ZnMT, principally in the liver, which binds Cd by replacement of Zn and thus renders much of the challenge dose biologically inert (NORDBERG 1971; SUZUKI and YOSHIKAWA 1974; LEBER and MIYA 1976; SQUIBB et al. 1976; PROBST et al. 1977; SCHNELL et al. 1979). In apparent agreement with this mechanism, KLAASSEN (1978) observed that, soon after the administration of ^{109}Cd to Cd-pretreated rats, 75% of the ^{109}Cd in the liver cytosol was bound to MT whereas, in control animals, only 8% of the soluble ^{109}Cd was in this form. Addition of Cd to solutions of (Cd,Zn)MT (isolated from the livers of Cd-dosed rats) was shown by TANAKA et al. (1977) to cause a "dose-dependent" replacement of protein-bound Zn (Table 9). The results of these in vitro studies have two features of particular interest. First, the amount of Cd bound at each "dose level" was almost equal to the amount of Zn displaced and the total metal content (Σnmol Zn+Cd) of the MT remained constant. Thus in contrast to the contention of BELL (1979 a; see also KOCH et al. 1980), the Cd-induced (Cd,Zn)MT was not undersaturated with metallic ions. Second, saturation of the MT with Cd which, under the conditions of these experiments (Table 9), occurred between Cd concentrations of 72 and 143 μM, failed to displace all the bound Zn (calculations from the data of Table 9 show that 1.35 mol Zn per mol MT remained bound). BELL (1979 a) also has observed that 20% of the Zn in the ZnMT from neonatal rat liver (equivalent to 1.4 mol Zn per mol protein for a fully Zn-saturated MT) resists displacement by Cd in vitro and has inferred that the metal-binding sites may not be identical. Whilst this inference is difficult to reconcile with current

Table 9. In vitro replacement of Zn in (Cd, Zn) MT by Cd (TANAKA et al. 1977)[a]

Variable	Added Cd (nmol)					
	0	44.6	89.3	178.6	357.1	714.2
	MT-bound metals (nmol)					
Cd	63.5	83.8	91.8	125.5	144.3	153.3
Zn	118.3	87.5	85.0	63.5	35.5	35.3
Σ Cd+Zn	181.8	171.3	176.8	189.0	179.8	188.6
Δ Cd		+ 20.3	+ 28.3	+ 62.0	+ 80.8	+ 89.8
Δ Zn		− 30.8	− 33.3	− 54.8	− 82.8	− 83.0
Cd/Zn	0.54	0.96	1.08	1.98	4.06	4.34

[a] Equal volumes (5 ml) of the soluble fraction, obtained from the pooled livers of rats at 48 h after the subcutaneous injection of Cd (3.0 mg/kg), were incubated for 30 min at 37 °C with increasing amounts (0–80 µg; 0–714.2 nmol) Cd. Metallothionein was isolated from each of the reaction products and analysed for Cd and Zn

knowledge about the arrangements of these sites (see Sect. B), it is not without interest that studies on the relationship between Zn status and the occurrence of (Cu,Zn)MT in the livers of pigs, led BREMNER (1976) to suggest that Zn may be essential for the stabilization of the MT molecule.

Isolation of MT from the livers of Cd-pretreated rats at 30 min after a second intravenous injection of 0–3 mg Cd, enabled TANAKA et al. (1977) to demonstrate in vivo replacement of Zn in (Cd,Zn)MT by Cd. At this early time, the total content of MT-bound metals (Σ mol Cd + Zn) remained almost constant, but the Cd : Zn ratio increased with the dose over the range 0.5–2.0 mg Cd per kilogram body weight. Ion exchange chromatography, although accompanied by some loss of Zn from the initial MT preparation, showed clearly that Cd was substituted for Zn in both isoMT-1 and isoMT-2. In earlier work, SUZUKI and YOSHIKAWA (1974) observed that, at 2 h after the intraperitoneal injection of Cd (3 mg/kg) into male rats that had been pretreated 24 h previously with 0.3 mg/kg, the incorporation of each Cd atom into the hepatic MT was accompanied by the loss of only 0.76 atom Zn. This difference from the 1 : 1 ratio, which was observed in vitro, indicates that once the mechanism of synthesis is induced by Cd, additional MT synthesis can occur rapidly in response to a subsequent dose.

As discussed in Sect. E, pretreatment with an oral dose of Cd increases the uptake of a subsequent intragastric dose of ^{109}Cd and thus preinduction of MT in the intestinal mucosa does not limit the absorption of the toxic metal. Pretreatment of rats with an intragastric Cd dose of 20 mg/kg, for example, increases the uptake, relative to the nonpretreated control, by the liver, kidney and testis of Cd from a second oral dose (100 mg/kg) when administered 24 h later (SQUIBB et al. 1976). In the livers of the predosed and control animals, newly incorporated Cd is located mainly in the soluble fraction. In the former, however, the Cd in this fraction is associated solely with MT at all times, presumably because, as already outlined, the preinduced MT contains replaceable Zn and also additional MT synthesis can occur with little or no lag phase. In the nonpretreated animal, in which the induction of thionein mRNAs must precede the formation of MT, the cytosolic Cd of the liver is bound initially to hmw proteins. SQUIBB et al. (1976) propose, therefore, that decreased toxicity in orally predosed animals can be explained, at least in part, by increased Cd uptake by MT-containing organs, relative to other organs. Extrapolation of conclusions drawn from observations on the liver to organs such as the kidney and testis, however, seems unjustified (see later in this section), particularly as the total and MT-bound Cd concentrations in these organs are unlikely to be increased appreciably at 24 h after an oral dose of 20 mg Cd per kilogram body weight. Furthermore, parenteral treatment of rats with Cd before the administration of ^{109}Cd increases the hepatic concentration of the isotope, relative to that in nonpretreated controls, because biliary Cd excretion is reduced by the pretreatment (see Sect. D). It does not affect the liver uptake, blood (or plasma) clearance and the concentrations of ^{109}Cd in other organs within the first 2 h (KLAASSEN 1978).

In earlier studies, WEBB and VERSCHOYLE (1976) had shown that a greater percentage of a challenge dose of Cd was retained in the livers of Cd-pretreated, than control rats, but uptake of the metallic ion by other organs (brain, pancreas, heart, spleen and kidney) was unaffected. It would appear, therefore, that protection by preinduced hepatic MT against a normally lethal dose of Cd would be a realistic hypothesis if the liver was the target organ of toxicity. In this connection it is relevant that high doses of diethyldithiocarbamate, when given to mice at 2 h after an acute intraperitoneal dose of Cd, increase the survival rate, without any decrease (relative to control survivors) in hepatic Cd concentration (JONES et al. 1982). Furthermore, the tissue distribution of Cd, when administered by continuous infusion over a period of 2–3 days from subcutaneously implanted mini-pumps in male rats, is not altered significantly by pretreatment of the animals with Cd, Zn and Hg, in doses sufficient to induce high hepatic, or renal concentrations of MT (JOHNSON and FOULKES 1980). Since an acute dose of Cd affects a multiplicity of organs, it seems that the reported correlations between hepatic concentration of MT and Cd tolerance (LEBER and MIYA 1976) or LD_{50} (PROBST et al. 1977) are fortuitous. As pretreatment with Cd is bound to cause a dose-dependent increase in hepatic MT concentration, experimental approaches such as those used by these authors can support the protective function hypothesis, but lack the ability to disprove it, should it be wrong. Contrary evidence that protection is not related to preinduced MT is provided by observations, which show that: (a) whereas Cd-pretreated rats retain their hepatic contents of (Cd,Zn)MT, the tolerance induced by the pretreatment is maximal at 1–3 days and then decreases with time (WEBB and VERSCHOYLE 1976); (b) food restriction, which increased the concentration of ZnMT in the liver, does not alter the Cd LD_{50} in rats (WEBB and VERSCHOYLE 1976); (c) newborn rats normally contain high concentrations of ZnMT in their livers, but are no more resistant than adult animals to parenterally administered Cd (see Sect. K); (d) other metals (e.g. Mn and In), which do not induce MT, also protect against Cd toxicity (YOSHIKAWA 1970); and (e) pretreatment of male rats with phenobarbital induces tolerance to Cd (as well as to Pb and Hg), increases the liver uptake and biliary excretion of Cd, but does not affect appreciably the induction of hepatic MT (YOSHIKAWA and SUZUKI 1976; OHSAWA and FUKADA 1976). Thus protection by Cd pretreatment seems more likely to be due to some other effect of Cd, possibly to render membrane systems more resistant to damage by a subsequent higher dose of this, or other toxic metal, than to preinduction of MT. A change in membrane susceptibility, for example, would be in accord with the uniformity of the toxic mechanism at the cellular level (see MORSELT et al. 1983) and could explain the resistance of the testes and placentae to Cd in pretreated animals.

It remains possible that the presence of hepatic MT may protect against the inhibition by Cd of metal-sensitive functions, specifically in the liver. Some evidence for this was produced by ROBERTS and SCHNELL (1981) from studies on Cd inhibition of hepatic oxidative drug metabolism. As Cd does not inhibit cytochrome P-450 directly in vivo, but appears to decrease the rate of synthesis and increase the rate of degradation of the haem protein (MEANS et al. 1979), ROBERTS and SCHNELL (1981) attributed the reduced effect of Cd on cytochrome P-450 in Cd-pretreated animals to the diversion of Cd from critical subcellular sites to preinduced MT. More recent observations (ROBERTS and SCHNELL 1982), however, show that the time dependence of MT synthesis in the liver is not wholly consistent with the development of drug tolerance and suggest that additional, unknown factors must be involved.

G. Kidney Uptake, Metabolism and Toxicity of Exogenous Metallothionein

There is abundant evidence that (Cd,Zn)MT and (Cd,Cu)MT, when isolated from either the livers or kidneys of Cd-exposed rats and rabbits and injected into animals of the same or different species, are potent nephrotoxins (NORDBERG 1972; NORDBERG et al. 1975; CHERIAN et al. 1976; WEBB and ETIENNE 1977; CHERIAN and GOYER 1978; SQUIBB et al. 1979; SUZUKI and TAKENAKA 1979; MURAKAMI et al. 1983 a). The more recent of these studies, however, have shown that renal damage, although extensive at 24 h after administration of a nephrotoxic dose, is followed within 4 days by regeneration, both structural and functional (SUZUKI and MAITANA 1979; MURAKAMI et al. 1983 a) and the earlier reports of death from renal failure (NORDBERG et al. 1975; WEBB and ETIENNE 1977) have not been confirmed.

In contrast with its inorganic salts, Cd injected as (Cd,Zn)MT accumulates selectively in the mammalian kidney (NORDBERG et al. 1975; TANAKA et al. 1975; CHERIAN and SHAIKH 1975; CHERIAN et al. 1976; WEBB and ETIENNE 1977). Although some replacement of the bound metals, particularly Zn, by Cu occurs in the blood (TANAKA et al. 1975; BREMNER et al. 1978; CAIN and HOLT 1983), the protein remains intact and retains most of its bound Cd. In contrast with the parenterally administered Cd ion, for example, little or none of the injected MT-bound Cd is accumulated by the liver (SUZUKI et al. 1979). Rat liver isoCdMT-2, when administered orally to starved mice, also seems to cross the intestine without appreciable degradation and to be transported in the blood to the kidneys (CHERIAN 1979). In these organs the metalloprotein is cleared rapidly from the circulatory system (of the rat, or rabbit) by filtration through the glomeruli and reabsorption in the proximal tubules (FOULKES 1978 a; SQUIBB et al. 1979). Reabsorption involves at least two processes, one of which is saturated more readily than the others (NOMIYAMA and FOULKES 1977; FOULKES 1978 a) and is inhibited by ZnMT (JOHNSON and FOULKES 1980) and by myoglobin (FOULKES 1978 a). The same transport system also reacts with haemoglobin and thus its affinity for substrates is determined by factors other than the size (and shape) of the protein molecules (FOULKES 1978 b).

In vitro [109]CdMT binds to isolated (rabbit) renal proximal tubular brush border membranes (BBM), an interaction that requires an additional bivalent cation (Ca or Zn) and has characteristics that resemble those of the reabsorption of CdMT in vivo in the following aspects: (a) BBM contain two classes of binding sites, one of high affinity constant $(2.2 \times 10^7 \ M^{-1})$ and low binding capacity (0.13 µg CdMT per milligram BBM) and the other of lower affinity constant $(6.5 \times 10^5 \ M^{-1})$ and higher binding capacity (1.07 µg CdMT per milligram BBM); (b) binding of CdMT to BBM in vitro is inhibited by myoglobin; and (c) BBM that are isolated from rabbits, chronically treated with Cd such that the renal cortex contains about 340 µg Cd per gram wet weight, and reabsorption of CdMT in vivo is depressed, exhibit a 36% reduction in their ability to bind CdMT (SELENKE and FOULKES 1981). It seems, therefore, that the initial step in the reabsorption of CdMT in vivo is likely to involve charge-dependent interactions of the metalloprotein with a limited number of binding sites on the BBM. This process is followed by invagination of the membranes with the formation of endocytotic vesicles (see, e.g. FOULKES 1982); i.e. reabsorption occurs by receptor-mediated endocytosis (BESTERMAN and LOW 1983). By analogy with the renal reabsorption of other proteins of both high (MAUNSBACH 1966) and low molecular weight (BOURDEAU et al. 1973; CHRISTENSEN and MAUNSBACH 1974) these endocytotic vesicles would be expected to fuse with lysosomes to form heterolysosomes, wherein the protein is degraded.

There is no doubt that reabsorption of exogenous CdMT in the kidney tubules is followed by the liberation of Cd, which then induces de novo synthesis of renal MT (WEBB and ETIENNE 1977; CHERIAN 1978; SUZUKI et al. 1979; CAIN and HOLT 1983). Injection of only one MT isomer (either hepatic isoMT-1, or isoMT-2) into the rat results in the accumulation of two isometallothioneins in the kidneys (SUZUKI and YAMAMURA 1979). These newly formed isoproteins contain more Zn than Cu and thus differ in metal composition from those of the renal isometallothioneins induced by the repeated administration of $CdCl_2$ (SUZUKI and YAMAMURA 1980 b, d). Furthermore, injection of rat kidney MT (atomic Cd:Cu:Zn ratio = 2.7:3.5:1) also leads to the accumulation of a renal MT, in which Cd and Zn are the major bound metals (SUZUKI and TAKENAKA 1979). Although on gel filtration of the renal cytosol, some Cu is found to be associated with the MT fraction at 1 day after treatment, the maximum concentration of this metal in the elution profile is not coincident with that of the order two (Cd and Zn). Also the Cu concentration in the MT fraction decreases during the next 24 h, whereas that of Zn increases. To explain these differences, SUZUKI and TAKENAKA (1979) suggest that Cu, liberated by degradation of the injected (renal) MT, behaves in the same way as Cu(II), when administered to the Cd-pretreated rat (SUZUKI and YAMAMURA 1979) and induces CuMT as a separate molecular species. As the half-life $t_{1/2}$ of this metalloprotein is considered to be much shorter than that of the (Cd,Zn)MT induced by the liberated Cd, the metal content of the MT fraction changes with time. CAIN and HOLT (1983) have confirmed that administration of a nephrotoxic dose of (Cd,Zn)MT (0.8 mg MT-bound Cd per kilogram body weight) results in the accumulation of (Cd,Zn)MT in the kidneys. Because of the partial replacement by Cu of Zn and, to a lesser extent, Cd in the injected MT in the blood, however, the Cu concentration in the kidneys initially increases. This additional Cu, which is liberated by degradation of the exogenous MT; is not retained, but is eliminated rapidly after 2 h. These authors consider that this loss of Cu, coupled with the increase in kidney weight, in consequence of the oedema, explains the decrease in renal Cu concentration observed by SUZUKI and TAKENAKA (1979).

Nephrotoxicity of (Cd,Zn)MT clearly depends upon the presence of the Cd ion in the molecule. High doses of ZnMT, for example, do not cause kidney damage in vivo (WEBB and ETIENNE 1977) although, apparently, this MT is toxic (but less so than CdMT) in primary cultures of rat kidney epithelial cells (CHERIAN 1982). Also SUZUKI et al. (1979) have shown that the renal damage which results from the injection of (Cd,Zn)MT with different Cd:Zn ratios, is correlated with the content of MT-bound Cd, not with the amount of protein. In apparent agreement with the suggestion by WEBB and ETIENNE (1977) that, in the interval between the (lysosomal) degradation of the exogenous MT in the renal tubular cells and the synthesis of new, endogenous CdMT, "free" Cd is responsible for the nephrotoxicity (see also FOWLER and NORDBERG 1978), SQUIBB et al. (1979) found the numbers of pinocytotic vesicles and small, dense lysosomal structures to be increased in these cells soon after the injection of a nephrotoxic dose of either isoCdMT-1 or isoCdMT-2. Subcellular fractionation of kidney homogenates at different times after injection of CdMT ^{3}H indicated an initial temporary association of Cd with the heavy lysosomal–mitochondrial fraction (an observation supported by the demonstration of Cd in lysosomes in situ by X-ray microanalysis), degradation of the labelled protein moiety within this fraction, accumulation of the liberated Cd in the cytoplasm and, at later times, binding of the metallic ion to newly synthesized thionein. SUZUKI and YAMAMURA (1980 d) also observed that at 3–6 h after the injection of CdMT, Cd in the renal cytosol was associated mainly with the hmw protein fraction and, by displacement of the native metallic ions, to some extent with the endogenous MT. By 12 h, when further thionein synthesis had been initiated, however, Cd had migrated from its initial binding sites to the MT fraction. Additional evidence to support both the lysosomal degradation of the reabsorbed CdMT and the association of nephrotoxicity with the liberation of Cd ions had been given by CAIN and HOLT (1983). These authors, in contrast to SQUIBB et al. (1979), however, found 70% of the total Cd and about 80% of the ^{3}H-labelled protein moiety to be concentrated in the heavy particulate fraction ("nuclei and cell membranes") very soon after injection of a nephrotoxic dose of (Cd,Zn)MT ^{3}H.

CHERIAN (1978) also finds that Cd, when administered as CdMT, becomes bound by newly synthesized thionein in the kidneys, but considers the intracellular lysosomal system to have a minimal role in nephrotoxicity since, at all times after dosing, at least 90% of the total renal Cd is bound as MT. According to CHERIAN's (1978, 1979, 1982) model, toxicity results not from "free" Cd ions, but from the intact CdMT molecules, which cause membrane damage during their entry into the renal tubular cells. In support of this hypothesis, ROGERS and CHERIAN (1981) and CHERIAN (1982) have shown that, in primary monolayer cultures of rat kidney epithelial cells, preloaded with 2-deoxyglucose ^{3}H, membrane leakage follows the addition of 10^{-5} M Cd as CdMT to the culture medium, whereas 10^{-4} M CdCl$_2$ is necessary to produce the same effect. Pretreatment of the cells with Cd (10^{-5} M) caused the development of resistance to ionic Cd, but not to CdMT. These findings are difficult either to interpret, or to extrapolate to the functional kidney in vivo. Furthermore, some of CHERIAN's (1982) arguments, for example "if degradation of CdMT was the main cause of toxicity, the CdMT synthesized within the cells in response to Cd exposure should be as toxic as the CdMT introduced into the cells" and "if Cd ions were formed intracellularly from (exogenous) CdMT, Cd-pretreated cells should have exhibited significant resistance to CdMT toxicity" seem individually of doubtful validity and mutually contradictory. The former implies unjustifiably (see, e.g. CAIN and HOLT 1983) that exogenous CdMT is metabolized in the same way as the endogenous metalloprotein, whilst the latter, although contrary to the observations on cultured cells, is true in vivo (WEBB and ETIENNE 1977; SELENKE and FOULKES 1982). Also it has been established that glucose transport in brush border vesicles, prepared from CdMT-treated rats, is unaffected even at 24 h after treatment. In vivo, however, renal RNA-polymerase activity, which is known to be inhibited by Cd ions, is reduced by 90% at 4 h after injection of CdMT (0.6 mg protein-bound Cd per kilogram body weight). Thereafter, with the synthesis of new thionein in the kidney and the consequent redistribution of Cd, the inhibition of this enzyme decreases with time (SQUIBB et al. 1982). It seems reasonable to conclude, therefore, that the nephrotoxicity of exogenous CdMT in vivo is due to the initial interactions of the liberated Cd ion with critical intracellular sites. This conclusion does not exclude the BBM as one of these critical sites, even though alterations in its structure have not been detected by electron microscopy of renal tissue from animals after treatment with a nephrotoxic dose of CdMT (SQUIBB et al. 1982).

After parenteral administration of a nephrotoxic dose of CdMT, the concentration of Cd in the whole kidney is low (i.e. 10–15 µg/g; WEBB and ETIENNE 1977; 17 µg/g CAIN and HOLT 1983). As this Cd is unlikely to be distributed uniformly either between, or within the renal tubules, it seems that biochemical fractionation studies, particularly when made on homogenates of the whole organ, need to be interpreted with caution. Some cells may contain appreciable amounts of Cd in various forms; others, possibly a larger fraction of the total, may contain significant amounts of $(Cu,Zn)MT$, but no Cd. Homogenization, therefore, could lead to artifacts through the redistribution of Cd. The electron microscopic autoradiographic studies of MURAKAMI et al. (1983 a, b) on the renal metabolism of ^{109}CdMT (195 µCi per µmol) and ^{125}I-labelled CdMT (24.5 mCi per milligram MT) in the rat, therefore, are of particular interest. These investigations have shown clearly that at 30 min after treatment only the protein moiety of the injected MT and/or its catabolic products are located in apical vacuoles and cytoplasmic bodies (heterolysosomes) of the endocytic systems of the lining cells of the proximal convoluted tubules. Even at the earliest times (10 and 30 min) ^{109}Cd is not localized in any specific organelle, but is distributed uniformly throughout the cytoplasm. Thus Cd must be liberated from the MT very early in the reabsorption process. In this connection it may be relevant that certain small peptides appear to be hydrolysed at the luminal surface of the brush border before absorption (membrane or contact digestion) of some, or all of the digestion products and, according to CARONE et al. (1980), it is possible that larger molecules are partially degraded in this way before, or during the endocytotic process.

H. Function of Metallothionein in the Transport of Cd from the Liver to the Kidney

Contrary to the opinions of some authors (e.g. CHERIAN 1978; KOTSONIS and KLAASSEN 1981; SUZUKI 1982) it is not a paradox that synthesis of MT protects against Cd toxicity, yet parenterally administered CdMT is nephrotoxic. The former operates at chronic exposure; the latter is an acute effect that occurs at dose levels unrealistic in relation to the concentrations of CdMT that can be detected immunochemically (see Sect. C) in the blood of animals (or human beings) environmentally exposed to Cd. Although after a single, acute dose of Cd, renal accumulation of the metallic ion initially is small (see Table 1), as discussed previously (Sect. F) the pattern of organ distribution can be altered by the simultaneous administration of an excess of a suitable chelating agent. Combination of

10 µmol $CdCl_2$ with 5 mmol L-cysteine per kilogram body weight, for example results in a Cd concentration in the kidney of 20 µg Cd per gram wet weight. This concentration, although low in comparison with the critical renal Cd concentration at chronic exposure (see Sect. E), is accumulated rapidly (i.e. before the tubular cells can respond by synthesis of MT) and leads to death from renal failure (MURAKAMI and WEBB 1981). If, however, a smaller dose (e.g. 1 µmol $CdCl_2$ per kilogram body weight) is given together with the same dose of L-cysteine, renal damage does not occur. Moreover, repeated administration of this dose combination at 48-h intervals results in the accumulation of an appreciable renal burden of Cd without tubular damage. This is true also at chronic low-level exposure to CdMT. Thus repeated administration of small doses of the latter leads to the progressive accumulation of Cd, mainly bound as the cytoplasmic CdMT (80% of the total soluble Cd), in the renal cortex. Although a critical concentration of Cd has yet to be achieved under these conditions, renal burdens in excess of 100 µg Cd per gram wet tissue weight, unaccompanied by tubular dysfunction, have been obtained in the rat after 40 doses of 50 µg MT-bound Cd per kilogram body weight (M. WEBB and D. HOLT 1982, unpublished work).

In horses the hepatic and renal Cd concentrations are correlated ($r = 0.81$), the relationship being

$$\text{Kidney cortex Cd (mmol/kg)} = \text{liver Cd (mmol/kg)} \times 12.2 + 0.13$$

(ELINDER et al. 1981). In long-term experiments with animals that have been exposed to either a single acute dose, or multiple low doses of Cd, the concentration of Cd decreases in the liver and increases in the kidneys with time (see, e.g. WEBB 1979 a). Furthermore if, after termination of dosing, the hepatic burden is sufficiently high, renal damage may develop at a considerable time thereafter, apparently because the critical Cd concentration in the kidney is exceeded as a result of the interorgan transfer (KAWAI and KIMURA 1975). As the results of JOHNSON and FOULKES (1980) suggest, this transfer is a slow process: 0.08 and 0.7 µg Cd per day in rats that are maintained with 5 and 50 ppm Cd in their drinking water (FRAZIER 1982), 0.09 µg Cd per day in parenterally dosed rats with an initial hepatic content of 150 µg Cd (WEBB 1979 c). Although the synthesis of (metallo)-thionein on free hepatic polysomes (SHAPIRO and COUSINS 1980), as well as the absence of an extra signal (NH_2 terminal) peptide fragment from the ZnMT, formed by the cell-free translation of its mRNA (HEW and PENNER 1979), are considered to militate against a secretory function of MT, these values are equivalent to the transport of approximately 1–8 ng MT per minute (calculated as $(Cd_4,Zn_3)MT$) and thus are compatible with the plasma concentrations of MT (1–3 ng/ml in normal animals and 30–50 ng/ml in animals multiply dosed with Cd) that have been found by radioimmunoassay (VANDER MALLIE and GARVEY 1979; TOHYAMA and SHAIKH 1981; GARVEY and CHANG 1981; MEHRA and BREMNER 1983). Such concentrations might result from the normal turnover of hepatocytes coupled, perhaps with membrane damage or increased cell death if the liver Cd concentration is high. The observations of MEHRA and BREMNER (1984) that, in the plasma of newborn rats, the concentration of ZnMT is not only much higher than in the adult, but also is correlated with the hepatic ZnMT concentration, however, suggests that export of MT from the liver is a normal process. Nevertheless, in Cd-pretreated rats, increased cell death, due to exposure to aflatoxin, causes the release of CdMT from the liver in proportion to the loss in weight and results in increases in the content and concentration of Cd in the kidneys (CAIN and GRIFFITHS 1980). Similar observations have been made by TANAKA (1982) on Cd-exposed rats after treatment with other hepatotoxins (CCl$_4$, galactosamine, ethionine).

The transport (and excretory) function of MT, proposed originally by NORDBERG (1972) and TANAKA et al. (1975) from the results of experiments on animals given excessive doses of Cd and thus of questionable relevance to normal physiological processes, receives additional support from the immunohistochemical studies of DANIELSON et al. (1982) and BANERJEE et al. (1982), which demonstrated the extracellular localization of the metalloprotein in liver sinusoids and within the lumina of the renal tubules of Cd-exposed animals. It remains to be established, however, whether MT is the only protein involved in the transfer of Cd from the liver to the kidneys. The results of GARVEY and CHANG (1981), for example, indicate that MT is a major, but not the sole carrier of the small amount of Cd that is present in the serum of rats at 24–48 h after a single injection of 0.8 mg Cd per kilogram body weight.

J. Normal Functions of Metallothionein and the Interactions of Cd with these Functions

The defence function of MT at chronic exposure to Cd probably is fortuitous, since evolution would be expected to favour a mechanism that either limited the uptake, or enhanced the elimination of the toxic metal (WEBB 1982). It is possible that MT synthesis is not related to any specific process, but is a general response to increased intracellular concentrations of certain essential metals, perhaps to provide a temporary storage mechanism and to prevent toxic interactions, if the tolerable physiological limits are exceeded (see, e.g. BREMNER 1982). As on transfer from dietary excess to dietary deficiency of Zn, the accumulated ZnMT in the liver of the rat is depleted rapidly, whilst urinary and faecal Zn excretion are increased, CHEN et al. (1977) consider that MT is involved in the accumulation of excess Zn, rather than in the storage of the metal for later utilization. EVANS et al. (1975), however, conclude that the increased hepatic content of ZnMT, which results from starvation, or restricted food intake, probably represents a conservation mechanism since, although the liver weight decreases markedly, the hepatic Zn concentration increases. The presence of at least two isomers in the major organs of MT synthesis (Sect. B), the complex arrangements of the metal-binding sites into clearly defined clusters in each isoprotein (Sect. B), the occurrence of high concentrations of these metalloproteins in certain tissues of the foetus and newborn (Sect. K) and the demonstration by radioimmunological techniques of low endogenous levels of MT in other tissues and organs (Sect. D) suggest more fundamental, if unestablished functions. BRADY (1982), for example, considers MT to have a central role in Cu- and Zn-dependent macromolecular syntheses. Interaction of Cd with endogenous metallothioneins, as well as the induction by this metal of additional MT synthesis, thus not only may prevent the interaction of Cd at functional metal-sensitive cellular sites, but also may interfere with the metabolism of these essential metals.

A physiological role for ZnMT as a cation donor in the terminal step in the biosynthesis of various Zn metalloenzymes has been inferred from the ability of this metalloprotein to reactivate the apoforms of aldolase, carbonic anhydrase, thermolysin and alkaline phosphatase (UDOM and BRADY 1980; LI et al. 1980). Similar findings have been reported for CuMT and the metal-free forms of several Cu proteins, at least under certain conditions. Although HARTMANN et al. (1983) have described the transfer of Cu(I) from yeast CuMT to apostellacyanin both aerobically and anaerobically, the transfer reaction usually seems to be dependent upon the oxidation state (GELLER and WINGE 1982; BELTRAMINI and LERCH 1982; MORPURGO et al. 1983). From these in vitro studies it seems that native CuMT either forms a highly specific Cu(I) donor (HARTMANN et al. 1983; MORPURGO et al. 1983), or is unlikely to function in metal transfer in vivo unless it becomes oxidized, or degraded. Also there is no evidence that the intact ZnMT molecule donates Zn to apo(Zn)metalloproteins in vivo; such transfer, if it occurs could involve the degradation of the MT. Thus the observation (LI et al. 1980) that (Cd,Zn)MT reactivates Zn apoenzymes in vitro (i.e. the presence of Cd in the molecule has no significant effect on Zn exchange) may have little or no biological significance. More relevant in this connection may be the effect of Cd incorporation on the biological half-life $t_{1/2}$ of MT.

The half-lives of Zn-induced metallothioneins (in the rat) are about 20 h (COUSINS 1979), whilst those of the Cu-induced metalloproteins vary with Zn status (i.e. 16.9 ± 1 and 12.3 ± 0.5 h in the livers of Zn-sufficient and Zn-deficient rats; BREMNER et al. 1978). Irrespective of nutritional status, however, the release of bound metals (Zn,Cu) seems to occur simultaneously with the degradation of the MT protein moiety. In Cd-treated animals the $t_{1/2}$ values of protein degradation not only are longer than those of the Zn- or Cu-induced metallothioneins, but also vary with the Cd content of the MT (Table 10; CAIN and HOLT 1979).

The measurements shown in Table 10 refer to the protein moieties and there is only limited data on the turnover of the bound metals. The persistence of MT-bound Cd implies that essentially all this metal, liberated through degradation of the protein, re-binds to newly synthesized thionein. Thus the extremely low hepatic and renal turnover of Cd is not due to a highly stable form of MT, but to

Table 10. Degradation half-life of Cd-induced isoMT-1 and isoMT-2 in the livers of rats (CAIN and HOLT 1979)

Cd dose (mg/kg)	Isomer	Metal composition of MT (atomic ratio)		$t_{1/2}$ (days)
		Cd:Cu	Cd:Zn	
1.0	MT-1	4.6	0.63	2.2
	MT-2	9.4	0.57	3.1
6×1.0	MT-1	17.1	1.50	3.5
	MT-2	56.9	1.31	5.1

an inefficient mechanism of excretion of Cd from these organs (RIDLINGTON et al. 1981). Administration of ^{65}Zn to Cd-treated rats, however, results in a flux (i.e. incorporation and subsequent loss) of radioactivity in the hepatic (Cd,Zn)MT. Nevertheless, it seems that $t_{1/2}$ of Zn remains the same as that of the protein and thus increases with the Cd:Zn ratio. CHEN et al. (1975), for example, found identical $t_{1/2}$ values (4.2 days) for Zn and the protein moiety of the hepatic MT of Cd-doses rats. Thus any regulatory function of MT in Zn and, perhaps, Cu metabolism could be altered by the presence of Cd in the molecule. The available evidence, albeit obtained mainly with the rat, however, suggests that the inability of the liver and kidneys to eliminate Cd effectively does not lead to hepatic and renal traps for functional Zn and Cu. The decreased serum caeruloplasmin levels and appreciable changes (30%–70%) in the Cu concentrations in the livers and spleens of sheep, caused by the presence of low levels of Cd (5–15 ppm) in diets marginally sufficient in Cu (MILLS and DALGARNO 1972), probably result from interference by the former metal with the intestinal absorption of the latter. In rats with adequate intakes of Zn and Cu, prolonged exposure (36 weeks) to 100 ppm Cd in the diet increases the concentrations of MT-bound Zn and Cu, concomitantly with the accumulation of Cd in the livers and kidneys, respectively, but does not cause either systemic, or local deficiencies of these essential metals (STONARD and WEBB 1976). Furthermore, administration of Cd to Zn-deficient rats and mice significantly increases the activity of alcohol dehydrogenase in the liver (WINGE et al. 1978). On the assumption that the increase in enzyme activity is due specifically to the changes in hepatic Zn concentration, it seems that Zn, incorporated into the liver in consequence of the Cd-induced synthesis of MT, can be utilized to satisfy demands at other sites. If, however, (CdZn)MT can donate Zn to the apoform of the enzyme in vivo as well as in vitro, it could be argued that activation of alcohol dehydrogenase in the Cd-treated, Zn-deficient animal, is a consequence of MT synthesis.

From studies on the livers of (a) adult rats during regeneration after partial hepatectomy and (b) rat pups with time after birth, OHTAKI et al. (1978) and OHTAKI and KOGA (1979) consider that an increase in the concentration of one, but not both Zn isometallothioneins precedes and is essential for the synthesis of DNA, possibly because the metalloprotein regulates the levels, or activities of the Zn-dependent synthetic enzymes.

If, however, one isoform of ZnMT is required specifically for DNA synthesis, elevated concentrations of the metalloprotein might be expected in other tissues of the newborn in which, during the early period of development, growth occurs predominantly by an increase in cell number, rather than in cell size. The endogenous concentrations of either ZnMT in the kidneys, or of the analogous Zn-binding protein in the testes of the newborn rat, however, are much lower than in the liver and show no age-related changes that can be correlated with the growth pattern (BRADY and WEBB 1981). Furthermore, CAIN and GRIFFITHS (1983) have shown that both ZnMT isomers are synthesized in the residual liver of partially hepatectomized rats, although at different rates, the accumulation of isoZnMT-2 being much greater than that of isoZnMT-1 until 18 h after the operation, when the concentrations of both forms begin to decrease. It is interesting that the same pattern of response is observed after partial hepatectomy in Cd-pretreated rats and, because of the more rapid accumulation of isoMT-2, there is a redistribution of Cd between the two isomers (K. CAIN and B. L. GRIFFITHS 1982, unpublished work; see also WEBB and CAIN 1982). One important difference between the normal and Cd-pretreated rat after partial hepatectomy, however, is the persistence of MT-bound Zn in the latter. Nevertheless, neither this, nor the presence of (Cd,Zn)MT in the liver before operation, affects the rate of regeneration. In contrast, Ehrlich ascites tumour cells, when grown in Cd-dosed mice, show normal incorporation of uridine into RNA, but decreased uptake and incorporation of thymidine into DNA. In these cells Cd and Zn are bound to a low molecular weight protein with properties similar to those of MT. The same protein, but with Zn and Cu as the bound metals, however, is present in Ehrlich cells isolated from the normal host and seems to be a permanent cellular component, unaffected by the proliferative state of the population, or the segment of the cell cycle in which the cells are processed (KOCH et al. 1980).

K. Function of Metallothionein in the Reproductive Toxicology of Cd: Role in Perinatal Development

As discussed in Sect. F.I, the placenta is a target organ of Cd toxicity at acute exposure in late pregnancy. When administered earlier in gestation, i.e. during the critical period of organogenesis, a single acute dose of Cd, sublethal for the maternal animal, can be embryo/foetotoxic or teratogenic. Both the teratogenic dose and teratogenic response vary between and within species (see, e.g. GALE 1973; PARZYCK et al. 178; SAMARAWICKRAMA and WEBB 1981), but neither seem to be correlated with the uptake of a critical concentration of Cd in the embryo (see also LEVIN and MILLER 1980). Foetal toxicity of Cd in the pregnant animal also cannot be explained solely by a direct effect of Cd on the foetus and, as discussed elsewhere (WEBB 1983), is likely to be the result, either direct or indirect, of the inhibition of placental transport processes and other extrafoetal interactions. In the pregnant rat at 4 h after the intravenous injection of 1.25 mg Cd per kilogram body weight on the 12th and 20th days of gestation the Cd concentrations in the foetus are 15.7 ± 1.7 and 50 ± 4 ng per gram wet weight and in the whole placentae $2{,}010 \pm 62$ and $4{,}900 \pm 400$ ng/g, respectively (WEBB and SAMARAWICKRAMA 1981). These results are in accord with the earlier studies of SONOWANE et al. (1975), which demonstrated that, after intravenous injection of the dam, small amounts of Cd cross the placenta at all gestational ages, but the foetal concentration increases appreciably in late gestation, whilst the ratio of the placental : foetal concentration decreases with increasing dose. In rats given a single oral dose of Cd in different stages of pregnancy, a greater percentage of the absorbed Cd seems to be accumulated by the embryo before the formation of the functional placenta at about the 10th or 11th day of gestation, than by the foetus after placentation. Furthermore, under these conditions, the foetal Cd concentration decreases and placental accumulation increases with gestational age (AHOKAS and DILTS 1979). Thus the placenta appears to protect the foetus from both parenterally and orally administered Cd.

In the rat on the 12–14th days of gestation the Cd concentration in the foetal part of the placenta is 3–4 times greater than that in the maternal part, but in both (M. WEBB and D. HOLT 1980, unpublished work), as in the whole placenta (LUCIS et al. 1972), most of the soluble Cd is present as MT. HANLON et al. (1982) claim that at 24 h after injection of a teratogenic dose of Cd on day 9 of pregnancy in SWV-strain mice, much of the Cd in both the chorioallantoic and yolk-sac placentae is bound to dimers of MT, the normal function of which may be in the control of Zn transfer to the foetal system. Conclusive evidence for the existence of these dimers either in the placentae or, as reported by WOLKOWSKI (1974), in the blood of the foetal mouse, however, is lacking; their resolution into isoMT monomers by treatment with mercaptoethanol, for example, does not appear to have been investigated. Also, the earlier suggestion of LEYTON and FERM (1980), that the protection of C57BL/6J mice against a teratogenic dose of Cd on the 9th day of gestation by pretreatment with Cd or Hg within 3 weeks before pregnancy can be explained by preinduction of MT, seems unlikely to be true. Pretreatment with Cd and Hg before mating would induce significant MT synthesis in different organs (see Sect. D) and, therefore, would be unlikely to have similar effects on the organ distribution and binding of the subsequent Cd dose. Also stored Cd is not mobilized from the liver of the dam during pregnancy (WEBB 1972 b) and thus pretreatment with this metal would not be expected to enhance MT synthesis in the placenta during its development.

Whilst Cd exposure increases the placental concentration of MT and inhibits the transport of Zn (WEBB and SAMARAWICKRAMA 1981) and Cu (D. HOLT and M. WEBB 1982, unpublished work), there is no evidence of a causal relationship between these effects. Indeed placental synthesis of MT seems unlikely to affect the transfer of Cu to the foetus (see, e.g. Sect. E) and, as in the intestine (PETERING et al. 1979), cannot explain the inhibition by Cd of Fe transport, since all attempts to form Fe complexes with (Cd-induced) MT have been unsuccessful (KOJIMA et al. 1982). Furthermore dietary exposure of the dam to Cd throughout pregnancy appears to influence the transport of Fe and Cu to the foetus more than the transport of Zn (CHOUDHURY et al. 1978; WEBSTER 1979 a, b; PETERING et al. 1979; AHOKAS et al. 1980).

Normal foetuses and/or newborn of all mammalian species thus far studied, in contrast to adults, contain large amounts of MT in their livers. In some species, e.g. humans (RYDÉN and DEUTSCH 1978; RIORDAN and RICHARDS 1980) and sheep (BREMNER et al. 1977; BELL 1979 b), the concentration of MT, which contains both Zn and Cu in ratios that alter with age, is highest during gestation. In others, e.g. rats (WONG and KLAASSEN 1979; BELL 1979 a; BAKKA and WEBB 1981), rabbits, mice, Syrian and Chinese hamsters (BAKKA and WEBB 1981) the hepatic MT concentration is maximal at, or soon after birth. In the foetal rat, MT accumulates in the soluble fraction of the liver only after the 15th or 16th day of gestation (BAKKA et al. 1981; KERN et al. 1981). The concentration of the MT, which contains much more Zn than Cu, then increases in parallel with that of total hepatic Zn to a maximum at 1–2 days post-partum (BAKKA et al. 1981) and then falls to the low adult level at, or shortly after weaning (BELL 1979 a; MASON et al. 1981 a). For reasons yet to be explained, the presence of Cd (150 ppm) in the maternal diet prolongs the accumulation of ZnMT in the livers of newborn rat pups until about

20 days of age (OH and WHANGER 1979). Accumulation under these conditions cannot be due to the uptake of Cd by the neonate, since little or no Cd is secreted into the maternal milk (see NEATHERY 1981) and, as shown by OH and WHANGER (1979), Cd is not present in the liver of the newborn until after weaning.

The amount of translatable MT-mRNA is much greater in the liver of the neonatal rat than in the adult, but does not decrease concomitantly with the fall in MT concentration between 4 and 14 days and thus its function may be controlled by some mechanism other than at the transcriptional (MERCER et al. 1982), perhaps the translational (ANDERSEN et al. 1983) level. The MT from the livers of 1- to 4-day-old rats yields two MT isomers on ion exchange chromatography (cf. the conclusions of OHTAKI et al. 1978 discussed in Sect. J) which, although similar to the hepatic isoZnMT-1 and isoZnMT-2 of adult animals, differ from the latter in amino acid composition (Table 11; WONG and KLAASSEN 1979).

Administration of Cd (1.0 mg/kg i.p.) to the dam on the 18th day of gestation inhibits the placental transport of Zn and thus the accumulation of total and MT-bound Zn in the liver of the foetus (BAKKA et al. 1981). After birth, which eliminates the transport block, MT-bound Zn accumulates in the livers of the newborn pups to a maximum concentration, coincident with that of total Zn, at about 7 days of age, i.e. about 6 days later than in the newborn of normal dams. The increases in body weight is retarded in pups from the treated dams during the first

Table 11. Amino acid compositions of isoZnMT-1 and isoZnMT-2 from the livers of newborn (1- to 4-day-old) and adult rats (WONG and KLAASSEN 1979)[a]

Amino acid residue	Newborn		Adult	
	IsoZnMT-1	IsoZnMT-2	IsoZnMT-1	IsoZnMT-2
Lys	7.06 (7)	8.07 (8)	11.13 (11)	9.71 (10)
Arg	0.26 (0)	0.12 (0)	0.12 (0)	0.26 (0)
Asp	6.15 (6)	4.08 (4)	4.47 (4)	3.22 (3)
Thr	2.75 (3)	1.87 (2)	3.89 (4)	1.62 (2)
Ser	8.94 (9)	8.65 (9)	10.93 (11)	8.02 (8)
Glu	1.63 (2)	3.58 (4)	1.58 (2)	2.97 (3)
Pro	5.18 (5)	1.75 (2)	1.71 (2)	2.61 (3)
Gly	6.01 (6)	5.54 (6)	6.95 (7)	5.41 (5)
Ala	3.93 (4)	4.91 (5)	3.45 (3)	4.36 (4)
Cys	15.68 (16)	17.15 (17)	17.31 (17)	21.35 (21)
Val	2.63 (3)	1.22 (1)	2.13 (2)	1.04 (1)
Met	0.89 (1)	1.09 (1)	0.91 (1)	0.93 (1)
Ile	1.32 (1)	0.85 (1)	0.08 (0)	0.72 (1)
Leu	1.72 (2)	0.48 (0)	0.39 (0)	0.37 (0)
Phe	1.13 (1)	1.32 (1)	0.09 (0)	0.10 (0)
Total residues	66	61	64	62
Minimum molecular weight	6544	6132	6494	6332

[a] The results, expressed as residues/mol and, in parentheses, the "nearest integer values" were obtained by one analysis of each protein after oxidation with performic acid and hydrolysis with 6 M HCl for 24 h. The values for threonine and serine were corrected for losses in the hydrolyses

6–8 days post-partum and then parallels, but does not exceed that of normal pups. Thus, for at least 3 weeks after birth, the newborn of these dams remain "small for age". This and other evidence led MASON et al. (1981 b) to suggest that hepatic MT in the newborn rat functions to regulate the metabolism of Zn, before the development of the adult homeostatic mechanisms and to provide a source of Zn for the maintenance of appropriate concentrations of this metal at functional sites, particularly in the liver cytosol. Some support for these suggestions is provided by the observations of OH and WHANGER (1979) that the biological half-lives of Zn in the MT of the liver (and kidneys) of the young rat is about double that of the protein moiety; i.e. Zn must be retained by reincorporation into newly synthesized thionein during the turnover process. In rabbits, in apparent contrast to rats, administration of a single subcutaneous dose of Cd (0.25 or 0.5 mg/kg), 48 h before term, increases the concentrations of total cytosolic and MT-bound Zn in the foetal liver, these changes being coincident with a redistribution of Zn from extrahepatic sites (WAALKES et al. 1982). As, however, these doses of Cd produce significant reductions in foetal body, liver and kidney weights without either foetal lethality, or any significant change in foetal Zn content, it is possible that the increased hepatic MT concentrations are in accord with a conservation function.

In the liver of the newborn rat, the concentration of MT-bound Cu, in contrast to that of Zn, remains low throughout the first 2–3 weeks post-partum (MASON et al. 1981 b). Most of the Cu absorbed from the maternal milk seems to accumulate in the intestine, not in the liver. The major Cu-binding proteins from the small intestine of the newborn Long-Evans rat have been isolated and characterized as isoMT-1 and isoMT-2 by JOHNSON and EVANS (1980a). Those from the intestine of the neonatal Wistar rat, however, appear very heterogeneous and are obtained by gel filtration as a polydisperse "Cu complex", two minor components of which may be isometallothioneins (MASON et al. 1981 b). Both JOHNSON and EVANS (1980a, b) and MASON et al. (1981 b) consider these intestinal proteins, which decrease during the nursing period and are not detectable after weaning, to have the same function, i.e. to regulate the absorption of Cu before closure of the intestine, when uptake occurs by nonspecific pinocytosis of metal–protein complexes.

In the newborn rat, high absorption and intestinal retention are characteristic features of the uptake of various metals, both essential and nonessential, when administered intragastrically (see, e.g. WEBB 1983). The increased intestinal retention of Cd in neonatal rats (SASSER and JARBOE 1977), neonatal pigs and guinea-pigs (SASSER and JARBOE 1980), appears to correlate inversely with intestinal maturity. The intestinal Cu complex of the newborn Wistar rat in which, as in the intestinal MT of the Long-Evans rat (JOHNSON and EVANS 1980b), the $t_{1/2}$ of Cu is long (D. DINSDALE, D. HOLT and M. WEBB 1983, unpublished work), provides additional, immediately available, high affinity binding sites for certain foreign metals, such as Hg (WEBB and HOLT 1982) and Cd (HOLT and WEBB 1983). In particular, it seems probably that binding of Cd to this complex explains both the long retention time of Cd in the intestine of the newborn rat (SASSER and JARBOE 1977, 1980) and the limited transport of Cd to the carcass. The observation that systemic absorption of orally administered Cd is sixfold greater in 2-h-old than in 24-h-old rat pups (Sasser and Jarboe 1977) also seems to correlate with the rapid increase in the concentration of the Cu complex in the intestine from 17 µg protein-bound Cu at birth to 140 µg protein-bound Cu per gram wet weight at 2 days post-partum (Mason et al. 1981 b).

At high oral doses of Cd (e.g. 1.0 mg/kg) the content of the Cu complex in the intestine of the 8-day-old Wistar rat appears to be sufficient to bind only a fraction of the absorbed Cd; about 40% of the dose is transported to the body organs and intestinal retention at 18 h is reduced to about 50% of the body burden. In addition to the intestinal Cu complex, however, the endogeneous hepatic MT in these animals also provides high affinity binding sites for Cd (and Hg). In consequence, much of the Cd that reaches the liver either under these conditions, or after the intraperitoneal administration of Cd (0.1 or 1.0 mg/kg), binds to the endogeneous MT (Holt and Webb 1983). It is clear, however, that uptake of Cd by the neonatal liver is not promoted by the presence of MT therein (Wong and Klaassen 1980 a; Bell 1980; Asokan and Tandon 1981; Mason 1982; Holt and Webb 1983). Moreover, after parenteral administration, the LD_{50} of Cd seems to be lower (Bell 1980), whilst the concentrations of Cd in spleen, bone, brain, testis and muscle at 2 h (Wong and Klaassen 1980 a) and in the intestine and spleen at 24 h (Asokan and Tandon 1981) are higher in immature than in adult rats. In the kidneys, however, the Cd concentration increases with age, possibly because the number of nephrons also increases (Asokan and Tandon 1981). Thus the presence of the hepatic MT in the newborn rat, although seemingly protective against Hg toxicity (Webb and Holt 1982), seems to have no protective function at acute parenteral exposure to Cd and to be of much less significance than the intestinal Cu complex (or CuMT) in the regulation of Cd distribution at oral exposure. In this connection, comparisons of the oral toxicity of Cd in the neonatal rat and other species (e.g. the Syrian hamster), which do not contain Cu-binding proteins in their intestines, could be of interest. Possibly the loss of this Cu-binding protein fraction with the closure of the intestine contributes to the susceptibility of weanling rats to Cd-induced Cu deficiency, when the Cu intake is only marginally adequate for the maintenance of growth and normal plasma and tissue levels of Cu in control animals (Table 12; Campbell and Mills 1974).

Table 12. Concentrations of Cu and of caeruloplasmin in the plasma and of Cu in the livers of rats, fed Cd-supplemented diets for 9 weeks after weaning (Campbell and Mills 1974)[a]

Variable	Dietary Cd (mg/kg)			
	0.2 (control)	1.5	6.1	18.1
Plasma Cu (mg/l)	0.71	0.44	0.18	0.03
Plasma caeruloplasmin (units/l)	44.3	18.6	8.9	6.5
Liver Cu (mg/kg)	4.5	3.8	3.5	2.3

[a] The animals were maintained on a Cu-limited semisynthetic diet (Cu 2.6 mg; Zn 30 mg; Cd 0.2 mg/kg), supplemented with Cd to given the concentrations shown

L. Metallothionein: A Limiting Factor in the Chelation Therapy of Cd Intoxication

The use of chelation therapy in cases of chronic Cd poisoning is complicated by the high affinity binding of the metallic ion by the inducible protein, thionein (see SAMARAWICKRAMA 1979). Also certain chelating agents, if administered immediately after exposure to a single, parenteral dose, may decrease the body burden, but increase the renal uptake of Cd and thus potentiate the toxic hazard (cf., for example, the effect of coadministration of L-cysteine on the organ distribution and nephrotoxicity of Cd; Sects. F.I and H). Thus in experimental animals, mono- and dithiol chelating agents of low molecular weight (e.g. 2,3-dimercaptopropanol (BAL), DL-penicillamine, dithiothreitol), when given at 30 min after a single, acute dose of Cd (i.e. before the onset of MT synthesis), enhance the biliary excretion of the metallic ion, but also increase its concentration in the kidneys (CHERIAN 1980a). Carboxyl-containing chelating agents, e.g. ethylenediamine tetraacetate (EDTA), nitrilotriacetate, diethylenetriamine pentaacetate (DPTA), decrease the concentrations of Cd in the liver, kidneys and other organs and increase the urinary Cd excretion (CHERIAN 1980a), but are effective only before hepatic CdMT levels are less than half-maximal (CANTILENA and KLAASSEN 1982). Recently, however, CHERIAN and colleagues (CHERIAN 1980a, b; CHERIAN et al. 1982; CHERIAN and ROGERS 1982) have shown that high doses (e.g. 400 μmol/kg) of BAL and 1,2,3-trimercaptopropane, but not of other thiol-containing chelating agents, effectively mobilize Cd from the liver and kidney and thus from hepatic and renal MT, when administered either at 24 h after a single dose, or at 3 days after the last of four daily doses of Cd (1 mg/kg i.p.). In animals of the latter group, repeated administration (i.e. 5 days per week for 2 weeks) of BAL (50 mg/kg) either alone, or in combination with DTPA (50 mg/kg), reduced the whole body retention of Cd from 97% to 49%–52% of the dose. Total Cd and MT concentrations were reduced in both the liver and kidney (Table 13), without significant alterations in the concentrations of Zn and Cu in these organs. The latter, which may indicate increased (compensatory) absorption of these metals, is an important finding, since essential metal depletion usually is regarded as a hazard of chelation therapy.

The results of Table 13 suggest that the concentrations of MT, as determined polarographically (see Sect. C), are excessively high. It can be calculated, for example, that the concentration of MT in the control liver would be sufficient to bind almost all (83%) of the Cd, Zn and Cu present in the whole organ. Also the loss of 16 μg Cd per gram wet weight from the livers of the BAL + DTPA-treated animals, without any significant changes in the organ concentrations of Zn and Cu, is not stoichiometric with the loss of 300 μg MT per gram wet tissue weight. Thus the correlation between the loss of Cd and of MT (24.3% and 26.9%, respectively, after treatment with BAL and 33.6% and 32.3% after treatment with BAL + DTPA), which is apparent in Table 13, may not be as good as the results suggest. Nevertheless the incorporation of various correction factors does not alter the implication that the concentration of MT adjusts with the loss of Cd, possibly because (a) the distribution of Cd between the cytosol and other cellular components remains in equilibrium and (b) during the turnover process, the synthesis of new MT is proportional to the hepatic Cd concentration.

Table 13. Concentrations of Cd, Zn and Cu and of MT in the livers and kidneys of Cd-exposed rats after chelation therapy. (CHERIAN and ROGERS 1982)

Chelating agents (s)	Liver				Kidney			
	Cd	Zn	Cu	MT[a]	Cd	Zn	Cu	MT[a]
	(μg per gram wet tissue weight)							
None (control)	47.3 ± 3.4	49.1 ± 0.6	5.2 + 0.6	1,035 ± 91	23.7 ± 1.7	25.9 ± 2.7	11.7 ± 1.0	494 ± 51
BAL	35.8 ± 4.4	44.7 ± 1.3	4.3 ± 0.1	756 ± 115	16.3 ± 1.1	25.1 ± 1.1	8.9 ± 0.8	325 ± 22
DTPA	48.1 ± 2.2	46.4 ± 1.6	4.7 ± 0.1	862 ± 154	23.2 ± 1.9	30.9 ± 1.1	11.6 ± 0.6	522 ± 57
BAL + DTPA	31.4 ± 2.9	46.8 ± 0.8	4.9 ± 0.2	700 ± 65	14.7 + 1.7	27.2 + 1.6	10.6 ± 1.1	344 + 16

[a] Determined polarographically; liver values 7%–20% lower were obtained by analysis by the Cd-haem method (see Sect. C)

References

Abel J, Ohnesorge FK (1980) Energy-linked immunosorbent assay for metallothionein. Toxicol Lett SI No. 1:131

Ahokas RA, Dilts PV (1979) Cadmium uptake by the rat embryo as a function of gestational age. Am J Obstet Gynecol 135:219–220

Ahokas RA, Dilts PV, LeHaye EB (1980) Cadmium-induced fetal growth retardation: protective effects of excess dietary zinc. Am J Obstet Gynecol 136:216–221

Amacher DE, Ewing KL (1975) A soluble cadmium binding component in rat and dog spleen. Arch Environ Health 30:510–513

Andersen RD, Winter PE, Maher JJ, Bernstein IA (1978) Turnover of metallothioneins in rat liver. Biochem J 174:327–338

Andersen RD, Piletz JE, Birren BW, Herschman HR (1983) Levels of metallothionein messenger RNA in fetal, neonatal and maternal rat liver. Eur J Biochem 131:497–500

Anke M, Schneider H-J (1974) Trace elements of the human kidney in relation to age and sex. Z Urol Nephrol 67:357–363

Anke M, Klinger G, Grün M, Schneider H-J (1979) The dependence of the Cd-concentration in animals and human-beings on sex and age. In: Anke M, Schneider H-J (eds) Kadmium symposium. Friedrich Schiller University, Jena, pp 72–78

Asokan P, Tandon SK (1981) Effect of cadmium on hepatic metallothionein levels in early development of the rat. Environ Res 24:201–206

Bakka A, Webb M (1981) Metabolism of zinc and copper in the neonate: changes in the concentrations and contents of thionein-bound Zn and Cu with age in the livers of the newborn of various mammalian species. Biochem Pharmacol 30:721–725

Bakka A, Samarawickrama GP, Webb M (1981) Metabolism of zinc and copper in the neonate: effect of cadmium administration during late gestation in the rat on the zinc and copper metabolism of the newborn. Chem Biol Interact 34:161–171

Bakka A, Eriksen D, Rugstad HE, Bauer R (1982) Identification of cadmium binding sites within living human cells by perturbed angular correlation spectroscopy. FEBS Lett 139:57–60

Banerjee D, Onosaka S, Cherian MG (1982) Immunohistochemical localization of metallothionein in the cell nucleus and cytoplasm of rat liver and kidney. Toxicology 24:95–105

Barański B, Stetkiewicz I, Trzcinka-Ochocka M, Sitarek K, Szymczak W (1982) Teratogenicity, fetal toxicity and tissue concentration of cadmium administered to female rats during organogenesis. J Appl Toxicol 2:255–259

Bell JU (1979a) Native metallothionein levels in rat hepatic cytosol during perinatal development. Toxicol Appl Pharmacol 54:148–155

Bell JU (1979b) A renal : hepatic comparison of metallothionein in the sheep fetus. Toxicol Lett 4:407–411

Bell JU (1980) Induction of hepatic metallothionein in the immature rat following administration of cadmium. Toxicol Appl Pharmacol 54:148–155

Beltramini M, Lerch K (1982) Copper transfer between Neurospora copper-metallothionein and type 3 copper apoproteins. FEBS Lett 142:219–222

Benson JM, Henderson RF (1980) Isolation and characterization of a low molecular weight cadmium-binding protein from Syrian hamster lung. Toxicol Appl Pharmacol 55:370–377

Berliner AF, Jones-Witters P (1975) Early effects of a lethal cadmium dose on the gerbil testis. Biol Reproduct 13:240–247

Bernard A, Goret A, Buchet JP, Roels H, Lowerys R (1980) Characterization of the proteinuria induced by long term administration of cadmium in rat (Abstr). 19th Annual Meeting of the Society of Toxicology, A 280

Besterman JM, Low RB (1983) Endocytosis: a review of mechanisms and plasma membrane dynamics. Biochem J 210:1–13

Bordas J, Koch MHJ, Hartmann H-J, Weser U (1982) Tetrahedral Cu-S coordination in yeast copper-thionein: an EXAFS study. FEBS Lett 140:19–21

Boulanger Y, Armitage IM (1982) [113]Cd study of the metal cluster structure of human liver metallothionein. J Inorg Biochem 17:147–153

Bourdeau JE, Chen ERY, Carone FA (1973) Insulin uptake in the renal proximal tubule. Am J Physiol 225:1399–1404

Brady FO (1981) Synthesis of rat hepatic zinc-metallothionein in response to the stress of sham operation. Life Sci 28:1647–1654

Brady FO (1982) The physiological function of metallothionein. Trends Biochem Sci 7:143–145

Brady FO, Kafka RL (1979) Radioimmunoassay of rat liver metallothionein. Anal Biochem 98:89–94

Brady FO, Webb M (1981) Metabolism of zinc and copper in the neonate. (Zinc,copper)-thionein in the developing rat kidney and testis. J Biol Chem 256:3931–3935

Bremner I (1976) The relationship between the zinc status of pigs and the occurrence of copper and zinc-binding proteins in the liver. Br J Nutr 35:245–252

Bremner I (1979) Mammalian absorption, transport and excretion of cadmium. In: Webb M (ed) The chemistry, biochemistry and biology of cadmium. Elsevier/North-Holland, Amsterdam, pp 175–193

Bremner I (1982) The nature and function of metallothionein. In: Gawthorne JM, Howell JMcC, White CL (eds) Trace element metabolism in man and animals – 4. Springer, Berlin Heidelberg New York, pp 637–644

Bremner I, Davies NT (1974) Studies on the appearance of a zinc binding protein in rat pancreas. Biochem Soc Trans 2:654–656

Bremner I, Williams RB, Young BW (1977) Distribution of zinc and copper in the liver of the developing sheep foetus. Br J Nutr 38:87–92

Bremner I, Hoekstra WG, Davies NT, Young BW (1978) Effect of zinc status on the synthesis and degradation of copper-induced thioneins. Biochem J 174:883–892

Bremner I, Williams RB, Young BW (1981) The effects of age, sex and zinc status ont he accumulation of (Cu,Zn)-metallothionein in rat kidneys. J Inorg Biochem 14:135–146

Briggs RW, Armitage IM (1981) Evidence for site selective metal binding in calf liver metallothionein. J Biol Chem 257:1259–1262

Cain K, Griffiths BL (1980) Transfer of liver cadmium to the kidney after aflatoxin-induced liver damage. Biochem Pharmacol 29:1852–1855

Cain K, Griffiths BL (1983) A comparison of isometallothionein synthesis in rat liver after partial hepatectomy and parenteral zinc injection. Biochem J 217:85–92

Cain K, Holt DT (1979) Metallothionein degradation: metal composition as a controlling factor. Chem Biol Interact 28:91–106

Cain K, Holt DE (1983) Studies of cadmium-thionein induced nephropathy. Time course of cadmium-thionein uptake and degradation. Chem Biol Interact 43:223–237

Cain K, Skilleter DN (1980) Selective uptake of cadmium by parenchymal cells of liver. Biochem J 188:285–288

Cain K, Skilleter DN (1983) Comparison of cadmium-metallothionein synthesis in parenchymal and non-parenchymal liver cells. Biochem J 210:769–773

Cain K, Webb M (1983) Metallothionein and its relationship to the toxicity of cadmium and other metals in the young. In: Schmidt EHF, Hildebrandt AG (eds) Health evaluation of infant formula and junior food. Springer, Berlin Heidelberg New York, pp 105–111

Campbell JK, Mills CF (1975) Effects of dietary cadmium and zinc on rats maintained on diets low in copper. Proc Nutr Soc 33:15A–17A

Cantilena LR, Klaassen CD (1982) Decreased effectiveness of chelation therapy with time after acute cadmium poisoning. Toxicol Appl Pharmacol 63:172–180

Carone FA, Peterson DR, Oparil S, Pullman NT (1980) Renal tubular transport and catabolism of small peptides. In: Maunsbach AB, Olsen TS, Christensen EI (eds) Ultrastructure of the kidney. Academic, New York, pp 327–340

Carrasco L, Valquez D, Hernandez-Lucas C, Carbonero P, Garcia-Olmedo F (1981) Thionins: plant peptides that modify membrane permeability in cultured mammalian cells. Eur J Biochem 116:185–189

Cempel M, Webb M (1976) The time course of cadmium-thionein synthesis in the rat. Biochem Pharmacol 25:2067–2071

Chang CC, Vander Mallie RJ, Garvey SJ (1980) A radioimmunoassay for human metal-lothionein. Toxicol Appl Pharmacol 55:94–102

Chen RW, Ganther HE (1975) Relative cadmium binding capacity of metallothioneins and other cytosolic fractions in various tissues of the rat. Environ Physiol Biochem 5:378–388

Chen RW, Wagner P, Ganther HE, Hoekstra WG (1972) A low molecular weight cad-mium-binding protein in testes of rats. Possible role in cadmium-induced testicular damage. Fed Proc 31:699

Chen RW, Whanger PD, Weswig PH (1975) Biological function of metallothionein. I. Syn-thesis and degradation of rat liver metallothionein. Biochem Med 12:95–105

Chen RW, Vasey EJ, Whanger PD (1977) Accumulation and depletion of zinc in rat liver and kidney metallothionein. J Nutr 107:805–813

Cherian MG (1977) Biliary excretion of cadmium in rat. II. The role of metallothionein in the hepatobiliary transport of cadmium. J Toxicol Environ Health 2:955–961

Cherian MG (1978) Induction of renal metallothionein synthesis by parenteral cadmium-thionein in rats. Biochem Pharmacol 27:1163–1166

Cherian MG (1979) Metabolism of orally administered cadmium-metallothionein in mice. Environ Health Perspect 28:127–130

Cherian MG (1980 a) Biliary excretion of cadmium in the rat. III. Effects of chelating agents and change in intracellular thiol content on biliary transport and tissue distribu-tion of cadmium. J Toxicol Environ Health 6:379–391

Cherian MG (1980 b) Biliary excretion of cadmium in the rat. IV. Mobilization of cadmium from metallothioneins by 2,3-dimercaptopropanol. J Toxicol Environ Health 6:393–401

Cherian MG (1982) Studies on toxicity of metallothionein in rat kidney epithelial cell cul-ture. In: Foulkes EC (ed) Biological roles of metallothionein. Elsevier/North-Holland, Amsterdam, pp 193–202

Cherian MG, Goyer RA (1978) Metallothioneins and their role in the metabolism and tox-icity of metals. Life Sci 10:1–10

Cherian MG, Rogers K (1982) Chelation of cadmium from metallothionein in vivo and its excretion in rats repeatedly injected with cadmium chloride. J Pharmacol Exp Ther 222:699–704

Cherian MG, Shaikh ZA (1975) Metabolism of intravenously injected cadmium-binding protein. Biochem Biophys Res Commun 65:863–869

Cherian MG, Goyer RA, Delaquerriere-Richardson L (1976) Cadmium-metallothionein induced nephropathy. Toxicol Appl Pharmacol 38:399–408

Cherian MG, Goyer RA, Delaquerriere-Richardson L (1977) Relationship between plasma cadmium-thionein and cadmium-induced nephropathy. Toxicol Appl Pharma-col 41:145–146

Cherian MG, Goyer RA, Valberg LS (1978) Gastrointestinal absorption and organ dis-tribution of oral cadmium chloride and cadmium-metallothionein in mice. J Toxicol Environ Health 4:861–868

Cherian MG, Yu S, Redman CM (1981) Site of synthesis of metallothionein in rat liver. Can J Biochem 59:301–306

Cherian MG, Onosaka S, Carson GK, Dean PAW (1982) Biliary excretion of cadmium in the rat. V. Effects of structurally related mercaptans on chelation of cadmium from metallothionein. J Toxicol Environ Health 9:389–399

Chiquoine AD (1965) Effect of cadmium chloride on pregnant albino mouse. J Reprod Fertil 10:263–265

Chiquoine AD, Suntzeff V (1965) Sensitivity of mammals to cadmium necrosis of the testis. J Reprod Fertil 10:455–457

Choudhury H, Srivastava L, Murthy L, Petering HG (1974) Some observations on trace metal and endocrine relationships in male and female rats. Poultry Sci 53:1910

Choudhury H, Hastings L, Merden E, Brokman D, Cooper GP, Petering HG (1978) Effect of low level prenatal cadmium exposure on trace metal body burden and behavior in Sprague-Dawley rats. In: Kirchgessner M (ed) Trace element metabolism in man and animals – 3. Institut für Ernährungsphysiologie, Technische Universität München, Freising-Weihenstephan, pp 549–552

Christensen ET, Maunsbach AB (1974) Intralysosomal digestion of lysozyme in renal proximal tubules. Kidney Int 6:396–407

Colucci AV, Winge D, Krasno J (1975) Cadmium accumulation in rat liver. Arch Environ Health 30:153–157

Cousins RJ (1979) Regulatory aspects of zinc metabolism in liver and intestine. Nutr Rev 37:97–103

Cox CC, Waters MD (1978) Isolation of a soluble cadmium-binding protein from pulmonary alveolar macrophages. Toxicol Appl Pharmacol 46:385–394

Danielson KG, Ohi S, Huang PC (1982) Immunochemical detection of metallothionein in specific epithelial cells of rat organs. Proc Natl Acad Sci USA 79:2301–2304

Davies NT, Campbell JK (1977) The effect of cadmium on intestinal copper absorption and binding in the rat. Life Sci 20:955–960

Durnam DM, Palmiter RD (1981) Transcriptional regulation of the mouse metallothionein-1 gene by heavy metals. J Biol Chem 256:5712–5716

Durnam DM, Perrin F, Gahnon F, Palmiter RD (1980) Isolation and characterization of the mouse metallothionein-1 gene. Proc Natl Acad Sci USA 77:6511–6515

Elinder CG, Nordberg M, Palm B, Piscator M (1981) Cadmium, zinc and copper in horse liver and in horse liver metallothionein: comparison with kidney cortex. Environ Res 26:22–32

Engström B, Nordberg GF (1979) Factors influencing absorption and retention of oral ^{109}Cd in mice: age, pretreatment and subsequent treatment with non-radioactive cadmium. Acta Pharmacol Toxicol (Copenh) 45:315–324

Etzal KR, Shapiro SG, Cousins RJ (1979) Regulation of liver metallothionein and plasma zinc by the glucocorticoid, dexamethasone. Biochem Biophys Res Commun 89:1120–1126

Evans GW, Majors PF, Cornatzer WE (1970) Mechanism for cadmium and zinc antagonism of copper metabolism. Biochem Biophys Res Commun 40:1142–1148

Evans GW, Grace CI, Votana HJ (1975) A proposed mechanism for zinc absorption in the rat. Am J Physiol 228:501–505

Faeder EJ, Chaney SQ, King LC, Hinners TA, Bruce R, Fowler BA (1977) Biochemical and ultrastructural changes in the livers of cadmium treated rats. Toxicol Appl Pharmacol 34:473–487

Foulkes EC (1978a) Renal tubular transport of cadmium metallothionein. Toxicol Appl Pharmacol 45:505–512

Foulkes EC (1978b) Apparent competition between myoglobin and metallothionein for renal reabsorption. Proc Soc Exp Biol Med 159:321–323

Foulkes EC (1982) Tubular reabsorption of low molecular weight proteins. Physiologist 25:56–59

Fowler BA, Nordberg GF (1978) The renal toxicity of cadmium-metallothionein: morphometric and X-ray microanalytical studies. Toxicol Appl Pharmacol 46:609–623

Frazier JM (1980) Cadmium and zinc kinetics in rat plasma following intravenous injection. J Toxicol Environ Health 6:503–518

Frazier JM (1982) The role of metallothionein in the systemic distribution of cadmium. In: Foulkes EC (ed) Biological roles of metallothionein. Elsevier/North-Holland, Amsterdam, pp 141–153

Frazier JM, Puglese J (1978) Dose dependence of cadmium kinetics in the rat liver following intravenous injection. Toxicol Appl Pharmacol 47:153–166

Galdes A, Hill HAO, Bremner I, Young BW (1978a) ^{1}H-NMR investigations on the structure of sheep metallothioneins. Biochem Biophys Res Commun 85:217–225

Galdes A, Vašák M, Hill HAO, Kägi JHR (1978b) ^{1}H-NMR spectra of metallothioneins. FEBS Lett 92:17-21

Gale TF (1973) The interactions of mercury with cadmium and zinc in mammalian embryonic development. Environ Res 6:95–105

Garner CD, Hasain SS, Bremner I, Bordas J (1982) An EXAFS study of the Zn sites in sheep liver metallothionein. J Inorg Biochem 16:253–256

Garvey JS, Chang CC (1981) Detection of circulating metallothionein in rats injected with zinc and cadmium. Science 214:805–807

Geller BL, Winge DR (1982) Metal binding sites of rat liver copper-metallothionein. Arch Biochem Biophys 213:109–117

Gerson RJ, Shaikh ZA (1982) Uptake and binding of cadmium and mercury to metallothionein in rat hepatocyte primary cultures. Biochem J 208:465–472

Gick G, McCarthy KS, McCarthy KS (1981) role of metallothionein synthesis in Cd- and Zn-resistant CHO-KIM cells. Exp Cell Res 132:22–30

Glanville N, Durnam DM, Palmiter RD (1981) Structure of mouse metallothionein-1 gene and its mRNA. Nature 292:267–269

Gunn SA, Gould TC (1970) Cadmium and other mineral elements. In: Johnson AD, Gomes WR, Van Denmark NL (eds) The testis. Acadmic, New York, pp 378–481

Gunn SA, Gould TC, Anderson WAD (1965) Strain differences in susceptibility of mice and rats to cadmium induced testicular damage. J Reprod Fertil 10:273–278

Hall AC, Young BW, Bremner I (1979) Intestinal metallothionein and the mutual antagonism between copper and zinc in the rat. J Inorg Biochem 11:57–66

Hanlon DP, Sprecht C, Ferm VH (1982) The chemical status of cadmium in the placenta. Environ Res 27:89–94

Hart BA, Keating RF (1980) Cadmium accumulation and distribution in human lung fibroblasts. Chem Biol Interact 29:67–83

Hartmann H-J, Morpurgo L, Desideri A, Rotilio G, Weser U (1983) Reconstitution of stellacyanin as a case of direct Cu(I) transfer between yeast copper thionein and "blue" copper apoprotein. FEBS Lett 152:94–96

Hata A, Tsunoo H, Nakajima H, Kimura M (1978) Strain differences in susceptibility of mice to cadmium-induced metallothionein. Toxicol Lett 2:45–49

Hata A, Tsunoo H, Nakajima H, Shintaku K, Kimura M (1980) Acute cadmium intoxication in inbred mice: a study on strain differences. Chem Biol Interact 32:29–39

Hew CL, Penner PE (1979) Cell-free synthesis of rat liver zinc-thioneins. Can J Biochem 57:1050–1055

Hicks DJ, Miya TS, Schnell RC (1976) Sex-related differences in cadmium toxicity in rats. Toxicol Appl Pharmacol 37:156

Hildebrand CE, Cram LS (1979) Distribution of cadmium in human blood cultured in low levels of $CdCl_2$. Accumulation of Cd in lymphocytes and preferential binding to metallothionein. Proc Soc Exp Biol Med 161:438–443

Holt DE, Webb M (1983) Intestinal and hepatic binding of cadmium in the neontal rat. Arch Toxicol 52:291–301

Johnson DR, Foulkes EC (1980) On the proposed role of metallothionein in the transport of cadmium. Environ Res 21:350–356

Johnson WT, Evans GW (1980a) Isolation of a (copper,zinc)-thionein from the small intestine of normal rats. Biochem Biophys Res Commun 96:10–17

Johnson WT, Evans GW (1980b) Age dependent variation of copper in tissue and proteins of neonatal rat small intestine. Proc Soc Exp Biol Med 165:495–501

Jones SG, Basinger NA, Jones MM, Gibbs SA (1982) A comparison of diethyldithiocarbamate and EDTA as antidotes for acute cadmium intoxication. Res Commun Chem Pathol Pharmacol 38:271–278

Kägi JHR, Nordberg M (1979) Metallothionein. Experientia [Suppl] 34:1–378

Kägi JHR, Vallee BL (1960) Metallothionein: a cadmium and zinc containing protein from equine renal cortex. J Biol Chem 235:3460–3465

Kägi JHR, Vallee BL (1961) Metallothionein: a cadmium and zinc containing protein from equine renal cortex. II. Physicochemical properties. J Biol Chem 236:2435–2442

Karin MD, Herschman HR (1981) Induction of metallothionein in HeLa cells by dexamethasone and zinc. Eur J Biochem 113:267–272

Karin MD, Richards RI (1982) Human metallothionein genes: molecular cloning and sequence analysis of the mRNA. Nucleic Acids Res 10:3165–3173

Karin MD, Andersen RD, Herschman HR (1981) Induction of metallothionein m-RNA in HeLa cells by dexamethasone and by heavy metals. Eur J Biochem 118:527–531

Kawai K, Kimura M (1975) Renal lesion after single injection of cadmium in rabbit. Ind Health 13:261–265

Kello D, Dekanic D, Kostial K (1979 a) Influence of sex and dietary calcium on intestinal cadmium-absorption in rats. Arch Environ Health 34:30–33

Kello D, Sugawara N, Voner C, Foulkes EC (1979 b) On the role of metallothionein in cadmium absorption by rat jejunum in situ. Toxicology 14:199–208

Kern SR, Smith HA, Fontaine D, Bryan SE (1981) Partitioning of zinc and copper in liver subfractions: appearance of metallothionein-like proteins during development. Toxicol Appl Pharmacol 59:346–354

Klaassen CD (1978) Effect of metallothionein on hepatic disposition of metals. Am J Physiol 234:E47–E53

Klauser S, Kägi JHR, Wilson KJ (1983) Characterization of isoprotein patterns in tissue extracts and isolated samples of metallothioneins by reverse phase high pressure liquid chromatography. Biochem J 209:71–80

Koch J, Wielgus S, Shankara B, Saryan LA, Shaw F, Petering DH (1980) Zinc, copper and cadmium binding protein in Ehrlich ascites tumour cells. Biochem J 189:95–104

Kojima N, Young CR, Bates GW (1982) Failure of metallothionein to bind iron or act as an iron mobilizing agent. Biochim Biophys Acta 716:273–275

Kojima Y, Hamashima Y (1978) Immunohistological study of equine renal metallothionein. Acta Histochem Cytochem 11:205–211

Kotsonis FN, Klaassen CD (1977 a) Comparison of methods for estimating hepatic metallothionein in rats. Toxicol Appl Pharmacol 42:583–588

Kotsonis FN, Klaassen CD (1977 b) Toxicity and distribution of cadmium at sublethal doses. Toxicol Appl Pharmacol 41:667–680

Kotsonis FN, Klaassen CD (1978) The relationship of metallothionein to the toxicity of cadmium after prolonged oral administration to rats. Toxicol Appl Pharmacol 46:39–54

Kotsonis FN, Klaassen CD (1979) Increase in hepatic metallothionein in rats treated with alkylating agents. Toxicol Appl Pharmacol 51:19–27

Kotsonis FN, Klaassen CD (1981) Metallothionein and its interactions with cadmium. In: Nriagu JO (ed) Cadmium in the environment. II. Health effects. Wiley & Sons, New York, pp 595–616

Leber AP, Miya TS (1976) A mechanism for cadmium and zinc induced tolerance to cadmium thionein: involvement of metallothionein. Toxicol Appl Pharmacol 37:403–414

Levin AA, Miller RK (1980) Fetal toxicity of cadmium in the rat: maternal vs. fetal injections. Teratology 22:1–5

Leyton WM, Ferm VH (1980) Protection against cadmium-induced limb malformations by pretreatment with cadmium or mercury. Teratology 21:357–360

Li T-Y, Kraker AJ, Shaw CF, Petering DH (1980) Ligand substitution reaction of metallothioneins with EDTA and apocarbonic anhydrase. Proc Natl Acad Sci USA 77:6334–6338

Louwerys BR, Roels AA, Buchet J-P, Bernard A, Stanescu D (1979) Investigation of the lung and kidney function in workers exposed to cadmium. Environ Health Perspect 28:137–145

Lucis OJ, Lucis R (1969) Distribution of cadmium-109 and zinc-65 in mice of inbred strains. Arch Environ Health 18:307

Lucis OJ, Lucis R, Shaikh ZA (1972) Cadmium and zinc in pregnancy and lactation. Arch Environ Health 25:14–22

Madapallimatam G, Riordan JR (1977) Antibodies to the low molecular weight copper binding proteins from liver. Biochem Biophys Res Commun 77:1286–1293

Magos L, Webb M (1983) The influence of weight and other physiological changes during pregnancy and lactation on the toxicities of mercury and cadmium. In: Clarkson T, Nordberg G (eds) Reproductive and developmental toxicity of metals. Plenum, New York, pp 417–436

Margoshes M, Vallee BL (1957) A cadmium protein from equine kidney cortex. J Am Chem Soc 79:4813–4814

Mason R (1982) Metabolism of cadmium in the neonate: effect of hepatic zinc, copper and metallothionein concentrations on the uptake of cadmium in the rat liver. Biochem Pharmacol 31:1761–1764

Mason R, Bakka A, Samarawickrama GP, Webb M (1981 a) Metabolism of zinc and copper in the neonate: accumulation and function of (Zn,Cu)-metallothionein in the liver of the newborn rat. Br J Nutr 45:375–389

Mason R, Brady FO, Webb M (1981 b) Metabolism of zinc and copper in the neonate: accumulation of copper in the gastrointestinal tract of the newborn rat. Br J Nutr 45:391–399

Maunsbach AB (1966) Absorption of I-125 labelled homologous albumin by rat kidney proximal tubular cells. J Ultrastruct Res 15:197–241

McGivern J, Mason J (1979) The effect of chelation on the fate of intravenously administered cadmium in rats. J Comp Pathol 89:1–9

Means JR, Carlson SP, Schnell RC (1979) Studies on the mechanism of cadmium-induced inhibition of hepatic microsomal monooxygenase system in the male rat. Toxicol Appl Pharmacol 48:293–304

Mehra RK, Bremner I (1983) Development of a radioimmunoassay for rat liver metallothionein-1 and its application to the analysis of rat plasma and kidneys. Biochem J 213:459–465

Mehra RK, Bremner I (1984) Metallothionein-I in the plasma and liver of neonatal rats. Biochem J 217:859–862

Meisler M, Orlowski C, Gross E, Bloor JH (1979) Cadmium metabolism in cdm/cdm mice. Biochem Gen 17:731–736

Mercer J, Stevenson T, Camakaris J, Lazdins I, Danks DM (1982) Metallothionein-mRNA in neonatal and adult livers. In: Gawthorne JM, Howell JMcC, White CL (eds) Trace element metabolism in man and animals – 4. Springer, Berlin Heidelberg New York, pp 649–651

Mills CF, Dalgarno AC (1972) Copper and zinc status of ewes and lambs receiving increased dietary concentrations of cadmium. Nature 239:171–173

Minkel DT, Poulson K, Wielgus S, Shaw CF, Petering DH (1980) On the sensitivity of metallothioneins to oxidation during isolation. Biochem J 191:475–485

Morpurgo L, Hartmann HJ, Desideri A, Weser U, Rotilio G (1983) Yeast copper-thionein can reconstitute the Japanese lacquer-tree (Rhus vernicifera) laccase from the type-2-copper depeleted enzyme via a direct Cu(I) transfer mechanism. Biochem J 211:515–517

Morselt AFW, Copius-Peereboom-Stegeman JHJ, Puvion E, Maarschalkerweerd VJ (1983) Investigation of the mechanism of cadmium toxicity at the cellular level. Arch Toxicol 52:99–108

Murakami M, Webb M (1981) A morphological and biochemical study of the effects of L-cysteine on the renal uptake and nephrotoxicity of cadmium. Br J Exp Pathol 62:115–130

Murakami M, Cain K, Webb M (1983 a) Cadmium-metallothionein-induced nephropathy: a morphological and autoradiographical study of cadmium distribution, the development of tubular damage and subsequent cell regeneration. J Appl Toxicol 5:237–244

Murakami M, Tohyama C, Sano K, Kawamura R, Kubota K (1983 b) Autoradiographic studies on the localization of metallothionein in proximal tubular cells in the kidneys of rats. Arch Toxicol 53:185–192

Neathery MW (1981) Metabolism and toxicity of cadmium in animals. In: Nriagu JO (ed) Cadmium in the environment. II. Health effects. Wiley, New York, p 560

Nicholson JK, Sadler PJ, Cain K, Holt DE, Webb M, Hawkes GE (1983) 88MHz ^{113}Cd-nmr studies of native rat liver metallothioneins. Biochem J 211:251–255

Nomiyama K, Foulkes EC (1977) Reabsorption of filtered CdMT in the rabbit kidney. Proc Soc Exp Biol Med 156:97–99

Nomiyama K, Nomiyama H (1982) Tissue metallothioneins in rabbits chronically exposed to cadmium, with special reference to the critical concentration of cadmium in the renal cortex. In: Foulkes EC (ed) Biological roles of metallothionein. Elsevier/North-Holland, Amsterdam, pp 47–67

Nordberg GF (1971) Effects of acute and chronic cadmium exposure on the testicles of mice with special reference to the protective effects of metallothionein. Environ Physiol 1:171–182

Nordberg GF (1972) Cadmium metabolism and toxicity. Environ Physiol Biochem 2:7–36

Nordberg GF, Goyer R, Nordberg M (1975) Comparative toxicity of cadmium-metallothionein and cadmium chloride on mouse kidney. Arch Pathol 99:192–197

Nordberg M, Elinder C-G, Rahnster B (1979) Cadmium, zinc and copper in horse kidney metallothionein. Environ Res 20:341–350

Oberdörster G, Kördel W (1981) Metallothionein content in lung after chronic CdO and ZnO inhalation in rats. In: International conference heavy metals in the environment. CEP Consultants, Edinburgh, pp 502–505

Oh SH, Whanger PD (1979) Biological function of metallothionein. VII. Effect of age on its metabolism in rats. Am J Physiol 237:E18–E22

Ohsawa M, Fukada K (1976) Enhancement by phenobarbital of the biliary excretion of methylmercury and cadmium in rats. Ind Health 14:7–14

Ohtaki H, Koga M (1979) Purification and characterization of zinc-binding protein from the liver of the partially hepatectomized rat. Biochem J 183:683–690

Ohtaki H, Hasegawa K, Koga M (1978) Zinc binding protein in the livers of neonatal, normal and partially hepatectomized rats. Biochem J 174:999–1005

Olafson RW, Sim RG (1979) An electrochemical approach to the characterization of metallothioneins. Anal Biochem 100:343–351

Onosaka S, Cherian MG (1981) Induced synthesis of metallothionein in various tissues of rats in response to metals. I. Repeated cadmium injection. Toxicology 22:91–101

Onosaka S, Cherian MG (1982a) Comparison of metallothionein determination by polarographic and cadmium-saturation methods. Toxicol Appl Pharmacol 63:270–274

Onosaka S, Cherian MG (1982b) Induced synthesis of metallothionein in various tissues of rats in response to metals. II. Influence of zinc status and specific effect on pancreatic metallothionein. Toxicology 23:11–20

Otvos JD, Armitage IM (1979) [113]Cd NMR of metallothionein. Direct evidence for the existence of polynuclear metal binding sites. J Am Chem Soc 101:7734–7736

Otvos JD, Armitage IM (1980) Structure of the metal clusters in rabbit liver metallothionein. Proc Natl Acad Sci USA 77:7094–7098

Otvos JD, Olafson RW, Armitage IM (1982) Structure of an invertebrate metallothionein from Scylla serrata. J Biol Chem 257:2427–2431

Pařízek J (1964) Vascular changes at sites of oestrogen biosynthesis produced by parenteral injection of cadmium salts: the destruction of the placenta by cadmium salts. J Reproduct Fertil 7:263–265

Pařízek J (1965) The peculiar toxicity of cadmium during pregnancy – an experimental toxaemia of pregnancy induced by cadmium salts. J Reprod Fertil 9:111–112

Parzyck DC, Shaw SM, Kessler WV, Vetter RJ, Van Sickle DC, Meyer RA (1978) Fetal effects of cadmium in pregnant rats on normal and zinc-deficient diets. Bull Environ Contam Toxicol 19:206–214

Pence DH, Miya TS, Schnell RC (1977) Cadmium alteration of hexabarbital action: sex related differences in the rat. Toxicol Appl Pharmacol 39:89–96

Petering HG, Murthy L, Sorenson JRL, Levin L, Stemner KL (1979) Effect of sex on oral cadmium dose responses in rats: blood pressure and pharmacodynamics. Environ Res 20:289–299

Piotrowski JK, Bolanowska W, Sapota A (1973) Evaluation of metallothionein content in animal tissues. Acta Biochim Pol 20:207–215

Piscator M (1964) On cadmium in normal human kidney together with a report on the isolation of metallothionein from the livers of cadmium-exposed rats. Nord Hyg Tidskr 45:76–82

Piscator M, Lund B (1972) Cadmium, zinc, copper and lead in human renal cortex. Arch Environ Health 24:426–431

Post CL, Squibb KS, Fowler BA, Gardner DE, Illing J, Hook GER (1982) Production of low molecular weight cadmium-binding proteins in rabbit lung following exposure to cadmium chloride. Biochem Pharmacol 31:2969–2975

Prigge E (1978) Early signs of oral and inhalative cadmium uptake in rats. Arch Toxicol 40:231–247

Prins HW, Van den Hamer C (1981) Degradation of ^{35}S-labelled metallothionein in the liver and kidney of brindled mice; model for Menkes' disease. Life Sci 28:2953–2959

Prins HW, Van den Hamer C (1982) Copper metallothionein metabolism in the kidney of brindled mice. In: Gawthorne JM, Howell JMcC, White CL (eds) Trace element metabolism in man and animals – 4. Springer, Berlin Heidelberg New York, pp 645–648

Probst AS, Bousquet WF, Miya TS (1977) Correlation of hepatic metallothionein with acute cadmium toxicity in the mouse. Toxicol Appl Pharmacol 39:61–69

Raghaven SRV, Gonick HC (1980) Experimental Fanconi syndrome. IV. Effect of repeated injections of cadmium on tissue distribution and protein binding of cadmium. Miner Electrolyte Metab 3:36–43

Richards MP, Cousins RJ (1976) Metallothionein and its relationship to the metabolism of dietary zinc in rats. J Nutr 106:1591–1599

Ridlington JW, Winge DR, Fowler BA (1981) Long term turnover of cadmium-metallothionein in liver and kidney following a single low dose of cadmium. Biochim Biophys Acta 673:177–183

Riordan JR, Richards V (1980) Human fetal liver contains both zinc and copper-rich forms of metallothionein. J Biol Chem 255:5380–5383

Roberts SA, Schnell RC (1981) Tolerance development to cadmium-induced decrease in hepatic oxidative xenobiotic metabolism and cytochrome content in the male rat. Fundam Appl Toxicol 1:286–289

Roberts SA, Schnell RC (1982) Cadmium-induced inhibition of hepatic drug oxidation in the rat: time dependence of tolerance development and metallothionein synthesis. Toxicol Appl Pharmacol 64:42–51

Rogers K, Cherian MG (1981) Toxicity of cadmium metallothionein in rat kidney cell culture. Toxicologist 1:82

Rohrer SR, Shaw SM, Born GS, Vetter RJ (1978) The maternal distribution and placental transfer of cadmium in zinc-deficient rats. Bull Environ Contam Toxicol 19:556–563

Rydén L, Deutsch HF (1978) Preparation and properties of the major copper-binding component of human fetal liver. J Biol Chem 253:519–524

Sabbioni E, Marafante E (1975) Accumulation of cadmium in rat liver cadmium binding protein following single and repeated cadmium administration. Environ Physiol Biochem 5:465–473

Sabbioni E, Marafante E, Pietra R, Amantini L, Ubertalli L (1979) Long-term, low level exposure experiments by nuclear and radiochemical techniques. A two years accumulation study of cadmium in rat tissues. In: Anke M, Schneider H-J (eds) Kadmium symposium. Friedrich Schiller University, Jena, pp 111–116

Sadler PJ, Bakka A, Benyon PJ (1978) [113]Cd nmr of metallothionein. FEBS Lett 94:315–318

Samarawickrama GP (1979) Biological effects of cadmium in mammals. In: Webb M (ed) The chemistry, biochemistry and biology of cadmium. Elsevier/North-Holland, Amsterdam, pp 341–421

Samarawickrama GP, Webb M (1981) The acute toxicity and teratogenicity of cadmium in the pregnant rat. J Appl Toxicol 1:264–269

Sasser LB, Jarboe GE (1977) Intestinal absorption and retention of cadmium in neonatal rats. Toxicol Appl Pharmacol 41:423–431

Sasser LB, Jarboe GE (1980) Intestinal absorption and retention of cadmium in neonatal pigs, compared to rats and guinea-pigs. J Nutr 110:1641–1647

Sato M, Nagai Y (1980) Mode of existence of cadmium in rat liver and kidney after prolonged subcutaneous administration. Toxicol Appl Pharmacol 54:90–99

Sato M, Nagai Y (1982) Renal damage and form of cadmium in sub-cellular fractions. In: Foulkes EC (ed) Biological roles of metallothionein. Elsevier/North-Holland, Amsterdam, pp 163–179

Schmidt J (1936) Organic chemistry. Gurney and Jackson, London, p 670

Schnell RC, Means JR, Roberts SA, Pence DH (1979) Studies on cadmium-induced inhibition of hepatic microsomal drug biotransformation in the rat. Environ Health Perspect 28:273–279

Sciortino CV, Failla ML, Bullis DB (1982) Identification of metallothionein in parenchymal and non-parenchymal liver cells of the adult rat. Biochem J 204:509–514

Selenke W, Foulkes EC (1981) Binding of cadmium metallothionein to isolated renal brush border membranes. Proc Soc Exp Biol Med 167:40–44

Shaikh ZA, Hirayama K (1979) Metallothionein in the extracellular fluids as an index of cadmium toxicity. Environ Health Perspect 28:267–271

Shapiro SG, Cousins RJ (1980) Induction of rat liver metallothionein mRNA and its distribution between free and membrane-bound polyribosomes. Biochem J 190:755–764

Singh K, Nath R (1972) Studies on the identification of the cadmium-binding protein in rat testis. Biochem J 128:48P

Singh K, Nath R, Chakrarti RN (1974) Isolation and characterization of cadmium-binding protein from rat testes. J Reprod Fertil 36:257–265

Smith KT, Cousins RJ (1979) Quantitative aspects of Zn absorption by isolated vascularly perfused rat intestine. J Nutr 110:316–323

Sokolowski G, Pilz W, Weser U (1974) X-ray photoelectron spectroscopic properties of Hg-thionein. FEBS Lett 48:222–225

Sonowane BR, Nordberg M, Nordberg GF, Lucier GW (1975) Placental transfer of cadmium in rats: influence of dose and gestational age. Environ Health Perspect 12:97–102

Squibb KS, Cousins RJ, Silbon BL, Levin S (1976) Liver and intestinal metallothionein-function in acute cadmium toxicity. Exp Mol Pathol 25:163–171

Squibb KS, Ridlington JW, Carmichael NG, Fowler BA (1979) Early cellular effects of circulating cadmium-thionein on kidney proximal tubules. Environ Health Perspect 28:287–296

Squibb KS, Pritchard JB, Fowler BA (1982) Renal metabolism and toxicity of metallothionein. In: Foulkes EC (ed) Biological roles of metallothionein. Elsevier/North-Holland, Amsterdam, pp 181–192

Starcher BC (1969) Studies on the mechanism of copper absorption in the chick. J Nutr 97:321–326

Starcher BC, Glauber JC, Madaras JG (1980) Zinc absorption and its relationship to intestinal metallothionein. J Nutr 110:1391–1397

Stonard MD, Webb M (1976) Influence of dietary cadmium on the distribution of the essential metals copper, zinc and iron in tissues of the rat. Chem Biol Interact 15:349–363

Suda T, Horinchi N, Ogata E, Ezawa I, Otaki N, Kimura M (1974) Prevention by metallothionein of cadmium-induced inhibition of vitamin A activation reaction in kidney. FEBS Lett 42:23–26

Sugawara N (1977) Influence of cadmium on zinc distribution in the mouse liver and kidney: role of metallothionein. Toxicol Appl Pharmacol 42:377–386

Suzuki KT (1979) Copper content in cadmium exposed animal kidney metallothioneins. Arch Environ Contam Toxicol 8:255–268

Suzuki KT (1980) Direct connection of high speed liquid chromatograph, equipped with gel-permeation column, to atomic absorption spectrophotometer for metalloprotein analysis: metallothionein. Anal Biochem 102:31–34

Suzuki KT (1982) Induction and degradation of metallothionein and their relation to the toxicity of cadmium. In: Foulkes EC (ed) Biological roles of metallothionein. Elsevier/North-Holland, Amsterdam, pp 215–235

Suzuki KT, Maitana T (1979) Fate of i.p. injected liver metallothionein in rat kidney. Chem Pharm Bull 27:647–653

Suzuki KT, Takenaka S (1979) Fate of kidney metallothionein i.p. injected into the rat. Chem Pharm Bull 27:1753–1758

Suzuki KT, Yamamura M (1979) Gel and anion exchange chromatographic properties of copper-containing metallothioneins. Arch Environ Contam Toxicol 8:471–485

Suzuki KT, Yamamura M (1980a) Isolation and characterization of metallothionein dimers. Biochem Pharmacol 29:689–692

Suzuki KT, Yamamura M (1980b) Changes of metal contents and isometallothionein levels in rat tissues after cadmium loading. Biochem Pharmacol 29:2407–2412

Suzuki KT, Yamamura M (1980c) Induction of zinc-thionein in rat liver and kidneys by zinc loading as studied at isometallothionein level. Toxicol Lett 6:59–65

Suzuki KT, Yamamura M (1980d) Rat kidney metallothionein induced by injection of Cd-thionein: changes in chromatographic properties with time and their relation to copper content and kidney dysfunction. Toxicol Lett 5:131–138

Suzuki KT, Takenaka S, Kubota K (1979) Fate and comparative toxicity of metallothioneins with different Cd:Zn ratios in rat kidney. Arch Environ Contam Toxicol 8:85–95

Suzuki KT, Yamamura M, Yamada YK, Shimizu F (1981) Distribution of cadmium in heavy cadmium-accumulated rat liver cytosols: metallothioneins and related cadmium-binding proteins. Toxicol Lett 8:105–114

Suzuki S, Taguchi T (1970) Sex difference of cadmium contents in urine spot tests. Ind Health 8:150–152

Suzuki Y, Yoshikawa H (1974) Role of metallothionein in the liver in protection against cadmium toxicity. Ind Health 12:141–151

Taguchi T, Nakamura K (1982) Isolation and properties of cadmium-binding proteins induced in rat small intestine by oral administration of cadmium. J Toxicol Environ Health 9:401–409

Taguchi T, Suzuki S (1981) Influence of sex and age on the biological half-life of cadmium in mice. J Toxicol Environ Health 7:239–249

Tanaka K (1982) Effect of hepatic disorder on the fate of cadmium in rats. In: Foulkes EC (ed) Biological roles of metallothionein. Elsevier/North-Holland, Amsterdam, pp 237–249

Tanaka K, Sueda K, Okahara K (1974) Fate of heavy metals in animals: quantitative change of metallothionein in the liver, kidney and intestinal mucosa of rat after a single injection of ^{109}CdCl$_2$. J Hyg Chem 20:98–101

Tanaka K, Sueda K, Onasaka S, Okahara K (1975) Fate of ^{109}Cd labelled metallothionein in rats. Toxicol Appl Pharmacol 33:258–266

Tanaka K, Onosaka S, Doi M, Okahara K (1977) Substitution of zinc bound to metallothionein for cadmium in vitro and in vivo. J Hyg Chem 23:229–234

Taylor BA, Heiniger HJ, Meier H (1973) Genetic analysis of resistance to cadmium-induced testicular damage in mice. Proc Soc Exp Biol Med 143:629–633

Terhaar CJ, Vis E, Roudabush RL, Fassett DW (1965) Protective effects by low doses of cadmium chloride against subsequent oral doses in rats. Toxicol Appl Pharmacol 7:500

Tohyama C, Shaikh ZA (1978) Cross reactivity of metallothioneins from different origins with rabbit and rat hepatic metallothionein antibody. Biochem Biophys Res Commun 84:907–913

Tohyama C, Shaikh ZA (1981) Metallothionein in plasma and urine of cadmium exposed rats determined by a single antibody radioimmunoassay. Fundam Appl Toxicol 1:1–7

Tohyama C, Shaikh ZA, Nogawa K, Kobayashi E, Honda R (1982) Urinary metallothionein as a new index of renal dysfunction in itai itai disease patients and other Japanese women environmentally exposed to cadmium. Arch Toxicol 50:159–166

Tsunoo H, Nakajima H, Hata A, Kimura M (1979) Genetic influence on induction of metallothionein and mortality from cadmium intoxication. Toxicol Lett 4:253–256

Udom AO, Brady FO (1980) Reactivation in vitro of zinc-requiring apo-enzymes by rat liver zinc-metallothionein. Biochem J 187:329–335

Vallee BL (1979) Metallothionein: historical review and perspectives. Experientia [Suppl] 34:19–40

Vander Mallie RJ, Garvey JS (1978) Production and study of antibody produced against rat cadmium-thionein. Immunochemistry 15:857–858

Vander Mallie RJ, Garvey JS (1979) Radioimmunoassay of metallothioneins. J Biol Chem 254:8416–8421

Vašák M, Galdes A, Hill HAO, Kägi JHR, Bremner I, Young BW (1980) Investigation of the structure of metallothionein by proton nuclear magnetic resonance spectroscopy. Biochemistry 19:416–425

Vašák M, Kägi JHR, Hill HAO (1981) Zinc (II), cadmium (II) and mercury (II) transitions in metallothionein. Biochemistry 20:2852–2856

Waalkes MP, Thomas JA, Bell JU (1982) Induction of hepatic metallothionein in the rabbit fetus following maternal cadmium exposure. Toxicol Appl Pharmacol 62:211–218

Waalkes MP, Chernoff SB, Klaassen CD (1984) Cadmium-binding proteins of rat testes. Characterization of a low-molecular-mass protein that lacks identity with metallothionein. Biochem J 220:811–818

Wada O, Miyahara A, Manabe S, Matsui H, Ono T (1982) Effect of acute administration of cadmium on the distribution of zinc in the hamster. J Toxicol Environ Health 9:509–513

Waku K, Hayakawa F, Nakazawa Y (1980) Effects of Cd^{2+} and CdMT on the activities of phospholipid synthesizing enzymes of rat liver microsomes in vitro. Ann Biochem Biophys 204:288–293

Webb M (1972 a) Binding of cadmium ions by rat liver and kidney. Biochem Pharmacol 21:2751–2765

Webb M (1972 b) Persistence of stored Cd^{2+} in the livers and kidneys of female rats during pregnancy. J Reprod Fertil 30:99–103

Webb M (1979 a) The metallothioneins. In: Webb M (ed) The chemistry, biochemistry and biology of cadmium. Elsevier/North-Holland, Amsterdam, pp 195–266

Webb M (1979 b) Interactions of cadmium with cellular components. In: Webb M (ed) The chemistry, biochemistry and biology of cadmium. Elsevier/North-Holland, Amsterdam, pp 285–340

Webb M (1979 c) Cadmium-thionein and the nephrotoxicity of cadmium. In: Anke M, Schneider H-J (eds) Kadium symposium. Friedrich Schiller University, Jena, pp 101–107

Webb M (1982) Role of metallothioneins and other binding proteins in the renal handling and toxicity of metals. In: Bach PH, Bonner FW, Bridges JW, Lock EA (eds) Nephrotoxicity assessment and pathogenesis. Wiley, New York, pp 296–309

Webb M (1983) Endogenous metal binding proteins in the control of zinc, copper, cadmium and mercury metabolism during prenatal and postnatal development. In: Clarkson T, Nordberg G (eds) Reproductive and developmental toxicity of metals. Plenum, New York, pp 655–674

Webb M, Cain K (1982) Functions of metallothionein. Biochem Pharmacol 31:137–142

Webb M, Etienne AT (1977) Studies on the toxicity and metabolism of cadmiumthionein. Biochem Pharmacol 26:25–30

Webb M, Holt D (1982) Endogenous metal binding proteins in relation to the differences in absorption and distribution of mercury in newborn and adult rats. Arch Toxicol 49:237–245

Webb M, Magos L (1976) Cadmium-thionein and the protection by cadmium against the nephrotoxicity of mercury. Chem Biol Interact 14:357–369

Webb M, Samarawickrama GP (1981) Placental transport and embryonic utilization of essential metabolites in the rat at the teratogenic dose of cadmium. J Appl Toxicol 1:270–277

Webb M, Verschoyle RD (1976) An investigation of the role of metallothioneins in protection against the acute toxicity of the cadmium ion. Biochem Pharmacol 25:673–679

Webster WS (1979 a) Iron deficiency and its role in cadmium-induced fetal growth retardation. J Nutr 109:1640–1645

Webster WS (1979 b) Cadmium-induced fetal growth retardation in mice and the effect of dietary supplement of zinc, copper, iron and selenium. J Nutr 109:1646–1651

Weser U, Rupp H (1979) Physicochemical properties of metallothioneins. In: Webb M (ed) The chemistry, biochemistry and biology of cadmium. Elsevier/North-Holland, Amsterdam, pp 267–283

Whanger PD, Ridlington JW, Holcomb CL (1980) Interrelations of zinc and selenium on the binding of cadmium to rat tissue proteins. Ann NY Acad Sci 355:333–346

Winge DR, Miklossy KA (1982 a) Differences in the pleomorphic forms of metallothionein. Arch Biochem Biophys 214:80–88

Winge DR, Miklossy KA (1982b) Domain nature of metallothionein. J Biol Chem 257:3471–3476

Winge DR, Premakumar R, Rajagopalan KV (1975) Metal induced formation of metallothionein in rat liver. Arch Biochem Biophys 170:242–252

Winge DR, Premakumar R, Rajagopalan KV (1978) Studies on the zinc content of cadmium-induced thionein. Arch Biochem Biophys 188:466–475

Wolkowski RM (1974) Differential cadmium induced embryotoxicity in two inbred mouse strains. I. Analysis of inheritance of the response to cadmium and the presence of cadmium in fetal and placental tissue. Teratology 10:243–261

Wong K-L, Klaassen CD (1979) Isolation and characterization of metallothionein which is highly concentrated in newborn rat liver. J Biol Chem 259:12399–12403

Wong K-L, Klaassen CD (1980a) Tissue distribution and retention of cadmium in rats during post natal development, minimal role of hepatic metallothionein. Toxicol Appl Pharmacol 53:343–353

Wong K-L, Klaassen CD (1980b) Age differences in susceptibility to cadmium-induced testicular damage in rats. Toxicol Appl Pharmacol 55:456–466

Yoshida A, Kaplan BE, Kimura M (1979) Metal binding and detoxification, effect of synthetic oligopeptides containing three cysteinyl residues. Proc Natl Acad Sci USA 76:486–490

Yoshikawa H (1970) Preventive effect of pretreatment with low doses of metals on the acute toxicity of metals in mice. Ind Health 8:184–191

Yoshikawa H, Suzuki Y (1976) Cadmium distribution and metallothionein in the livers of mice treated with phenobarbital. Ind Health 14:103–108

CHAPTER 9

Immunotoxicity of Cadmium

J. H. Exon and L. D. Koller

A. The Immune System

During the past decade, a number of chemicals and drugs have been shown to alter immune functions inadvertently in animals and human beings. In fact, the immune system has been shown to be exquisitely affected at low levels of exposure to certain environmental toxicants before any other toxicologic manifestations are evident. The perturbation of immune responses by exogenous chemicals and drugs is not surprising considering the complex nature and delicate balances controlling these reactions. These types of immunomodulating effects have led government agencies and private industry to consider the incorporation of immunotoxicologic profiles into standard toxicologic assessment protocols for drugs and chemicals.

Immune responsiveness can be superficially separated into several general types of reactions that are mediated by specific types of immunocompetent cells. Humoral immunity, the production of antibodies, is mediated by B-lymphocytes, so named because of their maturation site in birds, the bursa of Fabricius, and their origin in mammals, the bone marrow. Cell-mediated immune (CMI) reactions are mainly due to the responses of T-lymphocytes which derive their name from the requirement of the thymus for normal maturation. The major subsets of effector T-lymphocytes are the cytotoxic T-cell (T_{CT}) and the T-cell-mediating delayed-type hypersensitivity (T_{DTH}). The major subsets of regulator T-lymphocytes include the T helper cells (T_H) and the T suppressor cells (T_S).

A third major immunocomponent cell is the tissue macrophage, which is a relatively large cell thought to be derived from circulating blood monocytes and capable of phagocytizing particles, substances, or cells foreign to the host. A fourth population of cells which have been only recently characterized are termed natural killer cells (NKC). These cells are thought to be important in first line defense against certain virus-infected or tumor cells. NKC are capable of attacking and lysing foreign or altered cells without having been previously exposed to these cells (i.e., natural immunosurveillance). NKC appear to be neither of T-lymphocyte or macrophage lineage and probably represent a separate line of lymphocyte differentiation.

The types of immune responses and cells described are by no means exclusive of each other in the production of immunity. Each cell type can have profound regulatory effects on the others through direct cell–cell contact or the production of soluble immunoregulating factors. For instance, although antibody production is mediated by B-cells, cooperation and interaction with macrophages and

T-cells is required for an optimal humoral immune response to complex antigens. Macrophages are required to "process" and "present" antigen to B-cells and T-cells in an immunorecognizable form. They also regulate T-cell functions by production of soluble factors such as interleukin 1 (IL1) and prostaglandins (PG), to name two. Subpopulations of T_H or T_S interact with B-cells to amplify or suppress ongoing antibody synthesis. T-cells also amplify the clonal expansion of other T-cells and NKC via the production of interleukin 2 (IL2) and gamma interferon (gIFN) and affect macrophage activation through lymphokines such as macrophage-activating factor (MAF) and migration-inhibition factor (MIF). These examples are but a few of the complex interrelationships of cells involved in the production and control of immune responses, but should serve to establish some appreciation of the potential for disruption of this delicate system by chemicals and drugs.

B. Immunoassays

When testing for immunomodulating potential of a chemical or drug, several types of immunoassay are employed which are designed to assess the integrity of major arms of the immune system. Several different assays are usually performed because it has been demonstrated repeatedly that chemicals can (a) selectively affect one major immune response without altering another or (b) affect separate types of immune responses differently. A typical immune profile would include assays for humoral immunity, CMI, macrophage function, host resistance to an infectious agent or tumor induction, and histopathology of lymphoid organs such as thymus, spleen, and lymph nodes.

Assays commonly used to assess humoral immunity could include quantitation of total immunoglobulins, antibody titers to specific antigens, the number of antibody-producing cells in spleens and/or lymph nodes (commonly called the plaque-forming cell assay PFC), hemagglutination or hemolysin titers, or quantitation of specific antibody production to T-cell-dependent and T-cell-independent antigens as measured by a radioimmunoassay (RIA) or enzyme-linked immunosorbent assay (ELISA). The lymphoproliferative response to the B-cell mitogen, lipopolysaccharide (LPS), has been used as a nonspecific in vitro assay for B-cell function.

CMI functions can be assessed in vivo by graft versus host reactions, rejection of tissue grafts, delayed-type hypersensitivity responses (DTH), antibody synthesis to a T-cell-dependent antigen or production of lymphokines such as IL2, gIFN, MAF, or MIF. In vitro assays for T-cell function include cytotoxic lympholysis (CTL), mixed lymphocyte responses (MLR), or lymphoproliferative responses to T-cell-specific mitogens such as concanavalin A (Con A) or phytohemagglutinin (PHA).

Macrophage function can be evaluated by their ability to phagocytize foreign particles such as xenogeneic blood cells, carbon or iron particles, latex beads, bacteria, or yeast cells. Other macrophage function assays include their ability to migrate (chemotaxis or chemokinesis), presence of surface receptors for the Fc portion of IgG or the C3 component of complement, and production of immunoregulator monokines such as IL1 or PG. NKC function is measured by their ability to lyse NKC-susceptible tumor cells in vitro without previous sensitization. Host susceptibility assays involve assessing resistance of toxicant-exposed animals to bacteria infection, bacterial endotoxins, virus challenge, parasite infestation, or induction of tumors. The endpoint measurement of these responses is usually percentage morbidity, mortality, or tumor growth.

C. Effects of Cadmium on Immune Responses

The effects of cadmium (Cd) on immune function are discordant. Cd-treated animals have been reported to be both more and less resistant to challenge with infectious agents. Antibody responses to antigens have been shown to be both enhanced and suppressed following exposure to Cd. The acute effects of Cd on immune function appear to be markedly affected by the duration of exposure, the dose, and temporal relationship between Cd treatment and administration of antigen. CMI responses have also been augmented or suppressed following Cd treatment. The effect of Cd on macrophages has varied from no effect to enhancement to depression. The effects of Cd on various immune functions are summarized in Tables 1–4 and are discussed in more detail in the following sections.

I. Host Resistance

Host resistance studies of rodents exposed to Cd at various doses and for various periods of time show variable effects (Table 1). Charles River rats were markedly

Table 1. Effect of cadmium on host resistance to infectious agents or tumors

Species	Cadmium form and route	Infectious agent/tumor	Resistance	References
Mouse	Acetate/oral	EMCV	I	Exon et al. (1979)
Mouse	Various salts/oral	EMCV	I	Exon et al. (1985)
Mouse	Oxide/air	*Orthomyxovirus*	I	Bouley et al. (1982)
Mouse	Chloride/oral	MOPC tumor	I	Gray et al. (1982)
Mouse	Chloride/oral	MSB sarcoma	I	Kerkvliet et al. (1979)
Mouse	Chloride/intraperitoneal	*Mycobacterium*	I	Bozelka and Burkholder (1979)
Chicken	Sulfate/oral	*Salmonella*	I	Hill (1979)
Mouse	Sulfate/oral	EMCV	D	Gainer (1977a, b)
Mouse	Chloride/oral	*Hexamita*	D	Exon et al. (1975)
Mouse	Oxide/air	*Pasteurella*	D	Bouley et al. (1982)
Mouse	Chloride/intraperitoneal	*Listeria*	D	Berche et al. (1980)
Mouse	Chloride/intraperitoneal	JEV	D	Suzuki et al. (1981)
Rat	Acetate/intravenous	*Endotoxin*	D	Cook et al. (1974)
Rat	Acetate/intravenous	*E. coli*	D	Cook et al. (1975)
Mouse	Chloride/intraperitoneal	*Klebsiella*	N	Berche et al. (1980)
Mouse	Chloride/intraperitoneal	*Pseudomonas*	N	Berche et al. (1980)
Chicken	Sulfate/oral	*E. coli*	N	Hill (1979)

D, decreased; I, increased; N, no effect

more susceptible to lethal effects of *Salmonella enteritidis* entotoxin or *Escherichia coli* after intravenous exposure to one dose of 0.6 mg Cd acetate given 3 days before challenge (Cook et al. 1974, 1975). Resistance to encephalomyocarditis virus (EMCV) was decreased in CD-1 mice given $CdSO_4$ chronically in drinking water at doses of 0.005 or 0.002 *M* in one study (Gainer 1977a, b) but was increased in Swiss–Webster mice exposed to 3, 30, or 300 ppm $CdCl_2$ or other Cd salts in the drinking water for 10 weeks as reported in two other studies (Exon et al. 1979, 1985). Swiss–Webster mice treated with 3, 30, or 300 ppm $CdCl_2$ in the drinking water for 2–3 weeks and infected with the protozoan, *Hexamita muris* had increased mortality rates compared with nontreated controls (Exon et al. 1975). Macrophages collected from C57BL/6J mice were inhibited from killing sarcoma I tumor cells in the presence of 10^{-5} or 10^{-6} *M* $CdCl_2$ in vitro (Nelson et al. 1982). Female SLC-ICR mice had significantly increased mortality rates and decreased time to death when injected with 0.09 mg $CdCl_2$ once and simultaneously inoculated intraperitoneally with Japanese encephalitis virus (JEV) (Suzuki et al. 1981). However, if mice were pretreated with $CdCl_2$ at the same dose at 10 days, or 3, 5, or 7 weeks prior to virus challenge or if JEV was given intracerebrally, no effect of Cd was observed. Susceptibility to bacterial challenge with *Klebsiella pneumoniae, Pseudomonas aeruginosa,* or *Listeria monocytogenes* was examined in Ham/ICR Swiss or C_3H mice treated by intraperitoneal injection of 10 µg $CdCl_2$ three times per week for 4 weeks (Berche et al. 1980). Only *L. monocytogenes* showed increased virulence in Cd-treated mice.

A good example of the dichotomous responses of Cd-exposed animals to infectious agents was recently demonstrated by Bouley et al. (1982). Groups of specific-pathogen-free mice were exposed to CdO 10 mg/m^3 by inhalation for a single 15-min period and then separate groups were challenged with either bacteria (*Pasteurella multocida*) or a virus (*Orthomyxovirus* influenza A) via the respiratory route. Bacterially exposed mice which received Cd had an increased death rate while virus-infected, Cd-treated groups had a decreased death rate as compared with controls.

BALB/c mice treated with low levels (0.01 ppm) of $CdCl_2$ in the drinking water for 5 weeks had significantly less MOPC-104E tumor-induced mortality rates than controls (Gray et al. 1982). However, tumor-induced mortality in mice from this same study that were treated with higher levels of $CdCl_2$ (0.1 or 1.0 ppm) were no different from controls. Exposure to $CdSO_4$ at levels of 20–400 ppm in feed has also been related to increased resistance of chickens to bacterial challenge with *Salmonella gallinarum* (Hill 1979).

II. Antibody Synthesis and B-Cells

The effects of Cd exposure on antibody synthesis is summarized in Table 2 and are also somewhat controversial. The IgG PFC response to sheep red blood cells (SRBC) challenge was significantly suppressed in Swiss–Webster mice given 3, 30, or 300 ppm $CdCl_2$ in the drinking water for 10 weeks and analyzed up to 42 days later (Koller et al. 1975). The IgM response was also suppressed, but appeared to be recovering by 14 days after cessation of Cd exposure. Chronic exposure (10

Table 2. Effects of cadmium on humoral immunity

Species	Exposure	Parameter	Effect	References
Mouse	Acute/oral	PFC	I	Koller et al. (1976)
Mouse	Chronic/oral	PFC	I	Cay (1981)
Mouse	Subacute/oral	Blastogenesis	I	Gaworski and Sharma (1978)
Mouse	Chronic/oral	Blastogenesis	I	Koller et al. (1979)
Mouse	Chronic/oral	Blastogenesis	I	Muller et al. (1978)
Rat	Acute/intraperitoneal	Ab titer	I–D	Jones et al. (1971)
Mouse	Chronic/oral	PFC	D	Koller et al. (1975)
Mouse	Acute/intraperitoneal	PFC	D	Koller et al. (1976)
Mouse	Chronic/intraperitoneal	PFC	D	Bozelka et al. (1978)
Mouse	Acute/air	PFC	D	Graham et al. (1978)
Mouse	Chronic/oral	C3 receptor	D	Koller and Brauner (1977)
Rabbit	Chronic/oral	Ab titer	D	Koller (1973)
Mouse	Chronic/oral	B memory	D	Koller and Roan (1980a)
Guinea pig	In vitro	MIF production	D	Kiremedjian et al. (1981b)
Mouse	In vitro	PFC	I–D–N	Fujimaki et al. (1982)
Mouse	In vitro	PFC	D–N	Lawrence (1981)
	Acute/intramuscular	PFC	N	Graham et al. (1978)
Mouse	Acute/subcutaneous	Neutralization	N	Suzuki et al. (1981)
Mouse	Chronic/oral	PFC	N	Muller et al. (1978)
Mouse	Acute/intraperitoneal	Hemagglutination	N	Kojima and Tamuar (1981)

D, decreased; I, increased; N, no effect

weeks) of rabbits to 300 ppm $CdCl_2$ reduced serum neutralizing antibody titers to pseudorabies virus challenge (Koller 1973). Borzelka et al. (1978) reported that both primary and secondary antibody synthesis of B10A2R mice chronically exposed to 2 ppm $CdCl_2$ by intraperitoneal injection for 40 days was also impaired.

Graham et al. (1978) also reported that CD-1 mice exposed to $CdCl_2$ 190 µg/m^3 in the air for 2 h had reduced ability to produce IgM antibody. However, if Cd was given by intramuscular injections in doses ranging from 0.148 to 11.81 µg/kg, no effect was observed. The antibody response in mice exposed to a single dose of 0.15 mg $CdCl_2$ by different routes showed that IgM and IgG responses were enhanced if Cd was injected intraperitoneally, but both were decreased if given orally (Koller et al. 1976). It has been reported that Sprague-Dawley rats injected with 0.6 mg $CdSO_4$ for 5 consecutive days beginning 7 days before antigenic challenge with human γ-globulin had reduced serum antibody levels, but if injections were started 14 days before antigenic challenge, antibody levels were enhanced (Jones et al. 1971).

Suzuki et al. (1981) showed no effect on antibody responses of SLC-ICR mice treated with one dose of 0.09 mg $CdCl_2$ given subcutaneously either simultaneously or before challenge with JEV. Another study showed that NMR-1 mice

treated with 30, 300, or 600 ppm Cd acetate for 10 weeks in the drinking water
had normal IgM and IgG antibody responses (MULLER et al. 1978).

CAY (1981) reported the primary PFC responses of BALB/c mice treated with
0.01, 0.05, 0.1, 1, or 5 ppm $CdCl_2$ in the drinking water for 5 weeks were significantly enhanced at all dosage levels. A more recent study has shown the primary
antibody response to SRBC was also augmented in cultures of BALB/c mice
spleen cells when incubated in vitro for 4 or 5 days with 4 or 8 μM $CdCl_2$, but
were suppressed in cultures receiving 20 or 40 μM $CdCl_2$ (FUJIMAKI et al. 1982).
Reconstitution studies of adherent and nonadherent cells and/or T- and B-cells
indicated that effects of Cd on B-cells were mainly responsible for enhancement
seen at the lower doses. No effects of in vitro Cd treatment were observed on the
secondary antibody response. The Cd levels used in those studies did decrease cell
viability. B-lymphocytes of mice given 160 ppm $CdCl_2$ in the drinking water for
30 days showed enhanced proliferative responses to LPS, a mitogen specific for
B-cells (GAWARSKI and SHARMA 1978). Similar results were observed in a different
study where Swiss–Webster mice were given 300 ppm $CdCl_2$ in the water for 10
weeks (KOLLER and ROAN 1980a). GALLAGHER et al. (1979) reported that $CdCl_2$
at 10^{-5} M was blastogenic ot BALB/c mice spleen cells in vitro, but did not alter
the LPS-induced response. SHENKER et al. (1977) found Cd enhanced LPS-induced mitogenesis of BALB/c mice splenocytes in vitro at levels of 10^{-7} and
10^{-6} M, but inhibited this response at higher concentrations.

KOLLER and ROAN (1980a) reported that the memory response was impaired
in Swiss–Webster mice given 300 ppm $CdCl_2$ orally for 10 weeks. Exposure levels
of 3 or 30 ppm, however, produced no effects on the secondary response. Another
study demonstrated that in vitro exposure of CBA/J mice spleen cells to 10^{-4} or
10^{-7} M $CdCl_2$ in cultures for 5 days significantly suppressed the primary PFC
response (LAWRENCE 1981). Primary PFC responses were not significantly altered, however, at 10^{-5} or 10^{-6} M $CdCl_2$ in the same study. Other studies relat-
ing to function of murine B-lymphocytes following exposure to Cd indicate that
this metal may impair the ability of complement components to bind with receptors (C3) on B-cells, thus reducing the effectiveness of antibody to destroy or in-
activate antigen (KOLLER and BRAUNER 1977).

III. Cell-Mediated Immunity and T-Cells

Cd-induced effects on T-lymphocyte-mediated immune responses (i.e., CMI) are
also varied according to the literature as summarized in Table 3. Inbred C57BL
mice given 3, 30, or 300 ppm $CdCl_2$ in drinking water for 10 weeks and challenged
with Moloney sarcoma virus-infected cells (MSB) developed fewer tumors or had
greater tumor regression rates than nontreated mice (KERKVLIET et al. 1979). In
vitro cytotoxicity to tumor cells by splenocytes of mice was also enhanced in this
study. The cytotoxic response was, however, inversely correlated to the level of
$CdCl_2$. Another study has shown that rejection of allografts is accelerated and
time to isograft acceptance increased in C57BL mice treated with 0.01, 0.1, 1.0,
or 10 ppm $CdCl_2$ in the drinking water for 4 weeks prior to grafting (BALTER et
al. 1982).

Table 3. Effects of Cadmium on cell-mediated immunity

Species	Exposure	Parameter	Effect	References
Mouse	Chronic/oral	Cytotoxicity	I	KERKVLIET et al. (1979)
Mouse	Subacute/oral	Graft rejection	I	BALTER et al. (1982)
Mouse	Chronic/oral	Blastogenesis	I	MULLER et al. (1978)
Mouse	In vitro	Blastogenesis	I–D	SHENKER et al. (1977)
Mouse	In vitro	Blastogenesis	I–D	GALLAGHER et al. (1979)
Mouse	Chronic/oral	Blastogenesis	I–D	KOLLER and ROAN (1980a)
Mouse	Acute/intraperitoneal	DTH	D	KOJIMA and TAMUAR (1981)
Mouse	Acute/intraperitoneal	Thymus weight	D	KOJIMA and TAMUAR (1981)
Mouse	Acute/intraperitoneal	T_H, T_S	D	KOJIMA and TAMUAR (1981)
Human	In vitro	Blastogenesis	D	KASTELAN et al. (1981)
Human	In vitro	MLR	D	KASTELAN et al. (1981)
Mouse	Chronic/oral	DTH	D	MULLER et al. (1978)
Mouse	Acute/intraperitoneal	Thymus weight	D	YAMADA et al. (1981)
Mouse	Subacute/oral	Blastogenesis	D–N	GAWORSKI and SHARMA (1978)
Mouse	Chronic/oral	MRL	N	KOLLER and ROAN (1980b)

D, decreased; I, increased; N, no effect

A more recent study showed that mice, given a single intraperitoneal injection of $CdCl_2$ 0.75 or 6 mg/kg within 2 days of immunization, had impaired DTH responses to ovalbumin as measured by a footpad swelling assay (KOJIMA and TAMUAR 1981). The Cd-induced suppression occurred in both the induction and progression phases of the DTH responses. Memory T-cell- and T_S-cell induction were also impaired and thymus weights reduced in these mice, but antibody titers to ovalbumin were not altered as measured by passive hemagglutination. MULLER et al. (1978) also reported that NMR-1 mice treated with 30, 300, or 600 ppm Cd acetate for 10 weeks in drinking water had a significantly reduced DTH response, but blastogenesis to PHA and Con A was enhanced. No effect was detected on antibody synthesis in this study.

In vitro studies involving lymphoproliferative responses to T-cell mitogens (Con A or PHA) or the MLR (the in vitro correlate of CMI) do not serve to clarify the in vivo data pertaining to exposure to Cd. Blastogenic responses of T-cells were reported to be enhanced at low doses of Cd, but inhibited at high doses (SHENKER et al. 1977; GALLAGHER et al. 1979). KOLLER et al. (1979) also reported a differential dose effect of $CdCl_2$ on CBA mice spleen cells exposed in vivo for 10 weeks. Responses to purified protein derivative (PPD) were enhanced at 300 ppm Cd, but were suppressed at 3 ppm. Neither dose affected Con A-induced lymphoproliferation or the MLR (KOLLER and ROAN 1980b). A depressed response to PHA was observed in a different study by KOLLER et al. (1979). Exposure of human lymphocytes in vitro to 1.6 or 3.3 µM $CdCl_2$ in culture significantly inhibited PHA-induced blastogenesis and MLR responses (KASTELAN et al. 1981). This suppressive action was most prominent if Cd was added at initiation of the cultures. GAWORSKI and SHARMA (1978) reported inhibition of PHA-, but not Con A-induced blastogenesis of spleen cells of mice given 160 ppm $CdCl_2$ for 30 days in the drinking water.

Production of the lymphokine, MIF, has been reported to be inhibited by Cd exposure in separate studies (BOZELKA and BURKHOLDER 1979; KIREMIDJIAN et al. 1981 a). The latter study also showed that Cd at doses of 10^{-3}–10^{-6} M lowered negative surface charge on guinea pig lymphocytes and interfered with the interaction of antigen with the cell membrane.

IV. Macrophage Function

Exposure to Cd has also been reported to affect various functions of macrophages as summarized in Table 4. In vivo intravascular clearance of lipid emulsions were increased, as was Kupffer cell localization of lipid in rats given a single intravenous dose of 0.6 mg/kg $CdCl_2$ (COOK et al. 1974). Similar effects were observed in vitro. Phagocytosis of SRBC was stimulated and acid phosphatase levels of macrophages increased in Swiss–Webster mice treated for 10 weeks with 300 ppm $CdCl_2$ in the drinking water (KOLLER and ROAN 1977).

The ability of reticuloendothelial cells of mice to bind and catabolize immune complexes in vivo was decreased following oral treatment with doses of $CdCl_2$ ranging from 10 to 300 ppm given in the drinking water for 3 months (KNUTSON et al. 1980). This effect was correlated to Cd levels in hepatic tissue and postulated to be due to Cd-induced perturbation of Fc or complement receptors on Kupffer cells, as similar effects were not seen in clearance of non-Ig molecules such as carbon or human serum albumin. Cd treatment has also been reported to impair rosette formation of alveolar macrophages which suggests the Fc receptor for Ig

Table 4. Effects cadmium on macrophage function

Species	Exposure	Parameter	Effect	References
Rat	Acute/intravenous	Liposome clearance	I	COOK et al. (1974)
Rat	In vitro	Liposome clearance	I	COOK et al. (1974)
Mouse	Chronic/oral	Phagocytosis	I	KOLLER and ROAN (1977)
Mouse	Chronic/oral	Acid phosphatase	I	KOLLER and ROAN (1977)
Mouse	Chronic/oral	Immune complex catabolism	D	KNUTSON et al. (1980)
Rabbit	In vitro	Fc receptor	D	HADLEY et al. (1977)
Mouse	In vitro	Phagocytosis	D	LOOSE et al. (1978a)
Rat	In vitro	O_2 consumption	D	CASTRANOVA et al. (1980)
Rat	In vitro	Glucose metabolism	D	CASTRANOVA et al. (1980)
Rat	In vitro	Oxygen radicals	D	CASTRANOVA et al. (1980)
Guinea pig	In vitro	Mobility	D	KIREMEDJIAN et al. (1981a,b)
Guinea pig	In vitro	Response to MIF	D	KIREMEDJIAN et al. (1981a,b)
Mouse	In vitro	Cytotoxicity	D	NELSON et al. (1982)
Rabbit	In vitro	Phagocytosis	D	GRAHAM et al. (1975)
Mouse	In vitro	Respiratory burst	D	LOOSE et al. (1977)
Mouse	In vitro	Viability	D	LOOSE et al. (1978b)

D, decreased; I, increased

may have been altered on these cells (HADLEY et al. 1977). Other studies have shown depressed phagocytic activity and microbial killing of macrophages of peritoneal or alveolar origin treated in vitro with 8×10^{-1}–8×10^{-3} mequiv./l $CdCl_2$ or Cd acetate for 30 min (LOOSE et al. 1978a, 1977). Cd also had a direct cytotoxic effect on these cells (LOOSE et al. 1978b). GRAHAM et al. (1975) has also reported reduced phagocytic activity of alveolar macrophages from rabbits exposed in vitro to 2.5 µg/ml $CdCl_2$.

The oxidative burst of rat alveolar macrophages during phagocytosis has also been shown to be depressed (CASTRANOVA et al. 1980). $CdCl_2$ or Cd acetate given in vitro for 15 min at a dose of 10^{-3} M significantly inhibited oxygen consumption, glucose metabolism, and release of active oxygen species from alveolar macrophages of Long-Evans rats. This cadmium-induced inhibition of oxidative processes of macrophages was postulated to diminish their antibacterial activity. More recent studies indicate that exposure to Cd may adversely affect macrophage functions such as mobility, response to macrophage-stimulating lymphokines, and cytotoxic activity (KIREMIDJIAN et al. 1981a, b). Peritoneal macrophages and splenic lymphocytes were collected from guinea pigs in these studies and exposed in vitro to doses of $CdCl_2$ ranging from 10^{-4} to 10^{-6} M in the media. The authors observed that ability of macrophages to migrate in an electric field was impaired and their capacity to react to MIF was decreased or abolished. These changes were attributed to Cd-induced membrane perturbation of macrophages and lymphocytes which resulted in decreased negative charges on cell surfaces as measured by altered cell electrophoretic mobility. A subsequent study revealed that murine macrophage-mediated cytotoxicity to sarcoma I tumor cells was inhibited following in vitro treatment with 10^{-5} or 10^{-6} M $CdCl_2$ (NELSON et al. 1982).

V. Other Immunologically Related Effects

Cd has been reported to inhibit the catabolism of light chains of antibody molecules, probably via a general inhibition of Zn-dependent aminopeptidases and carboxypeptidases. Antibody light chains are the major component of the proteinuria seen after chronic exposure to Cd (VIGLIANI 1969). Workers industrially exposed to Cd had up to 900 mg protein light chains in urine samples compared with a mean of 5 mg in controls. OHSAWA and KAWAI (1981) reported a cytologic shift in lymphocyte populations of Sprague-Dawley rats and ICR mice exposed to CdO 0.1 mg/m³ in the air for 4 weeks or injected subcutaneously with Cd doses of 2 mg/kg as $CdCl_2$ for 1–7 weeks. This effect consisted of a significant increase in large lymphocytes accompanied by a decrease in small lymphocytes. Splenomegaly was also observed in addition to anemia, neutropenia, and lymphopenia. Thymic atrophy and splenomegaly have also been observed in mice after single intraperitoneal injections of 1.8 mg/kg $CdCl_2$ (YAMADA et al. 1981).

It has also been reported that the formation of RNA, especially, and other phosphorylated intermediates are severely inhibited following in vitro exposure of murine (BALB/c) lymphocytes to Cd (GALLAGHER and GRAY 1982). Two recent studies using Sprague-Dawley rats that were either implanted with Cd wire

(Greenburg 1980) or orally exposed to 100 or 200 ppm $CdCl_2$ in drinking water for 30 weeks (Joshi et al. 1981) produced renal immune complex formation in these animals.

D. Summary

The effect of Cd exposure on immune responses of animals has been studied extensively over the past 10 years. Although results of these studies appear contradictory, in some instances, it is clear that exposure to Cd can alter certain immune responses. Host resistance to infectious agents or tumors may either be enhanced or suppressed, depending on the agent used and the strain or species of animal tested. Humoral immune responses appear to be enhanced or unaffected by low-dose acute exposure to Cd. Conversely, antibody production is usually suppressed in animals chronically exposed to moderate or high levels of Cd. CMI responses are not clearly altered by Cd treatment and have been shown to be either enhanced or depressed, depending on the parameter measured. A major toxic effect of Cd appears to be directed at macrophages. Various functions of macrophages are consistently suppressed following Cd treatment. This toxic effect of Cd could be significant to human and animal health, considering the central role of the macrophage in host defense reactions.

Part of the confusion surrounding the effects of Cd on immune responses stems from the myriad of variables between different studies, such as strain or species of animal, length and route of exposure, Cd formulation and dose, type of immunoassay, type, route, and dose of antigen, and the temporal relationship of antigenic challenge to quantitation of immune response. Additionally, in vitro effects of Cd on immune functions do not correlate well with in vivo exposures. As immunoassays are refined and standardized for immunotoxicologic/pharmacologic testing, the effects of Cd on overall immunocompetence will be clarified.

References

Balter N, Kaweki ME, Gingold B, Gray I (1982) Modification of skin-graft rejection and acceptance by low concentrations of cadmium in drinking water of mice. J Toxicol Environ Health 10:433–439

Berche P, Simonet M, Thevenin M, Fauchere JL, Prat JJ, Veron M (1980) Susceptibility of mice to bacterial infections after chronic exposure to cadmium. Ann Microbiol 131B:145–151

Bouley G, Chaumard C, Quero A-M, Girard F, Bouden E (1982) Opposite effects of inhaled cadmium microparticles on mouse susceptibility to an airborne bacterial and an airborne viral infection. Sci Total Environ 23:185–188

Bozelka BE, Burkholder PM (1979) Increased mortality of cadmium-intoxicated mice infected with the BCG strain of *Mycobacterium bovis*. J Reticuloendothel Soc 26:229–347

Bozelka BE, Burkholder PM, Chang LW (1978) Cadmium, a metallic inhibitor of antibody-mediated immunity in mice. Environ Res 17:390–402

Castranova V, Bowman L, Reason MJ, Miles PR (1980) Effects of heavy metal ions on selected oxidative metabolic processes in rat alveolar macrophages. Toxicol Appl Pharmacol 53:14–23

Cay BS (1981) The effect of cadmium on lymphocyte transformation. J Am Vet Med Assoc 36:143–147

Cook JA, Marconi EA, Diluzio NR (1974) Lead, cadmium, endotoxin interaction: effect on mortality and hepatic function. Toxicol Appl Pharmacol 28:292–302

Cook JA, Hoffman EO, Diluzio NR (1975) Influence of lead and cadmium on the susceptibility of rats to bacterial challenge. Proc Soc Exp Biol Med 150:741–747

Exon JH, Patton NM, Koller LD (1975) Hexamitiasis in cadmium exposed mice. Arch Environ Health 31:463–464

Exon JH, Koller LD, Kerkvliet NI (1979) Lead-cadmium interaction: effect on viral-induced mortality and tissue residues in mice. Arch Environ Health 34:469–475

Exon JH, Koller LD, Kerkvliet NI (1985) Tissue residues, pathology and viral-induced mortality in mice chronically exposed to different cadmium salts. J Environ Pathol Toxicol (in press)

Fujimaki H, Murakami M, Kubota K (1982) In vitro evaluation of cadmium-induced alteration of the antibody response. Toxicol Appl Pharmacol 62:288–293

Gainer JH (1977a) Effects of heavy metals and of deficiency of zinc on mortality rates in mice infected with encephalomyocarditis virus. Am J Vet Res 38:869–872

Gainer JH (1977b) Effects on interferon of heavy metal excess and zinc deficiency. Am J Vet Res 38:863–867

Gallagher KE, Gray I (1982) Cadmium inhibition on RNA metabolism in murine lymphocytes. J Immunopharmacol 3:339–361

Gallagher K, Mattarazzo WJ, Gray I (1979) Trace metal modification of immunocompetence: II. Effect of Pb^{2+}, Cd^{2+}, and Cr^{3+} on RNA turnover, hexokinase activity, and blastogenesis during B lymphocyte transformation in vitro. Clin Immun Immunopathol 13:369–377

Gaworski CL, Sharma RP (1978) The effects of heavy metals ^{3}H-thymidine uptake in lymphocytes. Toxicol Appl Pharmacol 46:305–313

Graham JA, Gardner DE, Water MD, Coffin DC (1975) Effect of trace metals on phagocytosis by alveolar macrophages. Infect Immun 11:1278–1283

Graham JA, Miller FJ, Daniel MJ, Payne EA, Gardner DE (1978) Influence of cadmium, nickel, and chromium on primary immunity in mice. Environ Res 16:77–87

Gray I, Arrieh M, Balter NJ (1982) Cadmium modification of the response in Balb/c mice to MOPC-104E tumor. Arch Environ Health 37:342–345

Greenberg SR (1980) Fluorescent studies on the potential existence of vascular metallic immune complexes. Arch Environ Health 35:148–151

Hadley JG, Gardner DE, Coffin DL, Menzel DB (1977) Inhibition of antibody-mediated rosette formation by alveolar macrophages: a sensitive assay for metal toxicity. J Reticuloendothel Soc 22:417–425

Hill CH (1979) Dietary influences on resistance to Salmonella infection in chicks. Fed Proc 38:2129–2133

Jones RH, Williams RL, Jones AM (1971) Effects of heavy metals on the immune response. Preliminary findings for cadmium in rats. Proc Soc Exp Biol Med 137:1231–1236

Joshi BC, Dwivedi C, Powell A, Holscher M (1981) Immune complex nephritis in rats induced by long term oral exposure to cadmium. J Comp Pathol 91:11–15

Kastelan M, Gerencer M, Kastelan A, Gamulin S (1981) Inhibition of mitogen and specific antigen-induced human proliferation by cadmium. Exp Cell Biol 49:15–19

Kerkvliet NI, Koller LD, Baecher LG, Brauner JA (1979) Effect of cadmium exposure on primary tumor growth and cell-mediated cytotoxicity in mice bearing MSB-6 sarcomas. J Natl Cancer Inst 63:479–485

Kiremidjian-Schumacher L, Stotzky G, Dickstein RA, Schwartz J (1981a) Influence of cadmium, lead, and zinc on the ability of guinea pig macrophages to interact with macrophage inhibitory factor. Environ Res 24:106–116

Kiremidjian-Schumacher L, Stotzky G, Likhite V, Schwartz J, Dickstein RA (1981b) Influence of cadmium, lead and zinc on the ability of sensitized guinea pig lymphocytes to interact with specific antigen and to produce lymphokines. Environ Res 24:96–105

Knutson DW, Vredevoe DL, Aoki KR, Havs EJ, Levy L (1980) Cadmium and the reticuloendothelial system (RES): a specific defect in blood clearance of soluble aggregates of IgG by the liver in mice given cadmium. Immunology 40:17–26

Kojima A, Tamuar SI (1981) Acute effects of cadmium on delayed-type hypersensitivity in mice. Jpn J Med Sci Biol 34:281–291

Koller LD (1973) Immunosuppression produced by lead, cadmium and mercury. Am J Vet Res 34:1457–1458

Koller LD, Brauner JA (1977) Decreased B cell response after exposure to lead and cadmium. Toxicol Appl Pharmacol 42:621–624

Koller LD, Roan JG (1977) Effects of lead and cadmium on mouse peritoneal macrophages. J Reticuloendothel Soc 21:7–12

Koller LD, Roan JG (1980a) Effects of lead, cadmium and methylmercury on immunological memory. J Environ Pathol Toxicol 4:47–52

Koller LD, Roan JG (1980b) Response of lymphocytes from lead, cadmium and methylmercury-exposed mice in the mixed lymphocyte culture. J Environ Pathol Toxicol 4:393–398

Koller LD, Exon JH, Roan JG (1975) Antibody suppression by cadmium. Arch Environ Health 30:598–601

Koller LD, Roan JG, Exon JH (1976) Humoral antibody response in mice after exposure to lead or cadmium. Proc Soc Exp Biol Med 151:339–342

Koller LD, Roan JG, Kerkvliet NI (1979) Mitogen stimulation of lymphocytes in CBA mice exposed to lead and cadmium. Environ Res 19:177–188

Lawrence DA (1981) Heavy metal modulation of lymphocyte activities. I. In vitro effects of heavy metals on primary humoral immune responses. Toxicol Appl Pharmacol 57:439–451

Loose LD, Silkworth JB, Warrington D (1977) Cadmium-induced depression of the respiratory burst in mouse pulmonary alveolar macrophages, peritoneal macrophages and polymorphonuclear neutrophils. Biochem Biophys Res Commun 79:326–332

Loose LD, Silkworth JB, Simpson DW (1978a) Influence of cadmium on the phagocytic and microbial activity of murine peritoneal macrophages, pulmonary alveolar macrophages, and polymorphonuclear neutrophils. Infect Immun 22:378–381

Loose LD, Silkworth JB, Warrington D (1978b) Cadmium-induced phagocyte cytotoxicity. Bull Environ Contam Toxicol 20:582–588

Muller S, Gillert K-E, Krause CH, Jautzke G, Gross U, Diamantstein T (1978) Effects of cadmium on the immune system of mice. Experentia 35:909–910

Nelson DJ, Kiremidjian-Schumacher L, Stotzky G (1982) Effects of cadmium, lead and zinc on macrophage-mediated cytotoxicity toward tumor cells. Environ Res 28:154–163

Ohsawa M, Kawai K (1981) Cytological shift in lymphocytes induced by cadmium in mice and rats. Environ Res 24:192–200

Shenker BJ, Matarazzo WJ, Hirsch RL, Gray I (1977) Trace metal modification of immunocompetence. I. Effect of trace metals in the cultures on in vitro transformation of B lymphocytes. Cell Immunol 34:19–24

Suzuki M, Simizu B, Yabe S, Oya A, Seta H (1981) Effect of Japanese encephalitis virus infection in mice. I. Acute and single dose exposure experiments. Toxicol Lett 9:231–235

Vigliani EC (1969) The biopathology of cadmium. J Am Ind Hyg Assoc 30:329

Yamada YK, Shimizu F, Kawamure R, Kubota K (1981) Thymic atrophy in mice induced by cadmium administration. Toxicol Lett 8:49–55

CHAPTER 10

The Effect of Dietary Selenium on Cadmium Cardiotoxicity

I. S. JAMALL and J. C. SMITH

A. Introduction

Research over the last decade or so has demonstrated that chronic exposure of laboratory animals to cadmium (Cd), at levels compatible with current environmental exposures, primarily via food, results in cardiotoxicity. Furthermore, the adverse effects of Cd on the heart occur in the absence of concomitant damage to the kidney. The relevance of elucidating the biochemical mechanism of Cd cardiotoxicity is underscored by the realization that the current acceptable daily intake (ADI) for Cd of approximately 70 µg/day is based on a critical concentration of 200 µg Cd per gram tissue (wet weight) in the renal cortex. If, as the data in this chapter suggest, the heart is vulnerable to Cd concentrations which are orders of magnitude lower than those in the kidneys and, if these low heart Cd levels are associated with injury in the absence of renal toxicity, then the while question of the ADI needs to be reevaluated in the light of these findings. Of course, Cd cardiotoxicity would first have to be established in exposed human populations.

In this chapter, we will confine ourselves to a critique of the literature on the cardiotoxic effects of Cd and the roles played by the essential trace elements, selenium (Se) and copper (Cu) in preventing Cd cardiotoxicity at the biochemical level. The cardiovascular effects of Cd are discussed in Chap. 7.

B. Cadmium and the Heart

The continuing debate over the occurrence and clinical relevance of Cd-induced hypertension has focused attention away from a growing body of evidence which suggests that Cd may exert a direct effect on the heart (PRODAN 1932; WILSON et al. 1941; DOTTA and FRUSCELLA 1963; KANISAWA and SCHROEDER 1969; STOWE et al. 1972; VOORS et al. 1973, 1979; AMACHER and EWING 1975; KOPP and HAWLEY 1978; KOPP et al. 1978a, b, 1980, 1982, 1983; KOPP and BARANY 1980; VOROBIEVA and EREMEEVA 1980). However, with only one exception, no evidence has been published to date on an increased incidence of cardiovascular disease (CVD) either in itai-itai patients exposed to high levels of Cd through environmental contamination of their food or in workers occupationally exposed to Cd (LAUWERYS 1979). VOROBIEVA and EREMEEVA (1980) reported a fourfold higher incidence of CVD among Cd-exposed workers in the Soviet Union compared with industrial workers not exposed to Cd.

Probably the most intriguing aspect of the recent research on the cardiotoxicity of Cd, and one that bears directly on the public health concern about environmental Cd exposures, is the relatively low levels of heart Cd concentrations that have been associated with cardiotoxicity in rats (KOPP et al. 1982, 1983; JAMALL and SMITH 1985 a). Both these groups reported observing cardiotoxicity in rats whose hearts contained approximately 5 ppm Cd (KOPP et al. 1982; JAMALL and SMITH 1985 a).

Could it be that rats are especially sensitive to the toxic effects of Cd on the heart or, perhaps, that the cardiotoxic effects of Cd in humans exposed to this metal have been overlooked, given the clinically more obvious effects on the kidneys?

C. Selenium Deficiency and Cardiomyopathy

Se is an essential trace element. Se deficiency has been shown to result in a wide spectrum of pathologic conditions in animals, including cardiomyopathy in rats, sheep, swine, and monkeys (GODWIN 1965; GODWIN and FRASER 1966; MUTH et al. 1971). Most of these conditions are characterized by, or associated with, the peroxidation of membrane polyunsaturated fatty acids. This discovery that Se is an integral part of glutathione peroxidase (GSH-Px), an enzyme responsible for the catalytic reduction of hydrogen peroxide (H_2O_2) and, possibly, toxic lipid hydroperoxides, provided a biochemical basis for the protective role of Se in ameliorating or preventing peroxidative tissue damage (ROTRUCK et al. 1973). The importance of Se in maintaining normal cardiac function in humans has been dramatically illustrated by the reports of Keshan disease, a cardiomyopathy endemic to certain regions of the People's Republic of China. Se supplementation of the "at risk" population, at levels of 0.5–1.0 mg sodium selenite per week, markedly reduced the incidence of this often fatal condition from 1.32 per 1,000 population in 1974 to 0.32 per 1,000 population in 1977 with no new cases being reported in the treated population since 1977 (CHEN et al. 1980). Cardiomyopathy associated with Se deficiency has also been reported in the United States (COLLIPP and CHEN 1981; JOHNSON et al. 1981; FLEMING et al. 1982).

Studies in animals and humans have established the importance of Se in maintaining normal cardiac function. However, the optimum levels of dietary Se for maintaining normal cardiac function have not been established. Furthermore, alterations in the optimum Se requirement in individuals exposed to toxic metals, such as Cd, known to interact with Se, are poorly understood.

D. Cadmium–Selenium Interactions

The study of the interactions between Cd and Se have been largely confined to acute studies with both agents being administered parenterally (KAR et al. 1960; PARIZEK et al. 1971). The mechanism of this interaction in plasma and red blood cells has been shown to involve the metabolism of Se, as sodium selenite (Na_2SeO_3) to selenide (Se^{2-}) by erythrocytes. This selenide (Se^{2-}) then complexes with Cd^{2+} and is associated with proteins of specific molecular weights.

The Cd in these Cd–Se–protein complexes is believed to be biologically inactive (GASIEWICZ and SMITH 1976, 1978 a, b, c).

Recently, MEYER et al. (1982) reported increases in specific heart weight (heart weight per 100 g body weight) in rats fed a basal low-Se diet or this diet supplemented with 0, 0.1, or 1.0 ppm Se and containing 0, 30, or 60 ppm Cd. The cardiomegaly observed at the end of the 30-day experimental period was most pronounced in rats fed the basal low-Se diet containing 60 ppm Cd and was minimal in rats fed this same level of Cd, but where the basal diet was supplemented with 0.1 or 1.0 ppm Se. No biochemical parameters were reported by these authors for the heart. MEYER et al. (1982) concluded that, since the dietary Se was able to protect against the Cd-induced anemia, this could explain the protective effects of Se, in agreement with a hypothesis put forward much earlier by WILSON et al. (1941).

Some epidemiologic studies have shown correlations between mortality from CVD and the ratios of Cd:Se and Cd:Se, Zn in the renal cortex. A significant positive correlation was found between CVD and high Cd:Se values (VOORS et al. 1979). In a study on the incidence of CVD in 25 countries, it was found that a positive correlation existed between the incidence of ischemic heart disease and dietary Cd intake while an inverse correlation was found between Se intake and ischemic heart disease (SHAMBERGER et al. 1975, 1976; SHAMBERGER 1983). The significance of these epidemiologic studies is unclear given the wide variations in Se content of foods grown in geographically different regions; nor does the bulk of our food come from a specific region which may be low in Se. Furthermore, correlations between Se concentrations in various indicator media (hair, blood, tissue, etc.) have not been firmly established, further complicating the interpretation of the epidemiologic studies of Cd–Se interactions and CVD.

E. Cadmium–Copper Interactions

Cd has been shown to affect the metabolism of the essential trace metal, Cu, and Cu supplements have been shown to protect against some of the toxic effects of Cd (BREMNER and CAMPBELL 1980). Recently, MINAMI et al. (1982) reported significant reductions in the activity of superoxide dismutase (SOD) in erythrocytes and lung lavage fluid taken from rats exposed to Cd fumes. SOD is responsible for the catalytic dismutation of the highly reactive and potentially toxic superoxide radical anion (O_2^-) to H_2O_2 (FRIDOVICH 1975). AMORUSO et al. (1982) demonstrated an enhancement of O_2^- production by human phagocytes exposed to Cd in vitro, thereby further implicating the involvement of this radical anion in Cd toxicity.

The interaction between Cd and Cu in the heart has not been investigated in biochemical terms, even though Cu deficiency per se, has been shown to affect the heart adversely (KLEVAY and VIESTENZ 1981) and Cd–Cu interactions have been studied in general terms (BREMNER and CAMPBELL 1980). Furthermore, the importance of the Cu-containing SOD in preventing Cd-induced peroxidative injury remains to be elucidated.

F. Cadmium–Metallothionein Studies

In the case of acute Cd toxicity, it is believed that Cd bound to metallothionein (MT), a low molecular weight cytosolic protein, is biologically inert. A corollary of this is that Cd toxicity occurs as a result of "free" or non-protein-bound Cd. In chronic Cd toxicity, the binding of Cd to MT facilitates its mobilization from tissues and reabsorption by the renal tubules, with gradual accumulation in the kidney. Chronic Cd toxicity therefore may result from the disruption of cellular activity owing to the sheer bulk of CdMT which accumulates in the kidney cytosol (Webb 1979). Support for a major role of CdMT in mediating Cd toxicity has come from studies on the intracellular distribution of Cd following its acute parenteral administration to laboratory animals. In these studies, much of the Cd in the cytosol of liver and kidney (between 70% and 90%) is bound to MT (Webb 1979). However, studies using chronic dietary Cd administration to rats fed a defined diet showed that less than 40% of total cytosolic Cd in kidney and liver was recovered bound to MT (Jamall and Smith 1985c). Heart CdMT was not investigated. These studies call into question the significance of MT as a detoxification mechanism in chronic Cd toxicity. No CdMT has been detected in the heart of rats following the acute administration of the metal (Chen and Ganther 1975). Also, no CdMT was detected in the heart of a human chronically exposed to Cd (Sato and Takizawa 1982).

There is very little information in the literature on the amount of CdMT in the heart and its significance when Cd is administered chronically at subtoxic levels. It is also not known if essential trace elements such as Se and Cu, known to offer protection against acute Cd toxicity, influence the binding of Cd to MT in situations involving chronic exposure to the toxic metal.

G. Investigations into the Mechanism of Cadmium Cardiotoxicity

I. The Idea

In the light of the known interactions between Cd and Se in acute toxicity studies, we decided to investigate the possibility that similar interactions between Cd and Se, under non-acute exposure conditions might result in a Se deficiency state. Such a deficiency of Se would be manifested as a decrease in the activity of the selenoenzyme, GSH-Px. Since GSH-Px is responsible for the catalytic detoxification of H_2O_2 and, possibly, toxic lipid hydroperoxides, the reduced activity of this enzyme in the heart would result in peroxidative injury in this organ. Furthermore, since Cd had been shown to result in increased O_2^- production in vitro and, since cytosolic SOD had been implicated in preventing oxidative tissue damage, we decided also to investigate the role played by SOD in Cd cardiotoxicity.

II. The Experiment

A three-pronged approach comprising biochemical, histopathologic, and functional parameters was taken to elucidate the mechanism of Cd cardiotoxicity.

Male, weanling Sprague-Dawley rats were randomly assigned to the various treatment groups. All animals were individually housed and were fed a basal low-Se, low-vitamin E diet or this diet supplemented with different levels of Se. The basal diet contained less than 30 ppb Se by analysis. The levels of other essential trace elements were also rigidly controlled (JAMALL and SMITH 1985a). Rats treated with Cd received 200 ppm Cd in their diet plus an additional 5 mg Cd (as $CdCl_2$) via osmotic minipumps (Alzet 2001) implanted subcutaneously on day 28 of the study and left in place for the remainder of the study. All animals were necropsied on day 56 of the experiment. The animals were pair-fed and had free access to deionized water.

The data in Tables 1 and 2 confirm that Cd treatment results in cardiotoxicity as demonstrated by increases in specific heart weight (Table 1) and histopathologic alterations (Table 2) in the rat. The assumption underlying this study was that this might be due to the production of a Se-deficient state as a result of the Cd treatment. Thus, rats rendered Se deficient by restriction of dietary Se intake would be expected to be particularly sensitive to the cardiotoxic effects of Cd. The data in Tables 1 and 2 show that Se deficiency per se causes cardiomegaly and histopathology and that this is accompanied by a marked reduction in the activity of the selenoenzyme, GSH-Px. This decrease in heart GSH-Px activity is associated with a significant increase in lipid peroxidation, measured as thiobarbituric acid-(TBA)-reactive substances (Table 1).

Table 1. Effect of cadmium administration on various heart parameters in rats fed different levels of selenium for 7 weeks

Dietary selenium (ppm)		0	0.1	1.0
Specific heart weight (heart weight/ 100 g body weight)	−Cd	0.349 ± 0.029^a	0.347 ± 0.015^b	0.356 ± 0.018^c
	+Cd	0.539 ± 0.094^a	0.460 ± 0.037^b	0.505 ± 0.068^c
Glutathione peroxidase (heart weight/ 100 g body weight)	−Cd	12 ± 1.6^a	92 ± 6.0^b	198 ± 45
	+Cd	9.3 ± 0.67^a	43 ± 11^b	165 ± 31
Lipid peroxidation (TBA-reactive, substances)^d	−Cd	0.131 ± 0.012^a	0.095 ± 0.008^b	0.117 ± 0.024
	+Cd	0.190 ± 0.028^a	0.148 ± 0.127^b	0.125 ± 0.011
Heart copper levels (µg Cu/g tissue dry weight)	−Cd	4.29 ± 0.459^a	4.85 ± 0.380^b	5.17 ± 0.819^c
	+Cd	2.14 ± 0.253^a	3.79 ± 0.993^b	2.58 ± 0.493^c
Superoxide dismutase (units/mg protein)	−Cd	18.5 ± 2.30^a	14.9 ± 2.24^b	15.9 ± 3.79^c
	+Cd	8.72 ± 1.43^a	10.5 ± 0.700^b	6.65 ± 0.663^c
Heart cadmium levels (µg Cu/g tissue dry weight)	−Cd	ND	ND	ND
	+Cd	3.88 ± 1.98	4.88 ± 1.86	2.40 ± 0.535

$^{a-c}$ All values are reported as the mean $\pm$ standard deviation of 5–6 rats per group. Groups having identical superscripts are significantly different from one another at $P < 0.05$ (one-way analysis of variance)
^{d} Thiobarbituric acid-reactive substances expressed as $A532 \times 10^3/20$ mg tissue

Table 2. Effect of cadmium administration on myocardial alterations in rats fed different levels of selenium for 7 weeks

Treatment		Pathology				
		N	O	+	++	+++
0 ppm Se	−Cd	5	0	3	2	0
0 ppm Se	+Cd	6	0	2	1	3
0.1 ppm Se	−Cd	6	3	3	0	0
0.1 ppm Se	+Cd	5	1	2	3	0
1.0 ppm Se	−Cd	5	1	3	1	0
1.0 ppm Se	+Cd	5	1	3	1	0

Rats fed the basal, low-Se diet and treated with Cd showed severe and extensive histopathologic changes relative to rats fed the same basal diet, but which received no Cd (Table 2). The Cd-treated rats also exhibited significantly elevated specific heart weights and TBA-reactive substances with lower heart GSH-Px activities (Table 1). The same effects are seen in rats fed the diet supplemented with 0.1 ppm Se plus Cd (Tables 1 and 2). These data support our initial hypothesis that Cd cardiotoxicity results in the production of a Se deficiency state characterized by increased lipid peroxidation and significant reductions in the activity of the selenoenzyme, GSH-Px.

However, the mechanism of Cd cardiotoxicity cannot be explained entirely by the "Se deficiency" theory. As can be seen from Table 1, Cd treatment also caused marked reductions in heart Cu levels and, as a consequence, reductions in the activity of the cytosolic, Cu-containing enzyme, SOD. This enzyme brings about the catalytic dismutation of the potentially toxic superoxide radical anion O_2^- to H_2O_2 and has been implicated in preventing oxidative tissue injury. It should be borne in mind that although O_2^- may be capable of causing tissue damage, the end product of the dismutation reaction, catalyzed by SOD, is H_2O_2 which, in the absence of adequate levels of GSH-Px can react with Fe^{2+} or with O_2^- and, perhaps other free radicals, to produce the potent hydroxyl free radical (OH$\cdot$), capable of initiating peroxidative tissue injury (FONG et al. 1973). Since our data show the reduction of both SOD and GSH-Px activities in the heart of Cd-treated rats (Table 1), we cannot at this point exclude either one from being relevant to the mechanism of Cd cardiotoxicity. This does not, in any way, detract from our essential finding, namely that Cd cardiotoxicity does, in fact, involve lipid peroxidation. And, what is especially striking is that the Cd-induced peroxidative injury was observed at heart Cd levels of approximately 5 ppm, on a dry weight basis (Table 1). KOPP et al. (1982) showed that heart Cd concentrations of about 5 ppm also caused cardiotoxicity in rats fed as little as 5 ppm Cd in the diet for approximately 18 months. It should be emphasized that, although both these groups (KOPP et al. 1982; JAMALL and SMITH 1985a) were able to demonstrate cardiotoxicity in rats containing about 5 ppm Cd in the heart, the data presented in Table 1 suggest that the absolute heart Cd concentration may be less relevant to cardiotoxicity than the concentration of this toxic metal relative to concentrations of Se and Cu.

Cd treatment of rats fed the basal diet supplemented with 1.0 ppm Se resulted in no significant reduction in the activity of GSH-Px nor was there any increase in TBA-reactive substances (Table 1). However, Cd treatment did bring about significant reductions in heart Cu levels and SOD activity (Table 1). The fact that Cd treatment in rats fed the high dietary Se (1.0 ppm Se) did not cause any increase in lipid peroxidation, even though there was a 50% reduction in SOD activity, supports our assumption (see earlier discussion) that GSH-Px may be more critical in preventing peroxidative tissue injury, since it is essential for detoxifying the H_2O_2 produced by the dismutation of O_2^- by SOD.

Cd treatment did, however, cause an increase in specific heart weight in rats fed the 1.0 ppm Se diet compared with rats fed the same level of Se, but which received no Cd treatment (Table 1). Histopathologic studies of the hearts from these animals show that 1.0 ppm Se caused cardiotoxicity when compared with rats fed 0.1 ppm Se without Cd. Cd treatment of rats fed the 1.0 ppm Se diet caused no further pathologic alterations (Table 2). Thus, the increase in specific heart weight with Cd treatment in the high dietary Se group (Table 1) appears inexplicable. In the studies described, vitamin E did not affect any of the parameters examined (data not shown). Also, the heart of the rats had no detectable Se-independent GSH-Px activity, in agreement with an earlier report (LAWRENCE and BURK 1978).

H. Physiologic Studies

In order to assess the functional significance of the observed Cd–Se interactions at the biochemical level, a study was conducted in 15 rats divided into three groups of 5 rats each. The groups consisted of animals fed the basal, low-Se diet with and without Cd treatment, the basal diet supplemented with 0.1–0.3 ppm Se without Cd treatment (controls), or this Se-supplemented diet with Cd treatment. The Cd dose employed was identical to that described for the biochemical studies described in Sect. G. All animals were necropsied during the 9th week of the experiment and the contractile force of isolated ventricular muscle strips studied as described (GRUPP et al. 1983). The basal contractile force was markedly diminished in Se-deficient rats with or without Cd treatment relative to the controls. A similar reduction in basal contractile force was also observed in muscle strips taken from Se-supplemented rats treated with Cd in comparison with the control group. Thus, Cd cardiotoxicity (defined here as a decrease in contractile force) clearly results from Se deficiency in the heart. In an effort to characterize the observed reductions in contractile force in myocardial strips from Se-deficient or Se-supplemented rats treated with Cd, the muscle strips were exposed in vitro to various concentrations of ouabain and a cumulative dose–response curve constructed. At the highest ouabain dose used (1.6×10^{-4} M), all three groups showed similar contractile force values. Since ouabain, an agent known to increase calcium delivery to the myocardial cell, is able to correct the functional alterations seen in Se-deficient or Se-supplemented hearts treated with Cd, it would appear that neither of these treatments, Se deficiency or Cd treatment, damages the contractile apparatus, but rather interferes with calcium delivery to it (GRUPP et al. 1983). It should be noted that in histopathologic studies of the heart from Se-deficient farm animals, a white subendocardial band shown by the von Kossa stain to consist of calcium has been reported. However, no attempt was made to describe the significance of this interaction between Se and calcium (CHEEMA and GILANI 1978).

The functional studies described are consistent with our biochemical and histopathologic findings that Cd cardiotoxicity involves the production of a Se-deficient state with consequent peroxidative tissue injury. What remains to be worked out is the precise quantitative relationships between heart Cd concentrations, GSH-Px and SOD activities, and the time course of the morphological and functional derangements observed (JAMALL and SMITH 1985a; GRUPP et al. 1983).

J. Conclusions

The data presented demonstrate that Cd cardiotoxicity is mediated via lipid peroxidation, secondary to conditioned deficiencies of Se and Cu, reflected by the significant reduction in the activities of the selenoenzyme, GSH-Px and the Cu-containing enzyme, SOD. The preliminary nature of the data and the design of the experiments do not allow for the evaluation of the quantitative roles of GSH-Px and SOD in Cd-induced peroxidative injury to the heart. It should be noted, however, that while the O_2^- species is extremely reactive and quite capable of initiating peroxidative tissue injury, the end product of the dismutation reaction catalyzed by SOD is H_2O_2 which can be detoxified effectively only by the selenoenzyme, GSH-Px. Thus, as far as protection against lipid peroxidation is concerned, a reduction of SOD activity may not be so serious as a reduction in GSH-Px activity while the simultaneous reduction in the activity of both these enzymes in a metabolically active organ, such as the heart, would have dire consequences as is evidenced by the data.

A most significant aspect of our findings is that the Cd-induced injury was observed at heart tissue Cd concentrations of approximately 5 ppm, in agreement with the findings of KOPP et al. (1980, 1982). Furthermore, the cardiotoxic effects of Cd were observed in rats without concomitant injury to the kidney, even though the Cd concentrations in the kidney were about 300-fold greater than those in the heart (KOPP et al. 1980, 1982). In our studies, we observed no lipid peroxidation in the kidney or liver of Cd-treated rats showing peroxidative injury of the heart, this in spite of the fact that the Cd concentrations in the kidney and liver were approximately two orders of magnitude greater than Cd concentrations in the heart (JAMALL and SMITH 1985a, b). A possible explanation for the greater susceptibility of the heart to Cd-induced peroxidative injury may be the relative absence of MT and the Se-independent GSH-Px activity relative to the liver and kidney (CHEN and GANTHER 1975; JAMALL and SMITH 1985a–c).

Acknowledgements. Experimental work described in this chapter was carried out in the Department of Environmental Health, University of Cincinnati, Cincinnati, Ohio and supported by Center Grant ES-00159 from NIEHS and a grant from the Selenium-Tellurium Development Association.

References

Amacher DE, Ewing KL (1975) Cadmium deposition in canine heart and major arteries following intravascular administration of cadmium chloride. Bull Environ Contam Toxicol 14:457–464

Amoruso MA, Witz G, Goldstein BD (1982) Enhancement of rat and human phagocyte superoxide anion radical production by cadmium in vitro. Toxicol Lett 10:133–138

Bremner I, Campbell JK (1980) The influence of dietary copper intake of the toxicity of cadmium. Ann NY Acad Sci 355:319–332

Cheema AH, Gilani SH (1978) Cardiac myopathies in neonatal lambs: histological and histochemical studies. Biol Neonat 34:84–91

Chen RW, Ganther HE (1975) Relative cadmium-binding capacity of metallothionein and other cytosolic fractions in various tissues of the rat. Environ Physiol Biochem 5:378–388

Chen X, Yang G, Chen X, Chen X, Wen Z, Ge K (1980) Studies on the relations of selenium and Keshan disease. Biol Trace Element Res 2:91–107

Collipp PJ, Chen SY (1981) Cardiomyopathy and selenium deficiency in a two year old girl. N Engl J Med 304:1304–1305

Dotta F, Fruscella R (1963) Le alterazioni miocardiche da intossicazione sperimentale da cadmio: Reperti istologici cardiopulmonari, reperti elletrocardiografici. Rassegna di Medicina Industriale e di Igiene del Lavoro 32:559–567

Fleming CR, McCall JT, O'Brien JF, Forsman RW, Lie JT, Petz J (1982) Selenium deficiency in long-term parenteral nutrition: a potentially fatal complication? Society for Environmental Geochemistry and Health. First Annual Scientific Meeting Greenville, NC October 31, 1982

Fong KL, McCay PP, Poyer JL (1973) Evidence that peroxidation of lysosomal membranes is initiated by hydroxyl free radicals produced during flavin enzyme activity. J Biol Chem 248:7792–7797

Fridovich I (1975) Superoxide dismutases. Ann Rev Biochem 44:147–159

Gasiewicz TA, Smith JC (1976) Interactions of cadmium and selenium in rat plasma in vivo and in vitro. Biochem Biophys Acta 428:113–122

Gasiewicz TA, Smith JC (1978 a) The metabolism of selenite by intact rat erythrocytes in vitro. Chem Biol Interact 21:299–313

Gasiewicz TA, Smith JC (1978 b) Properties of the cadmium and selenium complex formed in rat plasma in vivo and in vitro. Chem Biol Interact 23:161–183

Gasiewicz TA, Smith JC (1978 c) Interaction between cadmium and selenium in rat plasma. Environ Health Perspect 25:133–136

Godwin KO (1965) Abnormal electrocardiograms in rats fed a low-selenium diet. Q J Exp Physiol 50:282–288

Godwin KO, Fraser FJ (1966) Abnormal electrocardiograms, blood pressure changes and some aspects of the histopathology of selenium deficiency in lambs. Q J Exp Physiol 51:94–102

Grupp IL, Jamall IS, Millard RW, Grupp G (1983) Effects of selenium deficiency and selenium and cadmium supplementation on myocardial contractile force and ouabain sensitivity of the rat heart. IRCS Med Sci (Pharmacol) 11:22–23

Jamall IS, Smith JC (1985 a) Effects of cadmium on glutathione peroxidase, superoxide dismutase and lipid peroxidation in the rat heart: A possible mechanism of cadmium cardiotoxicity. Tox Appl Pharmacol 80:33–42

Jamall IS, Smith JC (1985 b) Effect of cadmium treatment on the activities of the selenium-dependent and selenium-independent glutathione peroxidases and lipid peroxidation in the kidney and liver of rats fed different levels of selenium. Arch Toxicol (in press)

Jamall IS, Smith JC (1985 c) The effects of dietary selenium on cadmium binding in rat kidney and liver. Arch Toxicol 56:252–255

Johnson RA, Baker SS, Fallon JT, Maynard EP, Ruskin JN, Wen Z, Ge K, Cohen HJ (1981) An occidental case of cardiomyopathy and selenium deficiency. N Engl J Med 304:1210–1212

Kanisawa M, Schroeder HA (1969) Renal arteriolar changes in hypertensive rats given cadmium in drinking water. Exp Mol Pathol 10:81–98

Kar AB, Das RP, Mukerji FN (1960) Prevention of cadmium-induced changes in the gonads of rats by zinc and selenium. Proc Natl Inst Sci (India) 26B:40–50

Klevay LM, Viestenz KE (1981) Abnormal electrocardiograms in rats deficient in copper. Am J Physiol 240:H185–H189

Kopp SJ, Barany M (1980) Influence of isoproterenol and calcium on cadmium or lead-induced negative inotropy related to cardiac myofibrillar protein phosphorylations in perfused rat heart. Toxicol Appl Pharmacol 55:8–17

Kopp SJ, Hawley PL (1978) Cadmium feeding: apparent depression of atrioventricular-His-Purkinje conduction system. Acta Pharmacol Toxicol 42:110–116

Kopp SJ, Fischer VW, Erlanger M, Perry EF, Perry HM (1978a) Electrocardiographical, biochemical and morphological effects of chronic low level cadmium feeding on the rat heart. Proc Soc Exp Biol Med 159:339–345

Kopp SJ, Baker JC, D'Agrosa LA, Hawley PL (1978b) Simultaneous recording of His bundle electrogram, electrocardiogram and systolic tension from intact modified Langendorff rat heart preparations I. Effects of perfusion time, cadmium and lead. Toxicol Appl Pharmacol 55:8–17

Kopp SJ, Perry HM, Glonek T, Erlanger M, Perry EF, Barany M, D'Agrosa L (1980) Cardiac physiologic-metabolic changes after chronic low-level heavy metal feeding. Am J Physiol 239:H22–H30

Kopp SJ, Glonek T, Perry HM, Erlanger M, Perry EF (1982) Cardiovascular actions of cadmium at environmental exposure levels. Science 217:837–839

Kopp SJ, Perry HM, Perry EF, Erlanger M (1983) Cardiac physiologic and tissue metabolic changes following chronic low level cadmium and cadmium plus lead ingestion in the rat. Toxicol Appl Pharmacol 69:149–160

Lauwerys R (1979) Cadmium in man. In: Webb M (ed) The chemistry, biochemistry and biology of cadmium. Elsevier/North-Holland Biomedical, Amsterdam, pp 433–455

Lawrence RA, Burk RF (1978) Species, tissue and subcellular distribution of non Se-dependent glutathione peroxidase activity. J Nutr 108:211–215

Meyer SA, House WA, Welch RM (1982) Some metabolic interrelationships between toxic levels of cadmium and nontoxic levels of selenium fed to rats. J Nutr 112:954–961

Minami M, Koshi K, Homma K, Suzuki Y (1982) Changes in the activity of superoxide dismutase after exposure to the fumes of heavy metals and the significance of zinc in the tissue. Arch Toxicol 49:215–225

Muth OH, Weswig PH, Whanger PD, Oldfield JE (1971) Effect of feeding selenium-deficient ration to the sub-human primate (Saimiri sciureus). Am J Vet Res 22:1603–1605

Parizek J, Ostadalova I, Kalouskova J, Benes I (1971) The detoxifying effects of selenium: interrelations between compounds of selenium and certain metals. In: Mertz WA, Cornatzer WE (eds) Newer trace elements in nutrition. Dekker, New York, pp 85–122

Prodan L (1932) Cadmium poisoning II. Experimental cadmium poisoning. J Ind Hyg Toxicol 14:174–196

Rotruck JT, Pope AL, Ganther HE, Swanson AB, Hafeman DG, Hoekstra WG (1973) Selenium: biochemical role as a component of glutathione peroxidase. Science 179:588–590

Sato M, Takizawa Y (1982) Cadmium binding proteins in human organs. Toxicol Lett 11:269–273

Shamberger RJ (1983) Biochemistry of selenium. Plenum, New York

Shamberger RJ, Tytko SA, Willis CE (1975) Selenium and heart disease. In: Hemphill DD (ed) Trace substances in environmental health, vol IX. University of Missouri Press, Columbia, Missouri, pp 15–22

Shamberger RJ, Gunsch MS, Willis CE, McCormack LJ (1976) Selenium and heart disease. II Selenium and other trace metal intakes and heart disease in 25 countries. In: Hemphill DD (ed) Trace substances in environmental health, vol X. University of Missouri Press, Columbia, Missouri, pp 48–52

Stowe HD, Wilson M, Goyer RA (1972) Clinical and morphological effects of oral cadmium toxicity in rabbits. Arch Pathol 94:389–405

Voors AW, Shuman MS, Gallagher PN (1973) Zinc and cadmium autopsy levels for cardiovascular disease in geographical context. In: Hemphill DD (ed) Trace substances in environmental health, vol VI. University of Missouri Press, Columbia, Missouri, pp 215–222

Voors AW, Johnson WD, Shuman MS, Blotcky AJ (1979) Adjusted cadmium levels in the renal cortex and heart weight at autopsy. In: Hemphill DD (ed) Trace substances in environmental health, vol XII. University of Missouri Press, Columbia, Missouri, pp 185–190

Vorobieva RS, Eremeeva EP (1980) Cardiovascular function in workers exposed to cadmium. Gig Sanit 10:22–25

Webb M (1979) The metallothioneins. In: Webb M (ed) The chemistry, biochemistry and biology of cadmium. Elsevier/North-Holland Biomedical, Amsterdam, pp 195–266

Wilson RH, Deeds F, Cox A (1941) Effects of continued cadmium feeding. J Pharmacol Exp Therap 71:222–235

CHAPTER 11

Cellular Resistance to Cadmium

M. D. Enger, C. E. Hildebrand, J. Seagrave, and R. A. Tobey

A. Introduction

This chapter focuses on the application of cultured cell systems to the study of cellular responses associated with exposure to Cd^{2+}. The scope of this review is limited to considerations of cellular metabolism of Cd^{2+} and the physiologic and genetic factors that modulate cadmium toxicity. Major emphasis is directed toward three areas: (a) the isolation or derivation of cells differing in Cd^{2+} cytotoxic response and utilization of such cells to define factors that play a role in cadmium resistance; (b) a consideration of the manifold environmental/physiologic conditions that affect cellular responses in culture; and (c) an evaluation of studies employing somatic cell and molecular genetic techniques to dissect in detail the molecular components of the response mechanisms. The chapter concludes with a discussion of directions and approaches to be pursued in the future to fill gaps in our current understanding of Cd^{2+} metabolism.

B. Cultured Cell Systems for Studying Cd Metabolism

Cultured cells offer significant advantages for studying certain aspects of Cd^{2+} metabolism. The experimenter can work with a homogeneous population free of complicating tissue, organ, and system responses, allowing one to focus on factors and mechanisms at the *cellular* level of response. Additives to the culture medium (e.g., metabolic precursors, inducers, inhibitors, effectors) may be precisely delivered and quantitated and the cells may be readily synchronized and shunted between proliferating and nonproliferating states under conditions of total cell accountability.

Variant cells may be isolated and produced in which important molecular components of Cd^{2+} metabolism have been altered (enhanced, lost, or modified). Such cells are employed to delineate protective mechanisms against cadmium toxicity and to examine modification of Cd^{2+} metabolism by other metals or by biochemical effectors such as hormones. Studies with these variant cells pave the way for both isolation of the genes involved in metal responses and determination of the mechanisms regulating their expression, and also suggest means for modulating their expression.

Once biochemical information is generated in a cultured cell system, attempts then may be made to ascertain whether comparable mechanisms also are operative in more complex entities such as intact animals and humans. In this manner, studies in cultured cells and intact animals are complementary in nature, and the combined system approach frequently leads to a more thorough understanding of the underlying physiologic processes.

I. Use of Cultured Cell Systems to Study the Roles of Metallothionein in the Cellular Response to Cd

A general discussion of the part played by metallothionein (MT) in Cd metabolism is presented in Chap. 8. In cultured cells, initial studies on the Cd^{2+} response showed that early passage human and animal fibroblasts and epithelial cells as well as transformed, established cell lines often respond as do cells in vivo, i.e., with the production of MT (LUCIS et al. 1970; HIDALGO et al. 1978; HILDEBRAND and ENGER 1980; RUDD and HERSCHMAN 1978; CHERIAN 1980; KOBAYASHI and KIMURA 1980; BAZZELL et al. 1979; SCIORTINO et al. 1982; HILDEBRAND et al. 1982). That MT plays an important role in Cd^{2+} detoxification in vitro was then established further by demonstrations of enhanced MT levels in cadmium-resistant cells derived by growth of various cultured cell populations in toxic levels of Cd^{2+} until resistant populations emerged (RUGSTAD and NORSETH 1975; HILDEBRAND et al. 1979; GICK et al. 1981; MAITI et al. 1982; ENGER et al. 1981, 1983 a; EVANS et al. 1983). In some instances, the parental, cadmium-sensitive cell (Cd^s) lacked the ability to produce MT (MT^-) or synthesized this protein at very low levels upon exposure to levels of Cd^{2+} that induced this protein in other cells (MT^+). Of particular utility were a series of variants derived from the CHO cell (HILDEBRAND et al. 1982), a tumorigenic cell line established from Chinese hamster ovary. The CHO cell is Cd^s and MT^-, derivatives are MT^+ and cadmium resistant (Cd^r), but differ in their levels of Cd^{2+} resistance and MT inducibility (Table 1). One variant, Cd^r 200T1, is constitutive (MT^c) for MT synthesis (ENGER et al. 1983 a). These variants were used as tools to facilitate isolation of the MT genes, to study the molecular bases for alterations in MT expression, to define the relationship between MT response and Cd^{2+} resistance, and to study the roles of MT in the modulation of Cd^{2+} response by other factors (HILDEBRAND et al. 1982; ENGER et al. 1983 a, 1979 a, b, 1980 b; GRIFFITH et al. 1981; WALTERS et al. 1981).

Early studies showed that the MT response is modulated in the CHO variants at the transcriptional level; thionein mRNA levels and synthesis rates correspond

Table 1. Metallothionein synthesis in CHO cells and Cd^r CHO variants

Cell line	Toxic threshold	Relative MT synthesis rate	
	(μM $CdCl_2$)	Uninduced	Maximally induced
CHO	0.2	UD	UD
Cd^r2C10	2.0	UD	28.3
Cd^r20F4	26	UD	60.6
Cd^r30F9	40	UD	41.7
Cd^r200T1	145	40	320

UD, undetectable by ^{35}S cysteine incorporation

during induction, deinduction, and "superinduction" of MT (ENGER et al. 1979 b). As was found to be the case in the mouse thymoma cell (COMPERE and PALMITER 1981), the MT genes are inactivated (in the parental, Cd^s CHO cell) by hypermethylation (ENGER et al. 1983 a). Further, as was shown in two other systems (BEACH and PALMITER 1981; MAYO and PALMITER 1982; GICK and MCCARTY 1982), the MT genes are amplified in the more resistant CHO variants (ENGER et al. 1983 a; HILDEBRAND et al. 1983; WALTERS et al. 1981). The levels of amplification do not correspond exactly, however, with the MT response (ENGER et al. 1983 a; WALTERS et al. 1981). The CHO variant showing constitutive MT synthesis is, however, the most highly amplified in MT gene content among the series of CHO-derived variants (ENGER et al. 1983 b). A detailed discussion of MT gene methylation and amplification is presented in Sect. C.I.

The component of the MT response determining the threshold level of Cd^{2+} tolerated following a single, acute exposure was defined by studying Cd^{2+} uptake and intracellular partitioning and the kinetics of MT synthesis in the CHO variants (HILDEBRAND et al. 1982, 1979; ENGER et al. 1981, 1983 a). As can be seen in Fig. 1, variants Cd^r 2C10 and Cd^r 2OF4, which differ in Cd^{2+} sensitivity ten-

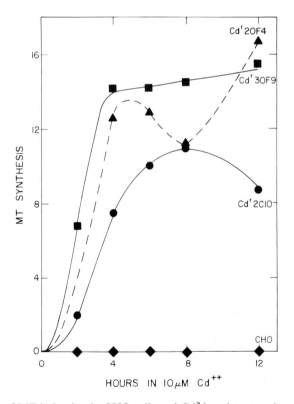

Fig. 1. Kinetics of MT induction in CHO cells and Cd^{2+}-resistant variants. MT synthesis was measured as a percentage of protein-incorporated cysteine ^{35}S in MT during a 1-h pulse at the time indicated

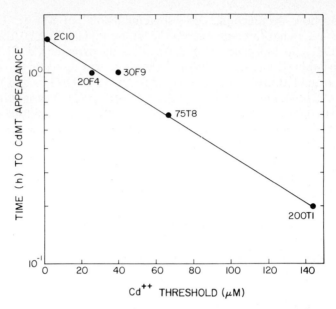

Fig. 2. Time of MT-bound cadmium (CdMT) appearance as a function of Cd resistance expressed as threshold for effects on survival. Cd^r cells were exposed to inducing levels of ^{109}CdCl$_2$. The accumulation of ^{109}CdMT was followed for 8 h. The linear accumulation of ^{109}CdMT was extrapolated back to the time of first CdMT appearance. These values are plotted in this graph against the maximum dose of Cd^{2+} tolerated by the variants

fold, have comparable MT synthesis rates when fully induced by 10 μM Cd^{2+}. However, the cells vary significantly in the rapidity with which they respond. This is most readily seen by observing the kinetics of MT-bound cadmium (CdMT) and non-CdMT accumulation in the variants. There are not large differences in the slopes of the CdMT accumulation curves. There are, however, significant differences in the points at which the CdMT accumulation curves intersect the time axes, the more resistant cells intersect closer to the origin (indicating a more rapid response). A plot of these intercepts against the cells' Cd^{2+} resistance thresholds shows a good semilogarithmic correlation of these parameters in Cd^{r}2C10, Ce^{r}20F4, Cd^{r}75T8, and Cd^{r}200T1 (Fig. 2), with Cd^{r}30F9 somewhat off the line for reasons to be presented later.

The effects of these CdMT kinetics are most importantly reflected in the non-MT and nuclear Cd burdens. In CHO, the non-MT and nuclear burdens continue to increase as intracellular Cd^{2+} accumulates (the Cd^s CHO and Cd^r variants accumulate at the same rates in general; Cd^{r}30F9 uptake is lower at low [Cd^{2+}], but comparable at its threshold dose). In the others, the non-MT and nuclear burdens plateau after a few hours exposure (Fig. 3). Thus, if a critical intracellular non-MT or nuclear concentration is necessary to kill the cells, this level must be reached within a few hours or not at all. As a consequence, the Cd^r variants are killed primarily during the first 6 h of exposure; thereafter the surviving cells repopulate the culture (Fig. 4) and growth rates return to normal, despite the con-

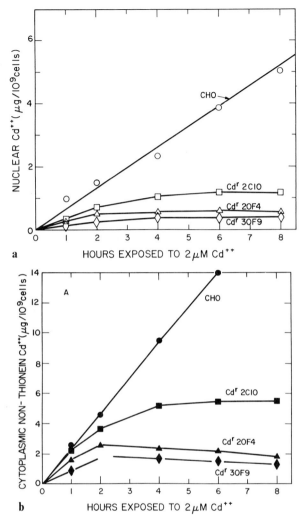

Fig. 3. a Kinetics of nuclear cadmium accumulation in CHO and Cd^{2+}-resistant variants. **b** Kinetics of non-MT cytoplasmic Cd^{2+} accumulation. (ENGER et al. 1981)

tinued presence of Cd^{2+}. These data suggest that the critical aspect of the MT response to acute Cd^{2+} exposure is not its eventual magnitude, but the *rapidity* with which the response is established.

That the MT response is not the only possible determinant of *differential* cellular response was also established using the CHO variants. The variant designated Cd^r30F9 is more resistant (40 μM vs 26 μM) than Cd^r20F4, yet produces MT no more rapidly, and has fewer MT genes (HILDEBRAND et al. 1982; ENGER et al. 1981, 1983a). That some *non-MT* resistance factor is enhanced differentially in these cells is obvious from the threshold non-MT level for toxic effects of Cd^{2+} in these cells (Table 2). The threshold non-MT level is that level of Cd^{2+} obtain-

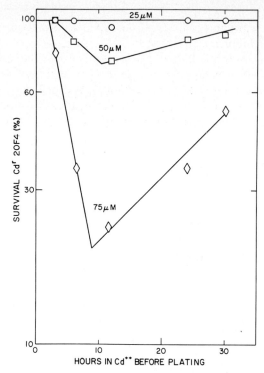

Fig. 4. Survival of Cd-resistant variant Cd^{r}20F4 as a function of time exposed to 25, 50, and 75 μM Cd^{2+}. (Enger et al. 1981)

ing in Cd^{r+} cells following exposure to the maximum concentration of Cd^{2+} tolerated by that cell for a period of time sufficient to reach a steady state level of non-MT-bound cadmium (cf. Fig. 3). It may be seen from the data in Table 2 that Cd^{r}30F9 cells can accumulate non-MT-bound cadmium to levels 4–8 times those of the other Cd^r variants before toxicity is evident. Possible non-MT mechanisms for conferring resistance in Cd^{r}30F9 are discussed in Sect. D.

In addition to employing resistant derivatives of a given cell, the correspondence of MT response, altered uptake, or other factors or mechanisms with Cd^{2+} cytotoxicity may be studied using cells of different origins (Kobayashi and Ki-

Table 2. Non-MT Cd^{2+} levels in cells exposed to maximum nontoxic Cd^{2+} levels for 8 h

Cell	Theshold level	Non-MT Cd^{2+} (μg/10^9 cells)	
	(μM CdCl$_2$)	Nuclear	Cytoplasmic
Cd^{r}2C10	2	1.2	5.4
Cd^{r}20F4	26	2.6	6.9
Cd^{r}30F9	40	9.5	39.6

MURA 1980; BAZZELL et al. 1979; ENGER et al. 1984a, b). Thus, human lymphocytes and mouse embryonic cells were found to have lower or more slowly inducible MT synthesis following exposure to Cd^{2+} at 2.5 µg/ml for 24 h than human
liver cells, HeLa cells, rabbit kidney cells, and mouse FRD cells (KOBAYASHI and
KIMURA 1980). There was however, no general correlation of resistance and MT
response. Further, a number of human tumor-derived cell lines were found to differ markedly in their ability to form colonies in the presence of Cd^{2+} (Fig. 5;
ENGER et al. 1984b). Some possessed no threshold for Cd^{2+} inhibition, others re-

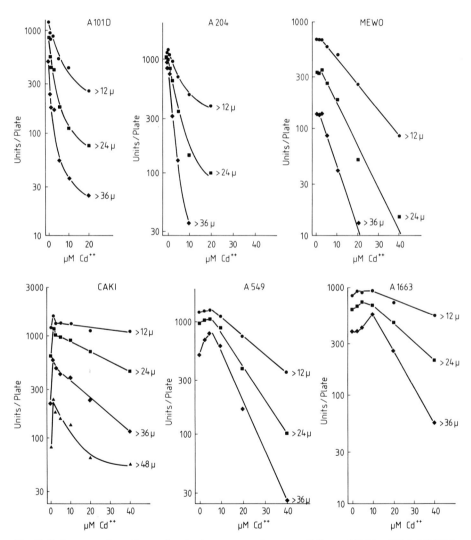

Fig. 5. Soft agar colony formation by human continuous cell lines *A101D, A204, MEWO,
CAKI-1, A549,* and *A1663* as functions of cadmium concentration. Cells were exposed continuously to Cd^{2+} during colony formation. Colonies with diameters exceeding indicated
values were scored using automated scanners. (ENGER et al. 1983d)

Table 3. Cd uptake and partitioning, and Cd-induced MT synthesis in MT$^+$ and MT$^-$ rodent cells and in normal and cancer-derived cadmium-sensitive (Cd^s) and resistant (Cd^r) human cells

Cell	Cd^{2+} uptake (µg/10^9 cells)[a] cytoplasmic				^{35}S cys MT, (% of total ^{35}S protein)[b]
	Total	MT	Non-MT	Nuclear	
Hamster MT$^+$ (Cd^{r}2C10)	62.5	16.3	40.7	5.5	13
Hamster MT$^-$ Cd^s (CHO)	60.1	0	46.9	13.2	0
Human skin fibroblast (HSF-7)	95.9	69.3	21.7	4.9	18
Human cancer line Cd^s (A204)	28.1	14.7	10.5	2.9	8
Human cancer line Cd^s (A101D)	92.3	49.9	28.3	14.1	11
Human cancer line Cd^r (CAKI)	84.4	48.0	25.8	10.6	9

[a] Following 6 h exposure to $2 \mu M$ CdCl$_2$; averages of duplicate determinations
[b] ^{35}S cysteine incorporated into MT as a percentage of total incorporation 4–6 h following exposure to $2 \mu M$ CdCl$_2$

sisted over 20 µM and were growth stimulated at lower doses. These cells have comparable MT responses, but their relative sensitivities do not in general correlate with differences in uptake or non-MT burdens (Table 3). These cells may thus provide additional systems useful in detecting and isolating non-MT factors responsible for Cd^{2+} resistance or sensitivity.

That factors other than MT may be effective in Cd^{2+} resistance was suggested also by studies of cultured human blood cells (HILDEBRAND and CRAM 1979; ENGER et al. 1983b). The most resistant blood cell population studied, the polymorphonuclear cells (granulocytes), showed no Cd^{2+}-induced CdMT or MT synthesis, but took up more Cd^{2+} than the other nucleated blood cells (lymphocytes and monocytes). A cadmium-binding protein (CdBP) not seen in the Sephadex G-75 profiles of other cells appeared in this instance. The position of the new CdBP corresponded with that of superoxide dismutase (SOD) although additional studies will be required to ascertain that the binding protein is, indeed, SOD. Thus, this cell system may also be useful in studying non-MT resistance factors.

That reduced MT response is not concomitant with Cd^{2+} sensitivity in many naturally occurring cell systems was shown by studies of Cd sensitivity and MT response in freshly cultured leukemic cells (ENGER et al. 1984a). These varied greatly in their cytotoxic responses to Cd^{2+}, but the Cd^s populations were MT$^+$. The Cd^s populations did however, in many instances show four- to fivefold enhanced Cd uptake, suggesting that altered uptake is an important parameter causing differential cytotoxic responses in these cells.

II. Cd Uptake

One might expect that cultured cells derived from different tissues and species could differ significantly in their uptake of Cd^{2+} as did the different leukemic populations already mentioned, and that this difference would be important in determining their relative cytotoxic responses to Cd^{2+}. Indeed, Cd^{2+}-resistant mutants of the CHO cell that have marked differences in Cd^{2+} uptake have been isolated from populations treated with ethylmethane sulfonate (CORRIGAN and HUANG 1981). On the other hand, no difference in uptake was found in Cd^r cells derived from three different Cd^s lines (one human epithelial and two mouse fibroblast lines) by exposure to Cd^{2+} (BAKKA and RUGSTAD 1981). It may be that uptake variants are more likely to be obtained following mutagenesis. The CHO uptake mutants should be useful in studying the factors responsible for Cd^{2+} uptake. The altered factors responsible for reduced uptake were not defined or isolated, although some aspects of Cd^{2+} uptake systems have been described (HART and KEATING 1980; STACEY and KLAASSEN 1980; FAILLA et al. 1979). It has been reported that Cd^{2+} uptake in primary cultures of rat liver parenchymal cells is effected by a temperature- and concentration-dependent process that requires sulfhydryl groups and is stimulated by dexamethasone (FAILLA et al. 1979). Uptake by isolated rat hepatocytes was found to be biphasic and insensitive to potassium cyanide and carbonyl cyanide-*m*-chlorophenylhydrazine, suggesting to the authors that an active process was not involved (STACEY and KLAASSEN 1980). In view of the fact that cultured CHO cells accumulate Cd^{2+} to concentrations that are 500- to 1,000-fold greater than the extracellular level, this conclusion is surprising (ENGER et al. 1978). In any event, further analysis of the uptake process is needed; cultured cell systems will be essential to such studies. Such studies may utilize not only cells that differ in uptake owing to mutation or differences in relevant gene expression, as with cells from different species or tissues, but also owing to the differences in uptake that occur in different growth states. Exponential and stationary phase L-cells, for example, differ twofold in uptake (OZAWA et al. 1976).

The extracellular factors that modulate Cd^{2+} uptake are, except for Zn^{2+} (HUANG et al. 1980 b), undefined. Their existence is inferred from the large differences in uptake that occur in different sera (DEAVEN and CAMPBELL 1980) and from the marked effect of stress factors on the metabolism of related metals such as Zn^{2+} in vivo (BEISEL et al. 1976). Cultured cells will be of obvious utility in such studies.

III. Use of Cultured Cell Systems to Study Cd Responses Other than Uptake or Cytotoxicity

Cd responses other than those involving direct cytotoxicity may be of overriding importance as determinants of the adverse health effects of this metal. These include transformation (carcinogenesis), effects on development (teratogenesis), and effects on the immune response. Cellular systems may be of great utility in studying these responses, but have not been applied to the extent that they have been for studying aspects of the cytotoxic responses to Cd^{2+}.

1. Genotoxic Effects

Epidemiologic studies on Cd-exposed humans and experiments with animals suggested the possibility that cadmium is a carcinogen (MALCOLM 1972; SUNDERMAN 1978; LAUWERYS 1979; SAMARAWICKRAMA 1979). The human studies showed higher incidences of renal, prostatic, and lung cancer in occupationally exposed humans. Because of the small numbers involved, however, the carcinogenicity of cadmium was not firmly established by these studies. Experiments with animals failed to elicit cancers subsequent to Cd ingestion or inhalation. Injection produced sarcomas at the sites of injection, but no metastatic cancers resulted.

That Cd is mutagenic was shown using a quantitative mammalian cell mutation system (HSIE et al. 1978). The ability of cadmium to produce chromosomal alterations in cultured cells was demonstrated in several laboratories (ROHR and BAUCHINGER 1976; DEAVEN and CAMPBELL 1980). These results are in accord with the observed mutagenic effects of Cd on oocyte chromosomes (WATANABE et al. 1979). However, no increase in dominant lethals or chromosome rearrangements were obseved in male mice injected with relatively high doses of Cd (GILLIAVOD and LEONARD 1975).

That Cd^{2+} may directly affect gene expression was indicated by studies which showed that exposure of cultured hamster cells to sublethal levels of Cd^{2+} altered RNA metabolism (ENGER et al. 1979a, 1978, 1976). In vitro studies showing Cd^{2+} to have clastogenic and mutagenic effects, as well as effects on gene expression support, but do not prove, the suggestion that Cd is a carcinogen. Such results are, however, usually considered a basis for further in vitro and in vivo studies.

2. Effects on the Immune System

Cadmium has varied and pronounced effects on the immune response in vivo (Chap. 9; JONES et al. 1971; KOLLER 1973; OHSAWA and KAWAI 1981; BOZELKA et al. 1978). Because of the complexity of immune responses, the many distinct cell types involved, and the multiplicity of their interactions in the development of cellular and humoral immunity, in vitro systems that allow dissection of the system and of the effects of Cd^{2+} on its component cell types are essential. These have been employed to define in part such effects. They have shown that Cd^{2+} affects the ability of both lymphocytes and macrophages to function appropriately (LAWRENCE 1981; KIREMIDJIAN-SCHUMACHER et al. 1981a, b; BOZELKA and BURKHOLDER 1982; LOOSE et al. 1977). Macrophages exposed to Cd in vitro showed decreased respiratory burst accompanying the phagocytic events, decreased mobility, and reduced response to migration factor. Cd also interfered with the interaction between lymphocytes and antigen and with the ability of lymphocytes to produce factors involved in the immune response.

IV. Use of Freshly Cultured Blood Cells to Study Variation in Human Response to Cd

An important, but largely unanswered question regarding the toxic effects of Cd^{2+} concerns the degree to which humans may vary in their sensitivity to this

Table 4. Cadmium cytotoxic responses of mononuclear cells cultured from human peripheral blood

Set	Threshold		LD_{50}		
	$\bar{X}$	SD	$\bar{X}$	SD	n
1	58.1	5.3	100.1	8.6	15
2	67.4	5.8	108.9	7.8	8
3	60.8	6.4	100.8	8.6	5
4	63.0	12.9	101.3	10.4	4
5	53.0	16.4	98.3	15.8	4
1–5	60.5	8.4	102.1	9.2	36

Threshold values for Cd^{2+} cytotoxicity were obtained by extrapolating survival values to 100%. The mean ($\bar{X}$) and standard deviation (SD) values for threshold and LD_{50} were determined for each set of subjects. Blood was drawn and mononuclear cell cultures were set up in Cd^{2+} on the same day for members of each set. One set of seven subjects showed exceptionally high values (without increased SD) and was not included. No individual differed from the set mean by more than 2 SD

element. Studies on different strains of laboratory animals indicate that large, genetically determined differences in sensitivity occur in animals (MEISLER et al. 1979).

An approach to the question of whether such genetically determined variations occur in humans involved analyzing the Cd^{2+} response of freshly cultured human mononuclear cells. As seen in Table 4, a study of the responses of cells derived from healthy human subjects did not show the kind of interindividual variation observed in animals.

C. Role of Metallothionein in Cellular Cd Resistance

As already noted, several lines of evidence, obtained in a variety of cultured mammalian cell systems, have shown that MT is a major factor in conferring cellular resistance to the cytotoxic effects of Cd^{2+} (reviewed in HILDEBRAND et al. 1982). Beginning with the studies of PISCATOR (1964), much evidence has accumulated implicating MT as an inducible protein involved in protection against Cd^{2+} toxicity. The high affinity, high capacity Cd^{2+}-binding property of mammalian MTs (WEBB 1975; NORDBERG and KOJIMA 1979) has suggested that these thiol-rich proteins can function to protect cellular targets of Cd^{2+} by sequestering the toxic ion in a nontoxic form (KOJIMA and KAGI 1978; JACOBSON and TURNER 1980). Thus, MT, by binding Cd^{2+} in a nontoxic form, can modulate the intracellular availability of the ion for association with other sensitive intracellular components. This concept is supported by analytic modeling of experimental results using Monte Carlo methods (HAYDEN et al. 1982). It should be mentioned that the cytotoxicity of MT-bound cadmium reported for exposure of kidney epithelial cells to *extracellular* (exogenous) CdMT is a separate phenomenon from the intracellular protection provided by endogenous MT (CHERIAN 1982).

Since it is well documented that MT plays a central role in conferring cellular resistance to Cd^{2+}, it is important to develop detailed understanding of how the protective MT response is regulated in cells. Multiple levels of control over MT production have been identified by investigators using a variety of biochemical analyses of MT regulation, both in cultured cells and in intact animals (SQUIBB et al. 1977; KARIN and HERSCHMAN 1979; ENGER et al. 1979 b; HILDEBRAND and ENGER 1980; BEACH and PALMITER 1981; COMPERE and PALMITER 1981; MAYO and PALMITER 1981; GICK and McCARTY 1982). The levels of control of MT produc-

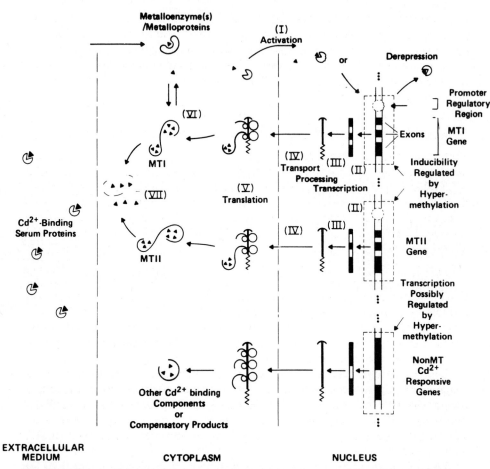

Fig. 6. Possible mechanisms regulating MT gene expression. Appearance of intracellular Cd^{2+} is recognized (*I*) either by an intracellular "receptor" which binds to a regulatory region of the MT gene(s) and activates transcription, or by causing a repressor component bound to a regulatory region of the MT gene(s) to be released from the region, leading to transcriptional activation (*II*). Transcription of MT genes is controlled by methylation of the MT-1 and/or MT-2 genes. The initial RNA transcripts are "processed" (*III*) in the nucleus and transported (*IV*) as mRNAs to the cytoplasm where they are translated (*V*) into protein which can bind metals and donate metals to other metalloproteins or metalloenzymes (*VI*). Turnover of MT proteins (*VII*) releases Cd^{2+} to the intracellular pool. Other non-MT metal-responsive genes are hypothesized

tion are summarized in Fig. 6. With the advent of recombinant DNA technology, it has become possible to isolate specific genes so that multiple levels of control of their organization and expression, as identified in Fig. 6, can be studied definitively. The following discussion focuses on the application of cellular and molecular biology approaches, including use of molecularly cloned MT gene sequences to define regulatory steps in MT production.

I. Metallothionein Production is Regulated at Several Levels

In an attempt to condense much of the published literature describing how MT production is controlled both in animal tissues and in cultured cells, Fig. 6 summarizes current understanding of the multiple levels of regulation of organization and expression of MT genes. The roles of these levels of control over MT production are discussed in relation to Cd^{2+} sensitivity and resistance both in cultured mammalian cells and in primary cell explants of human tissues.

1. Inducibility of Metallothionein Genes is Controlled by DNA Methylation

Several mechanisms have evolved to provide regulation of gene activity during development and differention (BURGER and WEBER 1982). One mechanism which is found in higher eukaryotes involves a specific chemical modification of one of the DNA bases. This modification, covalent linkage of a methyl group to the 5 position of specific cytosine residues (designated ^mC), does not alter the coding capacity of the modified cytosine, since the 5 position is not involved in hydrogen bonding interactions required for faithful DNA replication and RNA transcription (RAZIN and RIGGS 1980; DOERFLER 1983). In eukaryotes, ^mC residues are found predominantly in the dinucleotide $5'$-^mCG-$3'$. Numerous lines of investigation have implicated cytosine methylation as a factor in controlling transcription of DNA sequences (namely, specific genes) in which a high frequency of ^mC residue is found (DOERFLER 1983). In the majority of cases studied, increased methylation of cytosine residues within, or in regions neighboring specific genes results in suppressed expression of the genes.

Two approaches can be used to determine whether DNA methylation plays a significant role in controlling expression of specific genes. The first procedure used to determine whether specific genes are controlled by DNA hypermethylation is to grow the cells (with the genes of interest in an inactive, nonexpressed state) in the presence of the hypomethylating agent, 5-azacytidine (JONES and TAYLOR 1980).

This hypomethylating agent reduces maintenance methylation either (a) by being incorporated into the DNA during replication and, because it is blocked at the 5 position, causing a subsequent loss of methylation during subsequent rounds of DNA replication (JONES and TAYLOR 1980; DOERFLER 1983) or (b) by directly inhibiting maintenance methylases (DOERFLER 1983). In cases in which the genes of interest encode a selectable marker (e.g., for genes encoding Cd^{2+} resistance), it is possible to determine whether DNA methylation is a controlling factor in gene regulation by growing Cd^{2+}-sensitive cells in the presence of the hypomethylating agent for one population doubling time to allow one round of

DNA replication and then determining whether the hypomethylating agent has caused a high frequency of cells to become Cd^{2+} resistant.

Such analyses have been reported for both cultured mouse thymoma (W7) cells (Compere and Palmiter 1981) and for cultured Chinese hamster (CHO) cells (Hildebrand et al. 1982). In both mouse thymoma cells (Compere and Palmiter 1981) and CHO cells, MT genes are not expressed either in the absence or presence of Cd^{2+} (Hildebrand et al. 1979, 1982). However, following growth of thymoma cells in 5-azacytidine-containing medium, thymoma cells show a conversion from a Cd^s to a Cd^r phenotype with a corresponding switch of the MT-1 gene from a noninducible to an inducible state determined by measuring MT-1 expression (Compere and Palmiter 1981). Similarly, treatment of CHO cells with 5-azacytidine for one population doubling time resulted in a switch from a Cd^s to a Cd^r phenotype correlating with a switch from noninducibility to inducibility of both MT-1 and MT-2 proteins (Hildebrand et al. 1982). Although these studies raise the question of the relative roles of MT-1 and MT-2 in conferring Cd resistance, a role for DNA methylation in controlling MT inducibility is indicated.

A second method for defining the role of DNA methylation in regulation of specific gene expression involves molecular genetics approaches using molecularly cloned DNA sequences specific for the genes of interest (Compere and Palmiter 1981). Although space does not permit a detailed explanation of this latter procedure, the basic approach and the significance of the results can be summarized. Briefly, genomic DNA from cells whose DNA is to be examined for hypermethylation (or hypomethylation) in or near the gene (or genes) of interest is treated with methylation-sensitive DNA restriction endonucleases, designated HpaII or MspI. Both of these enzymes recognize and cleave double-stranded DNA at the sequence CCGG. However, if the internal C is methylated as in C^mCGG, HpaII does not cleave. MspI cleaves this sequence whether or not the internal C is methylated, but not if the external C (^mCCGG) is methylated. Typically it is methylation of the internal C that is involved in modulation of gene activity (Razin and Riggs 1980; Doerfler 1983). Following restriction endonuclease digestion, the resulting DNA fragments from Cd^s (MT noninducible) and Cd^r (MT inducible) cells are resolved electrophoretically, denatured, transferred to a nitrocellulose filter, and hybridized with radioactively labeled, molecularly cloned, DNA sequence probes specific for the gene (or genes) of interest. In the case of the DNA from Cd^s and Cd^r mouse W7 cells, the region of DNA containing the MT-1 gene was found to be resistant to HpaII cleavage in DNA from Cd^s (MT noninducible) cells, but in DNA from Cd^r cells this region was cleaved into several fragments (Compere and Palmiter 1981). Using Cd^s and Cd^r variants of Chinese hamster (CHO) cells, studies of HpaII and MspI sensitivity of genomic DNAs in the region of both the MT-1 and MT-2 genes showed that these genomic DNA regions are hypermethylated in Cd^s cells, but undergo a transition to a hypomethylated state in Cd^{2+}-resistant cells (Griffith et al. 1983; Hildebrand et al. 1982). In both mouse and Chinese hamster cells these observations are substantiated by the finding that the MT-1 gene in mouse, and both MT-1 and MT-2 genes in CHO cells, undergo the transition to the hypomethylated configuration in Cd^r cells derived by 5-azacytidine treatment (Compere and Palmiter 1981;

HILDEBRAND et al. 1982). While further studies are required to elucidate the molecular details of control of MT inducibility involving methylation of regions near or within the MT genes, it is clear that the level of methylation is an important factor in controlling MT gene expression.

2. Transcriptional Control of Metallothionein Expression

As discussed in the preceding section, the published literature suggests that a hypomethylated configuration of regions of DNA within or near MT genes is a prerequisite for inducibility of the MT genes. This inducible configuration of the MT genes permits modulation of transcriptional activity. Reports from several laboratories have demonstrated that both essential (Zn^{2+}, Cu^{2+}) and nonessential (Cd^{2+}, Hg^{2+}) trace metals and glucocorticoid hormones can regulate the level of MT gene transcription (SQUIBB and COUSINS 1977; ENGER et al. 1979 b; KARIN and HERSCHMAN 1979; DURNAM and PALMITER 1981; KARIN et al. 1981). As outlined in Fig. 6, multiple steps have been implicated in the transcriptional regulation of MT gene expression. Because of the dual nature of the control of MT gene expression (i.e., by metals and glucocorticoid hormones) indicated by studies in both cultured cells and mammalian tissues, several levels of recognition for these different inducers have been postulated.

In the case of modulation of MT expression by Cd^{2+}, intracellular mechanisms must exist for detection of elevated metal levels. Such a detection system could operate via an activation or a derepression mechanism. An activation process would require intracellular cadmium-binding proteins which detect elevated Cd^{2+} levels, translocate to the nucleus, and interact with specific control region (or regions) near the MT gene (or genes) to modulate (positively) MT gene transcription.

Alternatively, a derepression model would require a metal-binding repressor component which is normally associated with a DNA control (promoter) region near the MT gene (or genes) (Fig. 6, step I) to maintain a low level of MT gene transcriptional activity. According to this model, elevated intracellular Cd^{2+} levels would be detected by the metal-binding repressor, causing a change in its association with the DNA control region (or possibly, release from the promoter), and resulting in increased transcriptional activity. A role for apothionein (metal-depleted MT) or an apothionein fragment has been postulated in this regulatory model (KARIN and RICHARDS 1982). Other studies have provided several indirect lines of evidence indicating that a non-thionein regulatory repressor component is involved in controlling MT gene transcription (HILDEBRAND et al. 1982). Efforts are in progress in several laboratories to identify the regulatory molecule (or molecules) and to delineate the mechanism (or mechanisms) for modulation of MT gene transcriptional activity.

The DNA control regions involved in transcriptional modulation have been defined for the mouse MT-1 gene (MAYO et al. 1982) and the human MT-2 gene (KARIN and HOLTGREVE 1983) through a series of elegant studies utilizing combined recombinant DNA and somatic cell genetics techniques. In those studies, DNA fragments derived from regions near the 5' end of the respective MT gene (the regions containing the transcription start signal) were synthetically coupled to a gene encoding a viral thymidine kinase (TK) and then spliced into a plasmid vector. In one study (BRINSTER et al. 1982), mouse eggs were microinjected with the recombinant plasmid containing the MT promoter region sequence ligated to the TK gene and Cd^{2+}-regulated expression of TK activity was analyzed. In other investigations, transfection of cultured cells lacking TK with a recombinant plasmid containing the TK gene linked to various sequences from the human MT promoter region was followed by culture in a selective growth medium which allowed only cells with TK activity to survive (MAYO et al. 1982; KARIN and HOLTGREVE 1983). In addition to the selective growth condition, transfected cells were exposed to inducing concentrations of Cd^{2+} so that only cells which contained the necessary metal-regulated DNA transcription control region would be detected. The results of the studies of the microinjected mouse eggs showed that in the mouse MT-1 gene the metal-regulated DNA control sequences lie within 90 nucleotides of the 5′ side (upstream) of the transcription start site (BRINSTER et al. 1982). Similar results were found for the human MT-2 gene (KARIN and HOLTGREVE 1983). The identification of these regulatory sequences represents a major step in elucidation of the molecular details of the regulation of induction of MT transcription. It should be mentioned that in other genes additional transcriptional regulatory ("enhancer") signals have been found on the 5′ side (upstream) of the transcription start site (MARX 1983). Such signals have not yet been reported for the MT genes.

The kinetics of the Cd^{2+}-induced expression of MT genes and the appearance of cytoplasmic MT mRNA are rapid relative to most other inducible gene systems which have been characterized (ENGER et al. 1979b). In cultured mammalian cells which are maximally responsive to Cd^{2+} exposure, cytoplasmic MT mRNA concentration can be induced from a basal level to a maximally induced level more than 1,000-fold greater than basal level in a period of 4 h (GRIFFITH et al. 1981). As indicated in Fig. 6, the appearance of cytoplasmic MT mRNA can be regulated by several steps between transcription and nucleocytoplasmic transport. During these intermediate steps, the primary MT gene transcripts are processed to remove intervening sequences (introns), processed and modified at the 5′ (capped) and 3′ (polyadenylated) ends prior to transfer to the cytoplasm.

3. Translational Control of Metallothionein Expression

Metallothionein mRNA appears in the cytoplasm of mammalian cells in membrane-free (SHAPIRO and COUSINS 1980) polyribosomes – primarily in dimers through tetramers (HILDEBRAND et al. 1982). Although association of MT mRNA with cytoplasmic ribonucleoprotein (other than polyribosomes) has not been reported, it should be noted that translational control of another metal-binding, metal-regulated protein, ferritin, has been reported to involve storage of cytoplasmic ferritin mRNA in a translationally inactive form, e.g., as informosomes (DRYSDALE and MUNRO 1966).

While cytoplasmic storage of translationally inactive MT mRNA has not been observed, preliminary evidence for translational control of MT mRNA has been presented. These studies showed that, in one MT induction-proficient Cd^r cell line derived from Cd^s CHO cells, MT synthesis following Cd^{2+} induction rose rapidly, reached a peak rate of synthesis, and then decreased to < 50% of the peak rate while the level of translatable MT mRNA rose just preceding the rise in MT synthesis rate, but remained at a peak value while MT synthesis rate decreased (ENGER et al. 1980 a).

Since at least two major isoMTs are expressed in most cultured mammalian cell systems studied (HILDEBRAND et al. 1982), it will be of interest to explore in more detail the control of the relative synthesis of each of the MTs and their corresponding mRNAs. The accumulation of the MTs is controlled both by the rate of translation of MT mRNA and the turnover of the MTs. As noted in Sect. B.I, the rate of accumulation of MT is an important factor in cellular Cd^{2+} resistance, i.e., in general, Cd^{2+} resistance correlates with the rapidity with which a cell can respond to Cd^{2+} exposure by accumulation of Cd^{2+} into MT.

Finally, in the context of translational control of the MTs, it is important to consider the relative roles of the isoMTs in conferring cellular Cd^{2+} resistance. For example, does one of the isoMTs predominate in conferring the Cd^{2+}-resistant phenotype or are both (all) of the isoMTs involved? Recent studies from our laboratory suggest that in Chinese hamster cells both major isoMTs are coordinately expressed at approximately equal rates, suggesting that neither of the isoMTs predominates in conferring cellular Cd^{2+} resistance (HILDEBRAND et al. 1983).

4. Role of Metallothionein Gene Dosage in Cellular Cd Resistance: Metallothionein Gene Amplification

Mammalian cells can respond to environmental stress by a variety of compensatory or protective mechanisms. One primary mechanism of response is to increase the rate or amount of production of a specific cellular component which can ameliorate the action of a toxic agent. The most widely studied of such cellular responses is the development of resistance to the anticancer drug, methotrexate, which blocks single-carbon transfer reactions required for pyrimidine biosynthesis by inhibiting the enzyme dihydrofolate reductase (DHFR). In cultured cells selected for resistance to high levels of methotrexate, DHFR is overproduced (ALT et al. 1978). One of the mechanisms for achieving overproduction of DHFR is amplification of the genes encoding DHFR (ALT et al. 1978).

In the case of cellular Cd^{2+} resistance, the high affinity Cd^{2+}-binding MTs act to protect multiple potential intracellular targets from the cytotoxic action (or actions) of Cd^{2+}. Hence, cells which can overproduce MTs under culture conditions with elevated Cd^{2+} concentrations can accommodate increased Cd^{2+} burden and continue to proliferate.

Amplification of the MT-1 gene in both mouse (BEACH and PALMITER 1981) and Chinese hamster (GICK and McCARTY 1982; HILDEBRAND et al. 1983) cells has been correlated with increased production of MT-1 mRNA and increased resistance to Cd^{2+}. Studies from our laboratory with the Cd^r variants already described (HILDEBRAND et al. 1983) have demonstrated that overproduction of MT is a hallmark of development of the Cd^r phenotype. Application of molecularly cloned DNA sequence probes for Chinese hamster MT-1 and MT-2 gene sequences provided evidence that MT-1 and MT-2 genes are coordinately amplified up to 40-fold in MT-overproducing Cd^r cell lines (Griffith et al. 1983; Hildebrand et al. 1983).

Preliminary analyses of the organization of the amplified MT-1 and MT-2 genes of the Cd^r Chinese hamster cells indicate that these genes lie adjacent to one another in the genome. Further, cytogenetic approaches to the chromosomal localization of the amplified MT genes in the stably Cd-resistant, Cd^{r}200T1 cell line using in situ hybridization techniques showed that these genes were localized on a large submetacentric marker chromosome (Hildebrand et al. 1983). The localization of amplified genes to intact chromosomes is an indicator of stable integration of amplified gene sequences (reviewed in Schimke 1982). Thus, the results of the studies of the amplified MT-1 and MT-2 genes in Chinese hamster cells demonstrate that these genes can undergo amplification and remain stably amplified in the absence of continuous selective pressure.

II. Role of Metallothionein in Cellular Cd Resistance in Cultured Human Blood Cells

Previous studies have examined Cd^{2+}-mediated cytotoxicity in different cultured cell populations obtained from peripheral human blood (Enger et al. 1983b). As noted in Sects. B.I and B.IV, mononuclear blood cells showed a well-defined and reproducible (in both intra- and interindividual comparisons) cytotoxic response to Cd^{2+}. This class of blood cells also showed a proficiency for induction of MT and rapid accumulation of intracellular Cd^{2+} into CdMT (Enger et al. 1983b). In contrast, another population of leukocytes, polymorphonuclear leukocytes, or granulocytes, displayed an increased resistance to the cytotoxic action of Cd^{2+} compared with mononuclear cells (Enger et al. 1983b). The increased resistance of granulocytes relative to mononuclear cells could not be explained on the basis of a decreased Cd^{2+} uptake by granulocytes compared with mononuclear cells at iso-exposure Cd^{2+} concentrations. In fact, the granulocytes accumulated more Cd^{2+} per cell than did mononuclear cells. Analyses of the intracellular distribution of Cd^{2+} in granulocytes revealed no detectable CdMT. However, a larger cytoplasmic Cd^{2+}-binding species which appeared to be increased by Cd^{2+} exposure was observed in the granulocytes (Enger et al. 1983b). These findings suggest that non-MT Cd^{2+}-binding species may be implicated in protection against Cd^{2+} cytotoxicity in granulocytes.

D. Non-Metallothionein Mechanisms of Cellular Cd Resistance

While a variety of studies indicate that the induction of MT synthesis and subsequent binding of cadmium is an important mechanism for the cellular detoxification of cadmium, there are several lines of evidence which suggest that this is not the only mechanism for protection against the metal. First, when rats are pretreated with 1 mg/kg CdCl$_2$, the induced MT persists for 10 days. However, the protection against subsequent CdCl$_2$ challenge persists for only 3 days (Webb and Vershoyle 1976). On a cellular level, Cherian (1981) has shown that the induction of MT protects cells against CdCl$_2$, but not against extracellular CdMT, which is considerably more toxic than the chloride salt. Further evidence for a non-MT component of Cd resistance is given by a series of human cell lines all of which are competent to synthesize MT, but in which the threshold for Cd^{2+} toxicity ranges from 0 to $>40 \mu M$ (ENGER et al. 1984 b). As noted already, studies of MT production and cadmium resistance in cultured human blood cells showed that mononuclear cells (lymphocytes and monocytes) are fully competent to synthesize MT and sequester most of the intracellular Cd^{2+} as CdMT, whereas granulocytes (polymorphonuclear leukocytes) show no accumulation of CdMT, although both the Cd^{2+} content and Cd^{2+} resistance were greater than that observed for mononuclear cells (ENGER et al. 1983 b). Lastly, in a series of Cd-resistant variants of the Cd-sensitive CHO cell line, there is good correlation between Cd resistance and MT synthesis, with the exception that the $Cd^r 30F9$ cells (resistant to $40 \mu M$ CdCl$_2$) synthesize less MT than the $Cd^r 20F4$ cells (resistant to $24 \mu M$ CdCl$_2$) (HILDEBRAND et al. 1982).

One obvious factor influencing the toxicity of Cd^{2+} is the cellular uptake of the ion. This can be influenced by various conditions such as the salinity (ENGEL and FOWLER 1979), pH, the presence of competing cations or chelating agents, and the nutritional status of the cells (MULLER and OHNESORGE 1982). There are also genetic differences in the ability of different cell lines and tissues to take up the ion which can account for some of the variability in Cd^{2+} sensitivity (LUCIS and LUCIS 1969; HUANG et al. 1980a; HATA et al. 1980; ENGER et al. 1984a, b). However, the details of these systems have yet to be elucidated.

There are a number of indications that one or more non-MT proteins may be involved in Cd^{2+} resistance. Cd^{2+} treatment has been shown in chick embryo and human foreskin cells (LEVINSON et al. 1980), and in a line of Chinese hamsters fibroblasts (LI et al. 1982), to induce the synthesis of a small number of non-MT proteins which are very similar, if not identical, to the well-known heat shock or stress proteins. It was shown that CdCl$_2$ treatment will protect the hamster fibroblasts against a subsequent heat challenge (LI et al. 1982). However, at least in these cells, heat does not appear to induce protection against CdCl$_2$ (HAHN and LI 1982).

GRIFFITH et al. (1981) reported four translation products (including MT) of the polyadenylated mRNA from a Cd^{2+}-treated Cd^{2+}-resistant subline of CHO cells, not detectable in the Cd^{2+}-sensitive CHO cells. The relationship of these proteins to resistance has not been established, but their presence in only the Cd^{2+}-resistant subline is suggestive of a role in protection.

Another example is an 11,800 daltons Cd^{2+}-binding protein which accumulates in a human lung fibroblast cell line during treatment with Cd^{2+} (HART and KEATING 1980). Upon reaching confluency, the cells lose this protein and toxicity is observed. This protein may be related to the CdMT dimer of approximately the same molecular weight which appears specifically to protect the testes of mice (WOLKOWSKI-TYL and PRESTON 1979). The MT monomer, while present, is ineffective in protection. Progesterone appears to be required for the dimer formation. It is interesting that a gene controlling the protection against Cd^{2+}-induced testicular necrosis is a single, autosomal recessive gene (TAYLOR et al. 1973; HUNT and MHLANGA 1983), while somatic cell hybridization studies (CHEN et al. 1981) and animal studies (HUNT and MHLANGA 1983) have shown that the MT locus acts as a codominant gene.

Other thionein-related proteins were reported in rat kidney by Zelazowski et al. (1980). These authors found three proteins that: (a) bound Cd^{2+} and Cu^{2+}; (b) showed a partial reaction with antibody to MT-2 (but not with antibody to MT-1); and (c) exhibited a strong reaction with an antibody to MT-1+MT-2 polymerized with glutaraldehyde. While it is possible that the material isolated represents the native structures of these proteins, one must also consider the possibility of autooxidation of the cysteine-rich MTs during isolation (Minkel et al. 1980).

Higher molecular weight ($> 60,000$) Cd^{2+}-binding proteins have been observed in the livers of trout treated with low levels of Cd^{2+} (Roberts et al. 1979) and in cultured polymorphonuclear cells from human blood (Enger et al. 1983 b). MT was not present in either of these cases. However, again the relationship of these proteins to toxicity or resistance has not been unequivocally demonstrated.

One other factor which appears to play an important role in cellular protection against Cd^{2+} is the ubiquitous tripeptide, glutathione. Cd^{2+} has been shown to decrease the concentration of glutathione in both cultured cells (Stacey and Kappus 1982; Muller and Ohnesorge 1982) and in rat kidney and liver (Wong and Klaassen 1981). However, in several lines of cells derived from CHO on the basis of Cd^{2+} resistance, the initial decrease is followed by a recovery and the induction of increased glutathione levels up to 250% of the controls (Seagrave et al. 1983). In particular, in a cell line with a lower MT synthesis rate, but higher Cd^{2+} resistance (line Cd^r30F9, compared with Cd^r20F4) the initial concentration of glutathione is higher and the increase is especially rapid (Table 5). The known affinity of Cd^{2+} for sulfhydryl groups (as in MT) and for glutathione (Perrin and Watt 1971; Cherian and Vostal 1977) makes this an attractive mechanism for cellular resistance to cadmium.

Cell lines derived on the basis of cadmium resistance provide very powerful tools for the elucidation of the mechanisms of Cd^{2+} resistance as shown in the work of Huang et al. (1980a), Griffith et al. (1981), Chen et al. (1981), and Seagrave et al. (1983). With these techniques and with recent advances in trace metal analysis, high pressure liquid chromatography, and two-dimensional polyacrylamide gel electrophoresis, it seems likely that a more complete understanding of the mechanisms of cellular resistance to Cd will be achieved in the near future.

Table 5. Glutathione levels in cadmium-resistant CHO variants

Cell line 200T1	Threshold $CdCl_2$ toxicity (μM)	Maximum relative MT synthesis rate	Endogenous [GSH] (µg per milligramm protein)	Relative [GSH+GSSG] at 12 h	Time of first observed increase in [GSH+GSSG] (h)
CHO	0.2	0	8.0 ± 0.7	2.6	6
20F4	26	60	8.2 ± 0.8	2.5	6
30F9	40	40	14.5 ± 1.7	1.7	3
200T1	145	145	18.4 ± 1.2	1.0	

E. Models Describing Cd Metabolism and the Role of Metallothionein and Other Factors in Resistance and Sensitivity

Published models of Cd^{2+} metabolism have provided important new conceptual approaches to considering how Cd^{2+} interacts with cells to cause a toxic response. Models have been provided that describe cadmium uptake and retention and MT synthesis in experimental animals (PETERING and PETERING 1979; FOULKES 1982), in humans (KJELLSTROM and NORDBERG 1978), and in cultured cell systems (CHIN et al. 1978; HAYDEN et al. 1982). These models represent a variety of approaches to classification and quantification of the factors that modulate Cd^{2+} toxicity at the cellular and intact organism levels. They provide a rational basis for predicting critical organ levels of Cd^{2+} in exposed animals and humans and offer insight into the multiple factors that control cellular responses to Cd^{2+}. The studies of PETERING and PETERING (1979) and HAYDEN et al. (1982) are especially significant in this latter regard in their considerations of the molecular bioinorganic principles underlying heavy metal toxicology. As a measure of the complexity of current modeling, the approach of HAYDEN et al. (1982) considers roles of subcellular structures in Cd^{2+} metabolism and provides a basis for design of experimental cellular systems to evaluate relative roles of different subcellular structures in Cd^{2+} detoxification.

F. Future Directions

I. Models

The need for more detailed models focusing on cellular and molecular events is indicated by the multiplicity of potential cellular targets (JACOBSEN and TURNER 1980) (see Sect. F.II) and their interactions. The expanded application of modeling and theoretical analyses will have potential value in delineating the hierarchy of cellular factors and interactions among those factors involved in a toxic response as well as the hierarchy of cellular responses involved in conferring resistance to toxicity.

Also, as reviewed in Sect. B.I, the differential Cd^{2+} sensitivities of various classes of peripheral human blood cells, important in the immune response, suggest that organismal models of Cd^{2+} response should include considerations of the effects of Cd^{2+} not only at the level of critical organs, but also at the level of tissues involved in the immune response (see Chap. 9).

Finally, the usefulness of both cellular and organismal models will be increased as knowledge accumulates regarding genetic factors which alter uptake or cellular protective response (for example, control of MT inducibility and level of expression). Although much work will be required to identify in experimental animal and human populations the precise genetic factors responsible for altered sensitivity to Cd^{2+}, the experimental basis and significance of such studies has been demonstrated (MEISLER et al. 1979).

II. Cd Toxicity Targets

Although a considerable amount of information has been gathered regarding the MT mechanism for detoxifying Cd^{2+}, little is known about the actual targets of Cd^{2+} toxicity. There are at least four levels at which Cd^{2+} could interfere with cellular functioning. At the simplest level, Cd^{2+} could affect the cell surface, altering membrane structure and function in the manner of zinc (BETTGER and O'DELL 1981) or by altering transport mechanisms, especially those for zinc, copper, and other divalent cations. It is known that Cd^{2+} is associated with increased lipid peroxidation. However, work by STACEY and KAPPUS (1982) indicates that membrane lipids may not be a primary target for toxicity. Cadmium is also known to alter the activities of a large number of enzymes involved in such functions as nucleic acid metabolism (JACOBSEN and TURNER 1980), collagen metabolism (NAGAI et al. 1982), detoxification of xenobiotics (DIERICKX 1982), redox reactions, and electron transport (EATON et al. 1980; MAINES et al. 1982; DIAMOND et al. 1973; ASOKAN et al. 1981; JACOBSEN and TURNER 1980) and proteinase/antiproteinase balance (CHOWDHURY et al. 1982). Cadmium might further be expected to affect many other metalloenzymes. Cadmium may interfere with regulatory processes, such as the cyclic nucleotide/protein kinase/phosphatase systems (JACOBSEN and TURNER 1980) or the postulated "third messenger" glutathione (GILBERT 1982). Finally, Cd^{2+} might directly affect gene regulation through interactions with DNA itself, with RNA, with other components of chromatin (DEAVEN and CAMPBELL 1980; JACOBSEN and TURNER 1980; LEWIS and LAEMMLI 1982), or with the function of DNA methylases (CHAN et al. 1982). There is clearly much to be learned about the importance of the various interactions of this highly reactive metal with cellular functions and the relationship of such interactions with toxicity.

III. Gene Expression Domains

From the preceding discussion of the regulation of MT expression, it is apparent that although our understanding of the system has increased greatly in the last few years, there is still much to be learned both about the expression of MT itself and about the domain of other cellular responses to Cd^{2+}. It is believed that the MT-1 and MT-2 genes are linked, and, at least in CHO variants, expressed coordinately. But whether this is due to one promotor controlling both genes, or two promotors acting in concert, is not known. The mechanism of induced expression, whether by derepression or activation (or both) is not known. Presumably, either mechanism requires a Cd^{2+}-binding receptor (see Sect. C.I.2), the nature of which is not yet known. A suggestion that the receptor is MT itself, produced constitutively at very low levels (KARIN and RICHARDS 1982) could be tested using transfection of a variant cell line (whose MT genes are deleted or nonfunctional) with a plasmid containing the MT promotor linked to a viral TK gene. If metal-regulated expression of TK is unaltered in this transfectant (compared with that in a transfectant with a functioning MT gene), then MT, itself, is not the repressor. The promotor region of mouse MT-1 has been cloned; however, the interaction of this region with either Cd^{2+} receptors of glucocorticoid receptors is not understood. Part of the Cd^{2+} regulatory region becomes more sensitive to nuclease digestion in the presence of Cd^{2+} (SENEAR and PALMITER 1982), which suggests a derepression mechanism, but the authors point out the possibility that the binding of a Cd^{2+} activator complex could cause conformational changes leading to increased sensitivity.

Two other important questions relate to the induction of other proteins in the presence of Cd^{2+} (LEVINSON et al. 1980; LI et al. 1982; HEIKKILA et al. 1982) and alternate means of inducing MT (KARIN and HERSCHMAN 1980; OH et al. 1978; KOTSONIS and KLAASSEN 1979; WONG and KLAASSEN 1981). The former case may be similar to the heat shock system, with which, in fact, it shares considerable homology (LI et al. 1982; HEIKKILA et al. 1982). The genes for six heat shock proteins all have a very similar sequence less than 66 base pairs upstream from the mRNA initiation site (PELHAM 1982). Since it appears that several of the same proteins are induced by both heat shock and Cd^{2+}, it is of interest to determine if there is a common mechanism through which these two treatments affect the same promotor, or if two separate promotors are required – one sensitive to heat and the other to Cd^{2+}. Since MT is not induced by heat shock (HAHN and LI 1982; J. SEAGRAVE 1983, unpublished work) any Cd^{2+}-sensitive promotor for these genes would most likely be different from the MT promotor.

A similar problem occurs in explaining the induction of MT by other metals, by glucocorticoids (KARIN and HERSCHMANN 1980), and (possibly indirectly through glucocorticoid mediation) by such diverse treatments as cold stress, exercise, chloroform injection (OH et al. 1978), and alkylating agents (KOTSONIS and KLAASSEN 1979; WONG and KLAASSEN 1981) in animals. Glucocorticoids are known to induce a spectrum of proteins (IVARIE and O'FARRELL 1978), and the induction mechanism is thought to be similar to other known steroid-sensitive functions (O'MALLEY and MEANS 1974). The glucocorticoid-sensitive region of the MT gene has not been identified. The loss of glucocorticoid sensitivity in amplification (MAYO and PALMITER 1982) may provide a means for approaching this problem.

IV. Non-Metallothionein Protective Mechanisms

The previous discussion of non-MT protective mechanisms (Sect. D) indicated that MT is not the only means a cell has to modify the toxic effects of Cd^{2+}. In particular, some cells have altered uptake rates (HUANG et al. 1980a; CORRIGAN and HUANG 1981, 1983). Altered Cd^{2+} accumulation has also been observed in the tissues of genetically susceptible mice compared with resistant mice (LUCIS and LUCIS 1969). CORRIGAN and HUANG (1981, 1983) have begun to characterize the altered uptake in a resistant line of CHO cells, but little is yet known about the molecular basis for this phenomenon.

At least one non-MT Cd^{2+}-binding protein appears under some circumstances (ENGER et al. 1983b; ROBERTS et al. 1979), and the possibility exists for others (ZELAZOWSKI et al. 1980; HART and KEATING 1980). In few cases have the proteins been characterized and in none has the presence of the protein (or proteins) been unambiguously related to protection. Of further interest is the suggestion that MT dimers and polymers may play a role separate from that of the MT monomer in Cd^{2+} protection (WOLKOWSKI-TYL and PRESTON 1979; ZELAZOWSKI et al. 1980).

The induction by Cd^{2+} of proteins similar to heat shock proteins (LEVINSON et al. 1980; LI et al. 1982) implies a possible role in Cd^{2+} protection analogous to the induction of thermotolerance, which correlates with the induction of the heat shock proteins (HAHN and LI 1982; LANDRY et al. 1982; LI et al. 1982). The latter phenomenon is the subject of considerable research, but is not yet well understood. Current evidence suggests that despite the specificity of the induced proteins and their remarkable evolutionary conservation, the heat shock proteins play a relatively nonspecific role in stabilizing intracellular structure and function (MINTON et al. 1982; HENLE et al. 1983). Whether the same is true for the Cd^{2+}-induced proteins, or even whether these proteins are protective, remains to be seen. Improved two-dimensional gel electrophoresis and high pressure liquid chromatography will allow greater resolution of these proteins and perhaps identification of their functions.

Another mechanism for protection may be the induction of non-protein Cd^{2+}-binding elements, such as glutathione (SEAGRAVE et al. 1983). Glutathione has been shown to bind Cd^{2+} in vitro (PERRIN and WATT 1971) and is possibly involved in vivo in biliary excretion of Cd^{2+} (CHERIAN and VOSTAL 1977); however, this mechanism is not yet proven in intracellular protection.

A final possibility for protection against Cd^{2+} would be compensatory alterations in the targets. The synthesis of enzymes inhibited by the metal might be increased, perhaps by amplification of the genes; the level of unsaturation (and thus susceptibility to peroxidation) of membrane lipids might decrease; Cd^{2+}-resistant isozymes might appear, or mutations could occur rendering them less sensitive to Cd^{2+} effects. If metal-catalyzed oxidation of cellular components is an important mechanism of toxicity, then perhaps the redox state of the cell might be altered by increasing the activity of certain enzymes, for instance, glutathione synthetase, glutathione peroxidase, glutathione reductase, or the enzymes of the pentose phosphate pathway. These possibilities are all testable and could lead not only to identification of protective mechanisms, but also to an understanding of the targets of Cd^{2+} toxicity.

V. Role of Cd in Altered Gene Expression: Possible Involvement in Carcinogenesis

Considerable controversy has developed over the question of whether Cd^{2+} is a carcinogen (SUNDERMAN 1978). Conclusive evidence for a direct role in the multistep process of carcinogenesis (BARRETT et al. 1980; CRAWFORD et al. 1983) remains to be demonstrated. However, reports to date indicate that Cd^{2+} can perturb both the structural and functional organization of the mammalian genome (DEAVEN and CAMPBELL 1980; HSIE et al. 1978). These reports have indicated in cellular systems that Cd^{2+} can cause chromosomal damage (DEAVEN and CAMPBELL 1980) and increase mutation frequency at an X-chromosome-linked genetic locus (HSIE et al. 1978). The need for further study in the area of the carcinogenic potential of Cd^{2+} (or other forms of Cd) is indicated by the properties of Cd^{2+} which suggest interactions with multiple targets involved in maintenance of chromosome structure and control of gene expression.

VI. Extracellular Factors and Cd Responses

The roles played by extracellular growth factors, and by regulatory and stress factors, in modulating Cd^{2+} uptake and in influencing cell responses via the induction of specific cadmium-binding proteins are yet to be determined. Such determinations will be best made using cultured cell systems to allow assessment of the effects of individual factors as well as of defined combinations of factors.

VII. Role for Genetic Polymorphisms in Altered Cellular Responses to Cd

The advent of recombinant DNA technology has made possible high resolution analyses of the organization of a variety of genetic loci. Further, advances in biochemical analyses have improved capabilities to detect multiple isomorphic gene products (KLAUSER et al. 1983). The combined applications of these new experimental tools will be useful in identifying genetic polymorphisms which may cause functional alterations of the gene product. The MT locus is of special interest in this context since MTs are a major factor in Cd^{2+} detoxification.

Recent studies of the organization of human MT genes provide an example of the potential significance of a role for genetic polymorphisms in altered Cd^{2+} metabolism (KARIN and RICHARDS 1982). Those studies suggested the presence of multiple MT-1 or MT-1-like genes as well as a functional MT-2 gene in human cells. Independent studies from the laboratory of KÄGI (1984 and personal communications) have demonstrated multiple MTs from human tissue. Although studies in the area of genetic polymorphism in the MT locus and the potential functional significance of such polymorphisms are at an early stage, there is a well-defined need for further analysis of the MT locus in both experimental animals which display differences in MT expression (especially among the different MTs) and in human cases of diagnosed or suspected disorders in metal metabolism potentially related to abnormal MT gene function. As a prerequisite, studies of the MT loci of the species of interest (e.g., rodents and human) including chromosomal locations of the MT genes and their linkage (HILDEBRAND et al. 1983; COX and PALMITER 1983) will be important in understanding the significance of such genetic polymorphisms. Further delineation of the relative roles of each of the functional MT genes in conferring Cd^{2+} resistance will be possible through combined application of somatic cell and molecular genetics approaches.

An additional consideration in the context of MT gene polymorphisms concerns the potentially different functional roles of the different polymorphic (e.g., in different metal-binding domains) (OTVOS and ARMITAGE 1980) MTs in regulation of metals for which Cd^{2+} is antagonistic (e.g., $Cu^{+/2+}$ and Zn^{2+}). Is it possible, for example, that altered expression (e.g., by altered gene organization) of different polymorphic MTs changes the normal regulation of the essential trace metals, thereby altering the cell's sensitivity (or resistance) to Cd^{2+}? Answers to these questions await development of appropriate cellular and molecular tools.

VIII. Tissue-Specific Regulation of Expression of Metallothioneins and Other Factors

The role of control over MT gene inducibility by methylation of the regions adjacent to and/or within the structural gene sequences in both mouse and hamster cells was discussed in Sect. C.I (DOERFLER 1983). The phenomenon of DNA methylation appears to be a general mechanism for regulation of level of specific gene expression in higher eukaryotes. DNA methylation is involved in controlling tissue-specific gene expression of several differentiated functions (see DOERFLER 1983 for review). Although MT expression has been proposed to be a "housekeeping" function, i.e., an ubiquitous function in all tissues or cells of an organism, two lines of evidence suggest a tissue-specific control of MT expression, most likely by gene-specific DNA methylation. First, MT expression is regulated by DNA methylation in regions of MT genes in cultured cells derived from both mice and hamsters. Second, certain classes of peripheral blood cells of both rodents and humans are noninducible for MT. Further experiments will be required to determine whether this noninducible state for MT expression is due to MT gene methylation. Based upon these observations, it is likely that MT inducibility is under tissue-specific control. The multiplicity of MT genes, particularly as indicated in humans (KÄGI 1984), suggests that an important area for investigation will be definition of both tissue-specific methylation and expression of the various MT-1 and MT-2 genes. Further, as other specific genes and gene products which function in modulation of Cd^{2+} toxicity are identified and isolated, their tissue-specific expression and control by methylation will be important factors to examine.

The tissue-specific modulation of genes involved in Cd^{2+} metabolism is especially important in considerations of developmental pertubations by Cd^{2+}, possibly leading to teratogenic consequences. For example, does Cd^{2+} alter developmentally programmed DNA methylation patterns of not only genes involved in metal metabolism, but possibly also of other unrelated genes? Answers to these questions are accessible through combined application of modern toxicologic and cellular and molecular biology approaches.

IX. Strategies for Derivation of New Cell Systems to Define Mechanisms of Cellular Cd Resistance

Studies of cellular Cd^{2+} resistance in cultured Chinese hamster cells in our laboratory, together with investigations of the Cd^{2+} resistance phenomenon in mouse cells, have led us to propose a general strategy for pursuing further mechanisms which modulate cellular Cd^{2+} resistance. This strategy is presented schematically in Fig. 7. The central features of this strategy involve development of cellular Cd^{2+} resistance through: (a) derepression of potentially "silent" or transcriptionally repressed genes through application of a hypomethylating agent (e.g., 5-azacytidine); and (b) enhanced expression of factors conferring Cd^{2+} resistance by stepwise increases in Cd^{2+} concentrations in the growth medium.

Since, as reviewed in Sect. D, multiple factors participate in conferring cellular Cd^{2+} resistance in mammalian cells, the proposed scheme should provide a general approach for obtaining a variety of cell sublines with enhanced phenotypic expression of one or more of the specific factors conferring Cd^{2+} resistance. Characterization of the phenotypic expression (e.g., the spectrum of cytoplasmic and nuclear proteins produced, altered metabolic pathways, cross-resistance or sensitivity to other metals, etc.) would define gene products involved in conferring a resistance phenotype. Identification of the gene products would be the first step in isolating the genes involved in the Cd^{2+} responses.

In the proposed scheme for selection of Cd^{2+}-resistant cell lines, several paths for the selection process are indicated. The rationale for use of these multiple approaches is that different genes or sets of genes may become differentially activated and/or enhanced in level of expression. For example, pathway B in Fig. 7

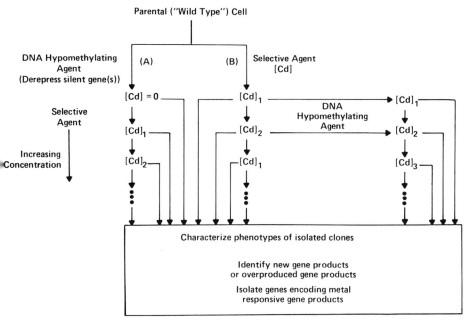

Fig. 7. General strategies for isolation of Cd^r variants. Multiple procedures are proposed for identifying Cd^{2+}-responsive gene products. In one pathway, treatment of the parental "wild-type" cell with the hypomethylating agent 5-azacytidine may cause derepression of genes involved in Cd^{2+} response. Cells which have such derepressed genes can be selected by continuing Cd^{2+}-selective pressure and cloning of isolated cells (A). To increase the efficiency of this response(s), the concentration of Cd^{2+} can be increased in a stepwise manner (*vertical arrows*) to select more responsive cells. Alternately, parental cells can be selected directly for increased Cd^{2+} resistance (B, *vertical arrows*) and further treated with 5-azacytidine (*horizontal arrows, C*) to derepress additional genetic mechanisms for response to Cd^{2+} toxicity. It should be noted that, although this is only a proposed scheme, two portions (A and B) of the scheme have been demonstrated to be useful in analysis of Cd^{2+} resistance (see text)

indicates direct selection of Cd^{2+}-resistant cells followed by stepwise increases in Cd^{2+} concentration to enhance expression of resistance factors. In addition to enhancement of expression of these specific resistance factors, an attempt to activate additional repressed cellular Cd^{2+} resistance factors can be made using a hypomethylating agent as indicated in pathway C (Fig. 7).

The usefulness of this scheme and modifications of this strategy are currently being evaluated in examining the multiple Cd^{2+} resistance factors involved in conferring resistance to both cultured human cells and variants of CHO cells. In this context, it should be reiterated that while MTs play a major role in Cd^{2+} detoxification, other factors are also implicated. In the case of certain human cells, it should be noted that cell lines have been identified and characterized that have a Cd^{2+}-sensitive phenotype, but express MT at a high level (see Sect. B.I). Such cells will provide ideal systems for activation of other cellular responses which operate in conferring resistance to Cd^{2+}.

X. Variation in Human Response

Preliminary studies on the Cd^{2+} responses of mononuclear cells cultured from the peripheral blood of normal (healthy) humans showed only small variations. However, the high level of exposure experienced by humans living in industrialized countries (which results in Cd^{2+} burdens one-tenth to one-half of those known to cause overt toxic effects in some individuals) may contraindicate detecting Cd^{2+} sensitivity in *healthy* adults. The study should be extended, using cells cultured from the blood of patients presenting with types of kidney dysfunction reflecting Cd^{2+} toxicity, i.e., with low molecular weight proteinuria and specifically enhanced excretion of β_2-microglobulin. Such a study would better delimit the possibility of cryptic Cd^{2+} toxicity in humans owing to reduced protective response to average Cd^{2+} exposure levels.

G. Summary

Based upon current data and indications of innovative experimental research approaches to be brought to bear on present day problems, the future for this research area is at once both exciting and highly promising. Within the next few years, a great deal of information should be generated that will increase greatly our knowledge and understanding of both trace element metabolism and eukaryotic gene regulation.

References

Alt FW, Kellems R, Bertino J, Schimke RT (1978) Selective multiplication of dihydrofolate reductase genes in methotrexate resistant variants of cultured murine cells. J Biol Chem 253:1357–1370

Asokan P, Dixit R, Mukhtar H, Murti CRK (1981) Effect of cadmium on hepatic mixed-function oxidases during the early development of rats: Possible protective role of metallothionein. Biochem Pharmacol 30:3095–3097

Bakka A, Rugstad HE (1981) Uptake and egress of cadmium in cultures of cadmium-resistant and the corresponding "wild-type" cells. Acta Pharmacol Toxicol 48:81–86

Barrett JC, Crawford BD, Ts'o POP (1980) The role of somatic mutation in a multistage model of carcinogenesis. In: Mishra N, Dunkel V, Mehlman M (eds) Mammalian cell transformation by chemical carcinogens, vol I. Advances in modern environmental toxicology. Senate, Princeton, New Jersey, pp 467–501

Bazzell KL, Coleman RL, Nordquist RE (1979) Induction of metallothionein-like protein in human breast tumor cells. Toxicol Appl Pharmacol 50:199–205

Beach LR, Palmiter RD (1981) Amplification of the metallothionein I gene in cadmium-resistant mouse cells. Proc Natl Acad Sci USA 78:2110–2114

Beisel WR, Pekarek RS, Wannemacher RW Jr (1976) Homeostatic mechanisms affecting plasma zinc levels in acute stress. In: Prasad S, Oberleas D (eds) Trace elements in human health and disease, vol I. Acadmic, New York, pp 87–106

Bettger WJ, O'Dell BL (1981) Minireview: a critical physiological role of zinc in the structure and function of biomembranes. Life Sci 28:1425–1438

Bozelka BE, Burkholder PM (1982) Inhibition of mixed leukocyte culture responses in cadmium-treated mice. Environ Res 27:421–432

Bozelka BE, Burkholder PM, Chang LW (1978) Cadmium, a metallic inhibitor of antibody-mediated immunity in mice. Environ Res 17:390–402

Brinster RL, Chen HY, Warren R, Sarthy A, Palmiter RD (1982) Regulation of metallothionein-thymidine kinase fusion plasmids injected into mouse eggs. Nature 296:39–42

Burger MM, Weber R (eds) (1982) Embryonic development, part A. Genetic aspects. IX Congress of the International Society of Developmental Biologists, Basel, Switzerland. Liss, New York

Chan JYH, Ruchirawat M, Lapeyre J-N, Becker FF (1982) In vitro inhibition of DNA methylase (DMase) by direct acting carcinogens and the protective ability of thiol reducing agents. Fed Proc 41:685

Chen DJ-C, Hildebrand CE, Walters RA, Griffith JK, Enger MD (1981) Somatic cell hybridization studies of the mechanism of cadmium resistance in Chinese hamster cells. J Cell Biol 91:383A

Cherian MG (1980) The synthesis of metallothionein and cellular adaptation to metal toxicity in primary rat kidney epithelial cell cultures. Toxicology 17:225–231

Cherian MG (1981) Comparative studies on mechanism of cellular toxicity of cadmium-metallothionein and cadmium chloride in rat kidney epithelial cell culture. Fed Proc 40:714

Cherian MG (1982) Studies of the toxicity of metallothionein in rat kidney epithelial cell culture. In: Foulkes EC (ed) Biological roles of metallothionein. Elsevier/North-Holland, New York, pp 193–202

Cherian MG, Vostal JJ (1977) Biliary excretion of cadmium in rat. 1. Dose dependent bilary excretion and the form of cadmium in the bile. J Toxicol Environ Health 2:945–954

Chin B, Lesowitz GS, Bernstein IA, Dinman BD (1978) A cellular model for studying accommodation to environmental stresses: A protective response to subtoxic exposure to cadmium. Environ Res 16:423–431

Chowdhury P, Lousia DB, Chang LW, Rayford PL (1982) Cadmium induced pulmonary injury in mouse: A relationship with serum antitrypsin activity. Bull Environ Contam Toxicol 28:446–451

Compere S, Palmiter RD (1981) DNA methylation controls the inducibility of the mouse metallothionein I gene in lymphoid cells. Cell 25:233–240

Corrigan AJ, Huang PC (1981) Cellular uptake of cadmium and zinc. Biol Trace Element Res 3:197–216

Corrigan AJ, Huang PC (1983) Cadmium and zinc flux in wild-type and cadmium-resistant CHO cells. Biol Trace Element Res 5:25–33

Cox DR, Palmiter RD (1983) The metallothionein-I gene maps to mouse chromosome 8: Implications for human Menkes' disease. Hum Genet 64:61–64

Crawford BD, Barrett JC, Ts'o POP (1983) Neoplastic conversion of preneoplastic Syrian hamster cells: rate estimation by fluctuation analysis. Mol Cell Biol 3:931–945

Deaven LL, Campbell EW (1980) Factors affecting the induction of chromosomal aberrations by cadmium in Chinese hamster cells. Cytogenet Cell Genet 26:251–260

Diamond EM, Jedeikin A, Kench JE (1973) Purification of tryptophan oxygenase and its interaction with cadmium. Biochem Biophys Res Commun 52:679–686

Dierickx PJ (1982) In vitro inhibition of soluble glutathione S-transferases from rat liver by heavy metals. Enzyme 27:25–32

Doerfler W (1983) DNA methylation and gene activity. Ann Rev Biochem 52:93–124

Drysdale JW, Munro HN (1966) Regulation of synthesis and turnover of ferritin in rat liver. J Biol Chem 241:3630–3637

Durnam DM, Palmiter RD (1981) Transcriptional regulation of the mouse metallothionein I gene by heavy metals. J Biol Chem 256:5712–5716

Eaton DL, Stacey NH, Wong K-L, Klaassen CD (1980) Dose response effects of various metal ions on rat liver metallothionein, glutathione, heme oxygenase and cytochrome P-450. Toxicol Appl Pharmacol 55:393–402

Engel DW, Fowler BA (1979) Factors influencing cadmium accumulation and its toxicity to marine organisms. Environ Health Perspect 28:81–88

Enger MD, Campbell EW, Barrington HL (1976) Stimulation of informosomal RNA synthesis in cultured Chinese hamster cells exposed to low levels of cadmium. FEBS Letters 70:43–47

Enger MD, Hildebrand CE, Jones M, Barrington H (1978) Altered RNA metabolism in cultured mammalian cells exposed to low levels of Cd^{2+}: correlation of the effects with Cd^{2+} uptake and intracellular distribution. In: Mahlum D, Sikov MR, Hackett PL, Andrew FD (eds) Developmental toxicology of energy-related pollutants. DOE symposium Series 47

Enger MD, Campbell EW, Ratliff RL, Tobey RA, Hildebrand CE, Kissane RJ (1979a) Cadmium-induced alterations in RNA metabolism in cultures of Chinese hamster cells sensitive to and resistant to the cytotoxic effects of cadmium. J Toxicol Environ Health 5:711–728

Enger MD, Rall LB, Hildebrand CE (1979b) Thionein gene expression in Cd^{2+}-variants of the CHO cell: correlation of thionein synthesis rates with translatable mRNA levels during induction, deinduction, and superinduction. Nucleic Acids Res 7:271–288

Enger MD, Griffith BB, Hildebrand CE (1980a) Differential patterns of thionein synthesis regulation in Cd^{2+}-resistant CHO variants. J Cell Biol 87:270a

Enger MD, Rall LB, Walters RA, Hildebrand CE (1980b) Regulation of induced thionein gene expression in cultured mammalian cells: effects of protein synthesis inhibition on translatable thionein mRNA levels in regulatory variants of the CHO cell. Biochem Biophys Res Commun 93:343–348

Enger MD, Ferzoco LT, Tobey RA, Hildebrand CE (1981) Cadmium resistance correlated with cadmium uptake and thionein binding in CHO cell variants Cd^r20F4 and Cd^r30F9. J Toxicol Environ Health 7:675–690

Enger MD, Hildebrand CE, Griffith JK, Walters RA (1983a) Molecular and somatic cell genetics analysis of metal metabolism in cultured cells. In: Rennert OM, Chan W (eds) Metabolism of trace metals in man: developmental biology and genetic implications. CRC Press, Boca Raton, pp 7–24

Enger MD, Hildebrand CE, Stewart CC (1983b) Cd^{2+} responses of cultured human blood cells. Toxicol Appl Pharmacol 69:214–224

Enger MD, Hildebrand CE, Walters RA, Seagrave JC, Barham SS, Hoagland HC (1984a) Molecular and somatic cell genetic analysis of metal resistance mechanisms in mammalian cells. In: Tashjian AH Jr (ed) Cellular approaches to understanding mechanisms of toxicity. Harvard University Press, pp 38–62

Enger MD, Tesmer JG, Hanners JL, Barham SS, Alley MC, Uhl CB, Tarara JE (1984b) Some cell lines derived from human cancers are cadmium-sensitive but produce metallothionein (in press)

Evans RM, Patierno SR, Wang DS, Cantoni O, Costa M (1983) Growth inhibition and metallothionein induction in cadmium-resistant cells by essential and non-essential metals. Molec Pharmacol 24:77–83

Failla ML, Cousins RJ, Mascenik MJ (1979) Cadmium accumulation and metabolism by rat liver parenchymal cells in primary monolayer culture. Biochim Biophys Acta 583:63–72

Foulkes EC (1982) Role of metallothionein in transport of heavy metals. In: Foulkes EC (ed) Biological roles of metallothionein. Elsevier/North-Holland, New York

Gick GG, McCarty KS Sr (1982) Amplification of the metallothionein-I gene in cadmium- and zinc-resistant Chinese hamster ovary cells. J Biol Chem 257:9049–9053

Gick G, McCarty KS Jr, McCarty KS Sr (1981) The role of metallothionein synthesis in cadmium- and zinc-resistant CHO-K1M cells. Exp Cell Res 132:23–30

Gilbert HF (1982) Biological disulfides: the third messenger? J Biol Chem 257:12086–12091

Gilliavod N, Leonard A (1975) Mutagenicity tests with cadmium in the mouse. Toxicology 5:43–47

Griffith BB, Walters RA, Enger MD, Hildebrand CE, Griffith JK (1983) cDNA cloning and nucleotide sequence comparison of Chinese hamster metallothionein I and II mRNAs. Nucleic Acids Res 11:901–910

Griffith JK, Enger MD, Hildebrand CE, Walters RA (1981) Differential induction by cadmium of a low-complexity ribonucleic acid class in cadmium-resistant and cadmium-sensitive mammalian cells. Biochemistry 20:4755–4761

Hahn G, Li GC (1982) Thermotolerance and heat shock proteins in mammalian cells. Radiation Res 92:452–457

Hart BA, Keating RF (1980) Cadmium accumulation and distribution in human lung fibroblasts. Chem Biol Interact 29:67–83

Hata A, Tsunoo H, Nakajima H, Shintaku K, Kimura M (1980) Acute cadmium intoxication in inbred mice: a study on strain differences. Chem Biol Interact 32:29–39

Hayden TL, Turner JE, Williams MW, Cook JS, Hsie AW (1982) A model for cadmium transport and distribution in CHO cells. Comput Biomed Res 15:97–110

Heikkila JJ, Schultz GA, Iatrou K, Gedamu L (1982) Expression of a set of fish genes following heat or metal ion exposure. J Biol Chem 257:12000–12005

Henle KJ, Peck JW, Higashikubo R (1983) Protection against heat-induced cell killing by polyols in vitro. Cancer Res 43:1624–1627

Hidalgo HA, Koppa V, Bryan SE (1978) Induction of cadmium-thionein in isolated rat liver cells. Biochem J 170:219–225

Hildebrand CE, Cram LS (1979) Distribution of cadmium in human blood cultured in low levels of $CdCl_2$: accumulation of Cd in lymphocytes and preferential binding to metallothionein. Proc Soc Exp Biol Med 161:438–443

Hildebrand CE, Enger MD (1980) Regulation of Cd^{2+}/Zn^{2+}-stimulated metallothionein synthesis during induction, deinduction, and superinduction. Biochemistry 19:5850–5857

Hildebrand CE, Tobey RA, Campbell EW, Enger MD (1979) A cadmium-resistant variant of the Chinese hamster (CHO) cell with increased metallothionein induction capacity. Exp Cell Res 124:237–246

Hildebrand CE, Griffith JK, Tobey RA, Walters RA, Enger MD (1982) Molecular mechanism of Cd detoxification in cadmium resistant cultured cells: role of metallothionein and other inducible factors. In: Foulkes EC (ed) The biological role of metallothionein. Elsevier/North-Holland, New York, pp 279–303

Hildebrand CE, Crawford BD, Enger MD, Griffith BB, Griffith JK, Hanners JL, Jackson PJ, Longmire JL, Munk AC, Tesmer JG, Walters RA, Stallings RL (1983) Coordinate amplification of metallothionein I and II gene sequences in cadmium resistant CHO variants. In: Hamer D, Rosenberg M (eds) Gene expression, vol VIII. UCLA Symposium on cellular and molecular biology. Liss, New York, pp 467–479

Hsie AW, O'Neill JP, SanSebastian JR, Couch DB, Fuscoe JC, Sun WNC, Brimer PA, Machanoff R, Riddle JC, Forbes NL, Hsie MH (1978) Mutagenicity of carcinogens: a study of 101 agents in a quantitative mammalian cell mutation system, CHO/HGPRT. Fed Proc 37:1384

Huang PC, Corrigan A, Smith B, Bohdan P, Moreadith R (1980a) Cadmium resistance in CHO mutants. Fed Proc 39:1680

Huang PC, Smith B, Bohdan P, Corrigan A (1980b) Effect of zinc on cadmium influx and toxicity in cultured CHO cells. Biol Trace Element Res 2:211–220

Hunt DM, Mhlanga T (1983) Genetic studies on metallothionein synthesis in the mouse: the induction of metallothionein by cadmium in inbred strains. Biochem Genet 21:609–625

Ivarie RD, O'Farrell PH (1978) The glucocorticoid domain: steroid mediated changes in the rate of synthesis of rat hepatoma proteins. Cell 13:41–55

Jacobsen KB, Turner JE (1980) The interaction of cadmium and certain other metal ions with proteins and nucleic acids. Toxicology 16:1–37

Jones PA, Taylor SM (1980) Cellular differentiation, cytidine analogs, and DNA methylation. Cell 20:85–93

Jones RH, Williams RL, Jones AM (1971) Effects of heavy metal on the immune response. Preliminary findings for cadmium in rats. Proc Soc Exp Biol Med 137:1231–1236

Kägi JHR, Vasak M, Lerch K, Gilg DEO, Hunziken P, Bernhard WR, Good M (1984) Structure of mammalian metallothionein. Environ Health Perspect 54:93–103

Karin M, Herschman HR (1979) Dexamethasone stimulation of metallothionein synthesis in HeLa cell cultures. Science 204:176–177

Karin M, Herschman HR (1980) Characterization of the metallothioneins induced in HeLa cells by dexamethasone and zinc. Eur J Biochem 107:395–401

Karin M, Holtgreve H (1983) Regulation of the human metallothionein II_A gene after transfection into rat fibroblasts. J Cell Biochem Suppl 7A:114

Karin M, Richards RI (1982) Human metallothionein genes – primary structure of the metallothionein-II gene and a related processed gene. Nature 299:797–802

Karin M, Andersen RD, Herschman HR (1981) Induction of metallothionein mRNA in HeLa cells by dexamethasone and by heavy metals. Eur J Biochem 118:527–531

Kiremidjian-Schumacher L, Stotzky G, Dickstein RA, Schwartz J (1981a) Influence of cadmium, lead, and zinc on the ability of guinea pig macrophages to interact with macrophage migration inhibitory factor. Environ Res 24:106–116

Kiremidjian-Schumacher L, Stotzky G, Likhite V, Schwartz J, Dickstein RA (1981b) Influence of cadmium, lead, and zinc on the ability of sensitized guinea pig lymphocytes to interact with specific antigen and to produce lymphokine. Environ Res 24:96–105

Kjellstrom T, Nordberg GF (1978) A kinetic model of cadmium metabolism in the human being. Environ Res 16:248–269

Klauser S, Kägi JHR, Wilson KJ (1983) Characterization of isoprotein patterns in tissue extracts and isolated samples of metallothioneins by reverse-phase high-pressure liquid chromatography. Biochem J 209:71–80

Kobayashi S, Kimura M (1980) Different inducibility of metallothionein in various mammalian cells in vitro. Toxicol Lett 5:357–362

Kojima Y, Kägi JHR (1978) Metallothionein. Trends Biochem Sci 3:90–93

Koller LD (1973) Immunosuppression produced by lead, cadmium, and mercury. Am J Vet Res 34:1457–1458

Kotsonis FN, Klaassen Cd (1979) The relationship of metallothionein to the toxicity of cadmium after prolonged oral administration to rats. Toxicol Appl Pharmacol 46:39–54

Landry J, Bernier D, Chrètien P, Nicole LM, Tanguay RM, Marceau N (1982) Synthesis and degradation of heat shock proteins during development and decay of thermotolerance. Cancer Res 42:2457–2461

Lauwerys R (1979) Cadmium in man. In: Webb M (ed) The chemistry, biochemistry and biology of cadmium. Elsevier/North-Holland, New York, pp 433–456

Lawrence DA (1981) Heavy metal modulation of lymphocyte activities. Toxicol Appl Pharmacol 57:439–451

Levinson W, Oppermann H, Jackson J (1980) Transition series metals and sulfhydryl reagents induce the synthesis of four proteins in eukaryotic cells. Biochim Biophys Acta 606:170–180

Lewis CD, Laemmli UK (1982) Higher order metaphase chromosome structure: Evidence for metalloprotein interactions. Cell 29:171–181

Li GC, Shrieve DC, Werb Z (1982) Correlations between synthesis of heat shock proteins and development of tolerance to heat and to adriamycin in Chinese hamster fibroblasts: heat shock and other inducers. In: Schlesinger MJ, Ashburner M, Tissieres A (ed) Heat shock from bacteria to man. Cold Spring Harbor Laboratory, New York, pp 395–404

Loose LD, Silkworth JB, Warrington D (1977) Cadmium-induced depression of the respiratory burst in mouse pulmonary alveolar macrophages, peritoneal macrophages and polymorphonuclear neutrophils. Biochem Biophys Res Comm 79:326–332

Lucis OJ, Lucis R (1969) Distribution of cadmium 109 and zinc 65 in mice of inbred strains. Arch Environ Health 19:334–336

Lucis OJ, Shaikh ZA, Embil JA Jr (1970) Cadmium as a trace element and cadmium binding components in human cells. Experientia 26:1109–1110

Maines MD, Chung AS, Kulty RK (1982) The inhibition of testicular heme oxygenase activity by cadmium. J Biol Chem 257:14116–14121

Maiti I, Mbikay M, Marengo C, Thirion JP (1982) Immunological characterization of metallothioneins in mouse LMTK cells and in a variant resistant to cadmium. J Cell Physiol 112:35–41

Malcolm D (1972) Potential carcinogenic effect of cadmium in animals and man. Ann Occup Hyg 15:33–36

Marx JL (1983) Immunoglobulin genes have enhancers. Science 221:733–734

Mayo KE, Palmiter RD (1981) Glucocorticoid regulation of metallothionein-I mRNA synthesis in cultured mouse cells. J Biol Chem 256:2621–2624

Mayo KE, Palmiter RD (1982) Glucocorticoid regulation of mouse metallothionein I gene is selectively lost following amplification of the gene. J Biol Chem 257:3061–3067

Mayo KE, Warren R, Palmiter RD (1982) The mouse metallothionein-I gene is transcriptionally regulated by cadmium following transfection into human or mouse cells. Cell 29:99–108

Meisler M, Orlowski C, Gross E, Bloor JH (1979) Cadmium metabolism in cdm/cdm mice. Biochem Gen 17:731–736

Minkel DT, Poulsen K, Weilgus S, Shaw CF III, Petering DH (1980) On the sensitivity of metallothioneins to oxidation during isolation. Biochem J 191:475–485

Minton KW, Karmin P, Hahn GM, Minton AP (1982) Nonspecific stabilization of stress-susceptible proteins by stress-resistant proteins: a model for the biological role of heat shock proteins. Proc Natl Acad Sci 79:7107–7111

Muller L, Ohnesorge FK (1982) Different response of liver parenchymal cells from starved and fed rats to cadmium. Toxicology 25:141–150

Nagai Y, Sato M, Sasaki M (1982) Effect of cadmium administration upon urinary excretion of hydroxylysine and hydroxyproline in the rat. Toxicol Appl Pharmacol 63:188–193

Nordberg M, Kojima Y (1979) Metallothionein and other low molecular weight metal-binding proteins. In: Kägi JHR, Nordberg M (eds) Metallothionein. Birkhäuser, Boston, pp 41–135

Oh SH, Deagen JT, Whanger PD, Weswig PH (1978) Biological function of metallothionein V. Its induction in rats by various stresses. Am J Physiol 234:E282–285

Ohsawa M, Kawai K (1981) Cytological shift in lymphocytes induced by cadmium in mice and rats. Environ Res 24:192–200

O'Malley BW, Means AR (1974) Female steroid hormones and target cell nuclei. Science 183:610–620

Otvos JD, Armitage IM (1980) Structure of the metal clusters in rabbit liver metallothionein. Proc Natl Acad Sci USA 77:7094–7098

Ozawa K, Sato A, Okada H (1976) Differential susceptibility of L cells in the exponential and stationary phases to cadmium chloride. Jpn J Pharmacol 26:347–351

Pelham HRB (1982) A regulatory upstream promotor element in the Drosophila hsp 70 heat-shock gene. Cell 30.517–528

Perrin DD, Watt AE (1971) Complex formation of zinc and cadmium with glutathione. Biochim Biophys Acta 230:96–104

Petering DH, Petering HG (1979) A molecular basis for metal toxicity. In: Bhatnagar RS (ed) Molecular basis of environmental toxicity. Ann Arbor Science, Ann Arbor, Michigan

Piscator M (1964) On cadmium in normal human kidneys together with a report on the isolation of metallothionein from livers of cadmium-exposed rabbits. Nord Hyg Tidskr 45:76–82

Razin A, Riggs AD (1980) DNA methylation and gene function. Science 210:604–610

Roberts KS, Cryer A, Kay J, de LG Solbe JF (1979) A high molecular weight cadmium-binding fraction isolated from the liver cytosol of trout exposed to environmentally relevant concentrations of the metal. Biochem Soc Trans 7:650–651

Röhr G, Bauchinger M (1976) Chromosome analyses in cell cultures of the Chinese hamster after application of cadmium sulphate. Mutat Res 40:125–130

Rudd CJ, Herschman HR (1978) Metallothionein accumulation in response to cadmium in a clonal rat liver cell line. Toxicol Appl Pharmacol 44:1–10

Rugstad HE, Norseth T (1975) Cadmium resistance and content of cadmium-binding protein in cultured human cells. Nature 257:136–137

Samarawickrama GP (1979) Biological effects of cadmium in mammals. In: Webb M (ed) the chemistry, biochemistry and biology of cadmium. Elsevier/North-Holland, New York

Schimke RT (ed) (1982) Gene amplification. Cold Spring Harbor Laboratory, Cold Spring Harbor, New York

Sciortino CV, Failla ML, Bullis DB (1982) Identification of metallothionein in parenchymal and non-parenchymal liver cells of the adult rat. Biochem J 204:509–514

Seagrave JC, Hildebrand CE, Enger MD (1983) Effects of cadmium on glutathione metabolism in cadmium sensitive and cadmium resistant Chinese hamster cell lines. Toxicology 29:101–107

Senear AW, Palmiter RD (1982) Expression of the mouse metallothionein-I gene alters the nuclease hypersensitivity of its 5' regulatory region. Cold Spring Harbor Symp Quant Biol XLVII:539–547

Shapiro SG, Cousins RJ (1980) Induction of rat liver metallothionein mRNA and its distribution between free and membrane-bound polyribosomes. Biochem J 190:755–764

Squibb KS, Cousins RJ (1977) Synthesis of metallothionein in a polysomal cell-free system. Biochem Biophys Res Commun 75:806–812

Squibb KS, Cousins RJ, Feldman SL (1977) Control of zinc-thionein synthesis in rat liver. Biochem J 164:223–228

Stacey NH, Kappus H (1982) Heavy metal toxicity and lipid peroxidation in isolated rat hepatocytes. Naunyn Schmiedebergs Arch Pharmacol [Suppl] 319:R27

Stacey NH, Klaassen CD (1980) Cadmium uptake by isolated rat hepatocytes. Toxicol Appl Pharm 55:448–455

Sunderman FW (1978) Carcinogenic effects of metals. Fed Proc 37:40–46

Taylor BA, Heiniger HJ, Meier H (1973) Genetic analysis of resistance to cadmium-induced testicular damage in mice. Proc Soc Exp Biol Med 143:629–633

Walters RA, Enger MD, Hildebrand CE, Griffith JK (1981) Genes coding for metal induced synthesis of RNA sequences are differentially amplified and regulated in mammalian cells. In: Brown D, Fox CF (eds) Developmental biology using purified genes. ICN-UCLA Symposium on molecular and cellular biology, vol XXIII. Academic, New York, pp 229–237

Watanabe T, Schimada T, Endo A (1979) Mutagenic effects of cadmium on mammalian oocyte chromosomes. Mutat Res 67:349–356

Webb M (1975) The metallothioneins. Biochem Soc Trans 3:632–634

Webb M, Vershoyle RD (1976) An investigation of the role of metallothioneins in protection against the acute toxicity of the cadmium ion. Biochem Pharmacol 25:673–679

Wolkowsky-Tyl R, Preston SF (1979) The interaction of cadmium-binding proteins and progesterone in cadmium-induced tissue and embryo toxicity. Teratology 20:341–352

Wong KL, Klaassen CD (1981) Relationship between liver and kidney levels of glutathione and metallothionein in rats. Toxicology 19:39–47

Zelazowski AJ, Szymańska JA, Cierniewski CS (1980) Immunological properties of low molecular-weight proteins binding heavy metals in rat kidney and liver. Chem Biol Interact 33:115–125

Subject Index

Absorption
  chemical factors   114
  dermal   76
  lungs   75
Absorption, intestinal   76
  age   91
  bile   91, 93
  brush border   78
  calcium-bindung protein   88
  and copper   89
  determinants   91
  dietary status   91, 94
  duodenum   77, 81
  fractional   75–76
  gastrointestinal secretions   93
  gestation   92
  ileum   77
  inhibition by milk   80
  interaction between metals   84, 89
  and iron   89, 92
  jejunum   77–78
  kinetic model   78–79, 81–83
  kinetic model, calcium effect   79, 87–88
  lactation   92
  membrane surface charges   90
  metallothionein   83, 94
  methods of study   79
  mucosal binding sites   90
  mucus   93
  in neonates   89, 92
  physiological variable   91, 92
  pinocytosis   91, 92
  and polylysine   90
  saturability   78, 83
  sex   91
  Vitamin D   87
  and zinc   85–86
Abundance in nature   1
Accumulation   183, 200, 202, 299
  background levels   57
  food chain crops   33, 57, 62
  liver   299
  plants   49, 53
  plants, metal interactions   52

  renal cortex   127
  vegetables   50
Acetyl choline   198
Adenosine triphosphate   216
ATPase activity   198
Aminoaciduria   156, 184
Analysis for cadmium   136–137, 140–141, 157, 160, 165–166, 181
Analytical methods   3
  atomic absorption spectrometry   4
  diethyl dithiocarbamate extraction   13
  dithizone extraction   12
  electrophoresis   179, 182
  isotope dilution   28
  neutron activation   26, 141, 143, 166, 181
  plasma emission spectrometry   14
  polarography   16
  x-ray fluorescence   23, 143
Anemia   147, 163
Animal disease model   110
  bone metabolism   111
Anosmia   146, 163
Antagonists
  calcium   137, 203, 212, 213
  cysteine   212, 226, 237
  glutathione   212
α-Antitrypsin   149
Atmospheric deposition   44

Biological half-life   77, 123, 143, 181, 316
Blood pressure   160
Body burden   75
  estimation   122, 141, 143, 156–157, 166, 181
Bronchitis   149
Brush border
  role in intestinal absorption   83, 86
  membrane vesicles   84

Cadmium-metallothionein   282, 284, 310–311, 313, 366
  effect on RNA polymerase activity   312
  toxicity   312
Cadmium oxide   203, 218

Cadmium-zinc-metallothionein   310–311
Calcium
  cardiac muscle contraction   204
  competitive effects   203, 208, 213
  inhibition of absorption   79, 87, 88
  intake   147
  intracellular levels   196
  mechanisms of cellular reaction   196
  renal stone content   185
  sarcolemma   196
  sarcoplasmic reticulum   196
  sequestration   196
  transport   216
Calciuria   147
Cancer
  lung   161
  prostate   161
Carcinogenicity   161, 372, 386
Cardiac function   220, 226, 228
Cardiac muscle
  phosphorylation reactions   208
Cardiodepressive action   200
Cardiotoxicity   205, 207, 213, 217, 221,
  240, 351–352, 354–358
Cardiovascular disease   159–160, 202
Cardiovascular system   159, 195, 202
Cells
  Chinese hamster ovary   364, 367, 376,
  378, 381–382
Cellular binding sites
  for essential metals   196
Cerebrovascular disease   149, 160
Chelating agents   323
  cysteine   323
  2,3-dimercaptopropanol   323
  1,2,3-trimercaptopropane   323
Chelation
  by antihypertensive drugs   201
Chemical properties   1
Cholinergic nerve fibers   198
Chromosomal aberrations   163
Cigarette smoke   75
Citrate   186
Complex formation   1
Concentrations
  ambient air   33
  cigarette smoke   33, 140
  contaminated soils   41
  domestic water supplies   33
  food chain crops   54
  fresh waters   46
  lithosphere   35
  marine sediments   35
  natural soils   39, 52
  ocean surface waters   46
  pH effects on soil   47
  rock   35

Consumption
  alloys   38
  batteries   36
  chemicals   38
  electroplating   36
  miscellaneous uses   38
  pigments   36
  stabilizers   36
Copper   351, 353, 356
Copper-metallothionein   311, 316
Creatinine clearance   155–156, 159
Critical concentration   122, 181
  non-metallothionein cadmium   127
  renal cortex   123, 126, 165–166
Cytotoxicity   366, 368, 373, 379–380

Daily intake   77, 78
  average, to age 50   53
Detoxification   298, 364
Dietary intake   60, 61, 135–136, 298
Distribution   142
DNA
  methylation   365, 375–376, 388
Dose relationships   164

Electrophoresis   153, 179, 182, 184,
  188–189
Electrocardiogramm   225–227, 230–232
Emphysema   76, 146–149, 164
Enterohepatic circulation   80
Environmental pollution
  Belgium   105
  blood pressure   111
  cerebrovascular disease   112
  clinical symptoms   109
  critical levels in rice   107
  England   105
  German Democratic Republic   105
  heart disease   112
  Holland   105
  Japan   106–110
  reversibility, renal effects   112
Epidemiology   200
Essential metals   196
Excretion   143
  bile   75–76, 289
  chelating agent effect   75–76
  feces   75–76
  intestinal secretion   75–76
  kidney   75
  metallothionein effect   289
  urine   120
Exposure   215, 219–220
  blood flow   201
  corticosterone levels   199
  environmental   135, 156
  human   135, 140, 143, 220

occupational   109, 137, 200, 218, 220
pulmonary   75
safety margin   77
testicular necrosis   201

Ferritin
  serum   140
  urine   154
Fumes, metal   144, 148, 164

Genes
  amplification   365, 379–380
  expression   371, 375, 376–377, 384, 386
Glomerular filtrate   180, 182, 184, 187,
  189–190
Glomerular function   153–155, 187
Glucose intolerance   199
Glucosuria   156, 180, 184, 189
Glutathione   382, 384, 386
Glutathione peroxidase   352, 354–358

Heart   204, 207, 228, 230, 351, 353–354,
  356–358
  atrial muscle   210, 212
  cell culture   210
  contractile function   200
  electrical stimulation   212
  force-frequency relationship   212
  metabolism   209
  papillary muscle   210, 212
  relaxation   212
  rhythmicity   200
  tension   212
  vascular effects   234, 240
  vasoconstriction   238
Humoral effectors   198
Hypertension   159–161, 201, 202, 244, 246
Hypoglycemia   199

Immune response   154, 341, 348
  antibody synthesis   342
  host resistance   341, 348
Immunity   339
  cell-mediated immune reactions   399,
  344
  immune complex binding   346
Inhalation   140, 144
Intake   164, 167–168
Interferon   340
Interleukin   340
Intestinal secretion   81
Iron storage   140
Isometallothioneins   282 283, 284, 285,
  298
  metal clusters   284
  structure   298

Itai-Itai disease   87, 92, 101, 146–147, 186
  osteomalacia   109
  renal dysfunction   109

Kidney   154, 159, 164–165, 180–181, 351,
  354, 358
Kupffer cells   346
  complement receptors   346

Laminin   154
Lethal concentrations   145
Lungs   140, 164
  cancer   149
  fibrosis   145, 148, 164
  obstructive syndrome   148, 164
Lymphocytes   141, 163
  B-Lymphocytes   339–340, 342, 344
  T-Lymphocytes   339–340, 344

Macrophages   339
  activating factor   340
  function   346
  inhibiting factor   340
  oxidative burst   347
Maximum permissible intake   77, 128
Metabolism   140, 281 ff., 363, 383
Metal coordination complexes   284
Metallothionein   83, 117, 141–142, 181,
  183, 281 ff., 316, 354, 358, 364, 373, 375,
  379–388
  analysis for metal content   285, 296, 300
  antibody formation   286
  detoxification of cadmium   298, 309
  effects on kidney   310
  effects on zinc   302–303
  exogenous   310
  expression   364, 376–378, 384
  function   315
  genes   365–367, 375–379, 387–388
  induced synthesis   287, 296, 298, 300,
    302, 304, 314, 364, 388
  mRNA   378–379
  radioimmunoassay   286, 294
  sex differences   299
  structure   283–284
  synthesis   364–365, 378, 381, 383
  tissue content   294–295, 298
  transport effects   313–314
Microglobulin, β_2-   105, 125, 153–158,
  160, 165, 167, 180, 182–183, 187–189
Monocytes   339
Mortality   108, 149, 156–159, 163, 202
Mucosal binding sites   83
Municipal sewage sludge   42
  disposal   42
  recycling   42
Mutagenesis   371–372

Myocardium   203–205, 218, 220, 222
Myoglobin   183
Myosin ATPase activity   218

Natural killer cells   339
Nephropathy   157–158, 179
   see also Urinary proteins
   diagnosis   188
   prevention   190
   prognosis   189
   phosphaturia   156
   tubular acidosis   186
   tubular dysfunction   158, 179, 182–183,
   187
Nervous system   163
Neural effectors   198
Nutritional factors   140, 147

Osteomalacia   109, 146–147, 180, 185
Osteoporosis   146–147

Peroxidation   352, 355–356, 358
Phosphorus fertilizers   43
Phosphorylation reactions   216
Phototoxicity   164
Phytotoxicity   53
Plasma proteins   182
Producer nations   35
Production   1
   annual   35
Prostaglandin   340
Proteins
   binding sites for cadmium   301–302
   binding sites for zinc   307
   complexes with cadmium, selenium
   352, 353
   phosphorylation   196
Proteinuria   146, 150, 153, 180, 182, 188,
   190
   see also Urinary proteins
Proximal tubule, see Nephropathy
Pulmonary edema   76, 145

Renal cortex   179, 181, 185–186, 188, 190
Renal tubular acidosis, see Nephropathy
Resistance to cadmium   363–365, 370,
   372–376, 379–383, 388–390
Retention of cadmium   76

Safety margin, see Exposure
Selenium   351–354, 356–357
Sensitivity to cadmium, see Resistance
Smoking effects   140, 148–149, 160, 181
Soil contamination   157
Superoxide dismutase   353–354, 356–358,
   370

Teeth, discoloration   146, 163
Teratogenicity   163
Tissue storage   141–142, 157
Toxicity   144–145, 163, 180, 305–306, 312,
   363, 373, 383–384, 388
   bone   146–147
   chronic   145
   effects of age   114
   effects of cadmium pretreatment
   306–307
   effects of malnutrition   116
   effects of metalothionein   298, 304
   effects of temperature   116
   effects of zinc pretreatment   307
   heart   196, 351
   kidney   150
   lung   145, 147
   see also Nephropathy
   reproductive effects   318, 322
   zinc, copper metabolism   117
Transport   142
   liver to kidney   292, 313–314
Tubular dysfunction, see Nephropathy

Uptake
   see also Absorption
   cellular   370–371
   zinc deficiency   287
Urinary proteins   154, 180, 182, 187
   N-acetyl-β-D-glucosaminidase   158, 189
   albumin   153–154, 159, 187–189
   alkaline phosphatase   158
   carbonic anhydrase   153
   ferritin   154
   δ-globulin   153–154
   immunoglobulin G   153–154, 180
   lysozyme   153, 180
   β_2-microglobulin   153, 180, 188
   retinol-binding   153, 158–159, 167, 180, 188
   ribonuclease   153, 180
   transferrin   153–154
Urine   180
   cadmium content   143, 160, 166–167,
   181, 190
   pH   182
   phosphate content   147, 180, 189
   proteinuria   150, 153, 156, 184

Vascular tissue   133, 135, 141–142
   elasticity   198
Vitamin D   87, 110
   deficiency   146

Water factor   202
Water hardness   160

Zinc   181
Zinc-metallothionein   284, 316

Handbook of Experimental Pharmacology

Continuation of
"Handbuch der
experimentellen
Pharmakologie"

Editorial Board
G. V. R. Born, A. Farah,
H. Herken, A. D. Welch

Springer-Verlag
Berlin Heidelberg
New York Tokyo

Volume 39
Antihypertensive Agents

Volume 40
Organic Nitrates

Volume 41
Hypolipidemic Agents

Volume 42
Neuromuscular Junction

Volume 43
**Anabolic-Androgenic
Steroids**

Volume 44
Heme and Hemoproteins

Volume 45: Part 1
Drug Addiction I

Part 2
Drug Addiction II

Volume 46
**Fibrinolytics and
Antifibronolytics**

Volume 47
Kinetics of Drug Action

Volume 48
Arthropod Venoms

Volume 49
**Ergot Alkaloids and
Related Compounds**

Volume 50: Part 1
Inflammation

Part 2
Anti-Inflammatory Drugs

Volume 51
Uric Acid

Volume 52
Snake Venoms

Volume 53
**Pharmacology of Gang-
lionic Transmission**

Volume 54: Part 1
**Adrenergic Activators and
Inhibitors I**

Part 2
**Adrenergic Activators and
Inhibitors II**

Volume 55
Psychotropic Agents

Part 1
**Antipsychotics and
Antidepressants**

Part 2
**Anxiolytics, Geronto-
psychopharmacological
Agents and Psychomotor
Stimulants**

Part 3
**Alcohol and Psycho-
tomimetics, Psychotropic
Effects of Central Acting
Drugs**

Volume 56, Part 1 + 2
Cardiac Glycosides

Volume 57
Tissue Growth Factors

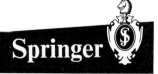

Handbook of Experimental Pharmacology

Continuation of
"Handbuch der
experimentellen
Pharmakologie"

Editorial Board
G. V. R. Born, A. Farah,
H. Herken, A. D. Welch

Springer-Verlag
Berlin Heidelberg
New York Tokyo

Volume 58
Cyclic Nucleotides
Part 1: **Biochemistry**
Part 2: **Physiology and**
Pharmacology

Volume 59
Mediators and Drugs in
Gastrointestinal Motility
Part 1: **Morphological**
Basis and Neuro-
physiological Control
Part 2: **Endogenous and**
Exogenous Agents

Volume 60
Pyretics and Antipyretics

Volume 61
Chemotherapy of Viral
Infections

Volume 62
Aminoglycoside Antibiotics

Volume 63
Allergic Reactions to Drugs

Volume 64
Inhibition of Folate
Metabolism
in Chemotherapy

Volume 65
Teratogenesis and
Reproductive Toxicology

Volume 66
Part 1: **Glucagon I**
Part 2: **Glucagon II**

Volume 67
Part 1
Antibiotics Containing the
Beta-Lactam Structure I
Part 2
Antibiotics Containing the
Beta-Lactam Structure II

Volume 68, Part 1+2
Antimalarial Drugs

Volume 69
Pharmacology of the Eye

Volume 70
Part 1
Pharmacology of
Intestinal Permeation I

Part 2
Pharmacology of
Intestinal Permeation II

Volume 71
Interferons and Their
Applications

Volume 72
Antitumor Drug Resistance

Volume 73
Radiocontrast Agents

Volume 74
Antiepileptic Drugs

Volume 75
Toxicology of
Inhaled Materials

Volume 76
Clinical Pharmocology of
Antiangial Drugs

Volume 77
Chemotherapy of
Gastrointestinal Helminths

Volume 78
The Tetracyclines

Volume 79
New Neuromuscular
Blocking Agents

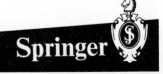

Springer